CLINICAL
NEUROSURGERY

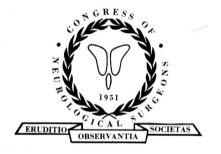

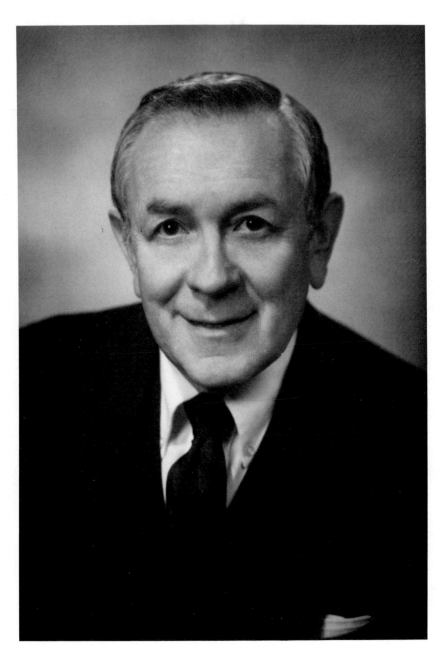

SIDNEY GOLDRING, M.D.

CLINICAL NEUROSURGERY

Proceedings

OF THE

CONGRESS OF NEUROLOGICAL SURGEONS

Honolulu, Hawaii

1985

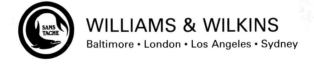

WILLIAMS & WILKINS
Baltimore • London • Los Angeles • Sydney

Copyright ©, 1986

Printed in the United States of America

Library of Congress
Catalog Card Number
S4-12666
ISBN 0-683-02028-5

The Library of Congress cataloged this serial as follows:
Congress of Neurological Surgeons.
    Clinical neurosurgery.   v. 1- 1953-
    Baltimore, Williams & Wilkins.
        v.   ill.   24 cm.
    Annual.
    "Proceedings of the Congress of Neurological Surgeons."
    Issues for 1954–70 include the Membership roster of the Congress
of Neurological Surgeons.
    Each vol. honors an individual scientist and presents a biographi-
cal sketch, bibliography, and some of his original papers.
    Indexes:
        Vols. 1–19, 1953–72, in v. 19.
    Key title: Clinical neurosurgery, ISSN 0069-4827.
    1. Nervous system—Surgery.   I. Congress of Neurological Sur-
geons. Proceedings. II. Congress of Neurological Surgeons. Membership roster. III. Title.
    [DNLM: W1 CL732]
RD593.A1C63   617.48   54-12666
                                                     MARC-S

                    86   87   88   87   90
        10   9   8   7   6   5   4   3   2   1

Preface

This volume constitutes the Proceedings of the 35th Annual Meeting of the Congress of Neurological Surgeons held in Honolulu, Hawaii from September 30 to October 4, 1985. Robert A. Ratcheson, M.D. (President); Steven L. Giannotta, M.D. (General Chairman); and Roberto Heros, M.D. (Chairman, Scientific Sessions) organized an outstanding scientific program upon which this volume is based.

Sidney Goldring, M.D. was the Honored Guest of the Congress. In two chapters, he discusses his experience with patients presenting with chronic seizures caused by gliomas and other lesions.

Neurosurgeons are not insulated from changing legal, social, and economic times. Accordingly, a group of experts, including playwright Brian Clark and economist Alain Enthoven, provide valuable insight into our prospects and responsibilities. Dr. Murray Goldstein, Director of NINCDS, presents his views on neurosurgery as a research discipline.

The main theme of the scientific program was "Controversies in Neurosurgery." Accordingly, experts with opposing viewpoints presented their arguments. Some of the topics discussed included the timing of aneurysm surgery, management of unruptured cerebral arteriovenous malformation, treatment of myelomeningocele, microdiscectomy, chemonucleolysis, and the neurosurgical treatment of vertigo. Dr. Sidney Peerless presented his views on cerebral bypass surgery in light of the EC/IC Bypass Study. His chapter will undoubtedly serve as a starting point for the impending discussion on this controversial procedure.

I would like to express my appreciation to the members of the Editorial Board for their superb effort in putting together this volume. My secretary, Ms. Marianne Lorini, is also to be congratulated for her help in this endeavor. A special thanks to Ms. Carol-Lynn Brown, Williams & Wilkins, for her guidance and support.

JOHN R. LITTLE, M.D.
Editor

Editorial Board

JANET W. BAY, M.D.	HOWARD H. KAUFMAN, M.D.
ARTHUR L. DAY, M.D.	WALTER J. LEVY, M.D.
MICHAEL J. EBERSOLD, M.D.	HAROLD L. REKATE, M.D.
STEVEN L. GIANNOTTA, M.D.	JON H. ROBERTSON, M.D.
STEPHEN J. HAINES, M.D.	JAMES WOODS, M.D.

Honored Guests

1952—Professor Herbert Olivecrona, Stockholm, Sweden
1953—Sir Geoffrey Jefferson, Manchester, England
1954—Dr. Kenneth G. McKenzie, Toronto, Canada
1955—Dr. Carl W. Rand, Los Angeles, California
1956—Dr. Wilder G. Penfield, Montreal, Canada
1957—Dr. Francis C. Grant, Philadelphia, Pennsylvania
1958—Dr. A. Earl Walker, Baltimore, Maryland
1959—Dr. William J. German, New Haven, Connecticut
1960—Dr. Paul C. Bucy, Chicago, Illinois
1961—Professor Eduard A. V. Busch, Copenhagen, Denmark
1962—Dr. Bronson S. Ray, New York, New York
1963—Dr. James L. Poppen, Boston, Massachusetts
1964—Dr. Edgar A. Kahn, Ann Arbor, Michigan
1965—Dr. James C. White, Boston, Massachusetts
1966—Dr. Hugo A. Krayenbühl, Zurich, Switzerland
1967—Dr. W. James Gardner, Cleveland, Ohio
1968—Professor Norman M. Dott, Edinburgh, Scotland
1969—Dr. Wallace B. Hamby, Cleveland, Ohio
1970—Dr. Barnes Woodhall, Durham, North Carolina
1971—Dr. Elisha S. Gurdjian, Detroit, Michigan
1972—Dr. Francis Murphey, Memphis, Tennessee
1973—Dr. Henry G. Schwartz, St. Louis, Missouri
1974—Dr. Guy L. Odom, Durham, North Carolina
1975—Dr. William H. Sweet, Boston, Massachusetts
1976—Dr. Lyle A. French, Minneapolis, Minnesota
1977—Dr. Richard C. Schneider, Ann Arbor, Michigan
1978—Dr. Charles G. Drake, London, Ontario, Canada
1979—Dr. Frank H. Mayfield, Cincinnati, Ohio
1980—Dr. Eben Alexander, Jr., Winston-Salem, North Carolina
1981—Dr. J. Garber Galbraith, Birmingham, Alabama
1982—Dr. Keiji Sano, Tokyo, Japan
1983—Dr. C. Miller Fisher, Boston, Massachusetts
1985—Dr. Hugo V. Rizzoli, Washington, D.C.
      Dr. Walter E. Dandy (posthumously), Baltimore, Maryland
1985—Dr. Sidney Goldring, St. Louis, Missouri

Officers of the Congress of Neurological Surgeons 1985

ROBERT A. RATCHESON, M.D.
President

JOSEPH C. MAROON, M.D.
President-Elect

DONALD O. QUEST, M.D.
Vice-President

MICHAEL SALCMAN, M.D.
Secretary

HAL HANKINSON, M.D.
Treasurer

Executive Committee

EDWARD R. LAWS, JR., M.D.
RONALD I. APFELBAUM, M.D.
ARTHUR L. DAY, M.D.
STEVEN L. GIANNOTTA, M.D.
ROBERTO C. HEROS, M.D.
J. MICHAEL MCWHORTER

FREMONT P. WIRTH, M.D.
PAUL CROISSANT, M.D.
LAWRENCE PITTS, M.D.
J. CHARLES RICH, M.D.
CHRISTOPHER SHIELDS, M.D.
JOHN M. TEW, JR., M.D.

STEVEN L. GIANNOTTA, M.D., *Chairman, Annual Meeting Committee*
ROBERTO C. HEROS, M.D., *Chairman, Scientific Program Committee*

Contributors

ADNAN A. ABLA, M.D., Department of Neurosurgery, Allegheny General Hospital, Pittsburgh, Pennsylvania (*Chapter 26*)

MICHAEL J. AMINOFF, M.D., F.R.C.P., Professor of Neurology, University of California Medical Center, San Francisco, California (*Chapter 13*)

JAMES I. AUSMAN, M.D. PH.D., Chairman, Department of Neurological Surgery, Henry Ford Hospital, Detroit, Michigan (*Chapters 19 and 20*)

ERIK J. BERTSTRALH, Department of Medical Statistics and Epidemiology, Mayo Medical School, Mayo Clinic, Rochester, Minnesota (*Chapter 36*)

PETER McL. BLACK, M.D., PH.D., Associate Professor of Surgery (Neurosurgery), Massachusetts General Hospital, Harvard University Medical School, Boston, Massachusetts (*Chapter 6*)

JOSE M. BONNIN, M.D., Division of Neurosurgery, University of Alabama at Birmingham, Birmingham, Alabama (*Chapter 37*)

LENNART M. BRANDT, M.D., Department of Neurosurgery, Lund University, Lund, Sweden (*Chapter 12*)

DEREK A. BRUCE, M.D., Department of Neurosurgery, University of Pennsylvania School of Medicine, Childrens Hospital of Pennsylvania, Philadelphia, Pennsylvania (*Chapter 23*)

LOUIS R. CAPLAN, M.D., Department of Neurology, Tufts University Medical School, Boston, Massachusetts (*Chapter 19*)

WILLIAM F. CHANDLER, M.D., Associate Professor of Neurosurgery, Section of Neurosurgery, University of Michigan Medical Center, Ann Arbor, Michigan (*Chapter 34*)

EDWARD B. CHARNEY, M.D., Department of Neurosurgery, University of Pennsylvania School of Medicine, Childrens Hospital of Philadelphia, Philadelphia, Pennsylvania (*Chapter 23*)

BRIAN CLARK, Playwright, Judy Daish Association, Limited, London, England (*Chapter 7*)

MARVIN B. CLIFTON, M.D., Department of Neurological Surgery, Mayo Medical, Mayo Clinic, Rochester, Minnesota (*Chapter 36*)

ROBERT M. CROWELL, M.D., Professor and Head, Department of Neurological Surgery, University of Illinois Medical Center, Chicago, Illinois (*Chapter 17*)

ARTHUR L. DAY, M.D., Associate Professor, Department of Neurological Surgery, University of Florida College of Medicine, Gainesville, Florida (*Chapter 24*)

FERNANDO G. DIAZ, M.D., PH.D., Department of Neurological Surgery, Henry Ford Hospital, Detroit, Michigan (*Chapters 19 and 20*)

GEORGE V. DIGIACINTO, M.D., St. Lukes-Roosevelt Hospital Center and Memorial Sloan-Kettering Cancer Center, New York, New York (*Chapter 30*)

MANUEL DUJOVNY, M.D., Department of Neurological Surgery, Henry Ford Hospital, Detroit, Michigan (*Chapter 20*)

MICHAEL S. B. EDWARDS, M.D., Associate Professor, Departments of Neurological Surgery and Pediatrics, University of California School of Medicine, San Francisco, California (*Chapter 21*)

ALAIN C. ENTHOVEN, PH.D., Graduate School of Business, Marriner S. Eccles, Professor of Public and Private Management, Professor of Health Care and Economics, Stanford University School of Medicine, Stanford, California (*Chapter 5*)

CHARLES A. FAGER, M.D., Neurosurgeon, Department of Neurosurgery, Lahey Clinic Medical Center, Burlington, Massachusetts (*Chapter 27*)

EUGENE S. FLAMM, M.D., Professor and Vice Chairman, Department of Neurosurgery, New York University Medical Center, New York, New York (*Chapter 11*)

WILLIAM A. FRIEDMAN, M.D., Assistant Professor, Department of Neurological Surgery, University of Florida College of Medicine, Gainesville, Florida (*Chapter 24*)

SIDNEY GOLDRING, M.D., Professor and Head, Department of Neurosurgery, Washington University Medical Center, St. Louis, Missouri (*Chapters 2 and 3*)

MURRAY GOLDSTEIN, DO, MPH, Director, National Institute of Neurological and Communicative Disorders and Stroke, National Institutes of Health, Bethesda, Maryland (*Chapter 8*)

ROBERT L. GRUBB, JR., M.D., Professor, Department of Neurology and Neurological and Division of Radiation Sciences, The Edward Mallinckrodt Institute of Radiology, Washington University School of Medicine, St. Louis, Missouri (*Chapter 16*)

STEPHEN J. HAINES, M.D., Associate Professor, Department of Neurosurgery, University of Minnesota Hospital, Minneapolis, Minnesota (*Chapter 39*)

E. CLARKE HALEY, M.D., Assistant Professor, Department of Neurology, University of Virginia School of Medicine, Charlottesville, Virginia (*Chapter 10*)

ROBERTO C. HEROS, M.D., Director of Cerebrovascular Surgery, Massachusetts General Hospital, and Associate Professor of Neurosurgery, Harvard Medical School, Boston, Massachusetts (*Chapter 14*)

JAMES E. O. HUGHES, M.D., St. Lukes-Roosevelt Hospital Center and Memorial-Sloan Kettering Cancer Center, New York, New York (*Chapter 30*)

WILLIAM E. HUNT, M.D., Professor and Chairman, Division of Neurologic Surgery, Ohio State University, Columbus, Ohio (*Chapter 29*)

PETER J. JANNETTA, M.D., Professor and Chairman, Department of Neurosurgery, University of Pittsburgh School of Medicine, Pittsburgh, Pennsylvania (*Chapter 40*)

DAVID L. KASDON, M.D., F.A.C.S., Associate Professor, Department of Neurosurgery, Tufts University Medical School, and Chief of Neurosurgery, St. Elizabeth's Hospital, Boston, Massachusetts (*Chapter 31*)

NEAL F. KASSELL, M.D., Professor, Department of Neurological Surgery, University of Virginia School of Medicine, Charlottesville, Virginia (*Chapter 10*)

EDWARD R. LAWS, JR., M.D., Professor of Neurological Surgery, Department of Neurologic Surgery, Mayo Medical School, Mayo Clinic, Rochester, Minnesota (*Chapter 36*)

BENGT LJUNGGREN, M.D., Professor, Department of Neurosurgery, Lund University, Lund, Sweden (*Chapter 12*)

THOMAS J. MAMPALAM, M.D., Department of Neurosurgery, University of California School of Medicine, San Francisco, California (*Chapter 38*)

JOSEPH C. MAROON, M.D., Clinical Professor, Department of Neurological Surgery, University of Pittsburgh School of Medicine, and Director of Neurological Surgery, Allegheny General Hospital, Pittsburgh, Pennsylvania (*Chapter 26*)

DAVID G. MCLONE, M.D., PH.D., Professor and Head, Division of Neurosurgery, The Childrens Memorial Hospital and Northwestern University Medical School, Chicago, Illinois (*Chapter 22*)

CAROLE A. MILLER, M.D., Associate Professor, Division of Neurologic Surgery, Ohio State University, Columbus, Ohio (*Chapter 29*)

AAGE R. MØLLER, PH.D., Associate Professor, Department of Neurosurgery, University of Pittsburgh School of Medicine, Pittsburgh, Pennsylvania (*Chapter 40*)

MARGARETA B. MØLLER, M.D., PH.D., Associate Professor, Department of Neurosurgery, University of Pittsburgh School of Medicine, Pittsburgh, Pennsylvania (*Chapter 40*)

RICHARD B. MORAWETZ, M.D., Professor of Neurosurgey, Division of Neurosurgery, University of Alabama Medical Center, Birmingham, Alabama (*Chapter 37*)

HARUO OKAZAKI, M.D., Department of Pathology, Mayo Medical School, Mayo Clinic, Rochester, Minnesota (*Chapter 36*)

SYDNEY J. PEERLESS, M.D., F.R.C.S. (C), Professor and Chairman, Division of

Neurosurgery, University of Western Ontario, London, Ontario, Canada (*Chapter 18*)

SELWYN PICKER, MB, BCH, Department of Neurosurgery, Washington University School of Medicine, St. Louis, Missouri (*Chapter 2*)

VINCENT G. PONS, M.D., Associate Clinical Professor, Department of Medicine/and Neurosurgery, Infectious Diseases University of California School of Medicine, San Francisco, California (*Chapter 38*)

DONALD O. QUEST, M.D., Associate Professor of Neurosurgery, The Neurological Institute, The College of Physicians and Surgeons of Columbia University, New York, New York (*Chapter 15*)

ROBERT A. RATCHESON, M.D., Professor and Chief, Division of Neurological Surgery, Case Western Reserve University School of Medicine, University Hospitals of Cleveland, Cleveland, Ohio (*Chapter 1*)

KEITH M. RICH, M.D., Department of Neurosurgery, Washington University Medical Center, St. Louis, Missouri (*Chapter 2*)

MARK L. ROSENBLUM, M.D., Associate Professor, Department of Neurosurgery, University of California School of Medicine, San Francisco, California (*Chapter 38*)

DOUGLAS F. SAVAGE, M.D., Department of Neurological Surgery, University of Florida College of Medicine, Gainesville, Florida (*Chapter 24*)

LALIGAM N. SEKHAR, M.D., Assistant Professor of Neurological Surgery, Department of Neurosurgery, Presbyterian-University Hospital, Pittsburgh, Pennsylvania (*Chapter 40*)

MICHAEL J. SCHLITT, M.D., Division of Neurosurgery, University of Alabama Medical Center, Birmingham, Alabama (*Chapter 37*)

DAVID E. SCHTEINGART, M.D., Section of Neurosurgery, University of Michigan Medical Center, Ann Arbor, Michigan (*Chapter 34*)

LUIS SCHUT, M.D., Department of Neurosurgery, University of Pennsylvania School of Medicine, Childrens Hospital of Philadelphia, Philadelphia, Pennsylvania (*Chapter 23*)

HENRY G. SCHWARTZ, M.D., Professor Emeritus of Neurosurgery, Department of Neurosurgery, Washington University Medical School, St. Louis, Missouri (*Chapter 4*)

GLENN E. SCHELINE, M.D., PH.D., Professor and Vice Chairman, Department of Radiologic Oncology, University of California at San Francisco, San Francisco, California (*Chapter 35*)

CHRISTOPHER B. SHIELDS, M.D., F.R.C.S.(C), Associate Professor, Division of Neurological Surgery, Department of Surgery, University of Louisville School of Medicine, Louisville, Kentucky (*Chapter 25*)

JOHN SHILLITO, JR., M.D., Associate Chief, Department of Neurosurgery, Childrens Hospital Medical Center, Boston, Massachusetts (*Chapter 32*)

NARAYAN SUNDARESAN, M.D., Assistant Attending Surgeon, Memorial Hospital and Assistant Professor of Surgery, Cornell University Medical Center, New York, New York (*Chapter 30*)

LESLIE N. SUTTON, M.D., Assistant Professor of Neurosurgery, University of Pennsylvania School of Medicine, Childrens Hospital of Philadelphia, Philadelphia, Pennsylvania (*Chapter 23*)

GEORGE W. SYPERT, M.D., C.M. and K.E., Overstreet Family Professor and Eminent Scholar, Departments of Neurological Surgery and Neuroscience, University of Florida College of Medicine, Veterans Administration Medical Center, Gainesville, Florida (*Chapters 24 and 28*)

EDWARD C. TARLOV, M.D., Neurosurgeon, Department of Neurosurgery, Lahey Clinical Medical Center, Burlington, Massachusetts (*Chapter 41*)

WILLIAM F. TAYLOR, PH.D., Medical Statistics, Mayo Medical School, Mayo Clinic, Rochester, Minnesota (*Chapter 37*)

JAMES C. TORNER, M.D., Department of Neurological Surgery, University of Virginia Medical School Charlottesville, Virginia (*Chapter 10*)

YONG-KWANG TU, M.D., Department of Neurosurgery, Harvard Medical School, Boston, Massachusetts (*Chapter 14*)

MARTIN H. WEISS, M.D., Professor and Chairman, Department of Neurological Surgery, University of Southern California Medical School, Los Angeles, California (*Chapter 33*)

RICHARD J. WHITLEY, M.D., Division of Neurosurgery, University of Alabama at Birmingham, Birmingham, Alabama (*Chapter 37*)

FREMONT P. WIRTH, M.D., Neurosurgeon, Savannah, Georgia (*Chapter 9*)

H. EVAN ZIEGER, M.D., Division of Neurosurgery, University of Alabama at Birmingham, Birmingham, Alabama (*Chapter 37*)

Biography of
Sidney Goldring, M.D.

Sidney Goldring was born April 2, 1923, in Kremnitz, Poland. His family immigrated to the United States and settled in St. Louis when Sidney was 3 months old. The Goldrings spoke not a word of English, but they had a passionate determination that their sons would be educated and have a profession. David, the first-born son, fulfilled his parents' dream by going to medical school. They, however, despaired of their second son, who was not distinguishing himself in school, and seemed more concerned about having fun and winning swimming meets for Soldan High School than getting serious about his studies. Sidney began college at Washington University in 1941, and entered the accelerated medical school program at Washington University, receiving his medical degree in 1947. He had finally become a serious scholar, and his parents had another son of whom to be proud.

Research has always been a driving passion in Dr. Goldring's life. During medical school he worked in the lab of Dr. Carl Harford, investigating the etiology of decreased cerebrospinal fluid glucose levels in meningitis, nurturing an early interest in the nervous system. His love of basic research continues today as he surrounds himself with anatomists, physiologists, and engineers working in his neurosurgery department, and he often encourages medical students and residents to consider working on doctorates in basic science.

During medical school Dr. Goldring's interest in the nervous system and the challenges of the developing specialty of neurosurgery confirmed his desire to enter this field. He did his internship and a year of residency in general surgery at the Jewish Hospital in St. Louis. In 1949, he became a Fellow in Neurology at Washington University working with Dr. James O'Leary. During this time he received his initial training in neurophysiology. In the laboratory he also came under the influence of the inquiring mind of Dr. George Bishop, one of the pioneers in the development of modern neurophysiology. Among Dr. Bishop's many achievements was the first recording of evoked potentials in experimental animals. Dr. Goldring was influenced not only by the scientific achievement of these men, but also by their strong moral character and sense of fairness, the same characteristics that today's generation sees in Dr. Goldring. His life-long interest and understanding in treating patients with severe seizure disorders began at this time, when every morning was spent reading electroencephalograms (EEGs) with Dr. O'Leary.

He began his neurosurgery training at Washington University and Barnes Hospital with Dr. Henry Schwartz in 1951. The influence of this superb surgeon and powerful personality has been a guiding force throughout Dr. Goldring's career. His residency was interrupted by eight months service in the U.S. Public Health Service as an Instructor in Neurosurgery with the Washington University Medical Unit in Thailand, an exchange program set up between Washington University and Chulalonkorn and Siriraj Universities in Bangkok. During this time Dr. Goldberg performed the first craniotomy for tumor ever done in Thailand. Returning home, Dr. Goldring entered the U.S. Army, spending one year at Walter Reed Hospital where he first met a future long-time associate, Dr. William Coxe, and worked with Dr. Ludwig Kempe. Dr. Goldring returned to St. Louis and finished his neurosurgical residency at Barnes Hospital in 1956.

Having completed his training Dr. Goldring became a member of the Washington University School of Medicine Faculty from 1956 to 1964. He then left Washington University to become Professor and Head of Neurological Surgery at the University of Pittsburgh. In 1966, he rejoined Washington University as Professor of Neurological Surgery. When a search committee was formed to find a new Head of Neurological Surgery to replace Dr. Henry Schwartz, the proverbial "legend in his own time," the job seemed herculean; but the answer kept coming back from all sources: "the best man is right there—search no further." In 1974, Dr. Goldring became Head of Neurological Surgery and Co-chairman of the newly created Department of Neurology and Neurological Surgery at Washington University School of Medicine, and Neurosurgeon-in-Chief at Barnes Hospital and St. Louis Children's Hospital. Dr. Goldring has continued the highly respected training program at Washington University in the tradition of Ernest Sachs and Henry Schwartz, encouraging and training neurosurgeons with a strong academic emphasis. In 1980, he was also appointed Director of the McDonnell Center for Studies of Higher Brain Function which was created with a large gift from the James S. McDonnell Foundation.

Dr. Goldring's research interests are in neurophysiology and experimental and clinical epilepsy. He has published extensively on these subjects and has developed a large experience in the surgical treatment of seizure disorders. Basic laboratory studies have focused on the steady voltage gradients that exist between the brain and an extracerebral reference, or across the cerebral cortex. These gradients (direct current [DC] potentials) were extensively studied during anoxia, asphyxia, hypoglycemia, focal brain injury, cerebral ischemia, anesthesia, and seizure discharge. Changes in DC potentials were shown to be due to sustained changes in the resting membrane potentials (RMP) of both neurons and glia; the RMP of glia reflecting fluxes in the extracellular K^+ concentration. The glial contribution of these potentials was definitively proven by simultaneous physiologic-morphologic studies in which the glial cells were marked intracellularly with horseradish peroxidase. Clinical research has dealt primarily with epilepsy. His most significant clinical contribution has been the development of a surgical method of treatment in which all surgical manipulation is carried out under general, rather than local, anesthesia. The sensori-motor region is identified in the anesthetized patient by recording cortical sensory evoked responses, and the epileptogenic focus is localized by the use of indwelling surface epidural electrode arrays for extraoperative electrocorticography which is carried out predominantly during spontaneously occurring seizures. This method has made it possible to extend surgical treatment of intractable seizure disorders to patients who heretofore could not as readily be considered for surgery, especially children.

Dr. Goldring has willingly given his time serving the National Institutes of Health and organized neurosurgery. He was a member of the Neurology Study Section of NINCDS from 1964 to 1968 and again from 1969 through 1973, serving as chairman of this section in 1972–1973. He was a member of the National Advisory Council of NINCDS from 1977 through 1981. Dr. Goldring was a member of the American Board of Neurological Surgery from 1971 through 1976, serving as chairman from 1974 through 1976. He was chairman of the Residency Review Committee for Neurosurgery from 1974 through 1976. In 1975, he was chairman of the Neurosciences Interdisciplinary Cluster of the President's Panel on Biomedical and Behavior Research. Currently he is chairman of the Scientific Advisory Committee for the Research Foundation of the American Association of Neurological Surgery (AANS) and has served since 1972, as a member of the Board of Trustees of the Grass Foundation. Dr. Goldring served as President of the Society of Neurological Surgeons in 1981–1982, the American Academy of Neurological Surgery in 1982–1983, and the AANS in 1984–1985.

Sidney Goldring met Lois Blustein when she was 15 years old. Showing characteristic good judgment, he fell in love with this young, beautiful redhead and married her in 1945, when she was a Washington University freshman. A lovely, vibrant, and outgoing woman, Lois has served as a strong complement to Sid while maintaining her own identity in important civic and cultural activities. The Goldrings have two children, James M. Goldring, a student at the Washington University School of Medicine, who completed a Ph.D. in Neurobiology before entering medical school, and a daughter, Kathryn Goldring Coryell, who lives in Iowa City, Iowa, with her psychiatrist husband, Bill, and children Matthew, age 5, and Julie, age 1, the special pride of grandparents Lois and Sid. This busy man has little time for hobbies, but vacation time usually finds Sidney and Lois waist deep in the best trout streams of Montana, and a hefty portion of Montana trout find their way to St. Louis deliciously prepared on the table for lucky family and friends.

The Congress of Neurological Surgeons is privileged to recognize Sidney Goldring as its Honored Guest.

Bibliography of
SIDNEY GOLDRING, M.D.

Effects of leucocytes and bacteria on glucose content of the cerebrospinal fluid in meningitis. (with C. Harford). Proc. Soc. Exp. Biol. & Med., *75:* 669–672, 1950.

Measurement of slow voltage changes under resting conditions and during convulsive therapy. Abst. (with G. Ulett and A. Greditzer). EEG Clin. Neurophysiol., *2:* 296, 1950.

Initial survey of slow potential changes obtained under resting conditions and incident to convulsive therapy. (with G. Ulett, J. L. O'Leary and A. Greditzer). EEG Clin. Neurophysiol., *2:* 297–308, 1950.

Roles of anterior commissure and thalamus interhemispheric spread of afterdischarge in the oppossum. (with F. Morin). J. Comp. Neurol., *93:* 229–240, 1950.

Experimentally derived correlates between ECG and steady cortical potential. (with J. L. O'Leary). J. Neurophysiol., *14:* 275–288, 1951.

Summation of certain enduring sequelae of cortical activation in the rabbit. (with J. L. O'Leary). EEG Clin. Neurophysiol., *3:* 329–340, 1951.

Maturation of evoked response of the visual cortex in the postnatal rabbit. (with W. E. Hunt). EEG Clin. Neurophysiol., *3:* 465–471, 1951.

Effect of malononitrile upon the electrocorticogram of the rabbit. (with J. L. O'Leary and R. L. Lam). EEG Clin. Neurophysiol., *5:* 395–400, 1953.

D.C. potentials. (with J. L. O'Leary). 3rd Int. EEG Cong., Symposium, 1953.

Correlation between steady transcortical potential and evoked response. I. Alterations in somatic receiving area induced by veratrine, strychnine, KCl and novocain. (with J. L. O'Leary). EEG Clin. Neurophysiol., *6:* 189–200, 1954.

Correlation between steady transcortical potentials and evoked response. II. Effect of veratrine and strychnine upon the responsiveness of visual cortex. (with J. L. O'Leary). EEG Clin. Neurophysiol., *6:* 201–212, 1954.

Cortical D.C. changes accompanying recruiting response. (with J. L. O'Leary). EEG Clin. Neurophysiol., *9:* 381, (Abst), 1957.

Cortical D.C. changes incident to midline thalamic stimulation. (with J. L. O'Leary). EEG Clin. Neurophysiol., *9:* 577–584, 1957.

The relation between spinoreticular and ascending cephalic systems. (with J. L. O'Leary and F. W. L. Kerr). Ford Hospital International Symposium on the Reticular Formation of the Brain, Detroit, Michigan, March, 1957.

Singly and repetitively evoked potentials in human cerebral cortex with D.C. changes. (with J. L. O'Leary and R. B. King). EEG Clin. Neurophysiol., *10:* 233–240, 1958.

Experimental modification of dendritic and recruiting processes and their DC after-effects. (with J. L. O'Leary and S. H. Huang). EEG Clin. Neurophysiol., *10:* 663–676, 1958.

Seizure discharges effected by intravenously administered convulsant drugs. ECG and DC changes in cerebrum and cerebellum of the rabbit. (with P. Vanasupa and J. L. O'Leary). EEG Clin. Neurophysiol., *11:* 93–106, 1959.

Pharmacological selectivity manifested by agents acting upon the cortical dendritic spike and its slow after-effects. (with J. Metcalf, S. H. Huang, J. Shields, and J. L. O'Leary). J. Nerv. Ment. Dis., *128:* 1–11, 1959.

Identification of a prolonged post-synaptic potential of cerebral cortex. (with J. L. O'Leary and D. Winter and A. Pearlman). Proc. Soc. Exper. Biol. Med., *100:* 429–431, 1959.

Steady potential changes during cortical activation. (with P. Vanasupa, J. L. O'Leary and D. Winter). J. Neurophysiol., *22:* 273–284, 1959.

Changes associated with forebrain excitation processes: D.C. potentials of the cerebral cortex. (with J. L. O'Leary). *Handbook of Physiology,* Chapter 13, American Physiological Society. Williams & Wilkins Co., Baltimore, Md., pp. 315–328, 1959.

Effects of convulsive and anesthetic agents on steady cortical potential. (with J. L. O'Leary). Epilepsia, *1:* 86–94, 1959.

Visually evoked slow negativity in rabbit cortex. (with A. L. Pearlman and J. L. O'Leary). Proc. Soc. Exper. Biol. Med., *103:* 600–603, 1960.

Pharmacological dissolution of evoked cortical potentials. (with J. L. O'Leary). Symposium on Physiology and Drug Action, Fed. Proc., *10:* 612–618, 1960.

Slow cortical potentials. Their origin and contributions to seizure discharge. (with J. L. O'Leary). Epilepsia, *1:* 561–574, 1960.

Comparison of nembutal and procaine effects on direct cortical responses in isolated cat cortex. (with M. J. Jerva, T. G. Holmes and J. L. O'Leary). Fed. Proc., (Abst), 19: #1, Pt. 1, March, 1960.

Altered activity at the margins of human epileptogenic foci. (with M. J. Jerva, T. G. Holmes and J. L. O'Leary). *Surgical Forum,* 46th Annual Clinical Congress, *XI:* 388–389, 1960.

Comparison of direct cerebral and cerebellar cortical responses in isolated cat cortex. (with A. Rhoton and J. L. O'Leary). Am. J. Physiol., *199:* 677–682, 1960.

Hypothermia and electrical activity of cerebral cortex. (with W. Weinstein, J. H. Kendig, J. L. O'Leary and H. Lourie). Arch. Neurol., *4:* 441–448, 1961.

Experimental evidence relating to the pathogenesis of post-traumatic epilepsy. (with J. L. O'Leary and W. S. Coxe). Epilepsia, *2:* 117–122, 1961.

Physiological and pathological aspects of the direct cortical response in man. (with M. J. Jerva, T. G. Holmes, J. L. O'Leary and J. Shields). EEG Clin. Neurophysiol., (Abst) *13:* 308, 1961.

Direct response of human cerebral cortex. (with M. J. Jerva, T. G. Holmes, J. L. O'Leary and J. R. Shields). Arch. Neurol., *4:* 590–598, 1961.

Simultaneous recording of direct cortical, pyramidal and muscle response, with reference to Adrian's "deep response." (with S. Mingrino, W. S. Coxe and J. L. O'Leary). Excerpta Medica. VIIth International Congress of Neurology, Rome, Italy, *38:* 75, 1961.

Investigation of the direct response in cerebral cortex of man. (with W. S. Coxe, S. Mingrino and J. L. O'Leary). Excerpta Medica, 2nd International Congress of Neurological Surgery, Washington, D.C., No. 36: E80, 1961.

Observations on selective brain heating induced by regional brain perfusion in dogs. (with A. B. Harris, J. H. Kendig and S. Mingrino). Excerpta Medica, 2nd International Congress of Neurological Surgery, Washington, D.C., No. 36: E80, 1961.

Direct response of isolated cerebral cortex of cat. (with J. L. O'Leary, T. G. Holmes and M. J. Jerva). J. Neurophysiol., *24:* 633–650, 1961.

The character of cortical activity (with J. L. O'Leary). *Psychosomatic Medicine. The First Hahnemann Symposium.* Eds.: J. H. Nodine and J. H. Moyer, Lea and Febiger, Philadelphia, Pa., Chapter 24, pp. 169–185, 1962.

Observations on selective brain heating in dogs. (with A. B. Harris, L. Erickson, J. H. Kendig and S. Mingrino). J. Neurosurg., *19:* 514–521, 1962.

The direct cortical response: associated events in pyramid and muscle during development of movement and after-discharge. (with S. Mingrino, W. S. Coxe, R. Katz and J. L. O'Leary). Int. Colloquium on Specific and Unspecific Mechanisms of Sensory-Motor Integration. Prog. Brain Res., *1:* 241–257, 1963.

Negative steady potential shifts which lead to seizure discharge. (with J. L. O'Leary). In: *Brain Function: Cortical Excitability and Steady Potentials; Relations of Basic Research to Space Biology.* Ed., M. A. Brazier, UCLA Forum Med. Sci. No. 1, U of California Press, Los Angeles, pp. 210–236, 1963.

Patterns of unit discharge associated with direct cortical response in monkey and cat. (with P. E. Stohr and J. L. O'Leary). EEG Clin. Neurophysiol. *15:* 882–888, 1963.

Experimental cerebrovascular occlusion in the dog. (with L. U. Anthony, J. L. O'Leary, and H. G. Schwartz). Arch. Neurol., *8:* 515–527, 1963.

"Caudate-induced" cortical potentials: comparison between monkey and cat. (with L. U. Anthony, P. E. Stohr, and J. L. O'Leary). Science *139:* 772, 1963.

D.C. potentials of the brain. (with J. L. O'Leary). Physiol. Rev., *44:* 91–125, 1964.

Maturation of evoked cortical responses in animal and man. (with E. Sugaya and J. L. O'Leary). In: *Neurological and Electroencephalographic Correlative Studies in Infancy* (Int. Conf. & Symposium), Grune & Stratton, Inc., pp. 68–77, 1964.

Ectopic neural tissue of occipital bone. (with F. J. Hodges and S. Luse). J. Neurosurg., *21:* 479–484, 1964.

Intracellular potentials associated with direct cortical response and seizure discharge in cat. (with E. Sugaya and J. L. O'Leary). EEG Clin. Neurophysiol., *17:* 661–669, 1964.

Somatosensory cortex of man as revealed by computer processing of peripherally evoked cortical potentials. (with D. Kelly and J. L. O'Leary). Trans. Amer. Neurol. Assn., *89:* 108–111, 1964.

Seizure activity due to intravenous strychnine: An electron microscopic study of the cortex. (with S. A. Luse and J. L. O'Leary). Arch. Neurol., *11:* 296–302, 1964.

Behavioral, unit and slow potential changes in methionine sulfoximine seizures. (with W. L. Johnson and J. L. O'Leary). EEG Clin. Neurophysiol., *18:* 229–238, 1965.

Averaged evoked somatosensory responses from exposed cortex of man. (with D. L. Kelly, Jr., and J. L. O'Leary). Arch. Neurol., *13:* 1–9, 1965.

Trauma of the spinal cord. Closed spinal cord injuries: General considerations. (with H. G. Schwartz and W. S. Coxe). *Neurol. Surg. of Trauma,* Office of the Surgeon General, Department of the Army, Chapter 23, 1965.

Trauma of the spinal cord. Definitive treatment. (with H. G. Schwartz and W. S. Coxe). *Neurol. Surg. of Trauma,* Office of the Surgeon General, Department of the Army, Chapter 24, 1965.

Intracellular potentials from "idle" cells in cerebral cortex of cat. (with Y. Karahashi). EEG Clin. Neurophysiol., *20:* 600–607, 1966.

Intracellular potentials from experimental glial tumors. (with Y. Karahaski, P. Sheptak and J. Moosy). Arch. Neurol., *15:* 538–540, 1966.

Averaged responses from association areas in waking cat. (with P. Sheptak and Y. Karahaski). EEG Clin. Neurophysiol., *23:* 241–247, 1966.

Traumatic occlusion of the carotid artery: a case report. J. Neurosurg., *28:* 78–80, 1968.

The effect of radiofrequency current and of heat on nerve action potential of the cat. (with F. Letcher). J. Neurosurg., *29:* 42–47, 1968.

Steady potential and pathologic correlates of cerebrovascular occlusion in the dog. (with M. P. Heilbrun). Arch. Neurol., *19:* 410–420, 1968.

Osmotically induced changes in brain SP and auditory evoked responses. (with M. Feldman). EEG Clin. Neurophysiol., *26:* 588–596, 1969.

Origin of somatosensory evoked scalp responses in man. (with P. Stohr). J. Neurosurg., *31:* 117–127, 1969.

Contribution to steady potential shifts of slow depolarization in cells presumed to be glia. (with V. Castellucci). EEG Clin. Neurophysiol., *28:* 109–118, 1970.

Comparative study of sensory input to motor cortex in animals and man. (with E. Aras and P. Weber). EEG Clin. Neurophysiol., *29:* 537–550, 1970.

The role of prefrontal cortex in grand mal convulsion. Arch. Neurol., *26:* 109–119, 1972.

Human motor cortex: sensory input data from single neuron recordings. (with R. Ratcheson). Science, *175:* 1493–1495, 1972.

Ionic determinants of the membrane potential of cells presumed to be glia in cerebral cortex of cat. (with B. Ransom). J. Neurophysiol., *36:* 855–868, 1973.

Slow depolarization in cells presumed to be glia in cerebral cortex of cat. (with B. Ransom). J. Neurophysiol., *36:* 869–878, 1973.

Slow hyperpolarization in cells presumed to be glia in cerebral cortex of cat. (with B. Ransom). J. Neurophysiol., *36:* 879–892, 1973.

An ipsilateral input to the primary somatosensory (SI) area of raccoon cerebral cortex. (with C. L. Vera). Brain Res., *65:* 357–361, 1974.

Pathophysiology of epileptic discharge. *Neurological Pathophysiology,* Chapter 5, Oxford University Press, New York, pp. 155–167, 1974.

DC potentials recorded directly from the cortex. *Handbook of Electroencephalography and Clinical Neurophysiology.,* Ed., H. Caspers, Elsevier Scientific Pub. Co., Amsterdam, 1974.

Science and Epilepsy. (with J. L. O'Leary), Raven Press, New York, 1975.

Comparative study of motor potential in animal and man. (with C. Pieper). Abst. presented at Society for Neuroscience, 1976.

Management of seizure disorders: selected aspects (with W. E. Dodson, A. L. Prensky, D. C. DeVivo and P. R. Dodge). J. Pediatr., *89:* 527–540, 1976.

The effect of barbiturate and procaine on glial and neuronal contributions to evoked cortical steady potential shifts. (with B. R. Ransom). Brain Res., *134:* 479–499, 1977.

Surgical management of epilepsy in adults. *Neurological Surgery, 2nd. Ed.,* Ed., Youmans, J. R., Vol. VI: 3910–3926, Saunders, Co., Philadelphia.

A method for surgical management of focal epilepsy; especially as it relates to children. J. Neurosurg., *49:* 344–356, 1978.

The effect of local anesthetics on the potassium ion-selective electrode. (with R. Greenwood and W. E. Dodson). Brain Res., *165:* 171–176, 1979.

Intracellular marking with Lucifer yellow CH and horseradish peroxidase of cells electrophysiologically characterized as glia in the cerebral cortex of the cat. (with M. Takato). J. Comp. Neurol., *186:* 173–188, 1979.

Comparative study of cerebral cortical potentials associated with voluntary movements in monkey and man. (with C. Pieper, A. B. Jenny and J. P. McMahon). EEG Clin. Neurophysiol. *48:* 266–292, 1980.

Potassium activity and changes in glial and neuronal membrane potentials during initiation and spread of afterdischarge in cerebral cortex of cat. (with R. S. Greenwood and M. Takato). Brain Res., *218:* 279–298, 1981.

Glial membrane potentials and their relationship to $(K^+)_0$ in man and guinea pig: a comparative study of intracellularly marked normal, reactive and neoplastic glia. (with S. Picker and C. F. Pieper). J. Neurosurg., *55:* 347–363, 1981.

Electrophysiological properties of human glia. (with S. Picker). Trends in Neurosci., *5:* 73–76, 1982.

Surgical management of epilepsy using epidural recordings to localize the seizure focus: a review of 100 cases. (with E. M. Gregorie). J. Neurosurg., *60:* 457–472, 1984.

Epilepsy surgery. In *Clinical Neurosurgery*, Vol. 31, pp. 369–388. Williams & Wilkins, Baltimore, 1984.

Localization of function in the excision of lesions from the sensorimotor region. (with E. M. Gregorie). J. Neurosurg., *61:* 1047–1054, 1984.

Computed tomography in chronic seizure disorder caused by glioma. (with K. R. Rich and M. Gado). Arch. Neurol., *42:* 26–27, 1985.

The need to trace our roots in difficult times. Presidential Address, The American Association of Neurological Surgeons. J. Neurosurg., *63:* 485–491, 1985.

Contents

I

CHAPTER 1

CHAPTER 2

CHAPTER 3

II

PERSPECTIVES IN NEUROSURGERY

CHAPTER 4

CHAPTER 5

CHAPTER 6

―――――――――――― **III** ――――――――――――

CEREBROVASCULAR SURGERY

—————————— IV ——————————

PEDIATRIC NEUROSURGERY

—————————— V ——————————

SPINAL SURGERY

VI

INTRACRANIAL TUMORS

CHAPTER 36

VII

INFECTIONS

CHAPTER 37
CHAPTER 38
CHAPTER 39

VIII

NEUROSURGICAL TREATMENT OF VERTIGO

CHAPTER 40
CHAPTER 41

I

1

Presidential Address: Meeting the Challenges to Neurosurgical Education

ROBERT A. RATCHESON, M.D.

I would like to thank the members of the Congress of Neurological Surgeons (CNS) for the honor and privilege of serving as your President. I am very pleased to have with us today two of my teachers, Dr. Henry Schwartz and our honored guest, Dr. Sidney Goldring. I would like to acknowledge my great debt to them and also to Drs. William Coxe and Frank Nulsen. These gentlemen have served as exemplary models for a generation of neurological surgeons and have inspired the theme of this talk: the responsibility of teachers of neurosurgery to their students.

Neurosurgery, although practiced and taught by masters, is always practiced and taught by students. We remain far from our goal of perfection and our scholarship is never finished. In this regard, the purpose of the Congress of Neurological Surgeons—the education of present and future generations of neurological surgeons—is shared by all who practice our specialty.

Through the efforts of the American Board of Neurological Surgery, the Residency Review Committee, The Society of Neurological Surgeons, and the Joint Committee on Education of the AANS and CNS, neurosurgery has developed an effective and dynamic system of graduate medical education. However, today we are being asked to make changes, not for the purpose of improving the educational process for the benefit of society, but solely on the basis of economic considerations. How did this come about? I would like to review the challenges that face modern neurosurgical education and provide one perception of the historical events that have spawned today's challenges.

The medical profession differs from other occupations in part by its ability to set its own rules and standards. This became possible when members agreed upon criteria for belonging to the profession. As Paul Starr (11) points out in his book, *The Social Transformation of American Medicine,* in the early 19th century, the development of medical education was retarded by mutual hostility among practitioners, intense competition, differences in economic interests, and sectarian antagonism. These differences prevented mobilization of the profession for collective action or influencing public opinion. In 1893, the Johns Hopkins Medical School set rigid standards for medical education requiring all entering medical students to have college degrees and outlined a 4-year program based on the concept that medical education is a field of graduate study rooted in basic science. This marriage of science and research to clinical hospital practice revolutionized American medical education.

In 1904, the American Medical Association (AMA) formed a Council on Medical Education to elevate and standardize educational requirements. It required 4 years of high school, 4 years of medical school, and a licensing test (11). These actions, along with the Flexner Report of 1910 and the increased length of medical education demanded by state licensing boards, greatly influenced who attended medical school. Increasing the academic year from 4 to 9 months raised tuition costs. Lengthening training to 8 years after high school prevented anyone entering the field from making a living much before the age of 30. These changes effectively eliminated proprietary medical schools and limited enrollment.

The standardization and lengthening of medical education helped the profession gain favorable public opinion. Doctors related to patients as healers and benefactors. They gave care according to the needs of the sick and regulated fees according to the ability to pay. Physicians' economic security was not assured, but they could dictate their own practice conditions.

Before the Second World War, scientists opposed federal financing of research, which at that time was supported by private foundations and universities. After the war, medical research gained priority. A 1947 budget of 4 million dollars grew to 400 million dollars by 1960. Despite prewar concerns, science remained free from pressure groups and the need to produce immediate practical results. This was a time of immense growth in the medical establishment. From 1950 to 1970, the medical work force increased from 1.2 to 3.9 million people and health care expenditures grew from 13 to 72 billion dollars. Medical developments emphasized research, sophisticated technical development, and hospital construction, but the distribution of medical services was not addressed until the mid-1960s.

Although government money for research was sought, organized medicine held a different attitude toward aid to medical education. In 1949, Congress favored grants to increase the number of physicians, but AMA opposition allowed critical legislation to die. During the 1950s, funding for research aided medical school growth and enrollment enough to keep pace with population growth, but not with the increased demand for medical care.

At the same time, academic medicine was undergoing radical changes. In the 1920s and 1930s, faculty promotions had been slow and uncertain. Research money was scarce; National Institutes of Health (NIH) grants changed that. They supported new centers and stipends for large groups of investigators. Specialties grew allowing more individuals to rise to senior posts. Funds were primarily directed toward expanding internal medicine faculties. Students began entering specialties in increasing numbers and hospitals found it advantageous to have residency programs. House staff provided inexpensive professional labor, night and weekend coverage, and more thorough evaluations of patients. Hospitals expanded and there was competition for staff. Residency positions grew from 5000 in 1940 to 25,000 by 1955. Unfilled positions increased. In 1957, there were 12,000 internship positions and only 7000 American graduates (12). This shortage was one reason for increasing the number of medical students and ultimately led to eased governmental restrictions on foreign medical graduates who, by 1960, comprised 26% of house staff.

In 1959, nonuniversity hospitals provided 73% of approved residency training programs. Unable to recruit house staff competitively, these institutions sought medical school ties. By 1970, less than 10% of residencies were offered in unaffiliated hospitals.

A 1959 government report estimated that to keep up with population needs, the number of medical students should increase from the current 7400 to to 11,000 by 1975, and recommended even greater expansion to meet the demand for service, research, and teaching. This need became widely accepted. As medical care became more costly to the individual and society, recognition grew that whoever paid the cost of illness generated the gratitude and goodwill of the sick and their families. This realization created a powerful incentive for government and other institutions to intervene into the economics of medicine. In 1963, Congress initiated measures to expand education in the health profession. Lyndon Johnson's Great Society speech supporting Medicare made a crucial issue of providing money for the training of health professionals. In 1964, Medicare was introduced. It soon evolved from a program of compulsory hospital insurance to one that included government subsidization for physician bills and expanded assistance to states for medical care of the poor. Despite physicians' initial protests and boycott calls, within 1 year, Medicare was firmly established. Doctors discovered it to be a bonanza.

Part A of Medicare paid direct patient costs—plus depreciation—thereby favoring hospitals with the newest and most expensive facilities. Although in the 1970s some inequities remained, the poor's access to care improved. The Federal Government's desire to launch these new social programs created financial incentives (for both hospitals and physicians) that were likely irresponsible and poorly conceived. Starr (12) describes this as a policy of accommodation. Growth had continued haphazardly and, by the late 1970s, many believed reorganization was necessary. Today, it appears that government, doctors, hospitals, and our patients will pay the price for the lack of economic reality in the original planning.

In the 1970s, a loss of confidence in the method of practicing medicine occurred. It no longer was accepted axiomatically that Americans needed more medical care or that physicians and private voluntary institutions were best qualified to decide how to organize services. The public's attention shifted from scientific progress to economic problems, and public loyalty switched from providers to payers. The physician's image of affluence generated little public sympathy. In a setting of enormous cost increases, uncertain benefits, and unchecked excesses, the government intervened. We now face a medical system geared to expansion and a society and state demanding control over medical expenditures.

In neurosurgery, graduate medical education occurs in teaching hospitals, where the cost of medical care is significantly higher than in nonteaching hospitals (2b). Real costs associated with education include salary for residents and supervising faculty, clerical support, physical facilities, lowered productivity, and increased use of ancillary services. Teaching hospitals are located in urban settings with higher personnel costs. To retain teaching as we know it, these costs cannot be avoided.

Teaching hospitals perform other critical functions closely related to medical education, such as charity care. The 335 institutions of the Association of American Medical Colleges (AAMC) Council of Teaching Hospitals represent 5.8% of the nation's community hospitals, 17.7% of all admissions, 31.5% of the bad debts, and, in 1981, rendered 51% of the charity care (3). In general, teaching hospitals serve the most severely ill patients and provide regional stand-by services, such as transplantation and burn units, and carry on clinical research efforts to advance diagnosis and treatment. These increased costs have been financed primarily by patient service revenues consistent with private payer practices and the clearly established Congressional intent for Medicare. These hospitals provide the majority of the nation's residency training. Receiving the benefits of fully trained physicians—without incurring the costs of training them—are 4600 hospitals, Health Maintenance Organizations (HMOs), competitive medical plans, and Preferred Provider Organizations (PPOs). These nonteaching hospitals have an advantage in negotiating contracts with payers whose primary interest increasingly is the cost of the medical care that they subsidize. Teaching hospitals simply cannot compete on a price basis when third party payers and health care plans favor hospitals with low charges. They will be severely jeopardized as payers withdraw support. A system of medical reimbursement is evolving in which the payer only pays for immediate service, or predetermined payment replaces cost reimbursement, or the criterion for hospital selection is lowest price. Teaching hospitals will find it more difficult to incorporate the cost of education into the cost of patient care.

Currently before the U.S. Senate is a bill which limits federal funding for graduate medical education to 5 years and mandates preferential support for primary care trainees. If passed, the legislation would soon be followed by Veteran's Administration (VA) Hospitals and private payers. The growing number of HMOs will go to the lowest bidder. The high cost of the teaching hospital will mitigate participation in this form of providing care unless the hospital owns the HMO and is willing to run it at little or no profit. This legislation threatens to destabilize some outstanding neurosurgical training programs. Already beleagured teaching hospitals may be asked to support residents, in specialties such as neurosurgery, from professional fees, faculty/clinical income, endowments, gifts, or surplus (6). This plan would encourage hospital administrators to determine the need and appropriateness of training programs.

Plans to meet the pressures which will alter methods of graduate medical education, or at least payment for it, should be developed. However, those which force teaching hospitals to alter programs, cut back on residents or faculty, or decrease care to the indigent are not appealing. Ideally, payers would subordinate their self-interests to a broader social or ethical interest. Another alternative would be for society to impose a tax, theoretically allowing teaching hospitals to become competitive; but this tax would subject medical education to the uncertainties of annual Congressional debate. Our charge is to avoid a decrease in quality of care, educational ability, and different levels of care at a time of decline in physician influence, autonomy, and prestige.

I would like, at this point, to look at neurosurgical graduate education and how it might relate to the issues I have described. The origins of modern neurosurgery can be traced to a dedicated group of innovative scientific practitioners. Chiefly through the efforts of Harvey Cushing, the establishment of neurosurgery as a specialty attracted a select group of young men to this new and exciting field. That they must have been of a different breed is without question. In his history of the Society of Neurological Surgeons, Ernest Sachs lamented how difficult it was to find courageous young men who would consider entering the discouraging field of neurosurgery. He describes craniotomies without finding tumors and the need to keep a stiff upper lip (10). Yet, such men were found; many initially served Cushing for a year and then disbursed to plant the seeds of this fledgling specialty in their own students. Training requirements were informal, as was acceptance in a training program. The field grew and certain individuals became prominent educators. Among them were Sachs, Peet, Adson, Bailey, and later, Penfield.

In the late 1930s, the need for a certifying board became apparent. In October 1940, the American Board of Neurological Surgery held its first official meeting. Fifty neurosurgeons were certified without examination on the basis of holding professional rank as a neurosurgeon in the United States or Canada. Twenty-four candidates were examined. Although one of the founding members, Dr. Paul Bucy, assured me these individuals were chosen because they would surely pass the examination, three failed. There can be no doubt that the Board started on a firm and fair basis.

In 1942, the Board published the requirements necessary to become certified: graduation from an approved medical school, a 1-year surgical internship, and a period of study in neurological surgery of not less than 3 years (1). This training was designed to emphasize the relationship of the basic sciences to neurological surgery. In 1946, the Board began to accredit hospitals and institutions for neurosurgical training. It set requirements and supervised the selection and evaluation of residency programs. In 1950, the Board required progressive responsibility for trainees, prompting some programs to become associated with so-called "charity" hospitals where independent surgical experience could be obtained. In 1954, the Board established the Residency Review Committee (RRC) with representatives from the Board and the AMA. Actions of the RRC were subject to ratification by the Board, which continued to prescribe training requirements for certification and, in 1955, increased the length of training to 4 years.

Due to perceived Federal Trade Commission pressures, in the late 1960s, the AMA and the American College of Surgeons advocated a tripartite Residence Review Committee. During the early 1970s, the AMA Liaison Committee on Graduate Medical Education (LCGME) gained power to override the actions of the Board and the RRC. In 1980, the LCGME approved new special requirements that increased the period for certification to 5 years. In general, the mechanism through the Liaison Committee proved unsatisfactory and from it evolved the Accreditation Council on Graduate Medical Education (ACGME). Thus, accreditation of neurosurgical residency training passed from the American Board of Neurological Surgery to the RRC as delegated by the ACGME (2a). In 1985, the RRC enacted new plans for program evaluation that emphasized objective data and the educational environment of a program.

Historically, from an informal setting of early preceptorships, the neurosurgical residency program has developed into a structured period of training designed to meet the needs of the trainees. Today, the number of residents in a program is determined on the basis of clinical resources. Despite complicated legal issues, I believe the next major change should invoke prohibition of independent practice before board certification. Presently, active programs involving issues of academic policy, resident training, selection and evaluation, ethics, and research are being pursued by the Society of Neurological Surgeons and the Graduate Education Committee of the Joint Committee on Education. These organizations remain dedicated to improving the quality of neurosurgical training and its product.

Today, there are new problems that face neurosurgical education. Presently, many academic medical centers are in direct competition with community hospitals and other academic institutions. They are involved in price wars where discounts are given for elective surgery (7) and cash payment. Doctors receive bonuses for changing hospital staff. Prospective payment offers temptation for more and shorter hospitalizations. Third-party payers insist upon same-day testing or surgery, a practice that may endanger some patients, and that certainly denies house officers the opportunity to evaluate these patients, make preliminary decisions, and present well thought-out plans of work-up. If, as it appears, we cannot reverse this trend, then, by changing the traditional role of house officers from purely in-patient contact and by integrating them earlier into the evaluation and decision-making process, perhaps we can avoid presenting trainees with a body for which their only obligation is rapid preparation for operation.

Cost containment cannot be allowed to destroy our standards. Just as society must recognize and support the special contributions of teaching hospitals, there must be special consideration for supporting education. It has been suggested that neurosurgical programs should fund residencies. Most already do so, particularly for laboratory years. Academic neurosurgeons gain significant benefits from their association with residents, but not in the realm of personal financial reimbursement. Academicians are subject to malpractice insurance costs and, because of the patient mix, may be more vulnerable to suit. They support the dean's office and faculty practice plans. Residents desiring to pursue academic careers frequently require additional training, paid for by the residency program. Increased competition for NIH funds has forced programs to bear expenses prior to—or between—grants, in order to maintain a suitable academic environment with an ongoing laboratory program and provide security for laboratory workers and technicians. In some instances, patient-care facilities not provided by hospitals have been provided by training programs without Medicare reimbursement. Resident expenses such as meeting attendance, manuscript production, library maintenance, and computer resources are factors that seem not to be appreciated by some legislators and primary care advocates.

No one can deny the wisdom of public support for the education of future practitioners and researchers. Our training programs will have the most important influence upon the quality of future medical care. They will provide knowledge, skills, and standard of practice. These programs investigate and first apply complex and new technology and teach community responsibility to young physicians. It is in these programs that physicians learn that our profession is unforgiving, and that shortcuts for the purpose of personal convenience, decreased operating room time, or economic advantage for either the physician, hospital, or patient are unacceptable. Training programs have the unique responsibility to educate and train tomorrow's neurosurgeons. This alone is the reason for their existence.

Just as society cannot afford legislative and economic considerations to impinge upon our ability to educate future neurosurgeons and to affect the quality of those who enter our field, it cannot afford to keep residents out of research laboratories. To me, it is inconceivable that residents would not be exposed to the scientific method that is best gained in the laboratory. The development of all fully trained and critically thinking neurosurgeons should include opportunities for research. Governmental proposals to eliminate research from graduate medical education lack a sense of responsibility for the development of individuals who later will be the leaders in improving health care and scientific knowledge. Despite the contributions of residency programs, decreased federal funding for graduate medical education will affect residents' laboratory opportunities, participation in clinical protocols, and research carried out in conjunction with inpatient care. The financial stress placed upon teaching hospitals will deter cooperative research with industry and the development of new and expensive technology as installation costs, protocols, and technicians are often supported by the hospital.

The support of teaching hospitals as the major site of technological development is a reasonable expenditure in the form of indirect medical education costs. In many instances, the expense will be repaid to society in the form of cost-effective technology and improvement in the quality of care. Research experience is a vital part of the educational process. There is no worse alternative than stopping it. Industrial research and development is recovered per unit service. There is no logical reason why a hospital should not be allowed to recover its cost for "R&D"—which is performed for society's benefit—from patient care dollars. Funding from commercial sources has its dangers, particularly as it relates to directed research at the expense of basic research. Propietary hospitals are not an answer: it is important to remember that profits from these institutions will support traditional academic interests only to a limited contractual part and that the real profits will revert to investors.

Our role is to provide what society demands. I do not believe that society desires an industrial approach to medical care and the education of neurosurgeons. We are dealing with the future of the world's best health care system—one that has developed because of its educational excellence. The teaching hospital with its missions of patient care, education, and research must be protected. I believe the use of tax dollars toward this end is most appropriate and, therefore, we are obliged to communicate clearly the importance of what we are trying to do.

We are in an age when corporate medicine is developing. HMOs and investor-owned companies are growing rapidly, and nonprofit groups claim their aggressive tactics are necessary for survival. As Arnold Rellman has pointed out, health care—both for profit and nonprofit—is now marketed and sold like any other commodity, instead of being a service provided by dedicated people as one of civilization's critical social functions (9). Today, 35 million Americans are without any type of hospitalization insurance (8). If health care is distributed by income, people who cannot afford care will be denied access or dumped by both profit and nonprofit hospitals into fewer and fewer hospitals, mainly into underfunded public ones.

If trends continue, large companies and hospital-based HMOs will set the conditions under which we work and care is delivered. Economic power may influence our profession's values and ethics. The physician may become either the captive or partner of a corporation with direct impact on the quality of care delivered. No matter how good the equipment or how well technically trained the doctor, I see no place for graduate medical education in neurosurgery in this type of setting. I share Rellman's repulsion at the concept of the physician businessman and medical entrepreneurs who profit from decisions made about their patients. Residents must be taught, by example, that their obligation is to care for all patients.

Institutions cannot easily ignore the impact of economic reality, but physicians and students retain personal choices. The educator must be wary of actions performed in the name of competition. If there is to be competition, let it be on the basis of quality; not on the basis of physicians exploiting the media's desire for sensationalism by having the common appear extraordinary, or by turning a patient's good fortune into outlandish claims of individual or institutional excellence. The blame cannot be placed on the public or on the marketplace. It belongs squarely on the shoulders of hospitals and physicians who seek to gain from publicity. Certainly the academic, who may have greatest access to the press, must not fall prey to the "me too" era of competition among increasingly profit-and-publicity oriented health care institutions. Even at some of our finest academic institutions, human experimentation has been exploited and taken on the atmosphere of a freak show. Competition, advertising, and promotion are poor examples for future neurosurgeons.

I believe the mood of the public will change. Patient dissatisfaction with healing institutions that base care and relationships on finances, instead of individual dignity, will eventually awaken society to the effects of cost-containment and prospective payment. Our responsibility during this time is to maintain our educational values intact so there will be no danger of their being lost. Patient care and medical research cannot be separated. Training programs must have funds available to utilize for education and research. Teachers, alone, must set the standard of practice for themselves and their trainees. They must be allowed to remain independent and resist contemporary temptations.

In Longfellow's poem (5) Robert of Sicily is told by the angel that he can have his former glory if he pays the angel his due. At a time when success-ful training programs must provide technical skills in neurosurgery through a busy clinical practice, encourage high technology research, and maintain smooth interaction with hospital administrators, it will be neces-sary to pay homage only to the angels if we desire to retain our glory. Longfellow did not tell what happened to Robert of Sicily, but I am afraid that today's external forces are not the angels, and submission will not lead to an era of scientists and neurosurgeons dedicated to the advancement of our field. Sir Jeffrey Jefferson described Cushing as being "lucky" for being appointed to one of the great chairs in surgery from the age of 43 on—able to do as he pleased with ample facilities and great authority (4). I was unable to determine to which angels Cushing paid homage, but I believe it is important that we continue to learn from our forebearers—not only to keep tradition, but also because these men were brave, innovative, and uncompromising workers and investigators whose contributions were for the general benefit of the public.

A neurosurgical graduate educational system that has evolved through innovation must be allowed to evolve further, so that it may respond to the needs of society. It is our responsibility to see that these needs are met in a single tiered system that is free from the financial pressures of outside agencies or the financial aspirations of its practitioners. Future genera-tions of neurosurgeons must be allowed the same opportunities as the past. A neurosurgeon is a scientist, and science cannot flourish in an atmosphere of constraint brought about by outside influence, prescription, and protocols. Half a century ago, Cushing spoke against the concept of the Neurosurgeon as a plumber or carpenter operating at the bidding and instruction of the master nonsurgical brain (4). Today, our educational system faces the same threat. Neurosurgery should not function in response to bureaucratic demands, but within itself must design the future of its educational process. Residents must be isolated from the financial dictates of hospital administrators and bureaucrats who have little knowledge or concern of the unique demands and challenges of our field. We must take our case to the community so the public can understand that the issues of quality care and quality medical education are inseparable. Neurological surgery represents one of civilization's finest efforts, and remains an active and dynamic battle.

It has been said that when pessimism is in vogue, a belief in progress sounds dated. At the risk of appearing dated, we should remember that our history is one of progress. However, progress is interrupted when human beings submit to their own limitations and those imposed by the world about them. Perhaps our present rise will be temporarily interrupted now and there may be some pessimism for the short run. In fact, there may be problems beyond our solving. Yet, for the long run, neurosurgery will continue upward. In the words of John Trotwood Moore, "It is only the game fish that swims upstream."

ACKNOWLEDGMENT

The author would like to express his gratitude to his wife, Peggy, for her help and insightful comments during preparation of this manuscript and to Ms. Jean Jensen, who tirelessly prepared its many drafts.

REFERENCES

1. American Board of Neurological Surgery, Inc. Approved examining boards in medical specialties. J.A.M.A., *119:* 1352–1353, 1942.
2a. Courtesy of the American Board of Neurological Surgery, Inc. and Accreditation Council for Graduate Medical Education.
2b. Cameron, J. M. The indirect costs of graduate medical education. N. Engl. J. Med., *312:* 1223–1238, 1985.
3. Inglehart, J. K. Health policy report. N. Engl. J. Med., *312:* 1000–1004, 1985.
4. Jefferson, G. Harvey Cushing. In *Neurosurgical Giants: Feet of Iron and Clay,* edited by P. C. Bucy, Elsevier, New York, 1985.
5. Longfellow, H. W. Tales of a wayside inn. In *The Complete Poetical Works of Henry Wadsworth Longfellow.* Houghton Mifflin Company, The Riverside Press, Cambridge 215–218, 1893.
6. Petersdorf, R. G. A proposal for financing graduate medical education. N. Engl. J. Med., *323:* 1322–1324, 1985.
7. Petersdorf, R. G. Current and future directions for hospital and physician reimbursement. J.A.M.A., *253:*17 pp 2543–2548, 1985.
8. Reitemeier, R. J. Effects of Cost Containment on Graduate Medical Education in Proceed-

ings of Invitational Conference on Financing Graduate Medical Education in An Era of Cost Containment, Council of Medical Specialty Societies, Lake Forest, April, 1985.
9. Rellman, A. The new medical industrial complex. N. Engl. J. Med., *303:* 963–970, 1980.
10. Sachs, E. The early history of the society of neurological surgeons. In *The Society of Neurological Surgeons—Diamond Jubilee.* Hunter Publishing Co., Winston-Salem, 1984.
11. Starr, P. *The Social Transformation of American Medicine,* Book 1, Chapter 3. Basic Books, Inc., New York, 1982.
12. Starr, P. *The Social Transformation of American Medicine,* Book 2, Chapter 3. Basic Books, Inc., New York, 1982.

CHAPTER

2

Experience with Gliomas in Patients Presenting with a Chronic Seizure Disorder

SIDNEY GOLDRING, M.D., KEITH M. RICH, M.D.,
and SELWYN PICKER, M.B. B.Ch.

In a previous brief communication (9), we reported a series of patients with chronic seizure disorder who had an isolated lesion of unknown etiology on computed tomography (CT) scan. The past history of these patients did not reveal any preceding event such as trauma, infection, or stroke to account for the lesions. The mean interval from the onset of seizures to surgery was 11 years; yet it was known for a number of years that the CT scan was abnormal in many of these patients. The usual reason for the delay in obtaining surgical evaluation was interpretation of the abnormal scan as showing a non-neoplastic lesion. The delay was more likely if the abnormality was located in the vicinity of the sensorimotor or language cortex. The majority of these patients (26 of 32), however, proved to have a glioma, with seven showing anaplastic changes. Because of this finding, we recommended early surgical treatment in patients with chronic seizure disorder who have an isolated lesion of unknown origin on CT scan.

Our experience with such cases, both gliomas and lesions that mimic them, has now grown to 51. In this paper, we analyze further our experience with this group of patients. We sought to answer a number of questions. What effect does surgical management have on the seizures? What kind of surgical procedure is necessary to bring the seizures under control? Does one have to include in the resection the presumed epileptogenic cortex adjacent to the lesion or is only excision of the gross pathology necessary (8)? What about the patients in whom only biopsy and radiation is possible? Does this therapy have a beneficial effect on the seizures? What about lesions in the vicinity of sensitive areas, such as the sensorimotor region or parasylvian territory in the dominant hemisphere? Should surgery be deferred in those cases and considered only as a last resort? Finally, what about the patients who harbored benign, non-neoplastic lesions that mimicked gliomas? How did they fare with surgery?

Our experience will be presented in two installments. In this chapter, we will deal with the gliomas. In Chapter 3, we will discuss those lesions that

15

mimic gliomas and then focus on the utility of functional localization as an important adjunct in the surgical management of gliomas and related lesions.

METHODS AND CLINICAL MATERIAL

The patient population consists of 51 individuals who were referred primarily for treatment of seizure disorder. Forty proved to have a glioma; six had a vascular malformation; three had an arachnoid cyst; and two had miscellaneous lesions (Table 2.1). Their ages ranged from 6 to 56 years, with a mean age of 20 years. The duration of the seizure disorder ranged from 1 to 27 years with a mean duration of 11 years. Seizures were the only symptom. The neurological examinations were normal except for a right lower extremity monoparesis in one patient. None exhibited signs of an expanding intracranial lesion. With the exception of seven patients who had anterior temporal lobectomies and two patients with frontal and parietal lobe gliomas, respectively, surgical management consisted only of excision of the lesion or in addition, excision of only that amount of cortex that was necessary for gaining access to the lesion. Resection of presumed epileptogenic cortex adjacent to the lesion was not performed. Electrocorticography (ECG) was employed in only three patients and led to resection of epileptogenic cortex in the two patients with the frontal and parietal lobe gliomas mentioned above. In the seven patients who had anterior temporal lobectomies, the uninvolved adjacent anterior hippocampus and parahippocampal gyrus were resected because of the known propensity of

TABLE 2.1

Pathology of Lesions Discovered on CT Scan in Patients Presenting with Chronic Seizure Disorder

Pathology	Number of Patients
Glioma	
Astrocytoma (low-grade)	25
Glioblastoma	2
Ganglioglioma	5
Mixed glioma	5
Xanthoastrocytoma	1
Oligodendroglioma	1
Vascular malformation	7
Arachnoid cyst	3
Miscellaneous	
Epidermoid	1
Cysticercosis cyst	1
	Total 51

the hippocampus for developing epileptogenic foci. Other than proximity of the pathology to the medial structures, no set of criteria was used to determine which patients would have the hippocampus and adjacent cortex resected and which would not. In fact, close proximity of the lesion to the medial structures usually did not result in an anterior temporal lobectomy. Twenty-three other patients who had temporal lobe lesions, many of which were located medially, had only the lesion excised.

RESULTS: HISTORY RELATED TO CT SCANS

In 23 of the 40 patients with gliomas, a solitary lesion had been demonstrated on the CT scan, from 6 months to 6 years before being referred for surgery. In the remainder, a single scan had been obtained, which had been interpreted as negative, and no further scans were made, or they had never had a CT scan before being referred for surgery (Table 2.2).

In those patients who were known to have a lesion, the referring neurologist or neurosurgeon usually interpreted the abnormality as representing a heterotopia, calcified clot, old infarct, or encephalomalacia. Gliomas were not considered to be a likely possibility. Figure 2.1 shows some representative examples of the abnormal scans. Interpretation of the scans as showing a non-neoplastic lesion was reinforced when serial scans taken over the years showed no change in size or appearance of the lesion. The failure to find a change, however, was typical. In only two cases did serial scans demonstrate a change. In one, the lesion increased in size and, in the other, a hypodense lesion came to show enhancement with intravenous contrast injection; although it did not show any growth. Another factor that influenced delay in surgical referral was the location of the lesion. Either the involved cerebral area was considered to be incapable of giving rise to the seizure pattern and, hence, the lesion was considered asymptomatic, or the abnormality was presumed to reside within, or in close proximity to, the sensorimotor or language cortex.

TABLE 2.2

History Related to CT Scan in 40 Patients Who Had Chronic Seizure Disorder Caused by Gliomas

Description	Number of Patients
Knowledge of positive CT scan 6 months to 6 years before surgery	23
Early CT scan negative. No further CT scans before surgical evaluation	10
Failed to get CT scan before surgical evaluation	7

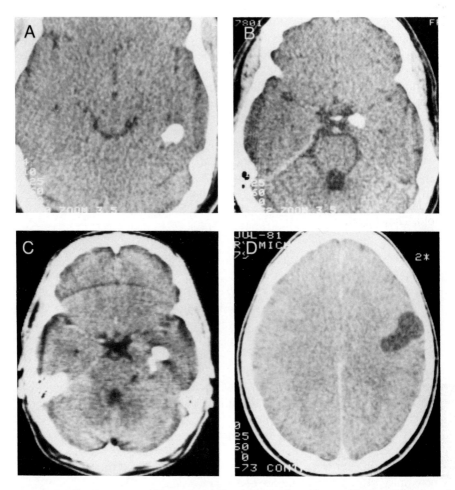

FIG. 2.1. Representative CT scans of solitary lesions in patients with chronic seizure disorder who proved to have gliomas. (*A*) Temporal lobe astrocytoma. (*B*) Temporal lobe astrocytoma with mild anaplastic changes. (*C*) Temporal lobe glioblastoma multiforme. (*D*) Parietal lobe, well-differentiated astrocytoma.

In all but one of the patients who were referred with a single negative scan, a lesion was clearly demonstrated in the routine scans we obtained for evaluation of epilepsy surgery. The most common explanation for the initial negative scan or the scan in which the presence of a lesion was equivocal was the quality of the image. The negative scans usually were obtained with early-generation scanners. In cases where the findings on the routine scan were equivocal, we found a high-resolution CT scan (axial slices made every 4 mm instead of 8 mm and a reduced field of view) helpful in clearly exposing the lesion. In only one of these cases, a ganglioglioma, did the preoperative CT scan, including a high-resolution one, fail to demonstrate a lesion. The tumor, however, was crisply demonstrated with a magnetic resonance image (MRI) scan. MRI scans also were helpful in defining more clearly the configuration and margins of some of the lesions and thus helped in planning the surgical approach. The following brief case histories will demonstrate the findings summarized above.

ILLUSTRATIVE CASE REPORTS

Case 1

M.C., a 14-year-old girl, developed focal seizures when she was 6 years old. They began with a feeling of numbness in her right leg. This aura was frequently followed by stiffening of both lower extremities and falling. She was experiencing four to five seizures a day. The outside CT scan was negative. She was admitted for surgical evaluation on March 8, 1981. Routine CT scans obtained during preoperative work-up suggested the presence of a lesion in the frontoparietal region near the midline. This finding was conclusively demonstrated with a high-resolution CT scan (Fig. 2.2). On March 10, 1981, she underwent a craniotomy with excision of a pilocytic astrocytoma. Functional localization showed the tumor to be nestled

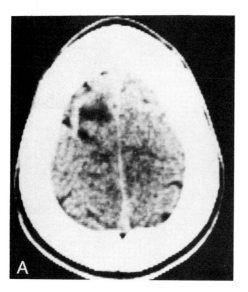 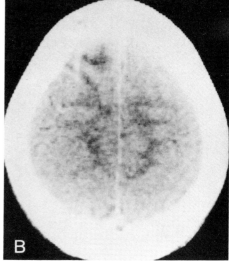

FIG. 2.2. Comparison of routine (*right*) with high-resolution (*left*) CT scan in patient with left posterior frontal astrocytoma.

against the anterior bank of the motor leg area (Figs. 2.3–2.5). She recovered without neurologic deficit and remains seizure-free 4 years after surgery.

COMMENT

This case demonstrates the value of obtaining a high-resolution CT scan and also the importance of not being dissuaded from proceeding with surgery when the seizure pattern and location of the abnormality suggest that the lesion resides in a sensitive area. During surgery, the lesion was found, for the most part, to be separable from the brain and could be totally removed without incurring a neurologic deficit. Functional localization precisely established the geographic relationship of the tumor to the motor cortex and provided the necessary information to deal knowledgeably and safely with removal of the lesion.

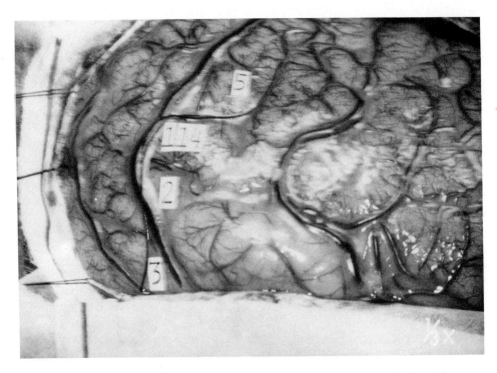

FIG. 2.3. Astrocytoma nestled against the motor gyrus. Anterior is to the right, the midline is at the bottom. Meandering black thread is central fissure. Numbered tickets relate to functional localization.

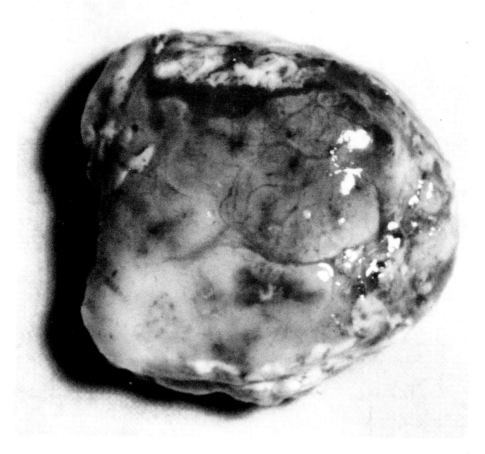

FIG. 2.4. Enucleated tumor shown in Figure 2.3.

Case 2

P.B., a 26-year-old woman, developed nocturnal generalized seizures in 1977. With anticonvulsant medication, seizures became focal, but were intractable to medical management. Seizures were characterized by extension of the right upper extremity followed by clonic jerking of the forearm and hand. A left hypodense frontoparietal lesion was demonstrated on CT scan in 1979, 5 years before surgery. Serial scans showed no change in the size or appearance of the lesion (Fig. 2.6). Because of the lesion's appearance and location, a debate ensued as to whether or not the patient should have only a needle biopsy or a craniotomy. An MRI scan provided much

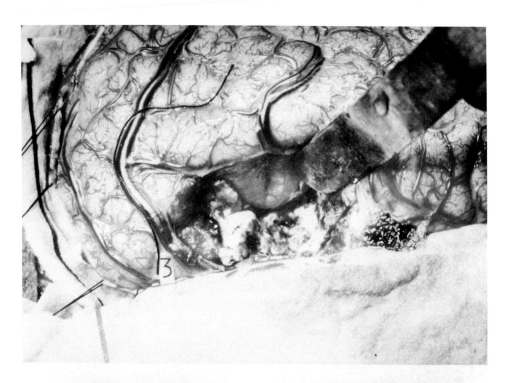

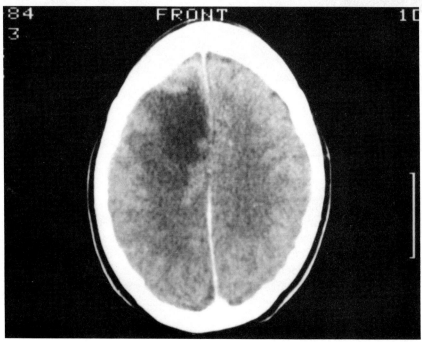

22

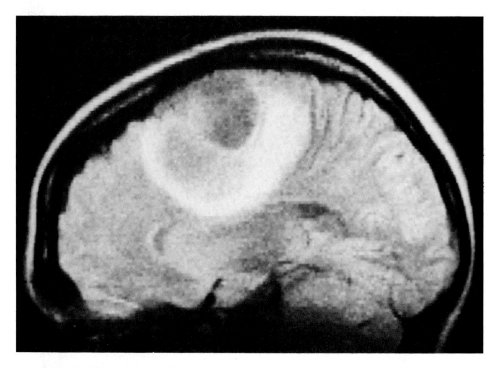

FIG. 2.7. MRI scan (proton density image) of same patient shown in Figure 2.6. Large, well-circumscribed, frontoparietal lesion with sharp margins. Note crowding and posterior displacement of the gyri posterior to the tumor. The central hypodense area does not represent a cyst and the surrounding hyperdensity does not represent edema. The entire lesion was solid tumor. The two different densities represent a change in tumor consistency with the central hypodense area having a more gelatinous and softer quality.

better definition of the lesion (Fig. 2.7). In contrast to the CT scan, the lesion appeared to be well circumscribed with sharp margins and did not indicate associated edema. The lesion occupied the frontoparietal region and appeared to be centered on the central sulcus. On October 30, 1984, the patient underwent craniotomy. A huge astrocytoma was encountered

---

FIG. 2.5. Tumor bed following removal of astrocytoma shown in Figure 2.3. Anterior is to the right and midline is at the bottom. Meandering black thread is the central fissure. Note the intact anterior bank of the motor gyrus. Numbered ticket 3 relates to functional localization.

FIG. 2.6. CT scan showing large, hypodense lesion without discrete borders in left frontoparietal region suggesting associated edema.

(Fig. 2.8). Functional localization showed that the tumor had displaced the motor strip posteriorly and could be peeled away from its anterior bank (Fig. 2.9). The tumor was entirely removed except anteriorly where it blended imperceptibly with normal brain tissue. Postoperatively, the patient exhibited a mild right hemiparesis and dysphasia, from which she recovered in several weeks. She has been seizure-free and without neurologic deficit since surgery 1 year ago.

COMMENT

This case demonstrates several important points. First, that the failure of serial CT scans to show a change in the size or appearance of a lesion is no assurance that the lesion is not a tumor. In this patient, serial scans over a 5-year period did not demonstrate any change. Second, the value of MRI scanning is in providing both better definition of the lesion and its relationship to the surrounding brain. Third, the importance of craniotomy

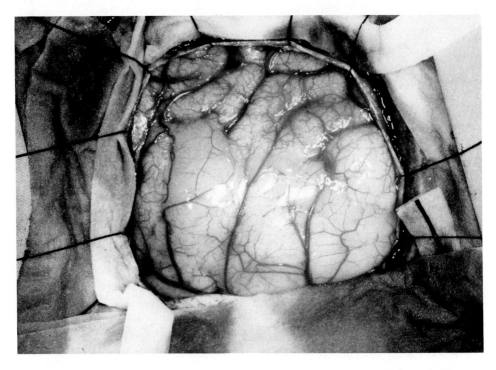

FIG. 2.8. Left posterior frontal astrocytoma. Same patient whose scans are shown in Figures 2.6 and 2.7. Anterior is to the right and midline is at the bottom. Tumor abuts an intact motor gyrus which has been displaced posteriorly.

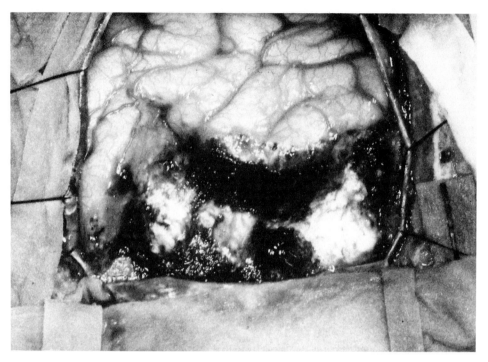

Fig. 2.9. Tumor bed after resection of astrocytoma shown in Figure 2.8. Tumor peeled away from the anterior bank of the motor gyrus which forms the posterior wall of the tumor bed. *Black areas* in tumor bed are surgical.

is to inspect the lesion directly and to carry out functional localization before deciding whether a lesion is inoperable. In this patient, both CT and MRI scans strongly suggested that the tumor could not be removed without producing a hemiparesis. Yet, functional localization demonstrated that the motor strip had been displaced posteriorly and was not involved, permitting gross, near-total removal.

Case 3

R.R., a 43-year-old male, experienced a grand mal seizure followed by transient postictal paralysis of his left face. In 1974, he developed complex partial seizures. Surgical evaluation failed to demonstrate a lesion or an electrical focus. The complex seizures disappeared, but left focal facial seizures continued to occur. In 1976, a CT scan showed a small, indistinct, right frontal hypodensity. In 1981, CT scan revealed a large, right frontal, hypodense, nonenhancing lesion (Fig. 2.10). On July 19, 1981, the patient

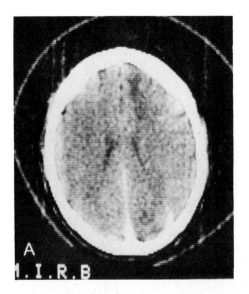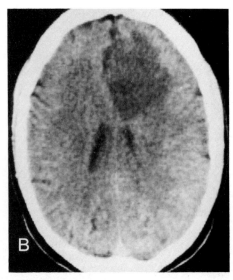

FIG. 2.10. CT scans showing growth of hypodense lesion (astrocytoma). CT scan on the *left* was taken in 1976; the one on the *right* in 1981.

underwent a right frontal craniotomy. The lesion did not lend itself to removal and only a biopsy was obtained. Histologic examination showed an astrocytoma with anaplastic changes. The patient underwent radiation therapy. Four years after radiation, he remains seizure-free and is neurologically normal.

COMMENT

This is the author's only case in which serial CT scans demonstrated tumor growth. The therapeutic response with respect to the seizures is also noteworthy. This aspect will be discussed in more detail later.

Case 4

W.G., a 30-year-old male, had two grand mal seizures in 1977. He was 23 years of age. Shortly thereafter, he began to have complex partial seizures that were poorly controlled with medication. Serial CTs, including a high-resolution scan, were normal (Fig. 2.11). On admission for surgical evaluation, the patient underwent an MRI scan that clearly defined a lateral lesion in the right anterior temporal lobe (Fig. 2.12). At surgery, the lesion occupied the inferior temporal gyrus. It was completely excised and proved to be a ganglioglioma. For the brief 1-year period since surgery, he remains seizure-free.

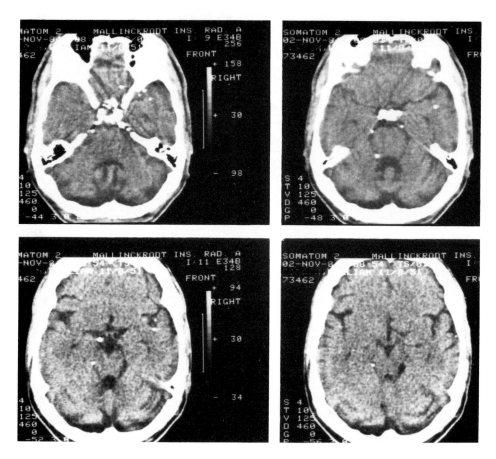

FIG. 2.11. Normal high-resolution CT scan in patient who proved to have a ganglioglioma of the right temporal lobe.

COMMENT

This is the only patient in this report whose lesion was not detected by CT scan but revealed by MRI scan.

Case 5

C.H., a 20-year-old woman, developed complex partial seizures at 5 years of age. The seizures were characterized by disorientation, loss of contact, and automatisms consisting of lip-smacking, fidgeting with her hands, and aimless walking. The seizures were poorly controlled. A cluster of four to six seizures a day occurred every few weeks. Serial CT scans showed a hypodense lesion in the right parieto-occipital area adjacent to the midline.

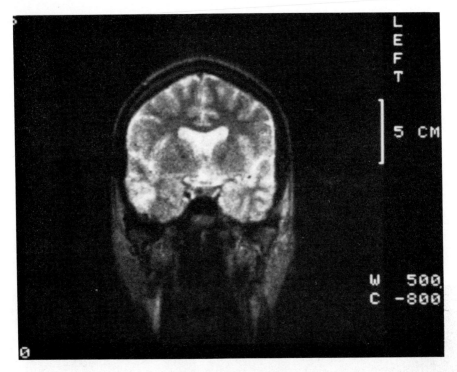

Fig. 2.12. MRI scan (T2 weighted image) of same patient whose CT scan is shown in Figure 2.11. Note lesion, ganglioglioma, occupying right inferiolateral temporal lobe. It was not detected by the CT scan shown in Figure 2.11.

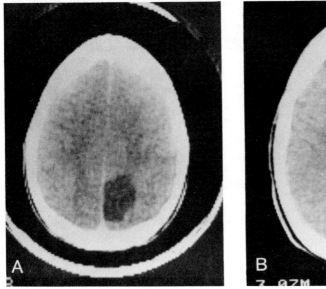
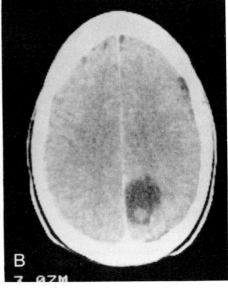

Fig. 2.13. Comparison of CT scans showing hypodense parietal lesion made in 1978 (*left*) and 1984 (*right*). No change in size, but 1984 scan shows hyperdense nodule not present in 1978.

The size of the lesion remained the same in the serial scans, but the preoperative scan showed an enhancing nodule that was not present earlier (Fig. 2.13). It was considered unlikely that the lesion was responsible for her seizures, which pointed to a focus in the temporal lobe. Because of the changing character of the lesion, however, it was decided to deal with the tumor first. If its removal did not achieve seizure control, which we believed would be the case, evaluation for an anterior temporal lobectomy would be considered at a later date. On June 5, 1984, a tumor was removed. It proved to be an astrocytoma with mild anaplastic changes. It presented on the medial surface of the hemisphere in the longitudinal fissure and extended inferiorly to the posterior cingulate gyrus. It separated from normal-appearing brain and was totally removed except anteriorly, where

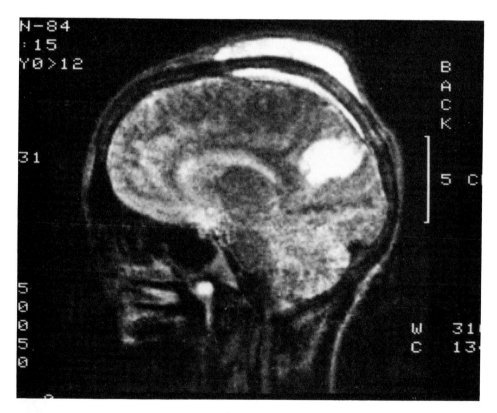

FIG. 2.14. Postoperative MRI scan (T2 weighted image) of same patient whose preoperative CT scans are shown in Figure 2.13. Note postoperative edema in tumor bed which extends to impinge on posterior cingulate gyrus. Edema also present in soft tissues in the vicinity of the craniotomy site.

it blended with normal-appearing tissue. That the tumor had abutted on the cingulate gyrus was supported by a postoperative MRI scan that showed postoperative changes extending to the cingulum (Fig. 2.14). In the early postoperative period, the woman had several seizures, but they were a different pattern from the preoperative seizures and were associated with drug abuse. Other than these several episodes, the patient remains seizure-free 1 year and 4 months since surgery and recently has been taken off all medication.

COMMENT

The finding that the lesion involved the cingulum was not appreciated until the patient was explored. The lesion was considered to reside in the posterior parietal lobe and probably to be unrelated to the seizures. Had not the latest CT scan shown a change in the appearance of the lesion, it is doubtful that the patient would have come to craniotomy. The fact that her seizures were brought under control after tumor removal implicates the lesion as the cause of her seizures.

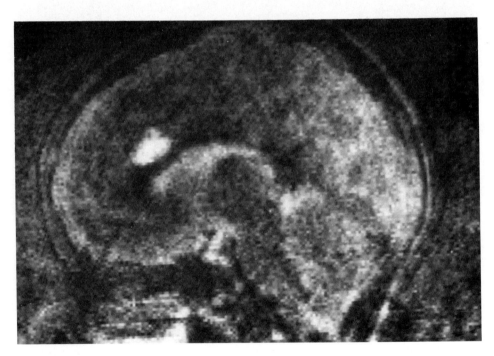

FIG. 2.15. MRI scan (T2 weighted image) showing hyperdense lesion (astrocytoma) embedded in anterior cingulate gyrus. The lesion gave rise to complex partial seizures.

Although the large majority of patients who suffer from complex partial seizures have their focus in the temporal lobe, production of complex partial seizures by extratemporal lesions is known, especially when they occur in the orbital and medial frontal lobes and cingulate gyrus (7, 11, 12). This is important to keep in mind, as demonstrated by this case. Indeed, two other patients in this series had complex partial seizures caused by lesions of the anterior cingulate gyrus. Both a 6-year-old child shown in Figure 2.15 and a 33-year-old woman shown in Figure 2.16 had astrocytomas.

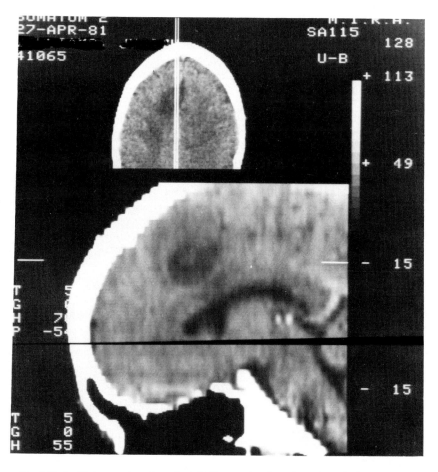

FIG. 2.16. Sagittal reconstruction of axial CT scan showing a hypodense lesion, an astrocytoma, impinging on anterior cingulate gyrus. As in the patients demonstrated in Figures 2.14 and 2.15, it gave rise to complex partial seizures.

Case 6

M.M., a 23-year-old male, had a febrile illness when he was 15 months old associated with coma and probably a generalized seizure. He was then asymptomatic until he was 5 years old when he exhibited absence attacks. Again seizures stopped until age 12 years, when he had a generalized status and subsequently developed complex partial seizures. The seizures were ushered in by a "weird" feeling followed by loss of contact, a grin, and automatisms consisting of lip-smacking, and clenching and unclenching his hands. The seizures occurred four to five times a day. CT scans demonstrated a hypodense, nonenhancing lesion in the parietal lobe (Fig. 2.17). This lesion was considered to be unrelated to the seizures. An MRI scan was obtained which more clearly defined the lesion and showed it residing in the parietal operculum and abutting on the posterior temporal lobe (Fig. 2.18). This finding increased the probability that the lesion was responsible for the complex partial seizures. At craniotomy, the tumor was

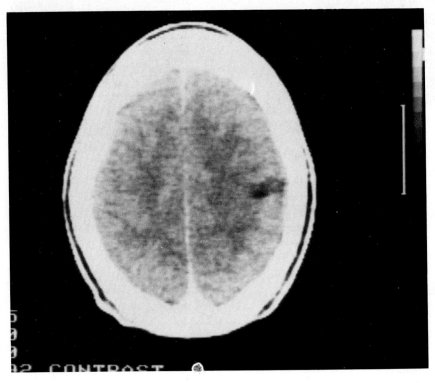

FIG. 2.17. CT scan showing a hypodense right parietal lesion which gave rise to complex partial seizures.

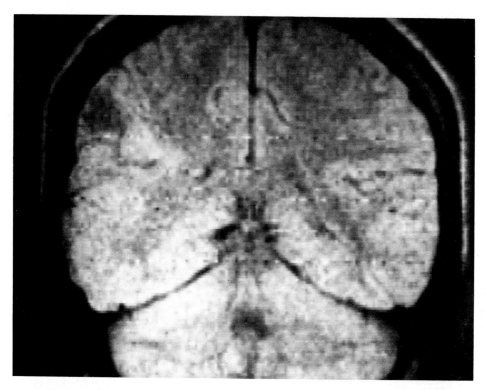

FIG. 2.18. MRI scan (T1 weighted image) of same patient whose CT scan is shown in Figure 2.17. Scan shows that the parietal lesion (*arrows*) abuts the posterior sylvian fissure.

found to present on the surface. Functional localization showed it to reside in the gyrus immediately posterior to the somatosensory zone in the region of the face representation. The tumor abutted on the buried surface of the superior temporal gyrus in the posterior temporal lobe (Fig. 2.19). The tumor could be readily peeled away from the cortex and it was entirely removed except in one small area of the superior temporal gyrus, which it had invaded and blended imperceptibly with normal brain tissue. Two months postoperatively, the patient had one seizure when he stopped taking his anticonvulsant medication regularly. Other than that episode, he has been seizure-free in the 1 year and 3 months since surgery.

COMMENT

This case is another example in which the location of the lesion on the CT scan made it seem unlikely that it was responsible for the seizures. The cause and effect relationship between the lesion and the seizure was made

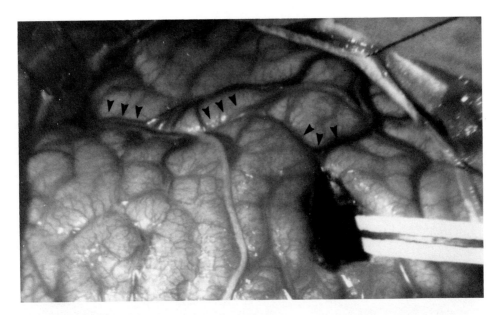

FIG. 2.19. Photograph showing tumor bed of the same patient whose scans are shown in Figures 2.17 and 2.18. Sylvian fissure is spotted by *arrows*. Thread identifies the central fissure. Cottonoid on the *right* rests in the tumor bed. As predicted by the MRI scan, the tumor impinged on the sylvian fissure. It superficially invaded the buried surface of the superior temporal gyrus and hence explained the complex partial seizures in this patient.

plausible by the MRI scan and surgical exploration. The seizure history also made it seem unlikely that the seizures and the lesion on CT scan were related. The seizures started in infancy during a febrile illness and there was a multiyear interval when the patient was seizure-free. Such a history is more characteristic of epilepsy of non-neoplastic origin.

SURGICAL OUTCOME

Results in Patients Who Had Surgery without Radiation

Thirteen patients did not receive postoperative radiation. In all but one, a gross "total" removal was achieved. With one exception, the seizures have been controlled from 6 months to 10 years after surgery with a mean follow-up of 3.3 years (Table 2.3). Three had one or several seizures in the early postoperative period. The others have been seizure-free since surgery. None show any evidence of tumor recurrence.

Results in Patients Who Had Surgery Followed By Radiation Therapy

In 23 patients, surgery was followed by radiation therapy. All but four have had their seizures controlled. Two had several seizures in the early

TABLE 2.3

Results in Patients Who Had Surgery Without Radiation

Patient	Age (yr) at Onset of Seizures/Surgery	Diagnosis	Follow-Up	Seizures*
B.G.	12/15	Temporal ganglioglioma	10 years	0
T.L.	6 mo/13	Frontal mixed glioma	8 years	X
L.F.	15/23	Temporal xanthoastrocytoma	4 years	0
M.H.	22/24	Temporo-occipital astrocytoma	4 years	0
W.B.	4/21	Temporal ganglioglioma	4 years	0
M.P.	5/14	Parietal astrocytoma	4 years	0^1
B.T.	9/13	Temporal ganglioglioma	2 years	0
D.S.	8/19	Occipital astrocytoma	2 years	0^1
J.P.	3/18	Temporal ganglioglioma	1½ years	0
C.H.	5/22	Parietal astrocytoma (AAF)	1 year	0
S.F.	6/17	Temporal astrocytoma (AAF)	1 year	0^1
W.G.	19/30	Temporal ganglioglioma	1 year	0
C.M.	6/18	Temporal astrocytoma	6 months	0^1

* 0 = no seizures; 0^1 = one or several seizures in early postoperative period; X = seizures; AAF = atypical or anaplastic foci.

postoperative period, but none thereafter. The others have been seizure-free since surgery. They have been followed from 3 months to 7 years with a mean follow-up period of 2.25 years (Table 2.4). One patient expired 1 year after surgery from recurrence of a xanthoastrocytoma that had malignant changes. She had complex parietal seizures for 7 years before surgery. During the year after surgery and before her death, she was seizure-free. All of the other patients in this group, including patient T.G. who had a glioblastoma multiforme, are well and have shown no signs of recurrence.

A gross total or near-total removal was achieved in all of these patients. As stated under Methods and Clinical Material, only three patients underwent electrocorticography for the purpose of localizing the epileptogenic focus and in two of these, recordings led to excision of the focus in addition to the tumor. In one (T.L.), the focus was in the attenuated shell of cortex overlying the tumor, a mixed glioma. This cortical shell was excised for the purpose of gaining access to the tumor, as well as eliminating the focus. This patient continues to have seizures, but their occurrence is related to failure to take anticonvulsant medication and drug abuse. The other patient (S.S.) had two types of seizures preoperatively. The most

TABLE 2.4
Results in Patients Who Had Surgery and Radiation

Patient	Age (yr) at Onset of Seizures/Surgery	Diagnosis	Follow-Up	Seizures*
B.S.	10/17	Temporal oligodendroglioma	7 years	0
J.D.	7/13	Temporal mixed glioma	5 years	0
S.S.	5/19	Temporal astrocytoma	5 years	0
M.C.	6/14	Parietal astrocytoma	4 years	0
R.L.	7/19	Temporal mixed glioma	4 years	X
B.H.	7/30	Temporal astrocytoma	4 years	X
J.P.	5/32	Temporal mixed glioma	4 years	0
J.W.	33/35	Frontal astrocytoma (AAF)	4 years	X
K.H.	6/10	Temporal astrocytoma	4 years	0
R.W.	18/23	Temporal astrocytoma (AAF)	3½ years	0
P.L.	11/25	Temporal astrocytoma	2½ years	0
T.G.	2/23	Temporal glioblastoma multiforme	2 years	0
J.J.	10/23	Temporal mixed glioma	1½ years	0^1
W.L.	11/18	Temporal astrocytoma (AAF)	1½ years	X
J.S.	1½/8	Temporal astrocytoma (AAF)	1½ years	0
N.H.	6/7	Frontal astrocytoma (AAF)	1½ years	0
M.M.	2/24	Parietal astrocytoma (AAF)	1 year	0^1
P.B.	19/26	Frontal astrocytoma (AAF)	1 year	0
D.B.	15/24	Temporal xanthoastrocytoma with malignant changes	1 year (expired)	0
H.B.	5/9	Temporal astrocytoma	4 months	0
J.M.	3/10	Temporal astrocytoma	4 months	0
P.D.	14/23	Temporal astrocytoma (AAF)	3 months	0
J.L.	2/19	Temporal ganglioglioma with malignant changes	3 months	0

* 0 = no seizures; 0^1 = one to several seizures in early postoperative period; X = seizures; (AAF) = atypical or anaplastic foci.

frequent seizure was focal, involving the left upper extremity. The other seizure was nonfocal, in which she lost contact and collapsed to the ground. Electrocorticography identified two foci, one in the gyrus immediately posterior to the somatosensory hand area and the other in prefrontal cortex. Only the parietal focus, which gave rise to the focal seizures, was excised. Both seizure types stopped. This patient remains seizure-free 5 years after surgery. Any explanation for the disappearance of the akinetic seizure related to the anterior focus would, at best, be speculative.

Results in Patients Who Had Only Biopsy and Radiation

There were four such patients (Table 2.5). All had frontal lobe tumors and, in all, the diagnosis was established by craniotomy. The tumors had no clear boundaries and did not lend themselves to surgical removal. All four have been followed for 4 years. Three have been seizure-free since radiation therapy. Two of these patients enjoy a normal neurologic status. The third has a mild ataxic gait, but CT scan shows no evidence of tumor recurrence. The fourth patient (M.V.), who continues to have seizures, has a right monoparesis in the lower extremity, which was present before radiation. This patient is the only one in the entire series who presented with a neurologic deficit in addition to seizure disorder. The most recent scan shows no evidence of recurrence.

Comparison Between Preoperative and Postoperative Seizure Record in Patients Who Continue To Have Seizures

Of the six patients who have postoperative seizures, the seizure frequency or intensity, or both, have been significantly reduced in three (R.L., B.H., J.W.), and they enjoy an improved quality of life (Table 2.6). In the remaining three, the seizure history is essentially unchanged in two (B.L. and M.V.) and in the third (T.L.), although the seizure frequency is much reduced, the breakthroughs associated with noncompliance and drug abuse are so disruptive that the patient remains dependent.

TABLE 2.5

Results in Patients Who Had Only Biopsy and Radiation (Frontal Lobe Tumors)

Patient	Age (yr) at Onset of Seizures/Surgery	Diagnosis	Follow-Up	Seizures*
R.R.	30/43	Astrocytoma (AAF)	4 years	0
D.W.	4/6	Astrocytoma	4 years	0
D.C.	32/44	Astrocytoma	4 years	0
M.V.	17/56	Astrocytoma	4 years	X

* 0 = no seizures; X = seizures; (AAF) = atypical or anaplastic foci.

TABLE 2.6

Comparison Between Preoperative and Postoperative Seizure Record in Patients Who Continue to Have Seizures

Patient	Preoperative	Postoperative
R.L.	Daily complex partial seizures with loss of contact and automatisms	Absence attack (several sec) about 2 a week
B.H.	2 to 3 complex partial seizures a day with loss of contact, automatisms, and urinary incontinence	2 to 3 daily absence attacks (several sec) a day
J.W.	Cluster of right focal seizure ushered in by complex partial phenomena (5 min) every 2 weeks	Several brief seizures a year
B.L.	3 to 4 complex partial seizures a day	After several weeks of being seizure-free, seizures returned and increased to preoperative frequency
M.V.	1 right focal seizure a month (leg), may generalize	1 right focal seizure a month
T.L.	10 to 20 left facial focal seizures a day, frequently generalizing	Breaks through with cluster of seizures several times a year, the latter related to noncompliance and drug abuse

Results, Regardless of Method of Treatment

In sum, if we consider all patients who have been followed for 1 or more years (mean follow-up of 3.3 years), regardless of the method of treatment, 29 of 35, or 82%, are seizure-free. If we add to the 29 seizure-free patients the three who have had a marked reduction in seizure frequency or intensity or both, (first three patients in Table 2.6), then 91% have benefited

TABLE 2.7

Resection of Temporal Lobe Tumor and Medial Temporal Lobe

Patient	Seizure	Follow-Up
W.B.	0	4 years
R.L.	X	4 years
B.H.	X	4 years
K.H.	0	4 years
T.G.	0	2 years
B.T.	0	2 years
J.P.	0	1½ years

0 = no seizures. X = seizures.

significantly from surgery. Spencer *et al.* report similar results in 15 patients with gliomas who presented with chronic seizure disorder (10).

It is also noteworthy that in five of the six patients who continue to have seizures, the postoperative seizures appeared within several weeks after surgery. This suggests that if seizures are going to continue to be a problem postoperatively, they usually appear soon after surgery. However, as shown earlier, the occurrence of a single or several seizures in the early postoperative course does not necessarily predict that the patient will continue to have seizures (Tables 2.3 and 2.4).

Comparison of Results in Patients Who Had Simple Excision of Temporal Lobe Tumors with Those Who Had an Anterior Temporal Lobectomy, Including the Tumor and the Uninvolved Hippocampus

Twenty-eight of these patients had temporal lobe tumors. In seven, the uninvolved and potentially epileptogenic medial temporal lobe (hippocampus and parahippocampus) was excised in addition to the tumor. The purpose was to provide greater protection against the occurrence of postoperative seizures. The results indicate, however, that excision of the medial temporal lobe may be unnecessary. Two of these seven patients continued to have seizures postoperatively (Table 2.7). In comparison, only one of 12 patients who had only the tumor excised and have been followed for a similar period (Table 2.8—B.G. through W.L.), continue to have seizures after surgery.

PATHOLOGY

With the exception of two tumors, a xanthoastrocytoma (Table 2.3, D.B.) and a glioblastoma multiform (Table 2.3, T.G.), the histologic features of these tumors are consistent with long survival times. Seventeen of the astrocytomas were well differentiated. The cell density was moderate, the cells were uniform, and mitosis was absent or very rare. Ten showed atypical or anaplastic foci (1). These tumors exhibited increased cellular density and pleomorphism of varying degrees, but none showed significant mitosis, vascular endothelial proliferation, or necrosis. The entire group of astrocytomas reported herein would fall into Kernohan's classification of grade I and II astrocytomas (5). In a recent review of 461 low-grade astrocytomas (grades I and II, Kernohan), Laws *et al.* (6) emphasized that long survival times after total or radical subtotal removal of tumor, with or without radiation, could be expected if the patients were young at the time of surgery (the most important determinant), had no neurologic deficit preoperatively, had a long duration of symptoms before surgery, seizures were the presenting symptom, and the patients were free of neurologic deficit following surgery (6). These conditions characterize most of the

TABLE 2.8

Resection of Temporal Lobe Tumor Only

Patient	Seizures*	Follow-Up
B.G.	0	10 years
B.S.	0	7 years
J.D.	0	5 years
L.F.	0	4 years
M.H.	0	4 years
J.P.	0	4 years
P.L.	0	2½ years
D.S.	0	2 years
J.S.	0	1½ years
R.M.	0	1½ years
J.J.	0^1	1½ years
W.L.	X	1½ years
S.F.	0	1 year
D.B.	0	1 year (expired)
W.G.	0	11 months
C.M.	0^1	6 months
J.M.	0	4 months
H.B.	0	4 months
P.D.	0	3 months
J.L.	0	3 months

* 0 = no seizures; 0^1 = one to several seizures in the early postoperative period; X = seizures.

patients with astrocytomas we report. The other tumors, ganglioglioma, mixed glioma, xanthoastrocytoma, and oligodendroglioma, are also associated with long survival times postoperatively (2–4).

CONCLUSIONS

The results of this study permit the following conclusions.

1. Given a patient with chronic seizure disorder who has a solitary lesion on CT scan which is not explicable by a prior encephalopathy, the likelihood is great that the patient harbors a low-grade glioma. If the tumor is removed, the seizures will probably stop and the prognosis for a long survival time is good. From a dependent and stigmatized existence, the patient may look forward to an independent and productive life after surgery. Also, it appears that even in some of the patients who have only biopsy and radiation therapy, the seizures will come under control and the patient may enjoy the same good results as the patients in whom the lesion

was extirpated. In other words, early diagnosis and definitive treatment in this entire group of patients makes a substantial difference!

2.   In the large majority of cases, simple excision of the tumor is all that is necessary to effect seizure control. Excision of the adjacent epileptogenic cortex, either presumed or identified by electrocorticography, is unnecessary.

3.   In addition to eliminating the seizures, early surgery is also important because the tumors in some patients who had seizures for many years before surgery showed anaplastic foci. In one patient with a 22-year history of seizures, the tumor showed the histologic features of a glioblastoma multiforme, and in another, a temporal lobe xanthoastrocytoma showed malignant changes. One year after surgery, the tumor recurred as a glioblastoma, from which the patient expired. The patient had had complex partial seizures for 1 year before surgery. It is possible that in both of these patients, early surgery would have found the tumors free of malignant features.

4.   The failure to demonstrate an increase in the size of these lesions on serial CT scans is no assurance that they are not tumors and should not delay surgery.

5.   MRI scans are important for earlier discovery and treatment of some of these lesions. In patients with focal seizures and normal or equivocally abnormal CT scans, MRI scans may clearly expose the lesion. Also, in some cases, MRI scans can give better definition of the lesion demonstrated on CT scan and provide the critically needed information for planning the surgical approach; e.g., needle biopsy vs. craniotomy and removal of the tumor.

6.   It is important to remember that complex partial seizures are occasionally caused by lesions of the cingulate gyrus. Awareness of this fact will prevent unnecessary delay in dealing definitively with these medially situated lesions.

7.   A history typical of either non-neoplastic or idiopathic seizure disorder is no assurance that the patient does not harbor a tumor. For example, the history of a generalized seizure with a febrile illness in infancy, subsequently followed by the development of complex partial seizures—a history typical of patients with temporal mesial sclerosis—was the history given by some of the patients who harbored temporal lobe gliomas. We also encountered patients who had seizure-free intervals of several years' duration.

8.   Finally, the apparent location of lesions either in or in the vicinity of sensorimotor or language cortex should not be a deterrent to proceeding with surgery. In contrast to what the seizure pattern and imaging studies predict, the tumors may be found to only abut or displace functional

cortex, and with the use of functional localization, lend themselves to safe removal.

In Chapter 3, we will discuss the other lesions which we encountered in this group of patients. We will focus on the method and utility of functional localization in dealing with both the gliomas and the lesions that mimic them. It will be demonstrated that with the use of functional localization even lesions that reside within the sensorimotor gyri may be safely extirpated in some cases.

REFERENCES

1. Fulling, K. H., and Nelson, J. E. Cerebral astrocytic neoplasms in the adult: contribution of histologic examination to the assessment of prognosis. Sem. Diag. Pathol., *1:* 52–163, 1984.
2. Hart, M. N., Petito, C. K., and Earle, K. M. Mixed gliomas. Cancer, *33:* 134–140, 1974.
3. Johannsson, J. H., Rekate, H. L., and Roewssmann, U. Gangliogliomas: Pathological and clinical correlation. J. Neurosurg., *54:* 58–63, 1981.
4. Kepes, J. J., Rubinstein, L. J., and Eng, L. F. Pleomorphic xanthoastrocytoma: A distinctive meningocerebral glioma of young subjects with relatively favorable prognosis. A study of 12 cases. Cancer, *44:* 1839–1852, 1979.
5. Kernohan, J. W., Mabon, R. F., Svien, H. J., and Adson, A. W. A simplified classification of the gliomas. Proc. Mayo Clinic, *24:* 71–73, 1949.
6. Laws, E. R., Jr., Taylor, W. F., Clifton, M. B. V., and Okazaki, H. Neurological management of low-grade astrocytoma of the cerebral hemispheres. J. Neurosurg., *61:* 665–673, 1984.
7. Mazars, G. Criteria for identifying cingulate epilepsies. Epilepsia, *11:* 41–47, 1970.
8. Rasmussen, T. Surgery of epilepsy associated with brain tumors. In: *Advances in Neurology,* edited by D. P. Purpura, J. K. Penry, and R. D. Walter, pp. 227–239, Raven Press, New York, 1976.
9. Rich, K. M., and Goldring, S. Computed tomography in chronic seizure disorder caused by glioma. Arch. Neurol., *42:* 26–27, 1985.
10. Spencer, D. D., Spencer, S. S., Mattson, R. H., and Williamson, P. D. Intracerebral masses in patients with intractable partial epilepsy. Neurology, *34:* 432–436, 1984.
11. Wieser, H. G. *Electroclinical Features of the Psychomotor Seizure.* Gustav Fischer, Stuttgart, 1983.
12. Williamson, P. D., Spencer, D. D., Spencer, S. S., Novelly, R. A., and Mattson, R. H. Complex partial seizures of frontal lobe origin. Ann Neurol. *18:* 497–504, 1985.

3

Experience with Lesions That Mimic Gliomas in Patients Presenting with a Chronic Seizure Disorder

SIDNEY GOLDRING, M.D., and ERIK M. GREGORIE, M.D.*

In the first part of this study (see Chapter 2), we reviewed our experience with the gliomas, by far the most common lesion discovered in this group of patients (40 of 51) (see Table 2.1, Chapter 2). The group was characterized by the following features. Except for one patient with a monoparesis, their neurologic status was normal and they presented with only one symptom—seizure disorder of long duration (mean duration = 11 years). None had had a previous encephalopathy. All had a solitary lesion on computed tomographic (CT) scan, except for one whose tumor was demonstrated only on magnetic resonance imaging (MRI) scan. In the majority, the presence of this abnormality was known from months to years before the patients were referred for surgery. The usual reason for delaying surgery was interpretation of the scan as showing a non-neoplastic lesion.

The response to surgery in these patients was excellent. With few exceptions, the seizures were brought under complete or significantly better control, and in the majority of patients only extirpation of the tumor was required; excision of presumed epileptogenic cortex or electrocorticography (ECG) for identification of the epileptogenic focus was unnecessary. The majority of these tumors were low-grade gliomas, and the prognosis for long survival times was good.

In this chapter we describe our experience with the other pathologic entities encountered in patients presenting with similar histories, and then focus on the role of functional localization in dealing with intrinsic brain lesions, of which the gliomas and the other lesions we describe are prime examples.

---

* Presently Erik M. Gregorie, M.D., Maj., M. C. Landstuhl Army Regional Medical Center, F.R.G.

Vascular malformation

The most common lesion we found, other than glioma, was an occult vascular malformation (Table 3.1). That is, the CT scan gave no clue of a vascular lesion and angiography was normal. Figure 3.1 illustrates examples of these lesions on CT scans. Microscopic examination showed them to be either arteriovenous malformations or cavernous angiomas. The vessels showed varying degrees of thrombosis and hemosiderin, the latter indicating previous hemorrhage. All were surrounded by a margin of gliosis. Table 3.2 summarizes our experience with six such patients. Three of these patients (D.W., J.H., M.B.), followed for 4 years, 1 year, and 8 months, respectively, have been seizure free since surgery. L.Z., the eldest patient, followed for 2 years and then lost to follow-up, continued to have seizures. Although seizures were less frequent, she had severe depressive disease, and the combination of depression and occasional seizure breakthrough left her quality of life unchanged. Patient D.B. has been lost to follow-up. The remaining patient (R.K.) has been followed for too brief a period to permit comment on the efficacy of surgery. With the exception of D.W., all had simple excision of the lesion. In D.W., the anterior uninvolved hippocampus was resected in addition to the cavernous angioma.

Arachnoid Cyst

There were three such lesions, all involving the temporal lobe (Fig. 3.2). In none did surgery improve the seizure disorder. Surgery consisted of

TABLE 3.1

Pathology of Lesions Discovered on CT Scan in Patients Presenting with Chronic Seizure Disorder

Pathology	No. of Patients
Glioma	
Astrocytoma (low-grade)	25
Glioblastoma	2
Ganglioglioma	5
Mixed glioma	5
Xanthoastrocytoma	1
Oligodendroglioma	1
Vascular malformation	7
Arachnoid cyst	3
Miscellaneous	
Epidermoid	1
Cysticercosis Cyst	1
Total	51

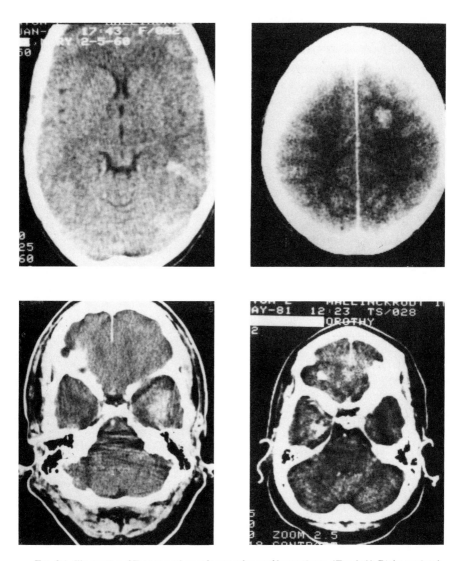

FIG. 3.1. Illustrative CT scans of occult vascular malformations. (*Top left*) Right parietal arteriovenous malformation. (*Top right*) Left posterior frontal cavernous angioma. Left is to the reader's right. (*Bottom left*) Left temporal arteriovenous malformation. Left is to reader's right. (*Bottom right*) Left temporal cavernous angioma.

TABLE 3.2

*Patients with Occult Vascular Malformations Presenting with Seizure Disorder**

Patient	Age (yr) at Onset of Seizures/Surgery	Diagnosis	Follow-Up	Seizures
D.W.	15/34	Temporal cavernous angioma	4 years	0
L.Z.	54/59	Frontal arteriovenous malformation	2 years	X
D.B.	8/10	Temporal arteriovenous malformation	Lost	?
J.H.	21/23	Temporal arteriovenous malformation	1 year	0
M.B.	23/24	Temporal arteriovenous malformation	8 months	0
R.K.	15/34	Temporal cavernous angioma	2 months	0

*0 = no seizures; X = seizures; ? = lost to follow-up.

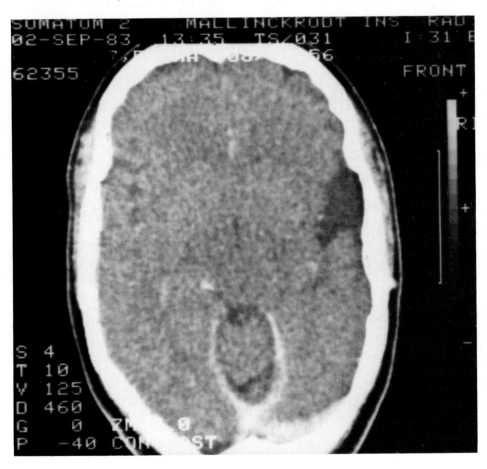

FIG. 3.2. CT scan showing temporal arachnoid cyst.

resecting as much of the cyst wall as possible and establishing communication with the basilar cisterns. In one of these patients who was subsequently monitored with indwelling electrodes during seizures, the monitoring showed that the ictus could originate in either temporal lobe, although it most frequently arose from the temporal lobe associated with the arachnoid cyst.

Miscellaneous Lesion

In the remaining two patients, one with a cysticercosis cyst (Fig. 3.3A) and the other with an epidermoid tumor (Fig. 3.3B), simple excision of the lesion eliminated the seizures. The patient with the parasitic cyst had suffered focal seizures of the left face and arm for 10 years prior to surgery at age 50. During the 5 years she has been followed since surgery, she has had no seizures. The patient with the epidermoid tumor had focal seizures for 6 years prior to surgery. He has been seizure free since surgery, 1½ years ago.

FUNCTIONAL LOCALIZATION

We used somatosensory evoked responses to localize the sensorimotor region. The procedure is carried out under general anesthesia (4). In ear-

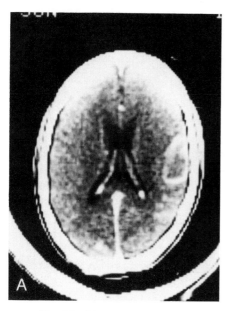 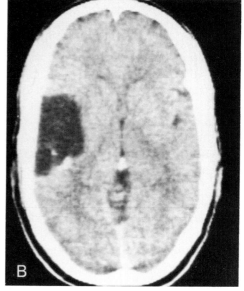

FIG. 3.3. CT scans showing parietal cysticercosis cyst (*left*) and temporal epidermoid tumor (*right*).

lier studies, we demonstrated that, under our conditions of recording, a cortical response to peripheral sensory stimulation appeared only in the contralateral primary somatosensory area and variably in the motor cortex (3, 6, 12). Responses in the vast surround of association cortex, like those observed in awake behaving animals, were not seen. It was these observations and the ability to readily record somatosensory evoked responses in the anesthetized patient that led us to begin using sensory evoked responses for localizing the sensorimotor region first in patients undergoing epilepsy surgery and, subsequently, in the removal of intrinsic brain lesions. Had responses also appeared in association cortex, the recordings from the primary somatosensory area probably would have lost their localizing significance and evoked responses could not have been used for functional localization.

The method requires the patient not to be paralyzed during functional localization. Therefore, the details of carrying out the general anesthetic are important. The patients are premedicated with atropine only. Induction of anesthesia is performed with halothane. Endotracheal intubation is carried out following administration of succinylcholine, a short-acting depolarizing muscle relaxant. Anesthesia is maintained with a combination of 50% nitrous oxide (N_2O) and O_2 and halothane up to 2% without neuromuscular paralysis. During functional localization, the halothane concentration is reduced to about 0.5%. It is usually possible to elicit movement with cortical stimulation in addition to recording somatosensory evoked responses. Upon completion of functional localization, the patient is paralyzed with pancuronium, artificially ventilated, and carried on the narcotic fentanyl for the remainder of the procedure.

After the brain is exposed, cortical sensory evoked responses are recorded to identify the sensorimotor region. A Silastic template, holding three rows of linearly oriented electrodes, is placed on the cortical surface in a plane parallel to the midline and spanning the presumed location of the sensorimotor region (Fig. 3.4). The interelectrode distance is 1 cm, and each row is separated by 1.5 cm. Simultaneous records are made from each adjacent pair of electrodes in the first row (that is, 1-2, 2-3, 3-4, etc.), while the contralateral median nerve is electrically pulsed transcutaneously (1/second) at the wrist. A special-purpose computer quickly exposes the sensory evoked response by "averaging" 25 to 50 post-stimulation epochs of electrical activity. If a response is not obtained, then recordings are made from the second row of electrodes, etc. A switching matrix controlled by a microprocessor is under keyboard command and it can select any row of recording sites in the time it takes to type a command, say "matrix A."

When a response is evoked only in the somatosensory area, the tracings

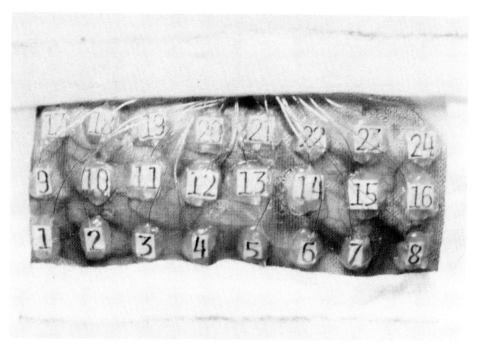

FIG. 3.4. Electrode array used to record somatosensory evoked responses. It overlies the cerebral cortex. Under each numbered ticket is an elliptical 1 × 2 mm pure platinum electrode disc. Teflon-coated wire exits from each electrode. The electrodes are embedded in a sheet of medical-grade Silastic.

from the row of linearly oriented electrode sites show responses from only two adjacent pairs or electrode combinations, and these responses are reversed in polarity (Fig. 3.5A). For example, simultaneous recordings made from the row of electrodes 1-2, 2-3, etc. show a response only from 5-6 and 6-7. The numbers identifying each trace correspond to the numbered tickets overlying each electrode site in row 1 of the epidural array shown in Figure 3.4. Tracings from all other electrode sites show either no response or inconsequential deflections. Since electrode sites 5 and 7 show a response only when they are paired with electrode 6, and not when they are paired with the other electrodes to which they are adjacent, electrode site 6 is identified as overlying the somatosensory area. When a response is evoked in the motor cortex in addition to the somatosensory area, responses are recorded from four adjacent pairs of electrode sites, rather than two, and there is a double phase reversal (Fig. 3.5B). The face area is similarly identified using a light tap to the upper or lower lip as the sensory stimulus.

A **B**

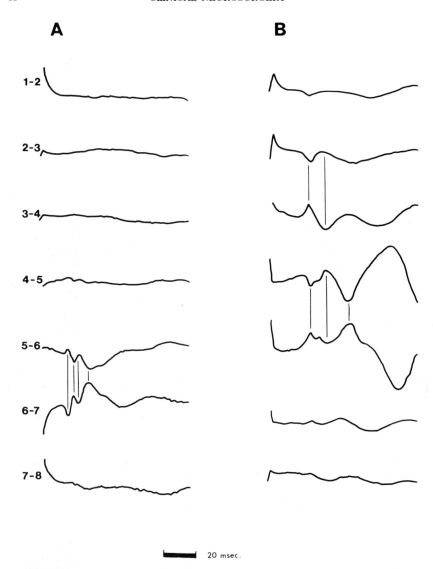

1-2

2-3

3-4

4-5

5-6

6-7

7-8

20 msec.

FIG. 3.5. Somatosensory evoked responses identifying the somatosensory and motor hand areas. Numbers to the left of each trace in *A* also apply to trace *B*. They correspond to the numbers overlying the recording electrodes shown in Figure 3.4. Vertical lines between traces indicate phase reversal of responses recorded from adjacent areas. Deflections at the beginning of each trace are shock artifacts. (*A*) Recordings in a patient in whom only the somatosensory area yielded a response. (*B*) Recordings in a patient in whom both the somatosensory and motor hand areas yielded a response. Time calibration is at bottom. (Modified from Gregorie, E. M., and Goldring, S. Localization of function in the excision of lesions from the sensorimotor region. J. Neurosurg., *61*: 1047–1054, 1984.)

After the sensorimotor region is identified, stimulation through the pair of electrodes just anterior to those overlying the sensory area can be used to produce movement and further verify the localization. The general anesthetic that we use usually permits the use of electrocortical stimulation to obtain motor responses. The preliminary recording of sensory evoked responses in these instances, then, may appear superfluous. However, under anesthesia the threshold for producing movement is raised. Much time usually is spent in varying stimulus intensities and exploring the cortical surface with the stimulating electrode. By contrast, recording sensory evoked responses quickly (within several minutes) identifies the sensori-

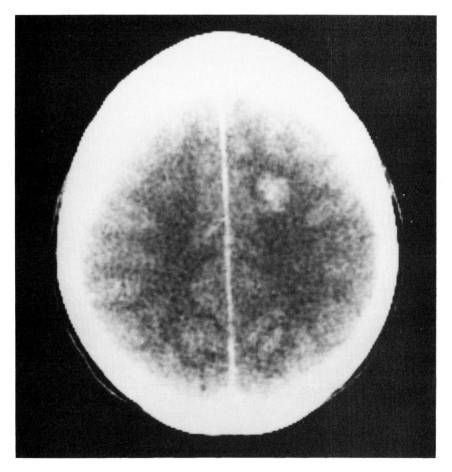

Fig. 3.6. CT scan showing hyperdense lesion in left posterior frontal lobe. Left is to the reader's right.

motor hand region. Even under local anesthesia it makes functional localization more efficient by quickly identifying the region of sensorimotor
representation for exploration with the cortical stimulating electrode.

In Chapter 2, we cited some examples demonstrating the usefulness of
functional localization in dealing with gliomas. The following cases will
demonstrate further its utility and emphasize the advantages of functional
localization when used in conjunction with MRI scanning and ultrasound
to guide the removal of subcortical lesions in the sensorimotor region.

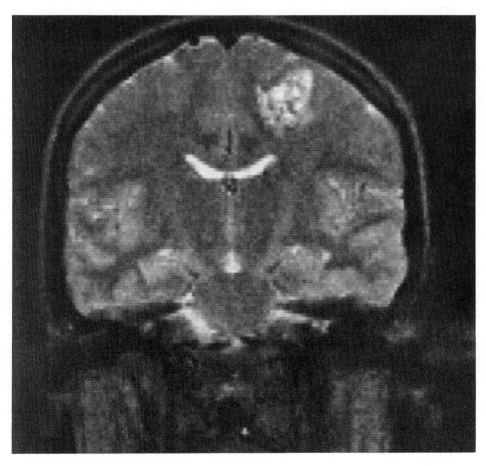

Fig. 3.7. MRI coronal scan of same patient whose CT scan is shown in Figure 3.6. Note shell
of cortex overlying the lesion. Left is to reader's right.

Case 1

This 24-year-old woman had experienced two nocturnal seizures. A CT scan showed a lesion in the left posterior frontal region (Fig. 3.6). The unenhanced scan showed some calcification; the scan following injection of intravenous contrast solution showed some enhancement. Angiography revealed no abnormal vascularity. The most likely diagnosis was considered to be a glioma. The MRI scan provided better definition of the lesion (Fig. 3.7). The scan showed the lesion to be located just subcortically, and the T1 weighted images with fast repetition times indicated that the lesion contained either fat or old blood, suggesting that the lesion was probably an occult vascular malformation. Upon exposing the brain during craniotomy, the cortical mantle appeared normal. The somatosensory and motor gyri were identified with functional localization (Figs. 3.8 and 3.9). We had

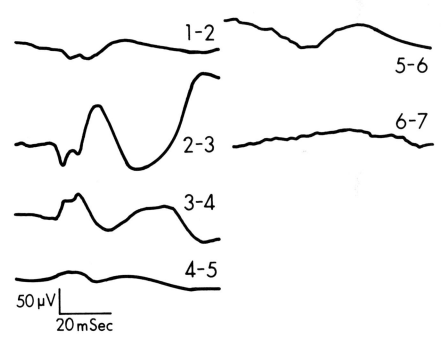

FIG. 3.8. Somatosensory evoked responses identifying the hand area in same patient whose CT and MRI scans are shown in Figures 3.6 and 3.7. The numbers to the right of each trace correspond to the electrode sites in the linear row of electrodes that were used to make the recordings. Responses appear in traces 2-3 and 3-4 and show phase reversal. Since electrode sites 2 and 4 show a response when they are paired only with electrode 3 and no other electrode, the recordings identify electrode 3 as overlying the somatosensory hand area. Time calibration is at *bottom left*.

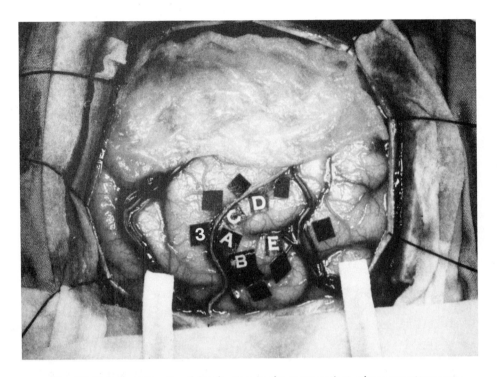

Fɪɢ. 3.9. Results of functional localization in the same patient whose somatosensory evoked responses are shown in Figure 3.8. Anterior is to the *right*, and midline is at the *bottom*. The numbered *ticket 3* corresponds to electrode site 3 shown in Figure 3.8, which the recordings identified as overlying the somatosensory hand area. The lettered tickets identify sites from which hand and forearm movements were elicited by cortical stimulation. The *black tickets* are areas which did not yield a response. The meandering thread identifies the central fissure. The two vertically oriented cottonoid strips were related to placement of the recording electrode array and are irrelevant to what this figure demonstrates.

guessed that the lesion might underlie the somatosensory gyrus, because it appeared somewhat fuller than the others. Examination with ultrasound (1), however, localized the lesion to the region of the sulcus separating the motor and premotor gyrus, with the bulk of the lesion lying just anterior to the precentral sulcus (Figs. 3.10 and 3.11). A cavernous angioma was found in the depth of the sulcus burrowing into the premotor gyrus, and it was removed (Fig. 3.12). It separated readily from the anterior bank of the motor gyrus, which it had dished out and displaced posteriorly. On the second postoperative day, the patient became dysphasic and developed a monoparesis of the right upper extremity. Both of these deficits cleared completely over the ensuing several days.

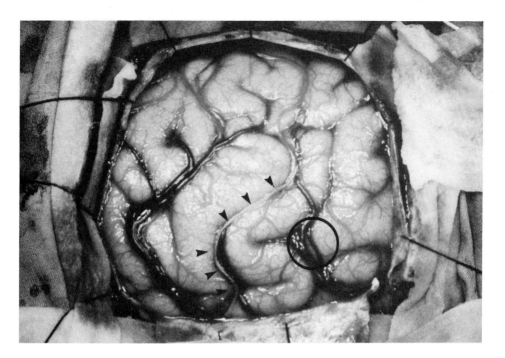

FIG. 3.10. Photograph of the brain of the same patient demonstrated in Figures 3.6 through 3.9. Anterior is to the *right*, and the midline is at the *bottom*. A meandering thread (*arrows*) identifies the central fissure. The *circle* identifies the subcortical location of a lesion detected by a sonogram.

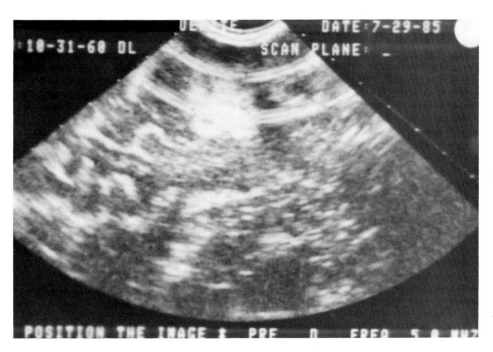

FIG. 3.11. Sonogram of the same patient illustrated in Figures 3.6 through 3.10. It shows a hyperdense, quasioval area that identifies the site of the subcortical lesion.

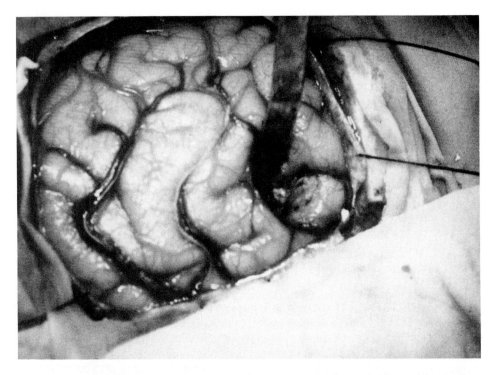

FIG. 3.12. Photograph of brain following removal of a cavernous angioma in the same patient illustrated in Figures 3.6 through 3.11. Anterior is to the *right*, and midline is at the *bottom*. A meandering thread is the central fissure. The retractor holds back the premotor gyrus.

COMMENT

This case demonstrates the two kinds of data that are needed to deal safely with any intrinsic lesion in a functionally sensitive area: (*a*) the subcortical location of the lesion and (*b*) the functional anatomy of the cortical mantle surrounding and overlying the pathologic entity.

Case 2

This 50-year-old woman had a 10-year history of focal seizures which began with tingling of the left side of her tongue followed by spread into her thumb and up into her left arm. Her neurological examination was normal. This patient had a cysticercosis cyst, as discussed above (Fig. 3.3). During craniotomy, the central fissure was identified with functional localization. The lower regions of both the somatosensory and motor gyri were swollen. The somatosensory gyrus, which showed the greatest swelling, was entered and the lesion removed in toto (Fig. 3.13). It occupied the territory of somatosensory face representation. Postoperatively, she had a mild left hemiparesis, including the face. The hemiparesis cleared in several days. The facial weakness completely resolved in several weeks. There was no sensory deficit.

Lesions from the motor face area can also be removed without producing a neurologic deficit, as shown by the next case.

Case 3

This 13-year-old boy (T.L.) had focal seizures involving his face which began in infancy (discussed in Chapter 2). At the onset of his seizure, he could not move the left side of his face. This then gave way to a clonic left facial seizure which spread to his left upper extremity and frequently generalized. At surgery, a mixed glioma was found to reside in the lateral portion of the motor gyrus. The gyrus, including the tumor, was resected from the sylvian fissure to the lower limit of the hand representation (Fig.

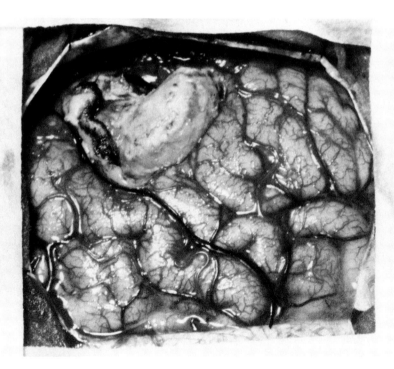

Fig. 3.13. Photograph of brain from which a cysticercosis cyst has just been removed from the somatosensory face area. Posterior is to the *right*, and the midline is toward the *bottom*. The black meandering line is the central fissure.

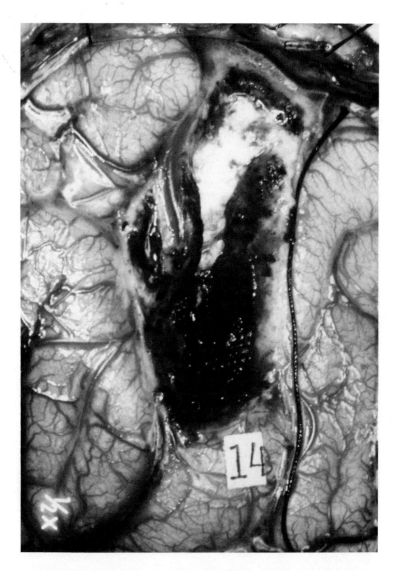

Fig. 3.14. Photograph of brain following removal of a mixed glioma and the motor gyrus in which it was embedded from the lower boundary of the hand representation to the sylvian fissure. Anterior is to the *left*. The numbered *ticket 14* marks the lower boundary of motor hand representation. A black thread identifies the central fissure.

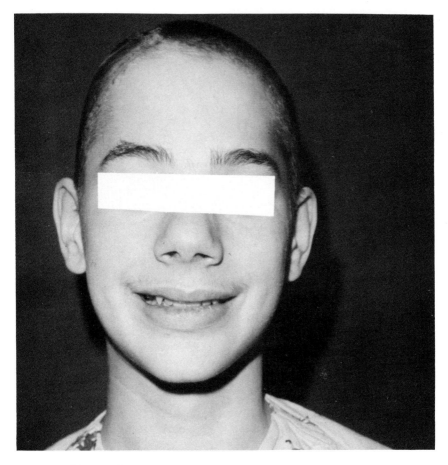

FIG. 3.15. Photograph of patient (case 3) showing normal motor function of facial musculature following excision of motor gyrus from the lower boundary of hand representation to the sylvian fissure.

3.14). Postoperatively, he had a mild left facial weakness and developed a dense left upper extremity paralysis on the first postoperative day. Both deficits completely cleared in 1 week (Fig. 3.15).

Combined resection of the motor and somatosensory areas of facial representation also may be carried out without producing a facial paralysis.

Case 4

Figure 3.16 shows the resection of an epileptogenic focus that occupied the somatosensory, motor, and premotor face representation in a patient

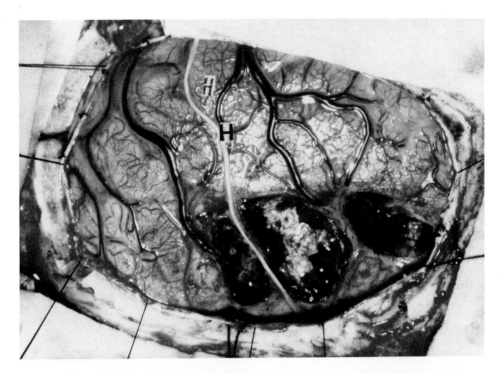

FIG. 3.16. Photograph of brain following removal of epileptogenic focus which occupied the premotor, motor, and seomatosensory gyrus. Anterior is to the *left*, and the midline is toward the *bottom*. The central fissure is identified by the meandering white thread. The lettered *ticket H* identifies sites from which electrical stimulation produced hand movements. Stimulation produced no response from the *upper H* (toward the sylvian fissure) to the upper margin of resection. Facial motor responses were obtained from the epileptogenic motor cortex that was resected.

with a 10-year history of focal seizure disorder. He did not have a space-occupying lesion and is not a case in the series we are reporting. He is presented because the result following his cortical resection is pertinent to this discussion. The intervening sulci between the gyri were left intact to avoid damage to any vessels in passage to the upper limb representation. There was no gross pathology. Histologic examination of the resected tissue showed subpial gliosis. Postoperatively, the patient has normal facial function.

COMMENT

In case 4, it is possible that some cortex concerned with facial representation still remained. Not all of the tissue beyond the lateral limit of the hand representation was excised. Nevertheless, in toto, the last three cited cases indicate that one should not be dissuaded from attempting total excision of a lesion occupying either the sensory or motor gyri in the area of facial representation. It is not known why facial function is unaffected when most, if not all, of the sensorimotor gyri concerned with facial representation are removed. One may speculate that there exists a significant ipsilateral facial representation that can take over, or that sensorimotor facial representation in the second somatosensory and motor areas, which lie buried in the sylvian fissure, is unaffected by the resections and is sufficient to ensure normal facial function. However, for now, whatever the explanation is, we can satisfy ourselves with the observation that it is possible to extirpate lesions occupying the facial domain of the sensorimotor gyri without incurring a neurologic deficit.

Case 3, the patient with the mixed glioma, also demonstrates how precise knowledge of the functional anatomy, in this instance the boundary between face and upper limb representation, permitted surgical excision of the tumor without incurring any paresis of the upper limb.

The next two cases have been reported before (5). They deal with removal of small metastatic lesions located within the somatosensory and motor gyri. Although the patients did not have chronic seizure disorder, and their medical problems are not germane to the thrust of this study, they each harbored a subcortical lesion that resided within the somatosensory and motor hand areas, respectively. The problems related to the removal of the lesions are the same as those for any intrinsic brain lesion, and hence, are presented here.

Case 5

This 48-year-old woman had a left upper lobectomy for carcinoma of the lung in 1976. In 1978, she experienced a focal seizure which began with twitching of her left index and middle fingers and spread to the arm and face. The clonic activity was associated with a feeling of pins and needles. A CT scan showed a solitary lesion associated with edema in the vicinity of the sensorimotor area. Neurological examination revealed a mild paresis of her left upper extremity; she had no cortical sensory loss.

At craniotomy, the brain was found to be swollen. Two contiguous gyri in the anterior half of the exposure were the most edematous. Otherwise, there was no surface clue to the subcortical location of the lesion, nor did gentle palpation of these gyri reveal an underlying lesion (Fig. 3.17). Without functional localization, the approach would probably have been to enter the brain through the anterior gyrus of this swollen pair, since it appeared well anterior to the sensorimotor region. This approach, however, would have entered the brain through the motor gyrus. Functional

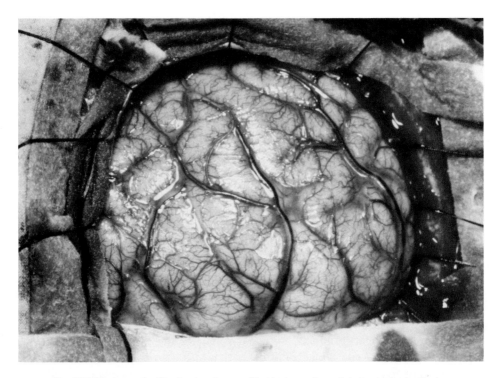

FIG. 3.17. Photograph of brain showing swelling in two adjacent gyri anterior to the large draining vein in center of exposure. Anterior is to the *left*, and the midline is toward the *bottom*.

localization showed the central fissure to lie between the two swollen gyri (Fig. 3.18). It had been displaced anteriorly by the tumor, which was found to reside in the area of hand representation in the somatosensory gyrus. Knowing the identity of the two swollen gyri, we chose to enter the posterior one of the pair from its buried posterior bank (Fig. 3.18, *arrow*). The reason for choosing the posterior gyrus was our impression that it appeared to be more swollen. Of course, today, we would use ultrasound to localize the subcortical tumor site. In 1978, we were not yet using ultrasound for localization of subcortical pathology. We entered the gyrus immediately posterior to the somatosensory one, just behind the sulcus separating the two. The posterior bank of the somatosensory gyrus was exposed, and the gyrus was entered through it. The tumor was encountered at a very shallow depth and was enucleated. The location of the tumor within the gyrus is shown in Figure 3.19. The cottonoid has been inserted through the posterior bank into the tumor bed where the lesion

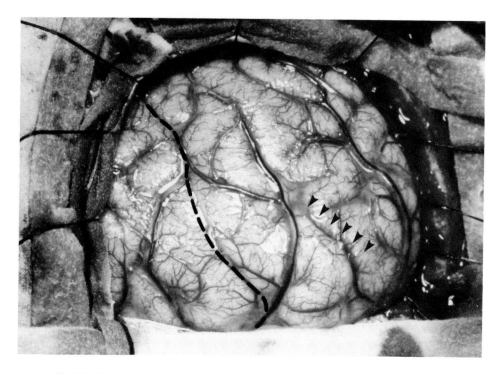

Fig. 3.18. Photograph of same brain shown in Figure 3.16 after functional localization. The black thread marks the central fissure. The *arrow* points to the posterior sulcus through which the posterior bank of the somatosensory gyrus was entered to gain access to the tumor.

resided. The tip of the bayonet forceps points to the location of the cottonoid tip within the tumor bed and demonstrates the extent to which the tumor nodule had invaded the gyrus. Postoperatively, she had an increase in the paresis of her left upper extremity and a cortical sensory deficit in the left hand. One month postoperatively, she exhibited only upward drift of her left upper limb on posture holding and mild astereognosis in her left hand. Over the ensuing months, she continued to improve. At 1 year after surgery, she had recovered normal neurologic function in her left upper extremity. She remained well for the ensuing 5 years and was free of any neurologic symptoms or deficits. In July, 1985, she developed further metastases and died.

COMMENT

The recovery of normal neurological function in this case might merely relate to the relatively small amount of cortex that was damaged in remov-

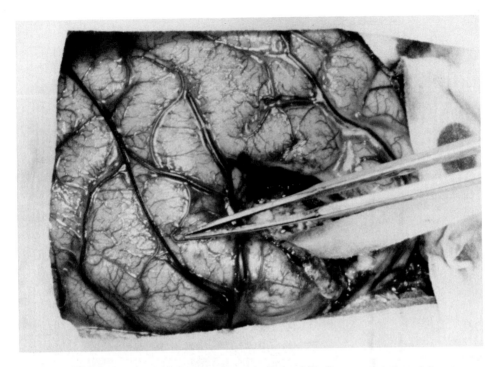

FIG. 3.19. Photograph of same brain shown in Figure 3.17 after a metastatic nodule was removed from somatosensory hand area. The black thread is the central fissure. Anterior is to the *left*, and midline is toward the *bottom*. For an explanation of bayonet forceps and cottonoid in tumor bed, see the text.

ing the tumor. That is, the amount of destroyed cortical tissue was perhaps less than the critical volume which must be destroyed before a neurologic deficit appears. Another explanation is found in recent studies of subhuman primates (5, 11). Multiple representations of the body have been demonstrated in the primary somatosensory cortex. There appear to be two complete and spatially separate representations of both cutaneous and deep body tissue. One is located anteriorly in areas 3a and 3b, and the other is located posteriorly in areas 1 and 2. Although there are probably differences in the sensory qualities subserved by the corresponding areas of the dual systems, it is possible that overlap of functional representation exists between each of the paired sensory representations. In this patient, the deep and cutaneous representations located anteriorly in areas 3a and 3b were left relatively undisturbed and may have been sufficient to subserve normal function.

Case 6

This 53-year-old man with renal cell carcinoma developed a paresis in his right upper extremity. A CT scan revealed a small left posterior frontal mass about 2.5 cm below the cortical surface in the region of the presumed central fissure (Fig. 3.20). Because of the location of the lesion, it was decided to treat him with radiation rather than surgery. The patient was referred to us 5 months later because there had been no improvement. An MRI scan was obtained, which provided two important pieces of information (Fig. 3.21). First, it showed the precise relationship between the lesion and the gyrus with which it was associated. Second, it showed that the involved gyrus was swollen and hence at surgery there would be a surface clue that would localize the gyrus that harbored the lesion. The missing information was the functional identity of the gyrus and its neighbors. At surgery, functional localization identified the swollen gyrus as the motor gyrus. Knowing this and knowing that the tumor was centered at the base of the gyrus, the precentral sulcus was opened and the anterior bank of the motor gyrus was exposed. It was entered at its base, and the tumor was carefully enucleated. Postoperatively, the patient exhibited a left hemiparesis. Over the ensuing months, he showed progressive recovery with

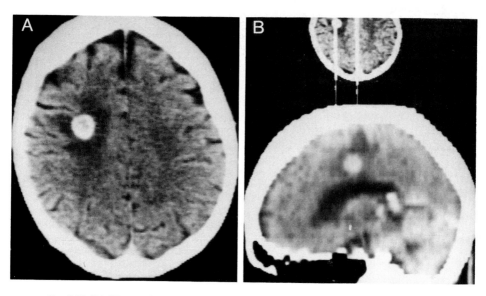

FIG. 3.20. (A) CT scan showing a subcortical lesion and adjacent edema in posterior frontal lobe. (B) Sagittal reconstruction of the CT scan shown on the *left*. (From Gregori, E. M., and Goldring, S. Localization of function in the excision of lesions from the sensorimotor region. J. Neuosurg., *61:* 1047–1054, 1984.)

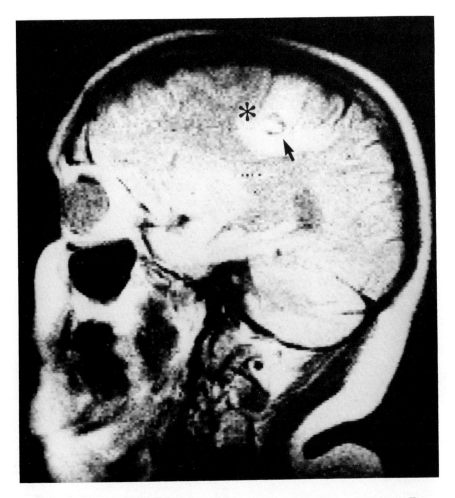

FIG. 3.21. MRI scan (T2 weighted image) of same patient whose CT scan is shown in Figure 3.19. Scan shows the tumor nodule (*arrow*) at the base of a swollen gyrus. Surrounding white matter and cortical edema are evident. The adjacent gyri appear normal. This finding was the only preoperative clue to indicate that we would find a landmark on the surface of the brain to guide us to the subcortical lesion. *Asterisk* identifies the base of the precentral fissure where the motor gyrus was entered to gain access to the tumor. (From Gregorie, E. M., and Goldring, S. Localization of function in the excision of lesions from the sensorimotor region. J. Neurosurg., *61:* 1047–1054, 1984.)

development of fine finger movements. Unfortunately, months after surgery, he died from the renal cell carcinoma. Therefore, the full extent of the recovery that he might have achieved is not known.

COMMENT

The motor cortex also has been shown to have a dual representation of the body situated anteriorly and posteriorly in the precentral gyrus of subhuman primates (7, 13, 14). However, the sensory input to each of these regions is different, the anterior region having a deep sensory input and the posterior area having a cutaneous one (8, 15, 17). These observations make it less likely that a "redundancy" of functional representation exists in spatially separate systems of motor control. The recovery of motor function where the motor gyrus was entered through its hidden anterior bank may be due to the relative sparing of the posterior region of the precentral gyrus. The apparent dominant role of this portion of the gyrus in eliciting movement is suggested by the observation that the lowest stimulus threshold for producing motor responses is found in the region bordering the central fissure.

DISCUSSION

The cases described in this study demonstrate that lesions that encroach upon the sensorimotor region, occupy the area of face representation, and in some instances, even reside within the area of limb representation may be removed without incurring a neurologic deficit. Comparison of cases 6 with cases 1 and 7 demonstrates other important information besides functional localization which the surgeon needs in order to safely extirpate subcortical lesions. In case 6 (the metastatic tumor in the somatosensory hand area), we knew the functional anatomy but did not know whether the tumor underlay the somatosensory or motor cortices, or both. Because the somatosensory gyrus was suggestively more swollen than the motor one, we reasoned that the tumor was situated more posteriorly and entered the brain through the gyrus and sulcus posterior to the somatosensory convolution. Fortunately, we guessed right. By contrast, in case 7, where the MRI scan clearly defined the configuration of the tumor and the swollen gyrus, which it underlay, we knew the precise subcortical location of the tumor when the brain was exposed. The same is true of case 1, in which ultrasound correctly localized the subcortical location of the cavernous angioma.

In sum, these cases demonstrate that to deal more knowledgeably with the removal of intrinsic brain lesions, one needs to know both their subcortical location and the functional anatomy of the gyri in which they are embedded. This is what MRI scanning, ultrasound, and functional localization provide, and their combined use adds a new dimension to the surgery of intrinsic brain lesions.

In the introduction to Chapter 2, we noted that the reason for the delay in some of the patients coming to surgery was the sensitive location of the lesion. We posed the following question. In patients with lesions in the vicinity of the sensorimotor region or in the parasylvian territory in the dominant hemisphere, should surgery be deferred and considered only as a last resort? Our experience indicates that such patients should have early surgical evaluation, including craniotomy, the same as the others. Until the true, not the presumed, relationship of the lesion to the functional areas is established at surgery, one cannot decide about operability. This is an especially important consideration in patients such as those we describe. They are incapacitated by both their seizures and their toxic menus of medication. Their families share the burden. Yet, their seizures are usually caused by relatively benign gliomas associated with long periods of postoperative survival, occult vascular malformations, and any one of a small miscellany of benign masses. The likelihood that surgery will eliminate their one and only incapacitating symptoms—seizures—is excellent; without it, they are destined to continue their dependent and stigmatized existence.

With respect to functional localization, our job is far from done. Language cortex can only be mapped by using electrical stimulation of the cortical surface to halt speech in the awake patient. It is a time-consuming procedure which is only available to those who can undergo surgery under local anesthesia. In the remainder, the boundaries of language cortex can only be mapped extraoperatively by stimulation through indwelling surface electrode arrays (2, 10).

The sensorimotor area is much more easily identified and can be accomplished under anesthesia, as demonstrated in this study. However, we need to do better. The method requires that the bone flap extend beyond the exposure needed to deal with the pathology, because localization requires the comparison of areas which give a response with those that do not (4). Also, consider that vast expanse of association cortex for which no methods of functional localization exist, primarily because the functional anatomy of the individual convolutions is relatively unknown. Information concerning the human association areas exists mainly in the neuropsychological literature. Those studies, however, have not provided the data base for developing pragmatic methods of functional localization during surgery.

An objective we have set for ourselves, and are currently pursuing, is to develop a profile of electrophysiologic signatures that could be used to identify the function with which a particular cerebral gyrus is concerned.

It is based on the hypothesis that architectonically distinct areas might have specific electrophysiologic markers. The proposition is supported by animal studies in which the direct cortical response, an electrical potential recorded in the immediate vicinity of a focal electrical stimulus applied to the cortical surface, exhibits a configuration in the primary sensory areas that is distinctly different from the ones evoked in association cortex (9, 16). There are undoubtedly other approaches to this problem; hopefully, studies will be done to test them.

As long as neurological surgeons must deal with intrinsic brain lesions and as long as we must manipulate and traverse the cortical mantle, our goal should be to reduce the risk of neurologic deficit to zero, if possible. Toward this end, we need to develop a method that can identify, in the anesthetized patient, language cortex, motor and primary sensory cortex, distinguish primary sensory from association cortex, and ultimately identify the function with which the particular association cortex being manipulated is concerned. Such identification should be possible through craniotomies of sufficient size to deal only with the pathology, and the method should be a practical one that can be used by all neurosurgeons who expose the brain (2). Implicit in the development of such a method is the acquisition of new knowledge about how the brain works. This, too, is the responsibility of the neurological surgeon.

REFERENCES

1. Dohrmann, G. J., and Rubin, J. M. Use of ultrasound in neurosurgical operations: a preliminary report. Surg. Neurol., 16: 362–366, 1981.
2. Goldring, S. Epilepsy surgery. In: Clinical Neurosurgery, Vol 31, pp. 369–388. Williams & Wilkins, Baltimore, 1984.
3. Goldring, S., Aras, E., and Weber, P. C. Comparative study of sensory input to motor cortex in animals and man. Electroencephalogr. Clin. Neurophysiol., 29: 537–550, 1970.
4. Gregorie, E. M., and Goldring, S. Localization of function in the excision of lesions from the sensorimotor region. J. Neurosurg., 61: 1047–1054, 1984.
5. Kaas, J., Sur, M., Nelson, R. J., et al. The postcentral somatosensory cortex: multiple representations of the body in primates. In: Cortical Sensory Organization, Vol 1: Multiple Somatic Areas, edited by C. N. Woolsey, pp. 29–45. Humana, Clifton, N.J., 1981.
6. Kelly, D. L., Goldring, S., and O'Leary, J. L. Averaged evoked somatosensory responses from exposed cortex of man. Arch. Neurol., 13: 1–9, 1965.
7. Kwan, H. C., MacKay, W. A., Murphy, J. T., et al. Spatial organization of precentral cortex in awake primates. II. Motor outputs. J. Neurophysiol., 41: 1120–1131, 1978.
8. Lamour, Y., Jennings, V., and Solis, H. Functional characteristics and segregation of cutaneous and noncutaneous neurons in monkey precentral motor cortex (MI). Soc. Neurosci. Abstr., 6: 158, 1980.
9. Landau, W. M., and Clare, M. H. A note on the characteristic response pattern in primary sensory projection cortex of the cat following a synchronous afferent volley. Electroencephalogr. Clin. Neurophysiol., 8: 457–464, 1956.
10. Lesser, R. P., Lueders, H., Dinner, D. S., et al. The location of speech and writing functions

in the frontal language area: results of extraoperative cortical stimulation. Brain, *107:* 275–291, 1984.

11. Merzenich, M., Sur, M., Nelson, R. J., *et al.* Organization of the S1 cortex: multiple cutaneous representations in areas 3b and 1 of the owl monkey. In: *Cortical Sensory Organization,* Vol 1: *Multiple Somatic Areas,* edited by C. N. Woolsey, pp. 29–45. Humana, Clifton, N.J., 1981.

12. Stohr, P. E., and Goldring, S. Origin of somatosensory evoked scalp responses in man. J. Neurosurg., *31:* 117–127, 1969.

13. Strick, P. L., and Preston, J. B. Multiple representation in the primate motor cortex. Brain Res., *154:* 366–370, 1978.

14. Strick, P. L., and Preston, J. B. Two representations of the hand in area 4 of a primate. I. Motor output organization. J. Neurophysiol., *48:* 139–149, 1982.

15. Strick, P. L., and Preston, J. B. Two representations of the hand in area 4 of a primate. II. Somatosensory input organization. J. Neurophysiol., *48:* 150–159, 1982.

16. Suzuki, H., and Taira, N. Regional difference of the direct cortical response. Jpn. J. Physiol., *8:* 365–377, 1958.

17. Tanji, J., and Wise, S. P. Submodality distribution in sensorimotor cortex of the unanesthetized monkey. J. Neurophysiol., *45:* 467–481, 1981.

II

Perspectives in Neurosurgery

4

A Clinician and Teacher's Overview of the Decision-Making Process

HENRY G. SCHWARTZ, M.D.

No probability formulas, no irrefutable mathematical equations, no transcending systems of philosophy, no algorithms, no unassailable randomized double-blind studies were involved in the magnificent sally of Athena as she sprang in regal splendor from the head of Zeus. Who or what were the decisive elements that entered into acceptance of such a universe-shaking event that captured and held the minds and hearts of thousands of undoubting worshippers for hundreds of years?

I assume that since the beginning of time, efforts have been made to expose and unravel the means by which we travel on our searching road to ultimate truth. Many concepts have grown and been accepted through reason or imagination, and man strives to enable the former to overcome the latter.

As one looks back, the centuries have been filled with towering figures who seem to have looked but failed to see. In basic anatomy, Aristotle's contributions were founded upon animal dissections from which arose speculations on the human body, some clarifications of which came in limited degree from human dissections by Herophilus. Galen's voluminous anatomical works went unchallenged for about 13 centuries until Leonardo da Vinci and then Vesalius substituted facts for fancy, incurring the vicious criticism of eminent traditional scholars who coincidentally at Padua made life so difficult for Copernicus. A century ago, Sir William MacEwen, a venerated member of the pantheon of neurosurgery, after presenting his historic address on surgery of the brain and spinal cord (8), commented philosophically that "they were so hampered by the inculcated physiological dogma of the time that their true significance never dawned on them."

Despite the best of intention, bias, prejudice, and fidelity to tradition are among the unmeasurable elements that affect the way we accept or deny concepts of the past and determine our responses to contemporary suggestions and recommendations. As a science, decision making in medicine has been and still is to a great extent relatively unprogrammed. As an art, like other forms, it holds many secrets and numerous characteristics that may vary in definition from one beholder to another and that challenge analysis.

As a glowing example of the difficulties that may beset decision making, I stand here now in a great quandary. Just what decision do I make with regard to the assignment that has befallen me as a participant in this colloquium? What am I to say that has not been said before and which undoubtedly will be said better and more convincingly by the speakers who follow. After considerable thought, I submit at the start that I do not know just what factors enter decision making, but I will comment regarding some events with which I have become familiar in my lifetime as a student, as a physician, and as a neurosurgeon. Perhaps such a recitation will provide some clues.

Experience of self and of others is certainly a great teacher and enters into any decision. At this late date it is almost incomprehensible to me to recall that in my days as a surgical house officer there were some questions regarding so straightforward a matter as treatment of appendicitis and peritonitis. Recent reading of Ravitch's (10) monumental history of the American Surgical Association reminded me of my own astonishment at that time when I was made aware of any divergence of opinion regarding surgical treatment. In a 1926 meeting, Le Grand Guerry (4) of Columbia, South Carolina, reported his impressive series of 2959 appendectomies with 16 deaths. It must be noted that almost all of the cases were "chronic appendicitis." In the discussion of Guerry's report were comments regarding the principles of management of diffuse peritonitis recommended by Albert J. Ochsner of Chicago, consisting of gastric lavage, morphine, and rectal feeding, with the expectation of localization of the infection and walling-off before proceeding with operation. Guerry was understandably convinced of the validity of his own personal experience with the deferred operation in cases of peritonitis, which he enlarged upon saying "the principle of deferred operation, broadly speaking, must be applicable in greater or lesser degree to the whole field of emergency surgery."

I cannot resist drawing a perhaps far-fetched parallel between the decision making by our surgical forebears and the questions which still arise periodically regarding the treatment of brain abscess and cerebritis. I might add further that our personal experience (11, 12) with delayed debridement of already heavily contaminated shell fragment war wounds fit with Guerry's broad statement. It would be inappropriate for me to pursue this specific matter in this presentation, but once again referring to the history of surgery, Jopson of Philadelphia in his paper on peritonitis noted that almost all American surgeons favored immediate operation in early appendicitis, but this was "not of universal adoption in some European countries" depending upon whether the surgical consultant was an "interventionist," an "abstentionist," or an "opportunist" (6).

To bring matters into sharper focus for ourselves as neurosurgeons, it is salutary to reflect upon the reception of what proved to be one of the outstanding contributions to clinical neurosurgery. All of us are familiar with Dandy and Blackfan's studies on hydrocephalus. Most older or middle group neurosurgeons are aware of pneumoencephalography and ventricular air injection. For practical purposes, these techniques have been superseded by less traumatic and more accurate diagnostic methods. In 1918, after trials in hydrocephalic patients, Dandy introduced ventriculography and proceeded to accumulate a large experience with the method. It is illuminating to review the abstract of his report and the star-studded discussion that followed his 1922 presentation to the members of the prestigious American Neurological Association (3). Harvey Cushing and Ernest Sachs were not at all charitable in their remarks, and among other distinguished commentators and decision makers, little praise was elicited from Adolf Meyer, Naffziger, or Ayer, but some measure of acceptance was acknowledged by Elsberg and Dowman. In his fairly lengthy remarks, Cushing (who was to assume the presidency the following year) was not at all gentle and expressed reservations about the figures presented by Dandy. The latter (who was not to become a member until 5 years later) responded to Cushing's critique in his characteristic, forthright manner; he defended the accuracy of his percentages and noted that "If one's experience is largely with pituitary tumors or those which are self-localizing, the percentage of necessary uses for ventriculography would be very much less." He added the additional rapier-like thrust: "I can readily see why everyone does not obtain results from the use of the procedure; for one can be misled easily in the interpretation of the plates, unless he has had sufficient experience in differentiating the phantom from the real shadows, and unless he knows every step taken in placing the patient's head correctly."

I cannot avoid an aside. In his comments regarding radical tumor removal, which was recommended by Dandy in his ventriculography report, another revered decision maker, Charles Frazier, stated: "I should be disposed to look on these deepseated infiltrating gliomas in which the definition is not sharp, in which the tumor tissue shades off into the neighborhood, as inoperable from the standpoint of eradication and of making a rapid recovery. I should be in favor of resorting to removal by decompression, followed by radium therapy by direct implantation and later by the indirect method." The wheels turn slowly. I recall the days in the 1930s when, following radical excision of a glioma, Dr. Sachs' patients were moved from the operating room into the adjacent radiology department and a massive dose of X-radiation was delivered into the open wound, under the direction of Dr. Sherwood Moore.

The 1930s saw the early reports of Mixter and Barr and the prompt acceptance of the concept of intervertebral disc disease with relatively little question of the indication for surgery and with very good results. Semmes was among the small number who advised against myelography, and he suggested that this, too, was a matter for decision making by individual surgeons. This has remained a gratifying type of surgery, for which only a few have limited reservations. Contemporaneously, we saw fairly wide acceptance of sympathectomy for hypertension with apparently good blood pressure control and protection against retinal hemorrhage. Fortunately, the several varieties of surgical sympathetic denervation could be displaced by appropriate medication.

The next decade saw the abandonment of choroid plexectomy in favor of shunts for hydrocephalus, without achieving the real solution to the problem. There then followed the burgeoning of vascular surgery and microsurgery. I need not remind this audience of the questions which arose regarding timing of aneurysm surgery, the studies of outcome, and the residual questions surrounding treatment that must influence our decisions today.

It is noteworthy that, as our surgical skills develop and make it possible to outshine our past achievements, we have begun to question the validity of what we are doing. The most recent report of the EC-IC Bypass Randomized Trial, presented at the meeting of the International Congress of Neurological Surgery in July, 1985, indicates that this attractive, fascinating surgical maneuver does not reduce the risk of stroke. The disappointing result of this carefully controlled study seems to negate numerous previously published case series and experimental reports that indicated effectiveness of the operation. At the moment it seems to me that we have a beautiful, technically gratifying, theoretically curative procedure looking for suitable indications. The pros and cons regarding its performance will place quite a strain upon the individual surgeon who recommends its use in a particular patient.

Numerous other conditions that require our best talents in making decisions readily come to mind. In the cerebrovascular area are the handling of tandem lesions, asymptomatic stenosis, aneurysms coexisting with carotid stenosis, multiple aneurysms, deep-seated anteriovenous malformations, and possibilities of radiation and stereotaxy. What should be our recommendations regarding malignant glial tumors, satisfactory treatment of which has really eluded us since the beginnings of our specialty? What data can we rely upon regarding the safety of effective radiation therapy, and what is the basis for recommending this in children?

Many are the areas which tax the judgment and wisdom of the neurosurgeon. Some are purely medical, some ethical, and most a combination in lesser or greater degree. Nowhere is the burden more difficult and heavier than in dealing with congenital defects or severe cranial or spinal trauma. In the latter part of my professional lifetime my interest in salvaging babies with severe craniofacial problems has frequently called forth what I hope have been correct decisions. There have been times when I could not help reflecting upon pertinent comments made by one of my plastic surgery friends, who, in discussing extreme efforts expended in the care of children with severe burns, commented: "Moral questions are constantly in mind, especially in the extensively burned child with hands and face involved and I emphasize hands and face. Are our efforts justified if the family is disrupted by the return of this severely handicapped, disfigured child to its midst? What will the suicide rate be in the teenaged disfigured child? One recalls the high rate of suicide in the cerebral palsy victims in their late teens. The answers are not ours to give, but society may ultimately have to make a decision about the salvage of these children (2).

Technological advances together with social, moral, ethical, legal, and economic factors play a tremendous role in the management of modern medical care. The past several years have seen increasing and important attempts by highly competent skilled physicians, educators, ethicists, and philosophers to analyze the elements which should go into the decision-making process, and these elements are bound to be elaborated and illuminated by the speakers who follow.

In the introduction to a recent paper, Siegler (13) put it quite simply: "Medical education and training should prepare physicians to make decisions, because that is what they do routinely in medical practice." Simplistically and traditionally the physician makes his examination, recommends needed tests, and comes to a diagnosis. He then weighs the prognosis along with the risks and benefits of treatment and presents the patient with his review and recommendations for management. These elements form the first of four categories which Siegler lists in his proposal for a systematic approach to clinical-ethical decisions. The others consist of patient preferences, quality of life considerations, and external factors. Medical indications take primacy but "now the public wants to participate in this process as informed shoppers" (7).

The increased complexity of contemporary practice has drawn so much attention that a Presidential Commission was established and presented its report on "Making Health Care Decisions" (9) in October, 1982. In reaching its objective of increased communication and shared decision making, and modifying the "professional dominance" view, the Commission discussed two possible means of influencing professional attitudes— namely, deliberately designed selection of specific types of individuals admitted into the health care professions and the content of professional training. I cannot take issue with these goals, but confess to having difficulty in setting valid identifying criteria for admission to medical school and to postgraduate training programs. There is no argument that we want to encourage broadly educated, highly motivated young people to come into the profession. The attributes of scientific competence and curiosity, along with integrity, the ability to endure the rigors of a medical curriculum, and maintenance of compassionate concern balanced by dispassionate evaluation of patients' problems are major requirements. With these as a start, that individual is well on his way to become a self-starting, self-stimulating learner, who needs only the opportunity to work and to expand his horizons. In the zeal for ensuring humanistic qualification, we should not withdraw from insistence upon high qualifications as a scientist and skill as a surgeon. Let us always keep our sights focused upon developing a galaxy of first class individuals rather than creating a category of second class specialists. We must adhere to the philosophy of the first rate.

Our parochial bias leads us to hope that interest in the nervous system will draw the bright students to a neurosurgical program in an institution that offers opportunity to perfect not only his craft but where resources are available for intellectual pursuit in associated areas. With discipline and a small amount of thoughtful guidance, such an individual will develop and expand his own talents and become the highly competent neurological surgeon in whose training the teacher will be proud to have had a share.

In reading a recent biography by a well-known industrialist I came across this interesting, somewhat hyperbolic comment: "You can use the fanciest computers and you can gather all the charts and numbers, but in the end you have to bring all your information together, set up a timetable, and *act*. Too many managers let themselves get weighted down in their decision making, especially those with too much education. The trouble with you is that you went to Harvard where they taught you not to take any action until you've got *all* the facts. You've got 95% of them, but it's going to take you another six months to get that last 5%. And by the time you do, your facts will be out of date because the market has moved on you. What constitutes enough information for the decision-maker? When you move ahead with only 50% of the facts, the odds are stacked against you. If that's the case, you had better be very lucky or else come up with some terrific hunches. There are times when that kind of gamble is called for, but it's certainly no way to run a railroad." "At the same time, you never know

100% of what you need. When you don't have all the facts, you sometimes have to draw on your experience" (5).

I applaud and urge persistent pursuit of applying the methods of science and logic to problem solving. The ideal neurosurgeon will bring to decision making his own unmeasurable and undefinable attributes. However much our information and data permit us to approach perfection in making decisions, let us always be alert and heed Robert Bridges, poet laureate of England a half-century ago in his *Testament of Beauty* (1):

> "Our stability is but balance, and wisdom lies
> in masterful administration of the unforeseen."

REFERENCES

1. Bridges, R. *The testament of beauty. A Poem in Four Parts*, Clarendon Press, Oxford, 1930.
2. Cannon, B. Cited in Ravitch, p. 1419.
3. Dandy, W. E. Ventricular radiography in the diagnosis of brain tumors. In: *Transactions of American Neurological Association*, edited by T. H. Weisenburg, Philadelphia, pp. 69–74, 1922.
4. Guerry, LeG. Cited in Ravitch, p. 636.
5. Iacocca, L. *An Autobiography*. Bantam Books, New York, 1984.
6. Jopson, J. H. Cited in Ravitch, p. 587.
7. Kiser, W. S. Buying and selling health care: A battle for the medical marketplace. Bull. Am. Coll. Surg., *70:* 2–7, 1985.
8. MacEwen, W. An address on the surgery of the brain and spinal cord. Br. Med. J., 302–309, August 11, 1888.
9. President's Commission for the Study of Ethical Problems in Medicine and Biomedical and Behavioral Research. *Making Health Care Decisions*. Vol. 1: Report. Washington, DC, U.S. Government Printing Office, October, 1982.
10. Ravitch, M. M. *A Century of Surgery: The History of the American Surgical Association*. J.B. Lippincott, Philadelphia, 1981.
11. Schwartz, H. G., and Roulhac, G. E. Craniocerebral war wounds. Med. Bull. N. African Theater of Operations, 22–23, 1944.
12. Schwartz, H. G., and Roulhac, G. E. Craniocerebral war wounds. Observations on delayed treatment. Ann. Surg., *121:* 129–151, 1945.
13. Siegler, M. Decision-making strategy for clinical-ethical problems in medicine. Arch. Intern. Med., *142:* 2178–2179, 1982.

5

The Changing Economic Context of Medical Decision-Making

ALAIN C. ENTHOVEN, PH.D.

INTRODUCTION

The U.S. health care economy is changing with remarkable speed from the noncompetitive guild system of the past 50 years to a competitive market system. A more efficient industry, more responsive to consumer preferences, is emerging.

THE OPEN-ENDED ERA OF HEALTH CARE FINANCE: 1960 TO THE EARLY 1980s

For 50 years, private health insurance was based largely on fee-for-service payment of physicians' so-called "usual, customary, and reasonable fees," and either retrospective cost reimbursement or fee-for-service for hospitals. Utilization was not seriously reviewed or controlled. Thus, providers got more money for doing more services and were at no financial risk for their use of resources. Medicare and, to some extent, Medicaid adopted the same model.

For 50 years, "free choice of provider" was a key element of our health care financing system. As interpreted by organized medicine, "free choice of provider" meant that every insurance scheme must, at all times, leave the patient completely free in choice of doctor. This so-called "freedom" is a medical-economic concept designed to assure that the payor has no bargaining power and that there will be no economic competition among doctors. The patients are not cost conscious because they are insured. And the payors have no bargaining power because they have no authority to direct patients away from costly doctors. The effect is to create a cost-unconscious demand, at least for those costly physicians' services that are insured. Martin Feldstein characterized this situation as "permanent excess demand" (6). This principle was enforced on insurance companies by boycotts of nonconforming insurers, and by the development of Blue Cross and Blue Shield insurance companies under provider sponsorship and control. In some states such as California, as well as in the Medicare and Medicaid programs, it was written into the law. The principle was enforced on nonconforming doctors by denials of referrals, denial of hospital medical staff privileges, and ostracism from professional societies. Charles Weller called this "guild free choice" to emphasize that it is, in fact, a restraint of trade (11). He contrasted it to "market free choice," a concept that I will be discussing later.

For about 20 years, federal subsidies to health care and health insurance were mostly in the form of open-ended subsidies of marginal costs. For example, if a Medicare beneficiary and his doctor agreed on a more, versus less, costly course of treatment, the government would pay most of the extra cost. If an employer and his employees agree on a more costly health insurance package, in effect the Treasury pays about one-third of the extra cost.

The combination of these characteristics was a sure prescription for rapid growth in health care spending. From 1960 to 1983, national health expenditures grew from $27 billion to $355 billion, from 5.3% of the Gross National Product (GNP) to 10.7%. Public sector spending grew from $7 billion to $149 billion. Private health insurance premiums (mostly, but not all, paid by employers) grew from $6.4 billion to $110.5 billion, from 13.4% of pre-tax corporate profits to 48.6%.

THE END OF THE OPEN-ENDED ERA

The health care financing system is now changing fundamentally and inexorably from cost-unconscious "free choice of provider" to cost-conscious choice among limited groups of selected providers contracting in advance. These limited provider organizations, which I shall refer to as "competitive medical plans" (whether or not they meet the Medicare definition), are reviewing provider performance and selecting cost-effective providers. They are also seeking to put providers at risk for their use of resources. At the same time, government is moving from open-ended subsidies of marginal cost to limited fixed-dollar global payments.

This change is occurring for three main reasons. First, the open-ended system got too expensive. Government and employers could no longer afford it. Starting about 1978, taxpayers revolted and signaled clearly that they wanted to stop the growth in taxes as a share of their incomes. At the same time, the Soviet military buildup, the invasion of Afghanistan, and the hostage crisis in Iran all led to public support for increased military spending. In the early to mid-1970s, the decline in military spending as a share of GNP made room for growth in health spending. By the 1980s, that was no longer the case. Public finances are obviously strained.

Second, attempts to solve the problem by price controls and similar regulatory restraints did not work. The 1970s were a decade of regulatory failure in health care.

Third, the idea that costs could be controlled through market forces caught on. Gradually, the evidence that health maintenance organizations (HMOs) really could cut cost while maintaining the quality of care became overwhelming. In the early 1970s, Dr. Paul Ellwood, in his famous paper "Health Maintenance Strategy," first put forward the idea of a socially desirable competition among HMOs (2). This led to the HMO Act of 1973. Through the 1970s, the idea picked up support while the national mood was increasingly disenchanted with regulation.

The generous increase in the supply of doctors helped. So did the wave of antitrust action that followed the Supreme Court's Goldfarb decision in which the Court ruled the learned professions were subject to antitrust.

Price competition is the normal way of doing business in America.

All this started a process of "falling dominos". In 1981, the Reagan Administration and the Congress sought to reduce the growth in federal outlays for Medicaid. The states were allowed to engage in selective competitive contracting for Medicaid providers. In 1982, Congress placed effective all-inclusive limits on the growth in hospital cost per case for Medicare patients. Allowable hospital costs per case could grow no faster than an index of the prices hospitals pay, plus 1%.

In 1982, California employers feared that they would be the victims of a massive "cost shift" if they remained on the open-ended system of health insurance for their employees. That is, they feared that hospitals would recover the revenues they lost under the new Medicare limits and Medicaid competitive contracting by simply raising the charges paid by cost-unconscious private insurance. So they teamed up with trade unions and the insurance industry to persuade the legislature to overturn the previous prohibition on selective contracting by insurance companies. This legislation was a signal event on the national health care financing scene. Employers and health insurers across the nation interpreted it to mean that organized medicine could no longer block selective contracting or what has come to be known as Preferred Provider Insurance (PPI).

In 1983, Congress enacted the Prospective Payment System (PPS) for Medicare inpatient hospital cases. Each inpatient hospital case is classified into one of 468 categories called Diagnosis Related Groups (DRGs). After a phase-in period, hospitals will be paid a uniform fixed prospective payment per case in each DRG, adjusted for each area's wage levels and for teaching costs. The original law provided that, at first, the payments would be adjusted annually in proportion to the index of the prices hospitals pay, plus 1%. However, in February, 1985, the Reagan Administration proposed that 1986 payments be kept at their 1985 levels without adjustment for inflation.

PPS represents a profound change from cost reimbursement and an important step in the direction of economic efficiency. It rewards providers for reducing costs per case. The PPS is forcing hospitals and their medical staffs to cooperate to control costs, to relate clinical and financial information, to consider cost-benefit tradeoffs, and to control quality. The surgeon who has a high complication rate can damage the financial health of the hospital.

I doubt that the PPS will be enough to bring the growth of Medicare outlays into line with the GNP. It works on too small a part of the problem, that is, the growth in cost per inpatient case. It leaves the faster growing outpatient costs uncontrolled, and, in itself, it does not control growth in numbers of cases. Ultimately, it will be necessary for the government to convert Medicare to a system of fixed prospective capitation payments for comprehensive care, paid to the participating competitive medical plan (CMP) of the patient's choice. Under this approach the government would effectively be able to limit the growth in its outlays to whatever it could afford. The 1982 changes in the Medicare law created an "HMO option" for Medicare beneficiaries. In the future, the per capita basis of payment (adjusted for age, sex, institutional status, and other factors) will have to become mandatory for all beneficiaries.

The last great open-ended entitlement in health care is the tax subsidy to health insurance, the fact that employer contributions to the health care of employees are excluded from the taxable incomes of employees. This cost the federal budget about $30 billion in 1984, an amount that is growing much faster than the GNP. As early as 1979, bills were introduced in the Congress to limit the amount of employer contributions that would be tax free to employees. In its 1984 budget, the Reagan Administration proposed a limit of $175 per family per month. Ultimately, the government will have to stabilize this source of revenue loss as a share of the GNP. And the simplest way would be a per capita limit on tax-free contributions. Powerful interest groups oppose this proposal, and it may not be enacted. But if and as this occurs and as Medicare is converted to a per capita contribution basis, the federal government will no longer be sharing in the extra costs when patients and providers choose more costly care, or when employers and employees choose more comprehensive insurance. For the most part, individual consumers will be bearing the extra cost. This will make them cost conscious in their choices. The open-ended era will yield to the era of market competition.

THE MARKET COMPETITION ERA

How can one reconcile widespread health insurance, which presumably makes consumers unconscious of cost, with economic competition in health care services, in the sense of cost-conscious buyers and sellers? The key is that the competition must take place at the point of an annual choice of comprehensive health care financing and delivery plan, and not at the point of receipt of individual medical services.

The concept of market competition is based on four ideas.

The first is the CMP that links insurance and a limited set of providers so that the insurance premium reflects the ability of those providers to control cost. CMP is a generic term that includes HMOs, PPI, and other similar concepts. The idea is to divide the physicians in a community into separate economic units that compete on the basis of price, quality of care and service.

The second idea is consumer choice: each consumer should have an annual choice among the health care financing and delivery plans serving his area. This is "market free choice," a different meaning of "free choice of provider." Each consumer may select the health care plan that includes the providers he prefers. But this interpretation of free choice permits economic competition among providers.

Third, the choice must be cost conscious. Whatever help each consumer receives toward the purchase of his health care plan membership must be in the form of a fixed payment, independent of his choice of plan. Thus, the consumer who chooses a more costly health plan pays the extra cost himself. The market free choice idea emphasizes cost consciousness at the time of the annual choice of health care plan, rather than cost consciousness at the time of need for individual medical services.

Fourth, market competition does not mean a "free market." A free market in health insurance would not be compatible with widespread health insurance. There need to be rules to make the competition equitable and effective. Rules are needed to assure that health plans prosper by giving better care at less cost, and not merely by selecting healthier people to insure. Health plans that serve people with greater expected medical needs should be compensated equitably for doing so.

HMOs are the prototypical competitive medical plans. HMOs provide (or arrange and pay for) comprehensive health care services for a fixed periodic per capita payment, set in advance, that is independent of the volume of services actually provided. The "product" of the HMO is comprehensive care for a person for a year, not lots of individual services. The HMO is paid for solving members' medical problems, not for doing more services. The HMO has a voluntarily enrolled population for which it plans resources, and a prospective budget within which to do it. HMO patients agree to obtain all their insured care from providers affiliated with their HMO. After years of slow growth, HMO membership growth has accelerated sharply in recent years. At the end of 1984, membership was 16.7 million, up 22.4% over a year earlier.

Growth is accelerating for several reasons that seem powerful and not likely to be reversed. First, at least in the case of the multispecialty group practice HMOs, the margin of economic advantage over "guild free choice" and fee-for-service is large and growing. A recent, randomized, controlled experiment in Seattle found that people cared for by a large HMO used about 40% less hospital days and 28% fewer total resources than the fee-for-service control group (7).

Second, perceptions of quality are changing. It used to be that the fee-for-service sector was the norm and that HMOs were suspected of under-serving their members. But in recent years, employers have come to suspect the fee-for-service sector of overutilization. The Mayo Clinic, often considered a symbol of excellence in American medicine, recently published hospital use rates for the people they care for in their home county. Adjusted for demography, their use was 38% below the national average and about the same as the large group practice HMOs (8). A literature review by a team at Johns Hopkins found that of 27 studies comparing quality of care, 19 found quality in the HMO to be superior, with no difference or inconclusive results in the other 8 (1).

A third reason for accelerating HMO growth has been a breakdown in the political and economic power of the medical profession. The growth in cost forced the development of countervailing political power. A fourth reason is that the increased supply of well-trained young physicians has made it much easier for HMOs to recruit doctors. At the same time, the fee-for-service sector is increasingly saturated. A fifth reason is the emergence of national HMO firms with the competence, the personnel and management systems, and the capital that enables them to enter new areas with assurance of success. There are now about 15 organizations with HMOs in more than one state.

Finally, after years of offering increasingly comprehensive coverages, employers are now moving to restore some cost consciousness among their employees—for example, by raising the share of medical bills paid by employees. This makes the comprehensive coverages of HMOs increasingly attractive to employees.

The past few years have seen the emergence of a new kind of CMP generally known as PPI. In this scheme, the insurer contracts selectively with providers on the basis of a negotiated fee schedule, which contracting providers accept as payment in full, and acceptance of utilization controls. Consumers are then given incentives to choose contracting providers, but they remain free to use other providers, though on less favorable terms.

PPI remains basically a fee-for-service concept. Providers do not take a financial risk with respect to the volume of services provided, as they do in HMOs. But hospitals do take the risk that they will be able to provide care at a cost that does not exceed the agreed prices. In principle, a preferred provider plan does not need to be linked to a cohesive provider organization that can control performance and allocate resources. For this reason, it is likely to be less effective than Prepaid Group Practice (PGP). However, under competitive pressures, perferred provider plans are likely to evolve into more cohesive organizations, probably based on hospitals and their medical staffs.

PPI is a way that employers can move quickly to control the health care costs of those of their employees now covered under fee-for-service arrangements. Large employers are requiring their insurance companies to create PPI plans for them. Some are doing it themselves. Patients' desire for free choice of provider is proving to be much less of a factor than leaders of organized medicine had implied. And both insurers and fee-for-service providers are participating because they need a way to compete with HMOs. The large insurance companies are marketing PPI aggressively.

These developments pose a serious economic threat to hospitals. Nationally we have about 4.4 acute beds per 1000 population. Efficient organizations can care for representative population groups with about half that many beds. In the past, cost reimbursement and cost-unconscious demand imposed no penalty on hospitals for being half empty. Now Medicare will not pay for excess overhead costs, nor will HMOs or PPI. So hospitals without patients are heading for serious economic trouble. Hospitals used to be deterred from contracting with HMOs or PPI by their medical staffs, who threatened to take their patients elsewhere. Now medical staffs are turning to their hospitals for help in the struggle to attract patients.

The four largest investor-owned hospital companies (controlling about 70,000 beds) have recently purchased insurance companies, and each is now offering PPI based on its own hospitals. In a typical arrangement, a company may offer an employer a reduced premium and an annual rate of increase limited by the Consumer Price Index provided the employees use the company's hospitals. By June, 1985, these companies had enrolled one million people in their PPI plans (9). At the same time, they are buying or starting HMOs. And they are investing in less costly substitutes for inpatient care. Some of the nonprofit hospital organizations are making similar moves.

There will be problems for hospitals as they attempt to make these changes. Their administrators have been trained to keep beds filled and to cater to physicians who order many tests and procedures. So these hospitals and their medical staffs will have to undergo a basic cultural change. But their eventual goal is emerging: to survive, they must become efficient comprehensive care organizations.

APPRAISAL: GOOD NEWS AND BAD NEWS

The likely outcome of the process I have described appears to be consolidation of the medical care system into comprehensive health care financing and delivery organizations serving, perhaps, several hundred thousand to several million people each. These organizations will be capable of controlling cost and quality of care. There are economies of scale in marketing, acquisition, and efficient use of capital, management systems, purchasing, and personnel development. So these organizations will seek to grow by enrolling subscribers and by mergers.

The competition of these organizations to serve subscribers who are conscious of both quality and cost is producing a new health care economy with many desirable features that were not present under the noncompetitive guild system. First, consumer satisfaction is beginning to get a higher priority. Second, in the HMOs, physicians accept major responsibility for controlling the quality and total cost of care. Strong effective peer review of the quality and economy of care is in the physicians' interest. Third, each CMP is under continuous pressure to improve quality of care and service while cutting cost. Cost-reducing innovation is encouraged (3). Fourth, various models of medical practice organization are being tested in the marketplace. Different models that suit the preferences of different providers and consumers are available. The best models will gradually emerge. And finally, the regulatory system governing the competition can be relatively simple and self-enforcing. Under guild free choice, provider incentives were to increase cost. Government efforts to control cost, in direct opposition to these incentives, became extremely complex and usually ineffective. Under market competition, the CMPs must control their own costs.

The developments I have described are likely to bring the growth of health care spending much closer to the growth rate of the GNP. And they are likely to improve quality control a great deal. But I see three large problems that they are leaving unsolved.

The first is the need for rules to make the competition equitable. Without rules, some health care financing schemes may succeed by skillfully selecting healthy people to insure, while dumping unhealthy people on other health plans. Today, the regulation of health care plans is needlessly complex. Some, such as federally qualified HMOs, are regulated by the federal government as well as by states, whereas others, such as insurance companies, are regulated by states. And insurance provided by employers who self-insure is regulated by neither. We need a uniform set of rules applicable to all health care financing and delivery plans.

Second, we have a major problem of uninsured people. One recent study found that about 9% of the under-65 population, or 19 million people, have no health insurance, public or private, all year; another 9.4% have no insurance for part of the year (5). In the past, uninsured people who could not pay got their care from public providers, such as county hospitals, or as charity patients at private hospitals. The economic competition I have described makes it increasingly difficult for hospitals to provide free care that is not paid for. In the past, they simply added these costs to their other costs and charged them to their cost-unconscious customers. Under competition to serve cost-conscious buyers, hospitals will not be able to do this.

Several states have adopted public utility regulation of hospitals to solve this problem. The controlled rates include allowances for uncompensated care, given to people unable to pay, and all the third-party payors are obliged to pay them. The alternative most compatible with market competition would be to make public subsidies for the purchase of health insurance available to all persons. As I noted earlier, through the income tax system, we subsidize the health insurance of employed people. What remains to be done is to make at least equally generous subsidies available to those who do not have employer-provided health insurance (4). This would need to be combined with state-supported agencies created to assure availability of health insurance to all people.

A third major problem concerns the role of university medical centers. The research and teaching missions of these organizations make the patient care they do more costly than it otherwise would be. In the past, these extra costs simply were passed on to Medicare in the form of cost reimbursement and to privately insured patients in the form of higher charges. With the advent of cost-conscious demand, university medical centers no longer will be able to do that. The CMPs will only be willing to pay for patient care in efficient hospitals.

Conceptually, it would seem easy enough to say that the extra costs of research and teaching should be separately identified and supported on their own merits, while the universities compete for patients. But as a practical matter, this will not be easy. The public sector is not in a position to absorb the extra costs, and university medical centers are far from being efficient producers of care. Their cultures and life styles are geared to research, not efficient patient care. Moreover, as CMPs refer increasing numbers of their patients to efficient community providers, only relatively more costly and complex cases will be referred to universities, cases that will not present a representative mix of patients for teaching purposes. Teaching may have to be moved into the settings used by the CMPs.

These problems are not without potential solutions. However, a considerable amount of adjustment will be required, and the end point is not clear.

SOME IMPLICATIONS FOR NEUROSURGEONS

As the system moves toward efficiency, cost effectiveness will become the way of life for surgeons. It will become increasingly important for you to measure and consider carefully your use of resources in producing medical care. Cost-reducing innovation will be rewarded.

A cost-conscious ethic will replace the cost-unconscious ethic. Under the "guild free choice" system, most insured people were not offered the choice of a less costly standard of care. For the most part, people were either covered by cost-unconscious insurance or not covered at all. In the economic environment of open-ended financing, it is easy to understand how the physician can be led to an ethic that demands he or she do everything that might help the patient, regardless of cost. After all, if the patient is not paying the bill, such behavior is in the patient's best interest.

In the market competition era, patients will have cost-conscious choices, and it is understandable that many will choose less than the most costly standard of care. At the margin, other things—such as food, shelter, sanitation, and education—may become more important for health than a more costly standard of medical care. When the patient must pay the extra cost if he chooses a more costly standard of care, he has an interest in cost containment. In this situation, the physician can quite ethically act as the patient's agent in delivering the standard of care the patient has chosen and contracted for. It will be very important, of course, that the physician cooperate in making this an informed choice.

It will be important for physicians generally to have a correct concept of cost. Their goal should not be to minimize the cost of medical care as such. It should be to minimize the total cost of illness and its treatment, including in the total cost of illness suffering, work lost, and disability. If, for example, you cut medical spending by $2000 by inflicting on a patient a 1 in 100 risk of avoidable disability that he would value at $500,000, then you have not reduced his cost of illness and its treatment. Competitive medical plans that cut spending merely by shifting such burdens onto patients are likely to gain a reputation for not being good bargains.

There are many ways in which efficient medical care organizations can cut cost without cutting the quality of care: controlling quality and doing it right the first time; appropriate physician incentives; matching resources used to the needs of the population served; regional concentration of specialized services such as neurosurgery; curtailing procedures and treatments of no marginal value, such as lengths of hospital stay; use of less costly setting such as outpatient surgicenters; use of evaluated technology; and others.

I think this will mean that we will see fewer neurosurgeons with fuller operating schedules as the work gets concentrated in efficient regional centers. There, the neurosurgeons will be able to make a good living at a low cost per case by treating a high volume of cases.

Outside such centers, I think we will see the demise of the fee-for-service solo practitioner. It used to be, not long ago, that a newly trained young surgeon could enter practice almost wherever he or she pleased. The open-ended financing system could always support another neurosurgeon. In the future, that will not be the case. HMOs and PPOs will channel their patients to the efficient high-volume centers with which they have contracted.

According to the 1980 Graduate Medical Education National Advisory Committee report, by 1990 we will have in this country nearly twice as many neurosurgeons as are needed (10). I think the likely consequence of the developments I have described will be to make that surplus even greater. Those of you who are about to consider practice opportunities now would do well to consider carefully the possibilities of practicing with HMOs or in medical centers that contract with HMOs and PPI organizations.

REFERENCES

1. Cunningham, F. C., and Williamson, J. W. How does the quality of health care in HMOs compare to that in other settings? Group Health J., *1:* 4–25, 1980.
2. Ellwood, P. M., Anderson N., Billings, J., *et al.* Health maintenance strategy, Med. Care, *291:* 250–256, 1971.
3. Enthoven, A. C. Shattuck lecture: cutting cost without cutting the quality of care. N. Engl. J. Med., *298:* 1229–1238, 1978.
4. Enthoven, A. C. A new proposal to reform the tax treatment of health insurance. Health Affairs, Spring, 1984.
5. Farley, P. J. *Who Are the Underinsured?* National Health Care Expenditures Study, National Center for Health Research, November, 1984.
6. Feldstein, M. S. The rising price of physicians' services. Rev. Economics Statistics, *52:* 121–133, 1970.
7. Manning, W. G., Leibowitz, A., Goldberg, G., *et al.* A controlled trial of the effect of a prepaid group practice on use of services. N. Engl. J. Med., *310:* 1505–1510, 1984.
8. Nobrega, F. T., Krishan, I., Smoldt, R., *et al.* Hospital use in a fee-for-service system. J.A.M.A., *247:* 806–810, 1982.
9. Private hospitals are now offering health insurance. New York Times, July 4, 1985.
10. Summary Report of the Graduate Medical Education National Advisory Committee to the Secretary, Department of Health and Human Services, Washington, D.C., September 30, 1980. DHHS Pub. No. (HRA) 81-651, April, 1981.
11. Weller, C. D. "Free choice" as a restraint of trade in American health care delivery and insurance. Iowa Law Rev., *69:* 1351–1392, 1984.

CHAPTER

6

Deciding Not to Treat—Medical, Legal, and Ethical Considerations

PETER McL. BLACK, M.D. PH.D.

A decision not to treat a patient in neurosurgery is usually made on the basis of the natural history of the disease and the risks and benefits of the proposed treatment. Most neurosurgeons have faced situations in which no easy answer about these factors comes from previous individual or group experience, however. Examples of such situations include:

1. A 58-year-old businessman remains in a chronic vegetative state after subarachnoid hemorrhage and vasospasm, now tracheostomized and ventilator dependent, with recurrent regurgitation from his gastrostomy feedings and subsequent great risk for pneumonia. His hospitalization has cost $400 per day for the last 6 months and there is little hope of chronic placement while he is on the ventilator. Should the gastrostomy be replaced by a jejunostomy requiring another operative procedure? Should his tube feedings be stopped because of the risk of aspiration? Should the pneumonias be treated when they occur or should the patient be allowed to die untreated? Should the ventilator be stopped?

2. An 82-year-old woman with increasing gait difficulty, barely able to walk unassisted, has what appears to be a spinal cord meningioma. She also has congestive heart failure. The medical consultant says there is a 10–15% risk of surgical death. Should the tumor be removed?

3. A 55-year-old woman executive has a glioblastoma multiforme in the nondominant parietal lobe, now recurrent for the third time in 18 months. She has continued doing part-time work, but now returns with increasing left hemiparesis and confusion. She has been on dexamethasone 16 mg per day for the past 3 months. Should the tumor be resected again?

4. A newborn is sent to the neonatal ICU 5 days after birth with hydrocephalus and an unclosed myelomeningocele. He has meningitis and is treated successfully with subsequent myelomeningocele closure and shunting. He begins having apneic spells with a demonstrable Arnold-Chiari malformation. Shunt revision and a posterior Cl–2 decompression are done without significant effect. He develops pneumonia and then candida sepsis. By this time, the newborn has been in the neonatal ICU for 10

weeks at approximately $600 per day and continues to be ventilator dependent. Should his candida sepsis be treated vigorously?

These cases are not unusual; they represent a kind of decision making that is not often talked about in neurosurgery, however. This paper will discuss the medical fact gathering, legal precedents, and ethical issues that are involved in making such decisions.

MEDICAL CONSIDERATIONS IN DECISIONS NOT TO TREAT

The best reason for withholding treatment from a patient is that the treatment does not work. The lack of efficacy of a particular treatment is determined by cumulative neurosurgical practice.

Careful reading of the literature is the first step in a surgical decision not to treat. A model of how "hard" data for making surgical decisions should be developed is provided by the history of extracranial to intracranial vascular anastomosis for treating cerebral ischemia (EC-IC bypass). The first anecdotal reports on EC-IC bypass emphasized the technical aspects of the surgery as well as its theoretical beneficial effects. A typical report implied the blood flow to the brain could be augmented, brain efficiency improved, and strokes averted.

Second in the evaluation of this treatment came retrospective reports. These presented large numbers of cases and detailed surgical results (4, 25). They had several deficiencies intrinsic to retrospective series: the patients were selected by varying and often uncertain criteria; there was no control group to establish efficacy over untreated cases; and the follow-up was often incomplete. Haines has described the difficulties of drawing conclusions from such retrospective studies (13).

The definitive evaluation of this procedure came from a single well-designed prospective study. This had control patients as similar as possible to treated patients except they did not receive the treatment; well-defined criteria for entry into the study and for evaluation of outcome; and statistically adequate numbers and design (8). The length and expense of the study is a telling example of the difficulty of doing a prospective study adequately; however, the data from one such study are many times more reliable than those from retrospective series. In the end, EC-IC bypass does not appear to reduce the risk of ischemic stroke (8).

The first step in deciding whether to treat is knowing the literature. However, not even published data provide all the relevant facts because of what might be called the "virtuoso effect." This is the tendency for only the best results from a particular procedure to be published. This is partly because the literature provides a standard for the practicing neurosurgeon and partly because reviewers tend not to accept what they consider mediocre results. It is a distorting characteristic of published reports, however, and one that amounts to group self-deception. Can the average neurosurgeon in his practice achieve the results of a virtuoso who has spent his surgical lifetime on a particular kind of procedure? It is unlikely. To a reading of the literature must be added a realistic appraisal of how applicable the reports are to the situation at hand.

Sometimes this will lead to a decision that one neurosurgeon should not do the procedure but that it might be possible in another surgeon's hands. This admission is difficult for a neurosurgeon, and yet is required if neurosurgeons are to be honest. This is as much a moral issue as dealing with a difficult decision whether to stop the ventilator; in a wider sense, it involves neurosurgical integrity as a profession.

Both reading the literature and knowing its relevance are therefore important in making a recommendation not to treat; surgeons may be misled into thinking they are making a major difference in the natural history when they are not. The rest of this chapter will discuss legal and ethical issues in the decision not to treat. Its general conclusions will be that once the facts have been gathered, the patient's decision is the important one. Both the law and medical ethics have adopted a principle of patient self-determination that significantly changes traditional approaches to decision making in this area.

LEGAL CONSIDERATIONS IN DECISIONS NOT TO TREAT

Legal decisions about withdrawing treatment emphasize patient self-determination. Generally speaking, a competent patient can legally decide to do what he or she wants to, including refuse life-saving treatment. In an incompetent patient, the law is not consistent. If there is doubt whether to treat, the law requires that appropriate procedures be carried out before implementing a decision not to treat.

Competent Patients

The right of the competent adult to refuse treatment even when it might save his or her life has been repeatedly established in case law. It stems first of all from general right to bodily integrity, the same right that prevents surgery without consent (16). This right was established by Justice Cardozo:

"Every human being of adult years and sound mind has a right to determine what shall be done with his own body; and a surgeon who performs an operation without his patient's consent commits an assault for which he is liable in damages" (29).

This is buttressed by the right to privacy, the same constitutional right used to argue for a woman's ability to terminate her pregnancy in the landmark abortion decision, Roe v. Wade (26). This right has been applied to decisions about refusing treatment. "By parity of reasoning, the constitutional right to privacy, we believe, encompasses the freedom of the terminally ill but competent individual to choose for himself whether or not to decline medical treatment" (9).

This right has been upheld in a number of cases: Lane vs. Candura, in which a 77-year-old woman's refusal to have her gangrenous leg amputated was supported by the appeals court of Massachusetts (14); Satz vs. Permutter, in which a 73-year-old man with amyotrophic lateral sclerosis petitioned a Florida court to have the ventilator removed despite his dependence on it (28); and similar decisions in New Jersey (23), Pennsylvania (15), Wisconsin (12), Illinois (11), and New York (10). If the patient has dependents, the situation is not as certain (16, pp 248–262, 18, 31).

In these decisions, the individual's right to refuse is paramount because the interests of the state are felt not to countermand it. There are four interests the state might have in forcing treatment: *(a)* it would be upholding the standards and values of the medical profession to do so; *(b)* it is preserving life; *(c)* it is preventing suicide; and *(d)* it is protecting dependents. The first three have not been found compelling; the last has had varying force in different circumstances and jurisdictions.

Incompetent Patients

For incompetent patients, several different procedures have been recommended by different jurisdictions in considering treatment withdrawal. Courts have generally used a model in which a surrogate represents the patient's interests. Incompetence is initially assessed as part of the court proceedings. Four factors of descending power are then considered: *(a)* the wishes the patient might have expressed in the past (here a "living will" or designation of surrogate may define the appropriate action); *(b)* the family's wishes; *(c)* the decisions of a hospital surrogate decision-making body; *(d)* the court's decision. As a general principle, the presumption is that life-sustaining therapy should continue. The courts have sensed an uncertainty within the medical profession on these matters and have subsequently increased explicit court involvement.

The legal approach to withdrawing lifesaving treatment for hopeless patients can best be understood by studying a group of landmark cases: Karen Ann Quinlan in New Jersey, Brother Joseph Fox in New York, and Joseph Saikiewicz, Sadie Dinnerstein, and Earl Spring in Massachusetts. They suggest a considerable range of decision-making procedures.

The decision favoring a hospital ethics committee is Re Quinlan in New Jersey (24). Karen Ann Quinlan was 21 years old when, on April 15, 1975, she had two 15-minute periods of apnea for unclear reasons. She remained in a vegetative state, which was ventilator dependent, for many weeks. Her father asked the court that he be appointed his daughter's personal guardian with a view to stopping her ventilator. The trial court initially denied his petition but the New Jersey Supreme court later upheld it. They found that the medical profession did not oppose cessation of artificial ventilation in this situation, that a reasonable person might have wished the ventilator to be disconnected in this situation, and that the state's interest in preserving life did not outweigh Karen's right to privacy. Her father was, therefore, given the legal right to remove her from the hospital and the ventilator. By this time she was able to support her own respirations and continue alive, but in a vegetative state, until the summer of 1985.

It should be emphasized that this decision has strict applicability only in New Jersey; there has not been a U.S. Supreme Court decision in this or other treatment termination case (3). However, the New Jersey court clearly suggested that its procedures for making treatment withdrawal decisions might have wider applicability. In summary, these procedures are: *(a)* if the physician and family agree that treatment withdrawal is appropriate, a second opinion should be sought; treatment can be withdrawn if consultant, physician, and family agree; *(b)* if there is a doubt about the patient's prognosis or accepted medical practice, a hospital ethics committee should be asked for advice; *(c)* if there is disagreement between physician and family or any other complicating feature, the courts may be used as a last adjudicating resort (16, p. 362).

This approach is in contrast to that advocated by the courts of New York and Massachusetts in the decisions Re Eichner, concerning Brother Joseph Fox (9), and Superintendent of Belchertown State School v. Saikewicz (30). Brother Joseph Fox was an 83-year-old man who had a cardiac arrest during a hernia procedure and was resuscitated, but entered into ventilator dependent vegetative coma. His superior, Father Eichner, petitioned for guardianship to remove him from the ventilator. Probably because Brother Fox had previously explicitly expressed his wish not to be placed on life-support systems, the petition was granted and upheld by the Supreme Court of New York. The court, however, rejected the Quinlan procedure, setting forth the following procedures to be followed where withdrawal of care is considered (16, p. 350).

1. The attending physician must certify that the patient is terminally ill and in irreversible, chronic, or permanent vegetative coma, and that prospects of regaining cognitive brain function are "extremely remote."

2. This diagnosis and prognosis is then presented to a hospital committee composed of at least three physicians for the purpose of confirming or rejecting the prognosis.

3. If the attending physician's prognosis is confirmed by a majority of the committee, judicial proceedings commence for the appointment of a "committee of the incompetent" (guardian) and for permission to have the life-sustaining treatment discontinued.

4. The District Attorney and Attorney-General are to be given notice and there should be an opportunity to have the patient independently examined before the hearing.

5. A guardian ad litem is appointed to protect the interests of the patient.

If, upon following this procedure, the court concludes that the petitioner has met the burden of proof with clear and convincing evidence, then "extraordinary life-sustaining measures" may be discontinued and no liability shall ensue.

The Court in Eichner concludes by saying that while the approved procedure may "at first blush" appear cumbersome and time-consuming, it is confident that it can be expeditiously complied with through the cooperation of all concerned.

The Massachusetts Experience

Joseph Saikewicz was a 67-year-old institutionalized retarded man with acute myeloblastic monocytic leukemia (30). A petition was made to forego chemotherapy and the Massachusetts state supreme judicial court concurred. In its decision, however, it specified that the courts must be consulted in any case in which usual treatment was not to be administered. The following procedure was to be required (16, p. 362).

1. Petition for appointment of a guardian is to be filed with the court; the time before a hearing will depend on the situation.

2. An appointed guardian ad litem is to present "all reasonable arguments in favor of administering treatment to prolong the life" of the patient.

3. A hearing will determine competency and the appropriate guardian.

4. "Applying the rules of 'substituted judgment' if the court finds that the patient would forego further treatment, the court shall enter such an order . . ."

The court, therefore, requires substantial proceedings before deciding not to administer full treatment to every patient. It confirms this intent in no uncertain terms:

"We take a dim view of any attempt to shift the ultimate decision-making responsibility away from the duly established court of proper jurisdiction to any committee, panel or group, ad hoc or permanent. Thus, we reject the approach adopted by the New Jersey Supreme Court in the Quinlan case of entrusting the decision whether to continue artificial life support to the patient's guardian, family, attending doctor, and hospital 'ethics committee' . . ." (30).

It should be recognized that this decision does not limit the requirement of a court proceeding to vegetative or dying patients, but applies it to any incompetent patient. Its harsh findings were perhaps softened by two subsequent decisions in Massachusetts, Matter of Dinnerstein and Matter of Spring. In Matter of Dinnerstein, the issue was whether a "no code" order could be written with family and physician approval but without prior court approval on a 67-year-old woman in a vegetative state from Alzheimer's disease (7). The appeals court concluded that the Saikewicz requirements could only hold for treatment having some expectation of cure or remission:

"Prolongation of life, as used in the Saikewicz case, does not mean a mere suspension of the act of dying but . . . a remission of symptoms enabling a return towards a normal, functioning, integrated existence" (7).

Thus, orders not to resuscitate at least could be written without prior court approval if the patient was terminally ill.

Earl Spring was a 78-year-old man with chronic renal failure who was mentally incapacitated and whose family petitioned the court for permission to stop his hemodialysis (27). In its decision, the Massachusetts appeals court affirmed the place of the physician and family in making these decisions . . . "the vast majority of treatment decisions relative to persons who are incompetent by reason of senility or retardation are made for them, by their family and the doctor, without court proceedings. This practice is sanctioned not merely by tradition but by the institutional limitations in the ability of courts to make day-to-day treatment decisions, even if restricted to treatments of a potentially life-saving or life-prolonging nature."

This reasoning was, however, overturned by the Supreme Court. In that overturning, they wrote the following:

"Neither the present case nor the Saikewicz case involved the legality of action taken without judicial authority, and our opinions should not be taken to establish any requirement of prior judicial approval that would not otherwise exist. The cases and other materials we have cited suggest a variety of circumstances to be taken into account in deciding whether there should be an application for a prior court order with respect to medical treatment of an incompetent patient. Among them are at least the following: the extent of impairment of the patient's mental faculties, whether the patient is in the custody of a state institution, the prognosis without the proposed treatment, the prognosis with the proposed treatment, the complexity, risk, and novelty of the proposed treatment, its possible side-effects, the patient's level of understanding and probable reaction, the urgency of decision, the consent of the patient, spouse, or guardian, the good faith of those who participate in the decision, the clarity of professional opinion as to what is good medical practice, the interest of third persons, and the administrative requirement of any institution involved . . ." (27).

These rather vague guidelines are presently what tell Massachusetts physicians whether a court order is necessary to stop treatment. These three different decisions in different jurisdictions demonstrate the variety of approaches the courts have used trying to deal with nontreatment decisions in medicine.

The problem of withdrawing care in vegetative patients has recently been complicated by the question of what constitutes minimal care. Tube feedings and intravenous fluids, not previously considered within the range of treatments that could be stopped, have been the subject of two decisions as well as of medical commentary (17, 19). In the Conroy decision in New Jersey, it was judged acceptable not to provide tube feedings for a patient who had expressed a wish not to remain in a vegetative state (5); in the Barber decision in California, a similar conclusion was reached on appeal, although initially, the physicians involved had been successfully prosecuted for murder (1).

The present relevance of these decisions is unclear for states other than those of the specific decision. However, as a group they indicate the way in which the courts have seen decisions about nontreatment as their concern. In part, court involvement is a means of guaranteeing individual liberty, but it may also reflect an attempt to assert legal power where there is medical uncertainty. It appears that the following guidelines should be satisfied in proposing nontreatment for an incompetent patient today:

1. It must be very likely that the patient's condition is irreversible by the proposed treatment or any other.

2. It is best if the patient is terminally ill. Patients in an apparently permanent vegetative state may constitute a second group of patients in whom nontreatment is permissible, but this is not well-established.

3. The family should agree with withdrawing whatever treatment is proposed.

4. The physician should be certain his view of the situation represents good medical practice. This is best achieved by obtaining a second opinion (*e.g.*, neurologic consultation) or, if there is doubt, opinion from an ethics committee within the hospital.

5. The facts of irreversibility and terminal condition along with discussions with family should be recorded in the chart.

6. The principle of substituted judgment should be used in determining the appropriate course of action whenever possible.

For children, the parents will usually be the spokespersons and may refuse treatment for the child in some cases. It is only where the parental treatment proposed is unreasonable that it may be overridden; this requires a court-appointed guardian.

The situation for newborns with severe congenital malformations has changed quite remarkably in the last 3 years and emphasizes the impact of factors outside of medicine or surgery in this field. "Baby Doe" regulations from the Department of Health and Human Services have mandated vigorous treatment for all children regardless of the severity of their congenital defect (26). This has been accomplished through regulation as a Medicaid provider that prevents discrimination, here discrimination against a child born with a handicap. As a result of these regulations every hospital had to have the following sign prominently displayed in the neonatal ICU, including its waiting rooms:

"Any person having knowledge that a handicapped infant is being discriminatorily denied food or customary medical care should immediately contact: Handicapped Infant Hotline . . ." (6).

At present the final status of Baby Doe regulations is uncertain, but it seems clear that nontreatment of severely defective newborns can only be undertaken with substantial risk in today's political-legal climate.

ETHICAL ISSUES IN DECISIONS NOT TO TREAT

The previous sections have presented the medical and legal considerations of decisions not to treat; they emphasize the problems of interpreting the medical literature to obtain an accurate prognosis and the contradictions that characterize legal decisions in this area. This section will discuss briefly some ethical issues that bear on these decisions, especially who should make them and what factors should be considered in making them.

Medical ethics can be seen as a balancing of four principles: self-determination, beneficence, knowledge, and justice (2). A generation ago, the major principles were beneficence, the principle that places the patient's interest before the physician's; and knowledge, the advancement of medical understanding. In the last two decades, the other two principles have become central: self-determination, which allows the patient primary decision making in his or her care; and justice, which attempts to equalize medical care to all. In this section, the conflict between the principles of beneficence and self-determination especially will be felt.

Like the law, medical ethics has focused primarily on the right of an individual patient to make a decision about treatment; in general, however, the emphasis has been on this process with medical and family help rather than with court decision making. The clearest and most influential statement has been from the President's Commission for the study of Ethical Problems in Biomedical and Behavioral Research, an 11-member panel which included the neurosurgeon, Dr. H. Thomas Ballantine. The two volumes published by the Commission on the issues involved here are the source of the following commentary (21, 22).

Who Should Decide?

Potential decision makers in withdrawing treatment include the physician, the patient, someone speaking for the patient, and the courts. The individual physician's role in this matter appears to be increasingly limited. It is his job to assess irreversibility of the illness, and prognosis with and without treatment; he should also be able to describe the risks of the treatment. He is no longer the authority who alone and unilaterally decides his patient's fate, however. ("He" used here means either "he" or "she.") There are several reasons for this: increasingly educated patients and their families demand to know more and have more to say about such decisions; the options of second opinions and changing physicians are usually available to them; neurosurgery is practiced in such an open fashion now that allied health professionals such as nurses often add their opinions. These features can be as important after the fact as during the treatment itself; a situation particularly unpleasant, for example, is one in which a family decides several months after treatment was stopped that their parent or child was not hopelessly ill and might have been saved. From the present ethical point of view the physician becomes a diagnostician, prognosticator, and advisor; his function is to explain, perhaps to persuade, but not to command.

If the patient is competent at the time of this decision making, the final choice is, therefore, his. This is not only unequivocally supported by legal decisions but also can be buttressed by an ethical belief in self-determination, the right of a patient to do what he wishes to do with his body. It is here that the tension between beneficence and self-determination is felt most strongly in neurosurgery. The paradigm of a fully informed patient, uncoerced and rational, selecting for himself what treatment best suits him, may be an impossible ideal. Its relevance for present practice is that patients and commentators on medical ethics are increasingly demanding a voice in medical care.

For the incompetent or incapacitated patient, the situation is parallel. Incompetence is suggested by the President's Commission to be characterized by three components (21, p. 121).

1. Incapacity to consider relevant alternatives with a stable set of personal values and life goals.

2. Inability to understand and communicate with health care givers about the decision.

3. Inability to reason and deliberate about one's choices.

The President's Commission applies the same paradigm as for competent patients but proposes that a surrogate speak for the patient. Usually the family member who would be asked to give autopsy permission will be surrogate. If the family is unsuitable or there is no family, the President's

Commission suggests that the hospital have some mechanism of appointing a surrogate decision maker and reviewing the decision making process (*e.g.*, a patient care representative or "ethics committee").

These recommendations about who should decide for an incompetent patient emphasize the importance of patient self-determination in the current development of ethical thinking. A neurosurgeon might ask where the insistence on patient self-determination as an ideal comes from. Is it the best principle for the patient? A popular reaction to overbearing medical paternalism? A result of application of moral principles to the medical field by well-meaning ethicists? An extension of the principles of the legal profession into this area? Whatever the source, it appears that this ideal will not change soon.

How Should Decisions Be Made?

There is a clear statement about the principles of decision making as well as about who should decide in the President's Committee report. Extending the concept of self-determination, the appropriate goal for the surrogate decision maker is to try to make the decision the patient would have made himself. This is called "substituted judgment"; it is not the same as deciding what is "best" for the patient. The latter would be a "best interests" decision; one that involves a societal concept of what is best but will not necessarily be the same as the patient's concept of what is best for him. The patient's choice may be expressed in some such document as a living will, which explicitly states his wishes, through the designation of a surrogate by the patient before his death, or by statements by family or friends about what the patient would have wished. Thus, even in decision making for incompetent patients, the principle of self-determination is crucial.

CONCLUSIONS

This paper has summarized some aspects of medical, legal, and ethical issues in deciding not to treat a patient with every means available. The major conclusion is that patient self-determination has primary importance in contemporary legal and ethical thinking. That this ideal is in the best interests of the patient appears to be assumed. In *The Second Career:* Wilder Penfield wrote: "The negative decisions that ease and shorten suffering have always been ours to make" (20). In the practice of neurosurgery, his concept may now be changing substantially.

REFERENCES

1. Barber v. Superior Court, 195 Cal Rpt 484 (1983).
2. Black, P. McL. Medical ethics in neurology and neurosurgery. Neurol. Clin., *3(2):* 215–227, 1985.

3. Cantor, M. Quinlan, Privacy, and the Handling of Incompetent Dying Patients. Rutgers L. Rev., *30:* (2) 243, 1977.
4. Chater, N., and Popp, J. Microsurgical vascular bypass for occlusive cerebrovascular disease; review of 100 cases. Surg. Neurol., *6:* 115–118, 1976.
5. In re Conroy (1983) 188 NJ Super 523, 457n A2d 1232.
6. Department of Health and Human Services. Nondiscrimination on the Basis of Handicap. Notice of Interim Final Rule, Office of the Secretary, Department of Health and Human Services, 48 Federal Register 9632, March 7, 1983.
7. Matter of Dinnerstein (1978, Mass App) 380 NE2d 134.
8. The EC/IC bypass study group. Failure of extra cranial-intracranial bypass to reduce the risk of ischemic stroke. Results of an International randomized trial. N. Engl. J. Med. *313:* 1191–1200, 1985.
9. Re Eichner (1980, 2nd Dept.) 73 App Div 2d 431, 426 NYS 2d 517.
10. Erickson v. Dilgard (1962) 44 Misc 2d 27, 252 NY S2d 705.
11. Re Estate of Brooks (1965) 32 111 2d 361, 205 NE2d 435.
12. Guardianship of Gertrude Raasch (1972) Co Ct for Milwaukee County, Probate Div., No. 455–996.
13. Haines, S. J. Randomized Clinical Trials in Neurosurgery. Neurosurgery, *12:* 259–264, 1983.
14. Lane v. Candura (1978, Mass App)m 1978 Adv Sheets 588, 376 NE2nd 1232, 93 ALR 3d 59.
15. Re Maida Yetter (1973) 62 Pa Dend C2d 619.
16. Meyers, D. W. Medico-legal Implications of Death and Dying. San Francisco, Bancroft-Whitney, 1981.
17. Micetich, K. C., Steinecka, P. H., Thomasma, D. C. Are intravenous fluids morally required for a dying patient? Arch. Int. Med., *143:* 975–978, 1983.
18. Re Osborne (1972, Dist Col App) 294 A2d 372.
19. Parris, T. J., Reardon, F. E. Court Responses to Withholding or Withdrawing Artificial Nutrition and Fluids. J.A.M.A., *253:* 2243–2245, 1985.
20. Penfield, W. *The Second Career*, with other essays and addresses. Boston, Little Brown, 1963.
21. President's Commission for the Study of Ethical Problems in Medicine and Biomedical and Behavioral Research; Deciding to Forego Life-Sustaining Treatment, U.S. Government Printing Office, 1982.
22. President's Commission for the Study of Ethical Problems in Medicine and Biomedical and Behavioral Research: Making Health Care Decisions. U.S. Government Printing Office, 1982.
23. Re Quackenbush (1978) 156 NJ Super 282, 383 A2d 785.
24. Re Quinlan (1976) 70n NJ10, 355 A2d 647, 79 ALR 3d 205, certden 429 US 922, 50 LEtd. 2d 289, 97 SCY 319.
25. Reichmann, O. H., Davis D. D., Roberts, T. S., et al. Anastomoses between STA and cortical branch of MCA for treatment of occlusive cerebrovascular disease. *Reconstructive Surgery of Brain Arteries*, edited by F. T. Marli, A. Kademel, Kiddo, Budapest, 1974.
26. Roe, v. Wade (1973) 410 US 113, 35 Lea2d 147, 93 SCT 705, cert den 410 US 959, 35 LED 2d 694, 93 SCt 1409.
27. Matter of Spring (1979, Mass App) 399 NE2d 493.
28. Satz v. Perlmutter (1978, Fla App D4), 362 So 3d 160, approved (Fla) 369 So 2d 359.
29. Schloendorf v. Society of New York Hospital (1914) 211 NY 125, 105 NE92.
30. Superintendent of Belchertown State School v. Saikewicz (1977) 373 Mass 728, 370 NE2d 417.
31. United States v. George (1965, DeConn) 239 F Supp 752.

CHAPTER

7

The Patient's Role in Medical Decision Making

BRIAN CLARK

It is difficult to decide at this moment which emotion is uppermost in my consciousness—pleasure resulting from the honor of being asked to contribute to such a distinguished congress, or fear resulting from the awareness of the difficulty of the subject. It seemed an easy enough topic—"The patient's role in making clinical decisions"—especially since Professor Shucart had given me such a clear brief: "The problem most of us have as surgeons is making certain that we are giving full consideration to the patient's needs and desires and actually taking into account quality as it affects any particular case. I think this applies not only to serious cases such as quadriplegia but probably also to much lesser disabilities which we as surgeons tend to disregard much of the time." I leapt at the chance of a trip to Hawaii thinking I had already thought out all of the implications of the topic and it should not take too long to assemble a paper to discharge my obligation. But over the months of thinking about it, I found that the topic kept dissolving in my mind as I had to reject one generalization after another. So to begin, let me share with you some of the difficulties I have encountered on the way to my final, if inconclusive, conclusions.

The first difficulty is, of course, that all medical decision making is culturally conditioned, if not determined. Consider an extreme example. A primitive tribesman goes to his local witch doctor, who proceeds to diagnose by disemboweling a chicken and to treat the patient by painting stripes of different colors on the patient's head. The only sensible contribution the patient can make is to give the doctor his blind faith that he knows enough magic to effect a cure. As a matter of fact, anthropological studies have shown that this faith is not always misplaced. Come to think of it, is that so remote an example from some accepted modern Western medical practices? There is surely not one physician who has not effected at least one "cure" by placebos. And certainly some allopathic doctors would consider that homeopathic doctors do it all the time.

So, we have to accept that a real—if scientifically unmeasurable—element in the patient's role is the faith he or she invests in his doctor's knowledge and skill. I do believe that this is an important element in the total therapeutic package. We may call this the art of medicine. It is an art because it is something that has to be engendered by the doctor. The seeds that will fertilize this faith are not only demonstrations of scientific knowledge and rigor, nor the subjection of the patient to batteries of tests, often by mysterious and complex machines, but also the perception by the patient of a sensitive and sympathetic awareness by the doctor of the patient's fears and hopes. To put it at its simplest the patient needs to believe that the doctor feels that the patient's views and feelings are important. And although strictly speaking this is outside my brief, perhaps you will permit me to say that this skill in interpersonal relationships is the least considered in the doctor's training. I would go further and say that if you had to devise a program that would most damage any inherent skills a student had in this direction, it would be hard to come up with a more destructive program than that of a typical medical school. As a result of some research I did for a film in some leading medical schools, I came to the conclusion that this consists of taking the best and brightest of a generation and, for the first 2 preclinical years, absurdly overloading the student with mental tasks, many of which have all the intellectual satisfaction of learning a telephone directory by rote. This may, as one psychologist claimed to me, amount to sensory deprivation. It certainly amounts to social deprivation, making relaxed relationships outside the medical school, at the very least, difficult. This overloading continues into the clinical period, though with more interesting material in a highly competitive environment. It speaks volumes for the resilience of the human psyche that doctors emerge able to communicate at all with nonmedical people, let alone achieve the rapport that many do achieve. I am sure that more doctors would be able to exercise the art of medicine with security and finesse if their immediate postadolescent years were not so stressed.

I am grateful for this opportunity to give my hobby horse a little canter. But it is important when considering the patient's role because the emotional and intellectual climate, the atmosphere in which the patient exercises his role in medical decision making, is created primarily by the doctor. Unless that atmosphere contains enough of the oxygen of sensitive awareness, the patient may be reduced to gasping; if after you have talked to the patient he or she still feels blue, the emotional cyanosis may be your fault.

Of course the atmosphere is not created entirely by the doctor, and this brings me to another culturally conditioned difference in medical decision making. America and Britain are different countries. The Declaration of Independence may have led to America's release from the tyranny of the British Crown but it does seem to have allowed other tyrannies to take its place. The Declaration claims for every citizen the absolute rights to life, liberty, and the pursuit of doctors through every court in the land. It is hard to see how the massive intervention of law into American medical practice can, in the large majority of cases, help the delicate decision-making process. The patient's role is exercised in relationship, and any relationship cannot be helped if one of the partners is constantly on his guard in case his words will later be repeated verbatim in a hostile environment. I cannot imagine that my marriage would be helped, for example, if when my wife asked, "What shall we do this evening," I had to phrase my answer bearing in mind how it could sound in a divorce court. There would be a certain loss of spontaneity to say the least. I am aware that with the ever-present specter of a malpractice suit, a doctor feels constrained to say too much to some patients and too little to others, for the optimum atmosphere for good decision making. However, except to note that this is a determinant in the American decision-making process, there is very little I can say or you can do about it. I can only suggest that if it becomes too bad, you could apply to rejoin the British Empire!

But let me come to what I think is the most interesting culturally determined difference—any particular culture's attitude about mortality and, of course, the differences between subgroups of the culture. The manifestations of the difference can be dramatically obvious. In India, for example, when a person dies, his body is carried on an open bier through the streets to a public ground where it is cremated openly on a wood fire. Any Indian child will have seen many dead bodies. In England, I know many adults who have never seen a human corpse and American funerary practice has been savagely dealt with by Nancy Mitford in "The American Way of Death" and brilliantly satirized by Evelyn Waugh in "The Loved One." It could be argued that it is a signal mark of failure in our culture that many—probably a majority of the members of it—never come to terms with their own mortality. We can claim a right to life but not to corporeal immortality and, if we live as though we can, we blight not only our deaths, but our lives as well. And it certainly interferes with proper medical decision making.

Surprisingly, this applies to some doctors as well as to patients. I remember talking to Dame Cicily Saunders, a wonderful woman and doctor, and the founder of our hospice movement. (Incidentally, her hospice, St. Christopher's, is the happiest hospital I have ever visited.) She told me she did not find it easy to find doctors who were relaxed with dying patients. "Doctors typically say," she said, "'I lost a patient,' as though the poor chap had fallen out of the back of the car on the way to the hospital. We never lose patients here; they die."

A very good indication of the way a culture copes with mortality is how hospitals cope with death. I once had a very interesting experience. My first job in the 1950s was as a teacher in a very poor East End district,

Stepney. It had been the first area to be settled by Jewish immigrants in the 19th century, and there were still many Jews living there. There was also a Jewish hospital. Its building was terrible, in the worst 19th-century daunting, intimidating, institutional style. But it was a real community hospital. I was taken ill at school with a lower back pain. So there I was, lying on boards, the only Gentile in the ward. Some days after I arrived, an old man died in a bed opposite mine. He was screened, washed, and put into a large black coffin. We were not screened when it was time to move him out. He was wheeled out and around the ward accompanied by two nurses carrying candles and preceded by a rabbi reading from the Bible. All the patients, who were mostly old, put on their shawls and prayed. After the old man was gone, everyone joined in an animated discussion about the deceased—how he had always misbehaved in schule, how his sister was no better than she ought to be, how his uncle was the first kosher butcher in Cable Street, and so on. The patients discussed a whole wonderful celebration of the man's life. There were many tears and much laughter. It was one of the most beautiful experiences I have ever had.

My back was slow to heal and after a few weeks I was moved nearer my home, to St. Margarets in Epping. This move made it easier for my visitors. When a patient died there, it was a different story. We were all screened and the body was whisked away like some unclean thing. When the screens were drawn back there was just the stripped bed, and the nurses who were extra cheerful with their polished professional smiles. In spite of all the Christian consolation that presumably the deceased was getting from St. Margaret—after all, he had just nipped up from her hospital—we all joined in the conspiracy that he had never existed. We devalued his death and his life and, by extension, our own lives. One other incident concerning the death in the Jewish hospital occurs to me. In the bed next to me was a very old rabbi, an immigrant from Poland. In the evening of that particular day, I said to him how well the hospital had handled the death. "Ah bubbala," he said, "They handle death so vell here, because they get so much practice at it." There was a man who would die as well as he had lived.

But you do not practice in the old Stepney Jewish Hospital that is no more, and we do not live in a culture that can see human life as a wonderful cycle and a natural human death as glorious and fitting as the death of the leaves in a New England autumn. We live in a culture where even to age is considered mildly antisocial behavior. We are allowed to get to 30 and then with the aid of gadgets, fitments, prostheses, disguises, dyes, even the surgeons knife, we have to hold the line there until, for some reason not overly gone into, we cease to appear in our usual haunts.

This widespread inability to come to terms with the natural progression of human life is at the root of the difficulties in decision making in many human activities and not least in the area of medical practice. If you, as a doctor, know that your patient cannot face the fact of his own death, it would be cruel in many circumstances to thrust it at him at a moment when he is the least prepared to cope with it. And so you fall back on euphemism, evasion, even perhaps at times, downright lying in an attempt to exercise the sensitivity that I indicated at the beginning was a prerequisite for exercising the art of medicine.

The final difficulty that I want to deal with is when, in the decision-making process, the decision is made in relationship between two parties. But there is not equality between the two. In a typical case, the power of making the final decision rests with one party, while the knowledge upon which a good decision is made resides in the other. The doctor may know, or believe he knows, what is best, but whether or not that knowledge is fully used—assuming it is properly communicated—is up to the patient.

We are coming to the nub of this question, so let me first get out of the way that little caveat I made—"assuming the knowledge is properly communicated." It will be obvious that the patient cannot exercise his role unless he is in possession of all of the relevant information. It is just one more example of how the doctor controls the decision-making process. Again we see how the doctor has to possess not only the sensitive awareness to perceive what his patient needs and can accept, but also the communication skills to be able to give this information. I wonder if enough work is done on this aspect of the doctor's skills. I do think we have seen an enormous improvement in this area in my lifetime. I seem to remember when I was young most doctors considered that a man had to be an M.B. Ch. B even to be able to pronounce "endocrinological," let alone know what it means. I also seem to remember an extreme reluctance to tell the patient what was wrong with him, as if the disease and its treatment were none of the patient's business. There has been an enormous change in this practice—possibly a beneficial side effect of the need to obtain informed consent, but also because there has been a marked rise in the level of understanding about our bodies and its workings in the population at large, and doctors have responded to this. Sometimes, of course, the difficulty is absolute. I remember going to see a wonderful old Scottish country doctor, Dr. Smith, who practiced in the Lake District in England. I showed him an ill-defined rash on my arm. He looked at it carefully, then took a hand glass and studied it closely. At length he put down the glass and looked at me, "It's a C.K. rash," he said. "What's that?" I asked him. "Christ Knows!" he said. Dr. Smith's communications skills were excellent, and I trusted him completely. When he did not know what was wrong he said so, colorfully—not to say blasphemously. So when he said he did know I believed him. Perhaps this statement indicates a new attitude that has gained ascendency in my lifetime—scepticism, healthy or unhealthy, according to one's view. Certainly I recall my parents' attitude to doctors as far more trusting, faith-based, than would be typical now. Again, I think we can look to a far higher awareness and knowledge in the population at large of the benefits and limitations of science.

We have now reached the core of the problem, only to discover it has largely disappeared. I told you at the beginning that the problem kept receding the longer I pondered it. It is now almost out of sight. I think there can be no doubt about who should make the final decision. I meant the question "Whose Life Is It Anyway?" to be purely rhetorical. It is the patient's life, and he must remain ultimately responsible for it; this is so for minor as well as major decisions. That was, really, the whole point of the play. Perhaps if I briefly sketch in the origin of the play, the point will be made. I was thinking about euthanasia. Why, I do not know. Perhaps I had read something in a newspaper, and I quickly came to the decision that I did not approve of it, certainly not if it involved committees of doctors and lawyers or any intervention of law at all, except insofar as it has already intervened in prescriptions against murder and so on. I thought if anyone really wanted to die, he could kill himself—it really is not all that difficult. I then thought—oh blessed moment—what if the person were a tetraplegic? I knew then I had a play because I had a situation where a man had to talk himself to death. But Ken Harrison, the patient in the play, did not ask for a doctor to kill him. He asked only to be discharged from the hospital. He wished to remain in as full control as he could; he knew his death was his responsibility and that it would be immoral to seek to give away that responsibility or for anyone else to accept it if offered. He did not ask anyone actively to kill him, merely to let nature take its course. The play is not a plea for mercy killing by doctors, but rather it seeks to make suicide a little more respectable in certain circumstances.

The patient's role, then, is, in optimum circumstances, that of the final decision maker, but it can only be exercised within the parameters set by the mores of the society in which the patient lives, the extent of his knowledge about himself and his body, the extent of the specific knowledge about his problem communicated by the doctor and, of course, within the limits of possibility itself. From this daunting list it will be seen that in any one specific case there is only one immediate variable and that is the role of the doctor. The decision is in fact—and I make no apology for repeating this—made in relationship.

So what of this relationship? How different should it be from any other important life relationship. Actually, I believe, less than is commonly supposed. We have to be aware, I think, of the tyranny of labels. If we label a doctor-patient relationship as *professional*, what limits does that set? Some obvious ones we may think. A doctor does not take advantage of his more powerful emotional position and the attraction that resides in some-one perceived to be powerful to seduce his patient. But that applies to any relationship in life. Obviously I am talking here morally not legally. A doctor must seek to act in such a way as to promote the physical and emotional well-being of his patient. Again, I would have thought that should apply to any relationship between two people, teacher-parent, brother-sister, parent-child, husband-wife. But here is a difficult question. Should a doctor remain sufficiently distant from his patient so that his personal decision making can be "objective," whatever that means? One hears it all the time. A doctor or nurse cannot become involved with each patient. It would be too painful. There is too much pain and suffering. The emotional burden would be too great. I do understand what is meant by this. I also know that it is sometimes used as an excuse. The point is that a doctor cannot be expected to bleed for every patient. It is his job to alleviate all of the pain and suffering he can, even at the end and with modern techniques of pain control, that is a great deal. However, he is not required to tear himself apart because he does not have the elixir of eternal youth to give to his patient. But then does anybody? I put this question to Dame Cicily. She dismissed it. This sometimes happens, she said, when the doctor has not come to terms with his own death so each terminal situation is perceived as a personal threat. The fact is there is a lot of pain and suffering all over the world and anybody, doctor or not, has to deal with it mentally, one way or another. It is hard to think that anyone's mental health is well served by refusing to face this—refusing to accept that it is part of human inheritance. To remain aloof from someone actu-ally experiencing at this moment what we all will experience is disabling, to the aloof individual and to the relationship in which he is the key member. But again, surely this applies to all relationships.

As I am here as the writer of *Whose Life Is It Anyway?*, perhaps you will forgive the vanity of quoting from the play because it sums up what many patients feel about professionalism. Ken is talking to a social worker who has shown herself very adept at sidestepping all of the patient's awkward statements and questions (Fig. 7.1). Our professional code, then, largely embodies the optimum behavior for any relationship. And the patient's role in the process is the same. He, too, must not make morally illegitimate demands, seek to throw responsibility on the doctor when this responsibil-ity actually is his alone. And it goes without saying, of course, that he should be truthful and open.

I am aware that all this is about as helpful as saying we should be against sin. The problem is that, bearing in mind many of the difficulties I have

KEN: All you people have the same technique. When I say something really awkward you just pretend I haven't said anything at all. You're all the bloody same . . . Well there's another outburst. That should be your cue to comment on the light-shade or the colour of the walls.

MRS BOYLE: I'm sorry if I have upset you.

KEN: Of course you have upset me. You and the doctors with your appalling so-called professionalism, which is nothing more than a series of verbal tricks to prevent you relating to your patients as human beings.

MRS BOYLE: You must understand; we have to remain relatively detached in order to help . . .

KEN: That's alright with me. Detach yourself. Tear yourself off on the dotted line that divides the woman from the social worker and post yourself off to another patient.

MRS BOYLE: You're very upset . . .

KEN: Christ Almighty, you're doing it again. Listen to yourself woman. I say something offensive about you and you turn your professional cheek. If you were human, if you were treating me as human, you'd tell me to bugger off. Can't you see that this is why I've decided that life isn't worth living? I am not human and I'm even more convinced of that by your visit than I was before, so how does that grab you? The very exercise of your so-called professionalism makes me want to die.

FIG. 7.1. Excerpt from *Whose Life Is It Anyway?*.

outlined, we are constantly, doctors and patients, working in a social and cultural climate that is often inimical to relaxed creative decision making. In any one concrete case, we can try to be as open, sensitive, and responsible as we can, but I am not here talking to an individual doctor but to a whole important section of the profession, a group that can and should have ambitions to alter the social and cultural climate in which we all live and make our decisions. It comes down, as always, to a matter of education. It is imperative that important bodies such as yours and the wider professional groupings of which you are a part, as the repository of so much experience, should claim a leading role in society to bring about those social and cultural values that will enhance all life as a by-product of seeking specifically to improve the climate in which doctors and patients have to make their decisions. A professional association is more than a trade union, seeking to raise the living standards of its members. But having been not entirely unsuccessful in this regard, may I suggest that you could, with even greater confidence, take on an even more active, more forceful role in the job of public education about medical decision making. This session is a good start. I am impressed that you have devoted such a large part of your congress to the topic and have invited a layman like me to express the patient's point of view, even if all I have been able to say is that it is up to you.

Of course, this is a congress of doctors; the debate needs to be much wider. It has to embrace the population at large. And as I have indicated, to do any good it will have to take on some pretty thorny subjects, like the question of mortality itself. I am not suggesting, of course, that you can achieve the change all by yourself, but you should not underestimate the authority you have, indeed that you have won. Changes in national consciousness can be made. I have been amazed at the effect of my play. I have been informed of conferences, using it as a starting point, taking place throughout Europe and Japan. It is used as a text in several schools of nursing and, I believe, of medicine. I participated in a very high-powered conference on teaching euthanasia organized by the ethical group of all the London hospitals. Sometimes it is enough to raise the question to release a spate of public participation. Not being a part of your country, I do not know exactly how you work in the field of public education, but I am confident that in such a participatory democracy as the United States, you could find ways to stimulate the debate about ways of raising the standards of medical decision making in which the patient would more and more be able to exercise his role with confidence.

It comes down to this. You have the onerous task, and great privilege, to be with us and share in some of the most important decisions we ever make. Such a great task needs preparation. It is too late—and I am aware that many of you are doctors of the last resort—to begin to think of many related questions when a major one is pressing, urgent. Time spent beforehand, when the mind is not clogged with pain or fear, will be time most valuably spent. The reward will be the great satisfaction of sharing in creative decision making in profound human relationship.

8

Neurosurgery as a Research Discipline

MURRAY GOLDSTEIN, D.O., M.P.H.

From its earliest developments in North America and abroad, neurosurgery has been identified as a "special" discipline—one on the forefront of the surgical sciences. Its early and contemporary leaders were not only persons of outstanding clinical skills but also were recognized as being among the world's leaders in scientific endeavors. Their contributions included the development of new clinical knowledge important both to the diagnosis and therapy of nervous system disease and basic knowledge explaining brain structure and function. Their names are part of the history of North American medicine.

In recent times, the neurosurgical community appropriately is expending a great deal of effort to take stock of its present status and its future potential. There are clearly important clinical issues to consider, including the scope of clinical practice, the number and distribution of neurosurgical clinicians, and the impact of changes in the organization of the health care system. These are all important to neurosurgery. I do not need to tell you how important.

However, there is another aspect of neurosurgery that is receiving focused attention and that is the future role and participation of the neurosurgeon in medical research. The reports I hear are ones of anxiety and frustration. They are often based upon three commonly held beliefs:

1. The number of research grants awarded to clinical investigators by the National Institute of Neurological and Communicative Disorders and Stroke (NINCDS) has declined significantly in the past decade;
2. At the present time, even if young clinicians receive adequate research training, they would not be able to compete at the NINCDS for research grant support against the recently trained basic neuroscientist; and
3. Unlike medical therapy, surgical results cannot be evaluated properly in randomized controlled clinical trials.

In order to evaluate these beliefs, let us examine the facts (Table 8.1).

Table 8.1 is a display of the success of the physician as compared to the Ph.D. in receiving research grant support from the NINCDS during the period 1970–1984. You will notice the spectacular increase in the number of research grant applications received from our Ph.D. colleagues during this period; you will also notice that the number of applications received from physicians has remained about the same. You can see quite clearly that the approval and funding rate for the M.D. applicant and Ph.D. applicant are quite similar for each year. Despite a substantial increase in the availability of research grant funds during this period, an increase from $46.9 million in 1970 to $209.1 million in 1984, the number of neuroscience applications has increased at a proportionately higher rate.

As a result, the number of research grants awarded to the physician has declined dramatically as a function of the number of applications from physicians and the declining proportion of all applications being supported. Approval rates and funding rates for both groups of scientists are nearly the same; the only significant difference is the size of the application pools. From these data, I must conclude that physician scientists are not receiving NINCDS research grant support because they are not applying for NINCDS research grant support. This is true whether they are medical neurologists or neurological surgeons.

Thus, the first generally accepted belief is true: physicians are not receiving as many NINCDS research grants as they did in the past. However, the reason is not because they do not compete successfully; the problem is that they do not apply. Despite a substantial increase in the number of neurological surgeons and a substantial increase in available research grant funds, there has been no increase in the number of applicants from the neurosurgical community.

Why? The acceptable methodologies of biomedical research have advanced so rapidly that it now takes extensive training before a physician can be an independent investigator. This is true whether the physician addresses a basic problem in the laboratory or a clinical problem in an experimental surgery. Is it worth the cost of training to the young physician—the time, the expense, the loss of income, and the uncertainties?

I am often told that physicians feel that it is a waste of time to receive in-depth research training since basic scientists are given preference in the National Institutes of Health (NIH) review process. To put it another way, young clinicians say, "Why bother? Despite our training we would not receive sympathetic review at the NIH."

Figure 8.1 examines the first aspect of this concern: how successful are young investigators who compete with their more senior colleagues for NINCDS research grant support?

TABLE 8.1
NINCDS Regular Research (R01, R23) Grants: FY 1970–1984

Fiscal Year	#	Applied		Approved Rate		Funding Rate (Approvals)		Funding Rate (Applications)	
		%M.D.	%Ph.D.	For M.D.	For Ph.D.	For M.D.	For Ph.D.	For M.D.	For Ph.D.
1970	787	39% (306)	61% (481)	62% (190)	61% (294)	79% (151)	77% (227)	49%	47%
1971	863	34% (295)	66% (568)	60% (177)	66% (375)	69% (123)	62% (231)	42%	41%
1975	984	32% (316)	68% (668)	73% (232)	79% (527)	69% (160)	63% (332)	51%	50%
1980	1233	24% (298)	76% (935)	69% (206)	78% (726)	56% (115)	50% (365)	39%	39%
1981	1511	24% (360)	76% (1151)	69% (247)	80% (925)	41% (101)	39% (361)	28%	31%
1982	1687	20% (342)	80% (1345)	81% (278)	84% (1129)	32% (88)	34% (388)	26%	29%
1983	1707	19% (318)	81% (1389)	82% (262)	87% (1204)	32% (83)	35% (424)	26%	31%
1984	1798	22% (390)	78% (1408)	85% (332)	89% (1250)	36% (118)	33% (411)	30%	29%

117

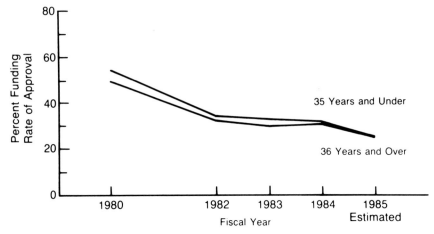

Notes: 1. This age was calculated as of the first day of the fiscal year.
       2. These data were not developed in accordance with NIH standards for the display
          of award rates, and should not be an indicator of the adequacy of appro-
          priations.
       3. Funding is defined as the Number of Awards divided by the Number of Council
          Recommendations for Approval.
       4. Age not reported in approximately 5 percent of the applications.

FIG. 8.1. NINCDS. Percentage of approved RO1 applications funded by age of investigator:
FY 1980–FY 1985.

If we accept as the definition of "young investigator," persons who have
not yet reached their 36th birthday, we see that in recent years age is not a
variable that predicts whether an approved NINCDS research project
grant application will be funded. This is not true in the case of program
project or research center applications, which usually have a well-established investigator as program director. In 1984, only 30% of active
NINCDS research grants in neurosurgery were to young investigators. The
reason for this is, again, the same relatively small number of applications
received from young neurosurgeons.

Another aspect of the concern about young investigators receiving
NINCDS research grant support is: if we are well-trained can we compete
against our well-trained basic science colleagues? Table 8.2 examines this
belief.

In 1970, the NINCDS established its Teacher-Investigator Development
Awards (TIDA) program as a research training base for neurological, neurosurgical, and otolaryngological fellows. The program provided 5 years of
research training and career development support to physicians complet-

TABLE 8.2

Research Grants Support of NINCDS Career Development Awardees and Graduates

TIDAs	TIDA Participants					Graduates	
Start date (FY)	1983	1982	1981	1980	1979	1978	1976–7	1970–5
Total number	29	21	28	26	26	16	14	24
Number with research support, FY 1983	7	6	13	9	13	10	9	17
Percent with research support, FY 1983	24%	29%	46%	35%	50%	63%	64%	71%
RCDAs	RCDA Participants					Graduates	
Start date (FY)	1983	1982	1981	1980	1979	1978	1976–7	1970–5
Total number	11	10	10	15	19	29	42	89
Number with research support, FY 1983	11	7	8	11	13	20	34	58
Percent with research support, FY 1983	100%	70%	80%	73%	69%	69%	81%	65%

ing their clinical training. The first graduating class was in 1975. How well did these clinical trainees do when competing against their Ph.D. colleagues for NINCDS research grant support? For comparison, we used post-Ph.D. neuroscientists awarded NINCDS Research Career Development Awards (RCDA). These RCDA recipients generally had already completed 2 to 3 years of postdoctoral research fellowship experience before receiving the 5-year RCDA. They are generally recognized as the cream of the crop, the basic neuroscientists who will clearly be the scientific leaders of the future.

The RCDA graduates are successful if one uses the ability to receive an NIH research grant as a measure of success. They do nearly twice as well as the total pool of NINCDS applicants. However, let us consider the physicians in training through the Teacher-Investigator Development Program. Within a 5-year period after finishing training, the physician-investigator is doing as well as the RCDA-trained basic scientist. The physician-investigator not only does twice as well as the total pool of applicants—most of whom are Ph.D.'s—but as well as the best of the Ph.D. basic scientists at similar levels of development.

Therefore, popular belief number 2 is not correct. Clinicians who have received research training can compete quite successfully with basic neuroscientists for NIH research grant support.

Clinical trials of medical methodologies—preventive, diagnostic, and therapeutic—are now an established part of the North American clinical research scene. The medical-surgical armamentarium has progressed over time from methodologies based on individual clinical judgments through case series to clinical trials. The "gold standard" is now established to be the randomized controlled clinical trial. I know we can all think of examples where a randomized clinical trial would probably not be necessary, for example, a cure for rabies; the first patient cured would be a miracle, the second, a conclusive end point. However, despite discussions of its relative appropriateness for a specific clinical evaluation, the controlled clinical trial is still a standard against which results arrived at by any other method must be evaluated. In medicine, including medical neurology, finely tuned methodologies for randomized trials have evolved and are applied regularly to important issues of patient care. Recent neurological trials in stroke, multiple sclerosis, diabetic neuropathy, and epilepsy are but a few examples.

However, it is also said that the methodology of the controlled clinical trial—particularly the randomized clinical trial—is not applicable to surgical procedures. To put it bluntly, we often hear the concerns: it would be unethical to deny the patient this procedure because *I* know it works; or you cannot pool *my* results with those of that other surgery.

I am not surprised that neurosurgery has now demonstrated to the entire surgical community that these concerns can be properly addressed; that controlled trials, which answer a therapeutic question ethically, can be instituted and the highest standards of surgical care can be maintained. Neurosurgery has now set the gold standard for the rest of the surgery.

I am referring to the recently completed, randomized, controlled clinical trial of the efficacy of extracranial-intracranial anastomosis for the prevention of stroke and stroke death. I know that some will question the interpretation of the data—but on what basis puzzles me. The data are unassailable; the results are crisp and not vague nor based on extrapolations from trends. Neurological surgery has demonstrated conclusively to the entire surgical community that controlled clinical trials of a surgical procedure are ethical and feasible. This was a job well done. But now that this has been demonstrated, do neurological surgeons also have the continuing responsibility to apply this methodology to other procedures which are based primarily on intuitive judgment and experience drawn from sequential case series?

Therefore, belief 3 is not true. Surgical results can be evaluated in randomized clinical trials. Neurosurgery has demonstrated that very clearly.

In conclusion, I put it to you bluntly. If neurosurgery dies as a research discipline, it will have died because of lack of attention. Whether neurosurgical research is to be done in the laboratory, the experimental surgery, or the clinic, I hope I have convinced you that you can compete successfully for research support, and that you can continue to set the pace for the community of surgical disciplines. As the Director of the NINCDS, I pledge to you our assistance. However, to paraphrase an old saying: The NINCDS can only help those who help themselves.

III

Cerebrovascular Surgery

CHAPTER

9

Surgical Treatment of Incidental Intracranial Aneurysms

FREMONT P. WIRTH, M.D.

Aneurysm-related subarachnoid hemorrhage constitutes a major public health problem despite advances in the diagnosis and treatment of this disorder (21). Data from the Framingham Study, the Mayo Clinic, and others suggest that in the United States alone each year 25,000 new cases of subarachnoid hemorrhage occur (6, 15, 17, 37). Estimated rates of hemorrhage range between 10 and 28 per 100,000 population (2, 31, 37, 43). Ruptured arteriovenous malformations account for only 4 to 5% of cases of subarachnoid hemorrhage (23, 31, 37, 40). No source of hemorrhage is discoverable in 14 to 22% of patients with subarachnoid bleeding (11, 31, 33, 40). The remaining 75 to 80% of hemorrhages which result from aneurysms constitute the cause of 8% of all strokes.

Although surgical techniques and management protocols for the treatment of subarachnoid hemorrhage have improved, the overall management outcome for subarachnoid bleeding remains poor. This is primarily due to the devastation wrought by the initial bleed. Whereas initial mortality may have decreased slightly from 50% in 1967 to 39% in 1985, the addition of significant morbidity in another 19% of patients resulted in a truly favorable outcome in only 42% of patients in Ljunggren's recent series (19, 31).

Even when only good risk patients are considered, the surgical treatment of aneurysms after subarachnoid hemorrhage is disappointing. Ropper and Zervas found that among 112 patients with no neurological deficit after aneurysm rupture less than half (46%) recovered fully (36). Only 44% were able to return to their former jobs. Management mortality for these patients was 11% at 1 year and morbidity was 20% due to persistent neurological deficits, primarily from vasospasm-induced strokes. Another series from Scandinavia has reported similar results with 8% mortality and 14% morbidity after early surgery in good grade subarachnoid hemorrhage patients (42).

It seems likely, therefore, that further reduction in morbidity and mortality of subarachnoid hemorrhage will depend on the reduction of risk factors for subarachnoid hemorrhage and the identification and obliteration

125

of unruptured aneurysms. Risk factors—including hypertension, cigarette smoking, oral contraceptives, and alcohol consumption—have been identified, but their elimination is not likely (21). Current advances in noninvasive testing, including high resolution computed tomography (CT) and digital subtraction angiography (DSA), promise to identify more incidental aneurysms (18). Surgical obliteration of these lesions has been recommended by some authors (5, 7, 9, 25, 26, 28, 34, 38, 39), but not all. In several series reported prior to 1974, surgery for these lesions was not endorsed (10, 24, 27, 32). With current and future imaging techniques the question of surgery for incidental aneurysms is expected to become a more frequent dilemma. Whether incidental aneurysms should be clipped depends upon a number of factors. These include the natural history of incidental aneurysms, specifically the rates of hemorrhage, and the safety of surgical obliteration of these lesions.

FREQUENCY OF INCIDENTAL ANEURYSMS

Estimates of the frequency of incidental intracranial aneurysms range between 5 and 10%. In 1971, McCormick suggested that aneurysms occurred in 10% of the general population (22). Chason and Hindman, however, in an earlier autopsy study estimated the incidence of aneurysms at 4.9% (3). In their study the incidence for males was 3.5% and for females was 7.2%.

The frequency of multiple aneurysms is a more established figure. Reports from 1964–1985 suggest that multiple aneurysms are present in 15 to 33.5% of cases of subarachnoid hemorrhage (20, 24, 28, 35, 41). An association has also been demonstrated between the sex of the patient, the presence of systemic hypertension, and the presence of multiple aneurysms (30). Both factors increase the likelihood of multiple aneurysms. In Ostergaard's recent series, 17.9% of cases demonstrated multiple aneurysms (30).

NATURAL HISTORY OF UNRUPTURED ANEURYSMS

Assessment of the rate of hemorrhage of incidental intracranial aneurysms is essential to any appraisal of the efficacy of surgery for these lesions. The analysis of data from the cooperative study in 1969 indicated an annual rate of bleeding of 6.25% (20). Jane, in 1977, reported a rate of 5% as the best approximation (14). Using decremental life table analysis of unruptured aneurysms, Dell has recently suggested a 16% lifetime risk of aneurysm rupture for a 20-year-old harboring such a lesion (4). This risk is estimated to fall to a 5% lifetime risk for a 60-year-old. These estimates are based on an assumption of a 5% incidence of aneurysms in the general population and may, therefore, be low.

More recent reports also have suggested a lower rate of hemorrhage. Jane and colleagues have revised their earlier estimate to a 1% yearly rate of hemorrhage for unruptured aneurysms whether discovered incidental to a study to evaluate some other disease, or in association with a ruptured aneurysm (13). Heiskanen, in a study of 61 aneurysms discovered during investigation of another ruptured aneurysm, found a rate of hemorrhage of 1.1%/year in a 10-year follow-up (9). This same group of patients experienced a mortality rate of 0.65%/year. In a 16-year follow-up, the mortality rate in this series reached 11.5%.

Incidental aneurysms may not be assumed to be static. They have been shown to enlarge on serial angiographic studies, and such enlargement has been associated with bleeding (45). Furthermore, enlargement and hemorrhage may occur after decades of clinical silence (8). Enlargement of aneurysms has been associated with increased risk of hemorrhage (44). That small aneurysms may bleed as well has also been documented (16). Thus all incidental aneurysms are at some risk of hemorrhage, although perhaps the risk is greater in those over 7 mm in size (29).

ASSESSMENT OF SURGICAL RESULTS

The results of several series of under 50 patients have been reported during the last 10 years (5, 12, 26, 27, 38, 39) (Table 9.1). Collectively these represent 141 cases with no surgical mortality; morbidity ranged from 0 to 16%. Because of a concern that only those series with optimal results might be published and that for this reason the neurosurgical literature might not present a valid estimate of the risks of surgery for incidental aneurysms, a multicenter retrospective study was carried out. This series of 119 surgically treated aneurysms in 107 patients has been reported (46). The data was collected from 12 different centers including both university and community hospital practices. While it is recognized that a retrospec-

TABLE 9.1
Surgical Results of Incidental Intracranial Aneurysm

Author	No. of Cases	Mortality	Morbidity
Jain (1976)	10	0	0
Drake (1976)	12	0	16%
Mount (1974)	20	0	5%
Moyes (1971)	21	0	9.5%
Salazar (1980)	29	0	10.3%
Samson (1977)	49	0	6.4%
Total	141	0	

tive study might have some limitations, it was felt that this would allow an assessment of the risks of surgery for incidental aneurysms.

A total of 119 aneurysms were clipped in 107 patients (46). These were drawn from a series of 1671 aneurysm operations at 12 institutions over a 6-year period (1975–1981). The criteria for inclusion in the study were: (a) aneurysms diagnosed at angiography for conditions other than subarachnoid hemorrhage, including the evaluation of cerebral ischemia, pituitary dysfunction, seizure disorder, or headache not due to subarachnoid hemorrhage; (b) aneurysms identified at the time of investigation of subarachnoid hemorrhage due to another aneurysm operated upon at a separate time through a different approach. Aneurysms 2.5 cm in diameter or greater were excluded, as were those aneurysms associated with a third nerve palsy, as these were not felt to be truly incidental aneurysms. Also excluded were aneurysms associated with arteriovenous malformations, hematomas, or brain tumors.

Surgical adjuncts included hypotensive anesthesia, corticosteroids, and the operating microscope. Some selection of patients did occur. Patients

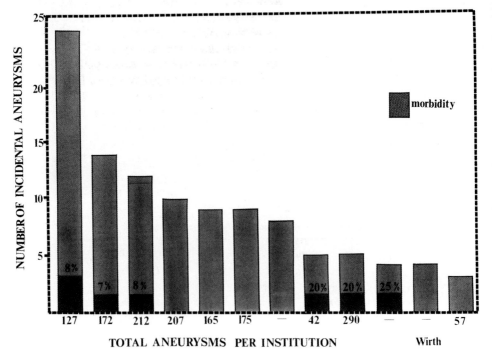

FIG. 9.1. Morbidity of incidental aneurysm surgery among individual institutions (46).

who were poor candidates for general anesthesia and major surgery were excluded. This was not felt to detract from the series in that such patients would not generally be considered for elective craniotomy. Although the number of aneurysms clipped at the different institutions varied from 3 to 24 during the period studied, there was no real difference in morbidity (Fig. 9.1) (46).

No mortalities were encountered. When combined with other reported series, surgical clipping of a total of 260 incidental aneurysms has been reported without mortality. Major morbidity, however, did occur in 6.5% of cases. This included left hemiparesis in three cases, moderate right hemiparesis and aphasia in two cases, left thalamic syndrome in one case, and mild memory deficit and altered affect in one case. The details of individual morbidities have been reported (46).

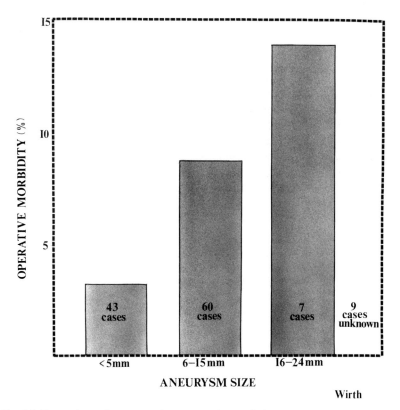

FIG. 9.2. Comparison of aneurysm size to operative morbidity indicates increasing morbidity with increasing aneurysm size (46).

Minor morbidity with complete resolution of symptoms occurred in 9 of 107 patients. This included one each of the following: wound infection requiring reoperation, transient fourth nerve palsy, transient third nerve palsy, ptosis, reoperation of clip replacement, phlebitis, transient sixth nerve palsy, transient aphasia and hemiparesis, and hyponatremia due to inappropriate antidiuretic hormone secretion (46).

Aneurysm size and location did influence operative safety (Figs. 9.2 and 9.3). Aneurysms less than 5 mm in diameter were associated with a 2.3% operative morbidity, those 6 to 15 mm with a 6.8% morbidity, and those 16 to 25 mm with a morbidity of 14%. The clipping of internal carotid–posterior communicating artery aneurysms resulted in a 4.8% operative morbidity, whereas middle cerebral artery aneurysms and internal carotid–ophthalmic aneurysms had operative morbidities of 8.1% and 11.8%, respectively. Anterior communicating artery aneurysms were among the most difficult and had a 15.5% risk of operative morbidity, and carotid bifurcation aneurysms had a 16.8% operative morbidity (46).

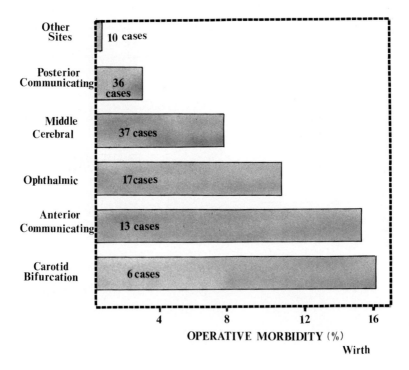

FIG. 9.3. Aneurysm location when compared to operative morbidity reveals a higher operative morbidity for aneurysms in less accessible locations, including the anterior communicating artery and carotid bifurcation (46).

TABLE 9.2

Relationship of Morbidity to Presenting Symptoms

Presenting Symptom	No. of Patients	Morbidity
Cerebral ischemia	37	10.8%
Headache	19	5.8%
Subarachnoid hemorrhage (other aneurysm)	41	2.4%
Dizziness (vertigo)	2	
Psychiatric illness	2	
Cranial nerve palsy (not third nerve)	3	
Family history of aneurysm rupture	2	50%
Visual loss	1	

Patients operated upon for an incidental aneurysm discovered at angiography for another ruptured intracranial aneurysm appeared to have less morbidity than those patients whose aneurysms were discovered at the time of evaluation of other problems, such as transient cerebral ischemia (Table 9.2). This may simply reflect the selection of the fittest patients.

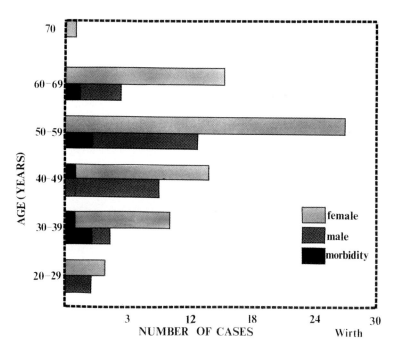

FIG. 9.4. Comparison of patient age and operative morbidity fails to reveal increasing morbidity of surgery with advancing age (46).

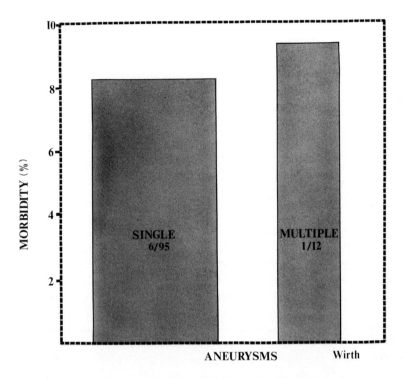

FIG. 9.5. Comparison of the morbidity of clipping single as opposed to multiple incidental aneurysms fails to reveal a difference (46).

These individuals had already survived subarachnoid hemorrhage and craniotomy and tolerated a subsequent craniotomy with minimal morbidity (46).

Neither the age of the patient nor whether single or multiple incidental aneurysms were treated at one operation could be correlated with operative morbidity (Figs. 9.4 and 9.5) (46). Advancing age in excess of 60 years has been demonstrated not to be a contraindication to surgery for ruptured intracranial aneurysms (1).

SUMMARY

It is clear that more incidental aneurysms will be encountered in the future. Approximately 5% or more of the population harbors these lesions, and advancing technology can be expected to demonstrate them with increasing regularity. Multiple aneurysms will also be found in at least 18% of patients with subarachnoid hemorrhage due to aneurysms. The best estimates suggest a rate of hemorrhage approximating 1%/year for incidental aneurysms and a 0.4 to 0.65% annual mortality rate for these lesions. It has also been shown that even small aneurysms may enlarge and bleed unpredictably with the passage of time.

Surgery for incidental aneurysms of the anterior circulation can be accomplished without mortality and with an operative morbidity of 6.5%. Higher morbidity occurs in surgery for aneurysms in more difficult locations as well as larger aneurysms. The increased risk of bleeding from larger aneurysms, however, may justify the increased morbidity of surgery for these lesions.

Surgery for incidental aneurysms can be recommended in healthy individuals whose anesthetic risk is acceptable and for aneurysms less than 1.5 cm in diameter arising from the middle cerebral and posterior communicating arteries. Advancing age alone is not a contraindication for surgery, nor is size greater than 1.5 cm in diameter; however, the latter factor increases the operative risk. Operations to clip aneurysms of the carotid bifurcation, carotid-ophthalmic, and anterior communicating arteries may also be recommended, but these aneurysms are more difficult to approach and surgery carries a higher morbidity. Larger aneurysms, greater than 1.5 cm in diameter, in patients over 60 years of age, and in less accessible locations may not benefit from operation because surgical morbidity for these lesions is high and with advancing age the lifetime risk of rupture has decreased. For incidental aneurysms of the posterior circulation there are insufficient data to make a recommendation regarding surgery, although it is anticipated that the counsel for anterior circulation aneurysms will apply.

If operative mortality and morbidity are to be maintained at acceptable levels, incidental aneurysm surgery should be the province of the accomplished aneurysm surgeon who has available to him the most modern techniques and equipment. With the clipping of incidental aneurysms, hopefully the number of patients suffering from subarachnoid hemorrhage with its high morbidity and mortality rates can be further reduced.

REFERENCES

1. Amacher, A. L., Ferguson, G. G., Drake, C. G., Girvin, J. P., and Barr, H. W. K. How old people tolerate intracranial surgery for aneurysms. Neurosurgery, 1: 242–244, 1977.
2. Bonita, R., Beaglehole, R., North, J. D. K. Subarachnoid hemorrhage in New Zealand: an epidemiologic study. Stroke, 14: 342–347, 1983.
3. Chason, J. L., Hindman, W. M. Berry aneurysms of the circle of Willis: results of a planned autopsy study. Neurology (NY), 8: 41–42, 1958.
4. Dell, S. Asymptomatic cerebral aneurysm: assessment of its risk of rupture. Neurosurgery, 10: 162–166, 1982.
5. Drake, C. G., Girvan, J. P. The surgical treatment of subarachnoid hemorrhage with multiple aneurysms. In: Current Controversies in Neurosurgery, edited by T. P. Morley, pp. 274–278. W. B. Saunders, Philadelphia, 1976.

6. Garraway, W. M., Whisnant, J. P., Drury, I. The continuing decline in the instance of stroke. Mayo Clin. Proc., 58: 520–523, 1983.
7. Graf, C. J., Nibbelink, B. W. Cooperative study of intracranial aneurysms and subarachnoid hemorrhage. Stroke, 5: 559–601, 1974.
8. Hashimoto, N., Honda, H. The fate of untreated symptomatic cerebral aneurysms: analysis of 26 patients with clinical course of more than 5 years. Surg. Neurol., 18: 21–26, 1982.
9. Heiskanen, O. Risk of bleeding from unruptured aneurysms in cases with multiple intracranial aneurysms. J. Neurosurg., 55: 524–526, 1981.
10. Heiskanen, O., Martilla, I. Risk of rupture of a second aneurysm in patients with multiple aneurysms. J. Neurosurg., 32: 295–299, 1970.
11. Ishii, R., Kuroki, M., Tanaka, R., Watanabe, M., Toyama, M., and Aria, H. Subarachnoid hemorrhage of unknown cause: clinical study. Neurol. Med. Chir. (Tokyo), 23: 262–266, 1983.
12. Jain, K. K. Surgery of intact intracranial aneurysms. J. Neurosurg., 40: 495–499, 1974.
13. Jane, J. A., Kassell, N. A., Torner, J. C., Winn, H. R. The natural history of aneurysms and arteriovenous malformations. J. Neurosurg., 62: 321–323, 1985.
14. Jane, J. A., Winn, H. R., Richardson, R. E. The natural history of intracranial aneurysms: re-bleeding rates during the acute and long term period and application for surgical management. Clin. Neurosurg., 24: 176–184, 1977.
15. Kagan, A., Popper, J. S., Rhoads, G. G. Factors related to stroke incidence in Hawaii Japanese men: the Honolulu Heart Study. Stroke, 11: 14–21, 1980.
16. Kassell, N. F., and Torner, J. C. Size of intracranial aneurysms. Neurosurgery, 12: 291–297, 1983.
17. Kurtzke, J. F. An introduction to the epidemiology of cerebrovascular disease. In: Cerebrovascular Diseases, edited by P. Scheinberg, pp. 239–253. Raven Press, New York, 1976.
18. Little, J. R., Furlan, A. J., Modic, M. T., Bryerton, B., Weinstein, M. A. Intravenous digital subtraction angiography: application to cerebrovascular surgery. Neurosurgery, 9: 129–136, 1981.
19. Ljunggren, B., Säveland, H., Brandt, L., and Zeygmunt, S. Early operation and overall outcome in aneurysmal subarachnoid hemorrhage. J. Neurosurg., 62: 547–551, 1985.
20. Locksley, H. B. Natural history of subarachnoid hemorrhage, intracranial aneurysm and arteriovenous malformations: based on 6,368 cases in the Cooperative Study, parts I and II. In: Intracranial Aneurysms and Subarachnoid Hemorrhage: A Cooperative Study, edited by A. L. Sahs, G. E. Perret, H. B. Locksley, and H. Nishioka, pp. 37–108. J. B. Lippincott, Philadelphia, 1969.
21. Longstreth, W. T., Jr., Koepsell, T. D., Yerby, M. S., and van Belle, G. Risk factors for subarachnoid hemorrhage. Stroke, 16: 377–385, 1985.
22. McCormick, W. F. Problems and pathogenesis of intracranial arterial aneurysms. In: 7th Conference: Cerebrovascular Diseases, edited by J. Moossy, and R. Janeway, pp. 217–231. Grune and Stratton, New York, 1971.
23. McKissock, W., and Paine, K. W. E. Subarachnoid haemorrhage. Brain, 82: 356–366, 1959.
24. McKissock, W., Richardson, A., Walsh, L., Owen, E. Multiple intracranial aneurysms. Lancet, 1: 623–626, 1984.
25. Mount, L. A., Brisman, R. Treatment of multiple intracranial aneurysms. J. Neurosurg., 35: 728–730, 1971.
26. Mount, L. A., Brisman, R. Treatment of multiple aneurysms, symptomatic and asymptomatic. Clin. Neurosurg., 21: 162–170, 1974.

27. Moyes, P. D. Surgical treatment of multiple aneurysms and of incidentally discovered unruptured aneurysms. J. Neurosurg., *35:* 291–295, 1971.
28. Nehls, D. G., Flom, R. A., Carter, L. P., Spetzler, R. F. Multiple intracranial aneurysms: determining the site of rupture. J. Neurosurg., *63:* 342–348, 1985.
29. Ojemann, R. G. Management of the unruptured intracranial aneurysm. N. Engl. J. Med., *304:* 725–726, 1981.
30. Østergaard, J. R., Høg, E. Incidence of multiple intracranial aneurysms. J. Neurosurg., *63:* 49–55, 1985.
31. Pakarinen, S. Incidence, aetiology, and prognosis of primary subarachnoid haemorrhage: a study based on 589 cases diagnosed in a defined urban population during a defined period. Acta Neurol. Scand. (Suppl. 29), 1–128, 1967.
32. Patterson, A., Bond, M. R. Treatment of multiple intracranial arterial aneurysms. Lancet, *1:* 1302–1304, 1973.
33. Phillips, L. H., II, Whisnant, J. P., O'Fallon, W. M., Sundt, T. M., Jr. The unchanging pattern of subarachnoid hemorrhage in a community. Neurology (NY), *30:* 1034–1040, 1980.
34. Poole, J. L., and Potts, D. G. *Aneurysms and Arteriovenous Anomalies of the Brain.* Harper and Row, New York, 1965.
35. Poppen, J. L., Fager, C. A. Multiple intracranial aneurysms. J. Neurosurg., *16:* 581–589, 1959.
36. Ropper, A. H., Zervas, N. T. Outcome one year after SAH from cerebral aneurysm. J. Neurosurg., *60:* 909–915, 1984.
37. Sacco, R. L., Wolf, P. A., Bharucha, N. E., *et al.* Subarachnoid hemorrhage and intracerebral hemorrhage: natural history, prognosis, and precursive factors in the Framingham study. Neurology (Cleveland), *34:* 847–854, 1984.
38. Salazar, J. L. Surgical treatment of asymptomatic and incidental intracranial aneurysms. J. Neurosurg., *53:* 20–21, 1980.
39. Samson, D. S., Hodosh, R. M., Clarke, W. K. Surgical management of unruptured asymptomatic aneurysms. J. Neurosurg., *46:* 731–734, 1977.
40. Shephard, R. H. Prognosis of spontaneous (non-traumatic) subarachnoid hemorrhage of unknown cause: a personal series, 1958–1980. Lancet, *1:* 777–779, 1984.
41. Stehbens, W. E. Intracranial arterial aneurysms. In: *Pathology of the Cerebral Blood Vessels,* pp. 351–470. C. V. Mosby, St. Louis, 1972.
42. Vapalahti, M., Ljunggren, B., Saveland, H., Hernesniemi, J., Brandt, L., and Tapaninaho, A. Early aneurysm operation and outcome in two remote Scandinavian populations. J. Neurosurg., *60:* 1160–1162, 1984.
43. Whisnant, J. P., Phillips, L. H., II, and Sundt, T. M., Jr. Aneurysmal subarachnoid hemorrhage: timing of surgery and mortality. Mayo Clin. Proc., *57:* 471–475, 1982.
44. Wiebers, D. O., Whisnant, J. P., and O'Fallon, W. M. The natural history of unruptured intracranial aneurysms. N. Engl. J. Med., *304:* 696–698, 1981.
45. Winn, H. R., Richardson, A. E., and Jane, J. A. The long term prognosis in untreated cerebral aneurysms. I. The incidence of later hemorrhage in cerebral aneurysms: a 10 year evaluation in 364 patients. Ann. Neurol., *1:* 358–370, 1977.
46. Wirth, F. P., Laws, E. R., Jr., Piepgras, D., and Scott, R. M. Surgical treatment of incidental intracranial aneurysms. Neurosurgery, *12:* 507–511, 1983.

10

Antifibrinolytic Therapy in the Treatment of Aneurysmal Subarachnoid Hemorrhage

N. F. KASSELL, M.D., E. C. HALEY, M. D., and J. C. TORNER, M.D.

INTRODUCTION

Rebleeding is the most irreversible and disastrous complication of aneurysmal subarachnoid hemorrhage (SAH). It ranks second only to vasospasm as a cause of death or disability in patients with ruptured aneurysms (9). If patients with ruptured aneurysms are treated with bed rest alone, approximately 20% will rebleed within 14 days, 30% in 30 days, 40% in 180 days, and thereafter patients will continue to rebleed at the rate of approximately 3%/year (10, 21). Thus, the patient who has had a ruptured aneurysm that has not been surgically corrected is continually at risk; furthermore, asymptomatic aneurysms which have not been surgically obliterated also confer risk of future rupture (7).

Recent evidence indicates that the rate of rebleeding is highest on the first 2 days following the initial hemorrhage. The rate then decreases fairly rapidly by the third or fourth day, and continues to decrease in a logarithmic fashion reaching a plateau at approximately 6 months (Fig. 10.1) (7). This recent evidence is in contrast to the previous notion that the peak of rebleeding is at the end of the first to the beginning of the second week following the initial hemorrhage (12). The latter concept was derived from data of the 1960s, where deterioration with vasospasm was confused with that of rebleeding. The time course of what was then called rebleeding is very similar to the time course of onset of ischemic neurological deficits from vasospasm (Fig. 10.2).

Rebleeding is a result of the transmural or "bursting pressure" of the aneurysm exceeding the strength of the wall. Following aneurysm rupture, the rent in the aneurysm is sealed by blood clot, probably both in the lumen of the aneurysm as well as in the subarachnoid space. Rebleeding can occur either as a result of an increase in the transmural pressure or as a result of weakening in the wall of the aneurysm. Weakening in the wall of the aneurysm occurs when the clot sealing the rent in the aneurysm lyses. SAH results in an increase in the fibrinolytic activity in the cerebrospinal fluid, which removes the subarachnoid portion of the clot. Evidence for

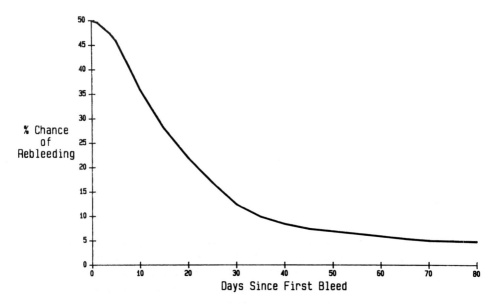

FIG. 10.1. Graph illustrating high rate of rebleeding initially seen, followed by rapid decline over 60 days to reach plateau rate of 3%/year.

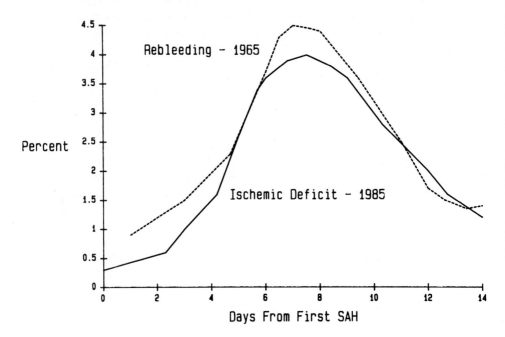

FIG. 10.2. Graph depicts rate of rebleeding from 1965 data of Locksley *et al.* (*dotted line*). Note similarity to rate of development of ischemic neurological deficits derived from 1985 Cooperative Aneurysm Study data (*solid line*).

activation of the systemic antifibrinolytic system (luminal side) is conflicting, but if it does occur, the effect is slight. Greater fibrinolytic activity is derived locally from the vessel wall (6). The rationale for use of antifibrinolytic agents is thus to inhibit this naturally occurring fibrinolytic process.

THE AGENTS

There are currently two antifibrinolytic agents in common use for the prevention of rebleeding following SAH. They are chemically related (Fig. 10.3) and act by similar mechanisms to inhibit the conversion of plasminogen to plasmin and to partially block the action of plasmin on the fibrin clot. ε-Aminocaproic acid (EACA), first identified and synthesized in Japan over 30 years ago, is the agent that is used most commonly in North America. Tranexamic acid (AMCA), introduced in the 1960s, has an antifibrinolytic activity approximately 10 times greater than that of EACA (13). It is in common use in the remainder of the world. Aside from the lower dose of tranexamic acid required to achieve the same level of antifibrinolytic activity, there appears to be no difference in the safety or efficacy of the two agents.

Another available agent is a naturally occurring protein, aprotinin. It has been proposed to exert antifibrinolytic action similar to its synthetic counterparts, but has a lower rate of thromboembolic complications. However, this lower rate of complications has not been proven.

Recently another synthetic cyclic aminocarboxylic acid, p-aminomethylbenzoic acid (PAMBA), has been safely administered intrathecally to patients with aneurysmal subarachnoid hemorrhage (6). No complications

	Relative Antifibrinolytic Activity
Epsilon - Aminocaproic Acid (EACA) H_2N -$(CH_2)_5$ - COOH	100
Trans-4-Aminomethylcyclohexane- carboxylic acid - (1) (AMCA) 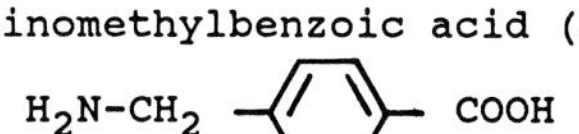 H_2N-CH_2 ⬡ COOH	1000
4-Aminomethylbenzoic acid (PAMBA) 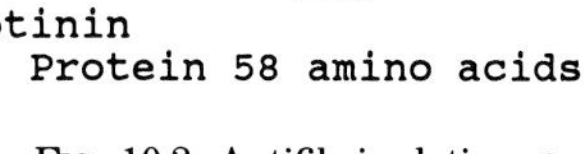 H_2N-CH_2 ⬡ COOH	500
Aprotinin Protein 58 amino acids	

FIG. 10.3. Antifibrinolytic agents. First three agents are synthetic aminocarboxylic acid derivatives. The last agent is a naturally occurring inhibitor.

were encountered in 25 patients, but its clinical efficacy remains to be determined.

HISTORICAL CONSIDERATIONS

EACA was first used clinically in patients with fibrinolytic states by Nilsson *et al.* and was reported in 1960 (17). This same group was the first to use EACA in intracranial bleeding disorders as well, reporting in 1961 on the use of the agent in two patients with presumed intracerebral hemorrhage (16). The clinical condition of the patients was not affected. Mullan *et al.* reported in 1964 that the duration of experimentally produced femoral artery thrombosis was prolonged by the administration of EACA and suggested that similar benefits might be obtainable in intracranial aneurysms (15).

In 1967, Gibbs and O'Gorman reported on the first series of patients with ruptured intracranial aneurysm treated with the antifibrinolytic agent EACA (3). Although their results showed no statistically significant benefit of treatment over controls, they opined that, "We are convinced that the future management of bleeding intracranial aneurysms will involve biochemical control of changes within them, surgery receding more and more into the background."

From 1967 through 1981, 24 additional studies were published dealing with the use of antifibrinolytic agents—either EACA, AMCA, or both—in aneurysmal SAH. The results of these studies have been reviewed elsewhere (5, 18, 20). To summarize, 12 uncontrolled series all reported reduced incidence of rebleeding. In 13 controlled series, seven reported decreased rebleeding, three showed no effect, and three reported a higher rebleeding rate in the treated group.

NEW OBSERVATIONS

By 1981, surgery clearly was not "receding . . . into the background." Based on the equivocal data, controversy continued to rage over the effectiveness of antifibrinolytic therapy in preventing rebleeding, as well as such therapy's contribution to a variety of complications, including hydrocephalus, deep vein thrombosis and pulmonary embolism, coagulation disorders, psychiatric abnormalities, rhabdomyolysis, and diarrhea. Moreover, as early as 1972, Kagstrom and Palma drew attention to the fact that antifibrinolytic therapy might be associated with an increase in the risk of vasospasm-induced cerebral ischemia (8). Other investigators subsequently made similar observations on small numbers of patients (2, 14). Perhaps part of the confusion, then, was attributable to the fact that many of the studies used rebleeding as the end point rather than considering the overall mortality and morbidity.

Two recent studies (1984), conducted by independent investigators using different study designs, have reached similar conclusions that perhaps clarify the issue. The first study was compiled from information derived from the Cooperative Aneurysm Study Timing of Surgery project (11). This nonrandomized, observational study included 672 patients from 68 participating centers who were admitted with aneurysmal SAH on days 0 to 3 following the ictus and who had their surgery planned for the period of 7 to 14 days after hemorrhage. Of these, 467 (69%) received antifibrinolytic therapy and 205 (31%) did not. Despite the lack of randomization, the two groups were virtually identical from the standpoint of prognostic factors for rebleeding (Table 10.1). Rebleeding rates, documented by either computed tomography (CT) or lumbar puncture, were compared between the two groups using life table techniques. Additionally, mortality rates and rates of development of focal ischemic neurological deficits, hydrocephalus, thrombophlebitis, and pulmonary embolism were compared.

The overall mortality rates were essentially the same in both groups at 14 and 30 days (13.2% and 22.3% for the antifibrinolytic group compared to 13.0% and 20% for the group not receiving antifibrinolytics). However, the rebleeding rate in the group not receiving antifibrinolytic agents was 19.4% at 14 days compared to only 11.7% in the group receiving antifibrinolytic therapy, a statistically significant difference ($p < 0.01$). The rebleeding rates on days 0 and 1 following the initial hemorrhage were essentially

TABLE 10.1
Comparison of Prognostic Factors*

Factors	Antifibrinolytic Therapy	No Antifibrinolytic Therapy
No. of cases	467	205
Interval to admission ≤ day	76.1%	79.7%
Consciousness: stupor or coma	12.4%	13.2%
Sex: female	60.4%	65.8%
Systolic blood pressure ≥170 mm Hg	17.1%	22.4%
Pre-existing hypertension	20.6%	20.0%
Subarachnoid blood on CT	80.0%	79.7%
Surgical treatment	78.4%	82.4%
Day of surgery (median days)	11	12
Age (years)	49.5	48.6

* None of the factors showed a significant intergroup difference.

Data derived from Cooperative Aneurysm Study Timing of Surgery project. Despite nonrandomized study design, prognostic factors for outcome were remarkably similar between patients receiving antifibrinolytic drugs and those who were not.

identical in the two groups. This might imply, as suggested by some, an inability to achieve therapeutic cerebrospinal fluid (CSF) drug levels of the antifibrinolytic agents during this interval.

On the other hand, patients receiving antifibrinolytic therapy were 50% more likely to develop focal ischemic neurological deficits by day 14 compared to the patients not receiving antifibrinolytic therapy (32.4% in the antifibrinolytic group versus 22.7% in the group without antifibrinolytic agents, $p < 0.01$). Also, hydrocephalus was twice as likely to occur in the group receiving antifibrinolytic agents. Thus, for this study, it appears that the reduction in mortality rate achieved from control of rebleeding by antifibrinolytic therapy is at the expense of an increase in mortality from ischemic neurological deficits. The rates of pulmonary embolism and deep vein thrombosis were not significantly different between the two groups.

The second study, a multicenter trial conducted in Rotterdam, Amsterdam, Glasgow, and London (RAGL), was a randomized, double-blind, placebo-controlled study of tranexamic acid (AMCA) in 479 patients enrolled between 1979 and 1982 (20). Again, mortality rates at 3 months were virtually identical (35% (AMCA) versus 37% (placebo)). Of the survivors, 44% of the control group had no neurological deficit compared to 42% of the AMCA group. However, the rebleeding rates were again seen to be substantially reduced in the treated (9%) compared to the control (24%) groups ($p < 0.001$), although they were nearly the same during the first 4 days after the initial hemorrhage. Likewise, the rate of infarction documented clinically or by CT scan was increased in the treated (24%) versus the control (15%) group ($p < 0.01$). Hydrocephalus developed more frequently in the treated group, but the difference did not reach statistical significance. Other complication rates were identical between the two groups.

The results of these two studies confirm that antifibrinolytic therapy does indeed effect a substantial decrease in the rebleeding rate following aneurysmal SAH in those patients not requiring early surgery. However, the cost is substantial in terms of morbidity and mortality from development of ischemic neurological complications.

THE FUTURE

The objective of the use of antifibrinolytic agents in the future is to optimize that aspect of the therapy which prevents rebleeding—particularly in the first 48 hours following SAH when rebleeding reaches its peak—and simultaneously to minimize the ischemic complications which may be related to a prolonged subarachnoid clot, increased arterial narrowing, and any tendency of these drugs to exacerbate intravascular thromboembolism.

Potential new approaches include the development of new agents such as the alpha chain of Factor XIII, or the intrathecal administration of more conventional agents. The use of antifibrinolytic therapy combined with measures to prevent ischemic neurological deficits is another potential development. However, considerable gains in the safety and efficacy of the use of ε-aminocaproic acid can probably be achieved by development of a more rational administration protocol.

At this time, there are few guidelines on how best to use this drug. It is interesting to note that, although the largest market for EACA in this country is in patients with SAH, there is no mention of how to use the drug on the package insert, since SAH from ruptured aneurysm is not a Food and Drug Administration-approved indication for use.

Many questions remain unanswered. When should therapy be started? What daily dose should be employed? Should the drug be given orally or intravenously? How should the effectiveness of therapy be monitored (e.g., drug levels versus clot lysis times, etc.)? What should the duration of therapy be following SAH? Should the therapy be discontinued abruptly, or should it be tapered? Is there a rebound hypocoagulability? Should the drug be discontinued when patients develop ischemic neurological deficits? Should the drug be discontinued prior to surgery or angiography? If so, how far in advance? What is the interaction with antihypertensive therapy or steroids? Approximately 75% of patients who receive antifibrinolytic therapy have a prolonged bleeding time as the result of the qualitative disturbance in platelet function (4). What is the significance of this clinically?

SUMMARY

At the present time, there remains considerable uncertainty regarding the safety and efficacy of antifibrinolytic therapy in the treatment of aneurysmal SAH. Furthermore, there is little to guide us on precisely how to employ the agents. Whether to continue to use antifibrinolytic therapy after considering the results of the 1984 Cooperative Aneurysm Study trial and the Glasgow-Rotterdam-Amsterdam-London trial remains very much a philosophical decision. However, rebleeding is instantly and permanently devastating and 70% fatal, while ischemic deficits from vasospasm have a gradual onset and are potentially reversible. Accordingly, our policy is to continue to use antifibrinolytic therapy in those patients in whom it is desired to delay surgery. Our feeling is that, while there is no demonstrated advantage in acute mortality in either of the previously mentioned series, hypertensive, hypervolemic therapy or calcium channel blocking agents might ameliorate the ischemic consequences of therapy. Accordingly, it is in the context of combined therapy that the reduction in rebleeding will significantly influence patient outcome.

ACKNOWLEDGMENTS

The authors gratefully acknowledge the assistance of Ms. Elizabeth Wright, who edited the manuscript, and Mrs. Lucille Staiger, who typed it.

REFERENCES

1. Adams, H. P. Current status of antifibrinolytic therapy for treatment of patients with aneurysmal subarachnoid hemorrhage. Stroke, *13:* 256–259, 1982.
2. Fodstad, H., Forssell, A., Liliequist, B., and Schannong, M. Antifibrinolysis with tranexamic acid in aneurysmal subarachnoid hemorrhage: a consecutive controlled clinical trial. Neurosurgery, *8:* 158–165, 1981.
3. Gibbs, J. R., O'Gorman, P. Fibrinolysis in subarachnoid haemorrhage. Postgrad. Med. J., *43:* 779–784, 1967.
4. Glick, R., Green, D., Chung-hsin, T., *et al.* High dose epsilon-aminocaproic acid prolongs the bleeding time and increases rebleeding and intraoperative hemorrhage in patients with subarachnoid hemorrhage. Neurosurgery, *9:* 398–401, 1981.
5. Haines, S. J. Are antifibrinolytic agents useful after subarachnoid hemorrhage? In: *Dilemmas in the Management of the Neurological Patient,* edited by C. Warlow and J. Garfield. Churchill Livingstone, New York, 1984.
6. Hindersin, P., Heidrich, R., and Endler, S. Haemostasis in cerebrospinal fluid: basic concept of antifibrinolytic therapy in subarachnoid hemorrhage. Acta Neurochir. (Supp. 34), 1984.
7. Jane, J. A., Kassell, N. F., Torner, J. C., and Winn, H. R. The natural history of aneurysms and arteriovenous malformations. J. Neurosurg., *62:* 321–323, 1985.
8. Kagstrom, E., and Palma, L. Influence of antifibrinolytic treatment on the morbidity in patients with subarachnoid hemorrhage. Acta. Neurol. Scand., *48:* 257–258, 1972.
9. Kassell, N. F., Sasaki, T., Colohan, A. R. T., and Nazar, G. Cerebral vasospasm following aneurysmal subarachnoid hemorrhage. Stroke, *16:* 562–572, 1985.
10. Kassell, N. F., and Torner, J. C. Aneurysmal rebleeding: a preliminary report from the Cooperative Aneurysm Study. Neurosurgery, *13:* 479–481, 1983.
11. Kassell, N. F., Torner, J. C., and Adams, H. P. Antifibrinolytic therapy in the acute period following aneurysmal subarachnoid hemorrhage. Preliminary observations from the Cooperative Aneurysm Study. J. Neurosurg., *61:* 225–230, 1984.
12. Locksley, H. B. Report on the Cooperative Study of Intracranial Aneurysms and Subarachnoid Hemorrhage: section V, part II. Natural history of subarachnoid hemorrhage, intracranial aneurysms, and arteriovenous malformation. Based on 6368 cases in the Cooperative Study. J. Neurosurg., *25:* 321–368, 1966.
13. Markwardt, F. Synthetic inhibitors of fibrinolysis. Handbook Exp. Pharm., *46:* 511–577, 1978.
14. Maurice-Williams, R. S. Prolonged antifibrinolysis: an effective non-surgical treatment for ruptured intracranial aneurysms? Br. Med. J., *1:* 945–947, 1978.
15. Mullan, S., Beckman, F., Vailati, G. *et al.* An experimental approach to the problem of cerebral aneurysm. J. Neurosurg., *21:* 838–845, 1964.
16. Nilsson, I. M., Björkman, S. E., and Andersson, L. Clinical experiences with epsilon-aminocaproic acid (EACA) as an antifibrinolytic agent. Acta Medica Scand., *170:* 487–509, 1961.
17. Nilsson, I. M., Sjverdsma, A., and Waldenström, J. Antifibrinolytic activity and metabolism of epsilon-aminocaproic acid in man. Lancet, *1:* 1322–1324, 1960.

18. Ramirez-Lassepas, M. Antifibrinolytic therapy in subarachnoid hemorrhage caused by ruptured intracranial aneurysm. Neurology, *31:* 316–322, 1981.

19. Vermeulan, M., Lindsay, K. W., Murray, G. D., *et al.* Antifibrinolytic treatment in subarachnoid hemorrhage. N. Engl. J. Med., *311:* 432–437, 1984.

20. Vermeulan, M., and Muizelaar, J. P. Do antifibrinolytic agents prevent rebleeding after rupture of a cerebral aneurysm? A review. Clin. Neurol. Neurosurg., *82:* 25–30, 1980.

21. Winn, H. R., Richardson, A. E., and Jane, J. A. The long term prognosis in untreated cerebral aneurysm. I. The incidence of late hemorrhage in cerebral aneurysm: a 10-year evaluation of 364 patients. Ann. Neurol., *1:* 358–370, 1977.

11

The Timing of Aneurysm Surgery 1985

EUGENE S. FLAMM, M.D.

The two major issues related to the management of subarachnoid hemorrhage (SAH) secondary to cerebral aneurysms that have monopolized most of our attention in recent years are the timing of surgical intervention and the control and management of ischemic events due to cerebral vasospasm (CVS). Although no resolution of these questions is possible, recent information makes it likely that the issues of timing and the treatment of CVS will be dealt with on a less empirical basis in the next decade. For the present time we must continue to be guided by anecdotal and experiential information strengthened by small bits of emerging data. To make categorical statements concerning these issues is at best difficult and more likely to be presumptuous.

A considerable amount of attention has been paid to the description of the natural history of cerebral aneurysms. This epidemiologic approach can be divided into two components—the natural history of the unruptured cerebral aneurysm and the incidence of rebleeding from an aneurysm that has already ruptured. From these investigations come the rationale for managing a large segment of the aneurysm population before subarachnoid hemorrhage occurs. Certainly agreement on one aspect of timing is secure, and that is to clip an aneurysm before it has bled.

DIAGNOSIS

In spite of the tremendous strides that have been made in terms of the intraoperative surgical management of cerebral aneurysms, the overall results in patients with this diagnosis remain disappointing. Before we congratulate ourselves on the technical advances of aneurysm surgery, we must critically evaluate a number of the outcome studies of case morbidity and mortality as opposed to surgical morbidity and mortality. After doing this one cannot help but come to the conclusion that cerebral aneurysms are dangerous and that our current approaches fall far short of a satisfactory result (Table 11.1). In 1977, we reported our experience with 100 consecutive patients with ruptured intracranial aneurysms (11). A good result, defined as the ability to return to previous activities, was achieved in 60% of patients; 25% had moderate to severe disability and the case

TABLE 11.1

Case Morbidity and Mortality of Cerebral Aneurysms

	Outcome		
	Good (%)	Impaired (%)	Dead (%)
NYU 1977	60	25	15
Adams 1981	56	15	29
Ljunggren 1983	38	23	37
Roper & Zervas 1984	46	43	11
CAS 1985	58	16	26

mortality was 15%, only half of which was due to surgical mortality. Adams *et al.* reported similarly discouraging results in 249 patients managed at 11 institutions (1).

In 1983, Ljunggren reported the outcome of 78 patients with SAH. In spite of the commitment to early surgery in Lund, only 33 patients (42%) were found suitable for operation within the first 72 hours of the SAH. Of the 29 grade I–III patients that underwent early surgery, 72% had a good result. Overall there were 45 grade I–III patients, only 47% of whom had a good result. Very clearly there are other factors that affect outcome that cannot be controlled by the timing of surgery alone. This is emphasized by the overall outcome results in this group of 78 patients of whom 38% had a good recovery, 23% were impaired, and 37% were dead (9). Kassell and Drake estimated that only 36% of an estimated 28,000 patients with subarachnoid hemorrhage annually in North America make a functional recovery (7). In a recent publication, Roper and Zervas reported the outcome of a group of 112 patients, 94% of whom were grade I or II on admission (13). Only 46% recovered fully; 26% were impaired, 17% dependent and 11% were dead at the 1-year follow-up.

The largest contemporary study is the International Cooperative Study on the Timing of Aneurysm Surgery (CAS), the preliminary results of which were reported this year (6). The course of 3500 patients admitted within 3 days of their SAH were carefully recorded. Six-month follow-up evaluations revealed that a good recovery occurred in 58%, 9% were moderately disabled, 7% severely disabled and 26% were dead (Table 11.2). It should be emphasized that these patients were cared for on neurosurgical services with documented interest and expertise in managing SAH. A critical reviewer would conclude that little advance had been achieved in almost a decade. What is the explanation of these findings and what can we hope to achieve in the future?

TABLE 11.2

Cooperative Study on the
Timing of Aneurysm
Surgery: Overall Management
Results

	%
Good recovery	58
Moderately disabled	9
Severely disabled	5
Vegetative	2
Dead	26

Several recent studies have been carried out to determine the natural history of cerebral aneurysms and the outcome from SAH (5). A significant goal for the future must be the application of the data obtained from these various studies to the management of patients harboring cerebral aneurysms. Although most neurosurgeons concentrate their efforts on improving the operative techniques and patient management in the perioperative period, a truly major improvement in the statistics of aneurysms must come from additional changes in our approach. It is unlikely that marked improvement in surgical morbidity or mortality will be made in the next 10 years. For this period of time the microsurgical approach has come close to its maximum efficacy. We must direct our attentions in the next decade to dealing with aneurysms before they have produced a SAH.

In Ljunggren's study, poor outcome could be attributed to damage from the initial hemorrhage in 58%, damage from rebleeding in 14%, surgical trauma in 11%, and delayed ischemia in 11% (9). In the current Cooperative Aneurysm Study (CAS), 25% of the total case morbidity and mortality was due to the effects of the initial hemorrhage (Table 11.3). This represents a large group of patients that will not benefit from the resolution of the

TABLE 11.3

Cooperative Study on the Timing of Aneurysm Surgery:
Causes of Death and Disability (N = 3521)

	Death (%)	Disability (%)
Direct effect of SAH	27	22
Vasospasm	28	40
Rebleed	26	5
Surgical complications	5	12

questions of timing of aneurysm surgery or the treatment of CVS (6). To improve the outcome of this large subset of patients we must look elsewhere.

Fortunately, there is information available about the probability of SAH in patients with unruptured aneurysms. It would appear that they bleed at a rate of 1–2% per year (18). Although Wiebers *et al.* suggested that there was little likelihood of an asymptomatic aneurysm less than 1 cm bleeding, experience of most aneurysm surgeons and that reported in the literature indicates that the majority of aneurysms that do bleed are less than 1 cm (17). A review of 1092 ruptured aneurysms reported to the CAS from 1970–1977 revealed a mean diameter of 8.2 mm with 71% having a diameter of less than 10 mm and 13% less than 5 mm at the time of rupture (8). Since the morbidity and mortality rates for surgery of unruptured aneurysms is less than 5%, these lesions should be corrected before SAH occurs.

Several developments in imaging techniques are likely to be of great importance in the next decade for diagnosing aneurysms prior to hemorrhage. In addition to the discovery of an incidental aneurysm on a CT scan performed for other reasons, dynamic CT as part of a screening work-up for cerebrovascular disease will lead to more frequent diagnoses. The wide application of digital intravenous angiography will also improve on the yield although the resolution of this type of study is not sufficient for definitive diagnostic studies.

We may anticipate the application of magnetic resonance imaging (MRI) to the diagnosis of cerebral aneurysms. At the present time, blood vessels are easily identified by their lack of signal on MRI if the flow is fast; a change in signal intensity is seen if the flow is slower. An aneurysm of sufficient size is seen as a black hole or with low- and high-intensity signals depending upon the amount of turbulence or thrombus within the lumen. With the development of paramagnetic contrast agents or tagging of red cells it is possible that enhanced MRIs will become applicable to the diagnosis of aneurysms. The use of surface coils and thinner sections may also prove applicable for imaging the retro-orbital region.

What is clear from the studies mentioned is that the most dangerous aspect of a cerebral aneurysm is the initial hemorrhage, not the surgery or the perioperative period. The salvage of the 40% of patients whose deficit and death are related to the damage at the time of the initial SAH will reduce greatly the morbidity and mortality of SAH, more so than any gain made from changes in the timing of aneurysm surgery following SAH. Armed with newer diagnostic methods and the knowledge that cerebral aneurysms, even less than 1 cm, bleed at an average rate of 1–2% per year, there exists a very real opportunity in neurosurgery for preventive surgery. The development of less formidable and less interventional diagnostic studies will improve our chances of reducing the high risk of intracranial aneurysms.

Pope *et al.* have suggested that there may exist in some patients a systemic marker for the presence of cerebral aneurysms (10). It has long been observed that there is a higher incidence of aneurysms in patients with a variety of conditions such as polycystic kidney disease, coarctation of the aorta, and some connective tissue disorders. Pope noted a type III collagen deficiency in skin biopsies and cultured fibroblasts in seven of 12 patients with cerebral aneurysms. This is the same deficiency found in Ehlers-Danlos syndrome in which vascular fragility and aneurysms occur. This may point the way to defining the etiology of cerebral aneurysms and may prove to be a method for the early identification of individuals likely to develop cerebral aneurysms.

CEREBRAL VASOSPASM AND CALCIUM

The evolution of ideas about mechanisms of CVS has been a search for the etiologic factors and for the final common pathway of vascular smooth muscle contractility. Whatever the cause of CVS, be it blood breakdown products, neurotransmitters, or alterations in prostaglandin synthesis, treatment will require control of the final common pathway in which calcium plays a critical role. To this end, the most recent approach to CVS following SAH has been the use of calcium channel blockers. A large group of agents share the property of being able to block the "slow channel" passage of extracellular calcium through the depolarized smooth muscle membrane. The most promising of these agents are the dihydropyridines, which include such drugs as nifedipine, nimodipine, and nicardipine. An initial study of nimodipine has been reported and the results of an expanded trial are soon to be released (2). What is not apparent from this report is whether the effect of nimodipine was on cerebral vasospasm itself or whether the calcium blockers act by limiting the influx of calcium into ischemic cells, which initiate a cascade of events that lead to cell death. In the nimodipine study there was no difference in the incidence of vasospasm between the treatment and control groups, although the outcome in the patients receiving the calcium channel blocker was better. New York University and The University of Iowa recently have begun a trial of another parenteral dihydropyridine, nicardipine, for the prevention of CVS (16). Before assuming that the regulation of calcium operates only on vascular smooth muscle, we must characterize the calcium-mediated events that occur when calcium enters an impaired cellular membrane (15). These include changes in neuronal and glial regulatory mechanisms as well as the initiation of abnormal changes in basic cellular components such as prostaglandins, arachidonic acid, and its other metabolic pathways. It will be important to study CVS as part of an overall problem of cerebral ischemia and not as an isolated smooth muscle event (3).

One of the major outcomes of the CAS concerns the occurrence of CVS in relation to the day of surgery. CVS occurs at a relatively fixed rate following SAH and is neither increased nor decreased in incidence or severity by early surgery. What does appear to increase the incidence of ischemic events is the prolonged use of antifibrinolytic agents.

TIMING OF SURGICAL INTERVENTION

Although there has never been agreement among neurosurgeons about the best time to operate on cerebral aneurysms, a recycling of the idea of early intervention developed in the late 1970s because of growing dissatisfaction with the regimen of delayed surgery and its seemingly high rate of rebleeding and vasospasm. This renaissance of early surgery was prompted by reports of Sano, Suzuki, and others, who suggested that the case morbidity and mortality was not worse with early surgery (4, 14, 19). Furthermore, they suggested that the risk of rebleeding was reduced and the incidence of spasm was reduced, or at least no greater, than with delayed surgery.

In response to the unanswered questions raised by these papers, a multicenter international study was organized under the direction of Kassell (6). Although this was not a randomized study, it sought to define the relationship between the timing of surgery and outcome. All patients were admitted to the 68 participating centers within 3 days of SAH and were assigned an anticipated date for surgery. One of the major stimuli for this study was the long held view based upon the experience of the CAS carried out in the 1960s that the peak incidence of rebleeding occurred on the 7th day. Data from the current CAS suggests that this peak occurs within the first 24 hours and that there is no delayed peak. Since it is unlikely that most major centers will be able to operate on all patients with aneurysmal SAH within the first 24 hours, we may have to reconsider the idea that early surgery will significantly impact on eliminating rebleeding as a cause of death and disability.

A 6-month follow-up evaluation has been completed in 3521 patients admitted to the study. The results in two groups of patients have been compared—patients selected for surgery on day 0–3 (early group, N = 1595) and those patients in whom surgery was planned from days 7–14 (delayed group, N = 1055). A further analysis of the results based on the day that surgery was performed has also been completed. After correction for differences in risk factors between the two groups, certain conclusions were reached.

TABLE 11.4

Cooperative Study on the Timing of Aneurysm Surgery:
Adjusted Mortality Rates

	Planned Surgery	
Admission Status	0–3 days (N = 1595) (%)	7–14 days (N = 1055) (%)
Alert	11	14
Drowsy	25	29
Stuporous	39	38
Comatose	57	65
Overall	20	24

1. There was a small difference in the overall mortality between the early and delayed planned surgery groups, 20% versus 24% (Table 11.4). Mortality was lowest in the alert patients operated upon from days 10–15; between days 4 and 9 mortality was higher than in the early or delayed surgical groups of alert patients. No such trend was noted in the patients who were drowsy on admission; as a group they had a higher mortality rate than the alert patients (Table 11.5).

2. There was a modest difference in the overall favorable outcome between the early and delayed planned surgery groups, 62% versus 56% (Table 11.6). When good recovery was examined in relation to the day of surgery, the best results were seen in the alert patients operated upon at

TABLE 11.5

Mortality (%) at Six Months

	Pre-op Status	
Day of Surgery	Alert	Drowsy
0–1	5.9	21.9
2–3	9.5	19.0
4–5	12.6	22.1
6–7	10.0	20.9
8–9	10.7	18.4
10–11	5.0	13.8
12–13	3.5	22.2
14–15	1.3	20.0

154 CLINICAL NEUROSURGERY

TABLE 11.6

Cooperative Study on the Timing of Aneurysm Surgery:
Causes of Death and Disability

	Planned Surgery	
	0–3 days (N = 1595) (%)	7–14 days (N = 1055) (%)
Direct effect of SAH	8	8
Vasospasm	14	15
Rebleed	6	13
Surgical Complications	4	4

either extreme of the 2-week period. Drowsy patients had a lower good recovery rate regardless of the day of surgery (Table 11.7).

3. There was no difference between the two groups with regard to the causes of death and disability with the exception of rebleeding. Specifically the direct effect of the initial hemorrhage, the incidence of cerebral vasospasm, surgical complications, and hydrocephalus were the same in the two groups. Only rebleeding was greater (13% versus 6%) in the delayed surgery group (Table 11.8).

4. Delayed surgery does not appear to be as unfavorable nor does early surgery seem to be as favorable as might have been anticipated before the study.

TABLE 11.7

Good Recovery (%) at Six Months

	Pre-op Status	
Day of Surgery	Alert	Drowsy
0–1	83.8	57.3
2–3	78.9	56.3
4–5	72.5	63.2
6–7	81.4	58.1
8–9	72.1	63.3
10–11	82.3	69.0
12–13	84.3	63.0
14–15	85.7	40.0

TABLE 11.8

Cooperative Study on the Timing of Aneurysm Surgery:
Favorable Outcome-Adjusted

	Planned Surgery	
Admission Status	0–3 days (N = 1595) (%)	7–14 days (N = 1055) (%)
Alert	78	73
Drowsy	54	53
Stuporous	34	33
Comatose	13	21
Overall	62	56

5. While early surgery shows a trend toward reducing rebleeding, there was no reduction in ischemic deficits or other complications in this group.

6. The analysis for specific aneurysm locations has yet to be completed and may impact on the interpretation of these results.

An analysis of the cases based on the day of actual surgery revealed some interesting surgical observations and showed some outcome patterns which can stimulate discussion but not establish any firm guidelines for all surgeons and all patients. The participating surgeons were asked to report certain aspects of the operative procedure. As might have been expected, the brains of patients operated upon early were noted to be more swollen or "tight" than the delayed cases. In spite of this, there was no greater need for major resections at the time of early surgery than in the delayed cases. Furthermore, brain contusions and lacerations were no greater in these swollen brains. With regard to the aneurysms themselves, the degree of difficulty reported in performing the dissection was the same in both groups. Interestingly, leak or rupture of the aneurysm was not greater with earlier surgery. Clearly these findings indicate that for the experienced aneurysm surgeons involved in the study, the technical aspects of clipping an aneurysm was no more difficult soon after the SAH than when performed 7–14 days later, even though they reported more brain swelling in the early cases. One can conclude that technically early surgery does not pose any serious obstacles to its performance.

A MODEST PROPOSAL

If the information that we currently have is correct, that the peak incidence of aneurysmal rebleeding occurs within the first 24 hours of SAH, there is a less compelling argument for proposing surgery during the 2nd to 5th day after SAH. There is no known advantage to surgery during this time with regard to cerebral function, the occurrence of vasospasm, the technical aspects of surgery, or the outcome of patients operated during this period.

The CAS has also supplied us with information about the effectiveness of antifibrinolytic therapy. Epsilon aminocaproic acid (EACA) clearly reduces the incidence of rebleeding. This advantage, however, seems to be offset by an increased incidence of ischemic events. Our own experience at New York University with over 600 patients indicates that rebleeding from aneurysms occurs at a rate of 6.5% during the preoperative period of 2 weeks. One approach that may become possible is the combination of antifibrinolytic therapy and an appropriate calcium channel blocker if these agents are found to be consistantly effective in reducing CVS. It may be possible in the near future to limit both rebleeding as well as vasospasm to permit surgery to be carried out on a clinically appropriate rather than an arbitrary day. Although this is a speculative approach at the present time, it is possible that enough information may become available in the next few years to either test this hypothesis with a randomized trial or in a study similar to the current CAS.

NAIVE ASSUMPTIONS

During the course of investigations over the past few years, many "naive" assumptions have been formulated. Perhaps by dispelling these we may begin to see a new approach emerge that will enable us to plan future studies.

1. The reason to regulate calcium is related only to its role in the contraction of vascular smooth muscle. This ignores the many other effects of this ion on cellular homeostasis. The many studies in progress that deal with the involvement of calcium in the processes leading to cell death from ischemia will clarify this issue in the coming decade.

2. Aneurysms will always be a "neurosurgical" problem. The recent advances made in interventional neuroradiology will undoubtedly impact on our future management of cerebral aneurysms (12, 20). This, together with earlier diagnosis and understanding of the etiology and natural history of aneurysms, may drastically change the technical aspects of aneurysm surgery in the coming decade.

3. There is one day that is most appropriate for surgical intervention for ruptured cerebral aneurysms regardless of size, site, condition of the patient, and experience of the surgeon. I suspect that the only unanimous position that can be reached in this regard is that aneurysms should always be operated upon the day before they are going to bleed. Further

analysis of the CAS data may direct us away from the gross oversimplification that timing of surgery can be answered with a single number.

For the present time my own plan is to delay surgery for 10–14 days after SAH in those patients who are not admitted to our Center and fully evaluated by 48 hours, have aneurysms that will require dissection in critical areas of the brain, or are not truly grade I. During this preoperative period we will continue to utilize our SAH regimen which includes antifibrinolytic therapy, volume expansion, and a calcium channel blocker. Although the CAS data allow one to follow either course with regard to timing of surgery, one must remember that this is a multicenter study that has averaged many different variables and not shown a statistically significant result. The study does provide us with a reference standard, but we must each utilize it with full knowledge of the variations that exist among centers, surgeons, aneurysms, and patients.

REFERENCES

1. Adams, H. P., Jr., Kassell, N. F., Torner, J. C., Nibbelink, D. W., Sahs, A. L. Early management of aneurysmal subarachnoid hemorrhage. A report of the Cooperative Aneurysm Study. J. Neurosurg., 54: 141–145, 1981.
2. Allen, G. S., Ahn, H. S., Preziosi, T. J., et al. Cerebral arterial spasm-a controlled trial of nimodipine in patients with subarachnoid hemorrhage. N. Engl. J. Med., 308: 619–624, 1983.
3. Demopoulos, H., Seligman, M., Schwartz, M., Tomasula, J., Flamm, E. Molecular pathology of regional cerebral ischemia. In Cerebral Ischemia, edited by Bes, A., Braquet, P., Paoletti, R., Siesjo, B. K. Excerpta Medica, Amsterdam, 1984, pp. 259–264.
4. Hunt, W. E., Miller, C. A. The results of early operation for aneurysm. Clin. Neurosurg., 24: 208–215, 1977.
5. Jane, J. A., Kassell, N. F., Torner, J. C., Winn, H. R. The natural history of aneurysms and arteriovenous malformations. J. Neurosurg., 62: 321–323, 1985.
6. Kassell, N. F. Cooperative Study on Timing of Aneurysm Surgery. Presented at the Annual Meeting, American Association of Neurological Surgeons, Atlanta, GA, 23 April, 1985.
7. Kassell, N. F., Drake, C. G. Timing of aneurysm surgery. Neurosurgery, 10: 514–519, 1982.
8. Kassell, N. F., Torner, J. C. Size of intracranial aneurysms. Neurosurgery, 12: 291–297, 1983.
9. Ljunggren, B., Saeveland, H., Brandt, L., Uski, T. Aneurysmal subarachnoid hemorrhage. Total annual outcome in a 1.46 million population. Surg. Neurol., 22: 435–438, 1984.
10. Pope, F. M., Narcisi, P., Neil-Dwyer, G., Nicholls, A. C., Bartlett, J., Doshi, B. Some patients with cerebral aneurysms are deficient in type III collagen. Lancet 1: 973–975, 1981.
11. Post, K. D., Flamm, E. S., Goodgold, A., Ransohoff, J. Ruptured intracranial aneurysms. Case morbidity and mortality. J. Neurosurg., 46: 290–295, 1977.
12. Romodanov, A. P., Shchegolov, V. I. Intravascular occlusion of saccular aneurysms of the cerebral arteries by means of a detachable balloon catheter. Adv. Tech. Standards Neurosurg., 9: 25–49, 1982.
13. Roper, A. H., Zervas, N. T. Outcome 1 year after SAH from cerebral aneurysm. Management morbidity, mortality, and functional status in 112 consecutive good-risk patients. J. Neurosurg., 60: 909–915, 1984.

14. Saito, I., Ueda, Y., Sano, K. Significance of vasospasm in the treatment of ruptured intracranial aneurysms. J. Neurosurg., *47:* 412–429, 1977.
15. Schanne, F. A. X., Kane, A. B., Young, E. E., Farber, J. L. Calcium dependence of toxic cell death. A final common pathway. Science, *206:* 700–702, 1979.
16. Takenaka, T., Handa, J. Cerebrovascular effects of YC-93, a new vasodilator, in dogs, monkeys and human patients. Int. J. Clin. Pharmacol. Biopharm, *17:* 1–11, 1979.
17. Wiebers, D. O., Whisnant, J. P., O'Fallon, W. M. The natural history of unruptured intracranial aneurysms. N. Engl. J. Med., *304:* 696–698, 1981.
18. Winn, H. R., Almaani, W. S., Berga, S. L., Jane, J. A., Richardson, A. E. The long-term outcome in patients with multiple aneurysms. Incidence of late hemorrhage and implications for treatment of incidental aneurysms. J. Neurosurg., *59:* 642–651, 1983.
19. Yosimoto, T., Uchida, K., Kaneko, U., Kayama, U., Suzuki, J. An analysis of follow-up results of 1000 intracranial saccular aneurysms with definitive surgical treatment. J. Neurosurg., *50:* 152–157, 1979.
20. Zubkov, Y. N., Nikiforov, B. M., Shustin, V. A. Balloon catheter technique for dilatation of constricted cerebral arteries after aneurysmal SAH. Acta Neurochirurg., *70:* 65–79, 1984.

12

Timing of Aneurysm Surgery

BENGT LJUNGGREN, M.D., and LENNART BRANDT, M.D.

"There seems to be something wrong with our bloody ships"—Admiral of the glorious Royal Navy, Earl David Beatty's comment on the disastrous outcome of the Battle of Jutland May 31–June 1, 1916. British mortality was 6097 young sailors and German mortality was 2551 young sailors.

In 1926, Sosman and Vogt presented the first report on intracranial aneurysms from a roentgenologic viewpoint (61) and in the following year, Egas Moniz performed the first cerebral contrast arteriography (43). Five years later he was able for the first time to visualize an intracranial aneurysm with this revolutionary new method (42). The stage was now set for establishing the diagnosis of intracranial aneurysms and for considerations on their possible surgical treatment.

Mid 1930s

Though Norman Dott had performed carotid ligation in a few cases of internal carotid artery (ICA) aneurysm and had even performed a direct surgical attack in one patient with a rewarding result (9), the attitude of this time toward surgical treatment of intracranial aneurysms was probably well reflected by Wardner Ayer's statement from 1934: "Can surgery offer anything? The possibility of clipping off a small berry aneurysm on one of the communicating branches might be considered, but it would be a most formidable procedure and exceedingly dangerous and, the writer fears, impracticable" (6).

Mid 1940s

Up to 1938 Dott, Hermann, and Obrador had performed carotid ligation in a total of 12 cases of intracranial aneurysms with a 50% success rate, 25% morbidity, and 25% mortality (43).

Walter Dandy first clipped a nonruptured ICA aneurysm in 1937 (7) and in his pioneering monograph of 1944 added two more cases of ICA aneurysms successfully treated by direct application of silver clips across the aneurysm necks (8). In ten cases of carotid artery aneurysms operated upon with a trapping procedure, he reported 90% success rate.

Dandy had no successfully operated case of berry aneurysm originating from the middle cerebral artery (MCA) or from the anterior communicating artery (ACoA) segments. Concerning MCA aneurysms he concluded that, "These aneurysms are always so intimately connected with the main trunk of the artery that it may not be possible to cure them without sacrificing this artery, and such a result would be worse than death and there is, therefore, probably less likelihood of curing an MCA aneurysm, at least in leaving a useful citizen" (8). Concerning anterior cerebral (ACA)-ACoA aneurysms, Dandy concluded that, "Since both of the anterior cerebral arteries lie very closely together, the risk of operative treatment is very great." When considering posterior fossa aneurysms, he stated, "I know of no successful outcome from operative attack upon such an aneurysm, but for those on the vertebral and posterior cerebellar arteries, which afford good exposure, cures will certainly come in time" (8).

Mid 1950s

In the period 1945–1955 Sjöquist (60), Falconer (12–14), Hamby (18), and Norlén (45–47) among others showed that MCA and ACoA aneurysms could also be approached, wrapped in muscle, and sometimes even closed off. In 1953, Norlén and Olivecrona published a landmark paper (47) comprising a series of 63 patients subjected to intracranial aneurysm operation in the "free interval quiescent period," that is 3 weeks or more after rupture with a 3% mortality rate (neck ligation in 48, wrapping in eight, trapping in two, and exploration only in five patients). In 15 patients (nine ICA, four ACoA, and two MCA aneurysm) who had been operated upon "in the acute stage," that is, between a few hours and up to 3 weeks after hemorrhage (47), the mortality rate was 53% (eight patients) and the success rate 40% (six patients). The authors concluded that the prognosis of cerebral aneurysms once they have started to bleed is so serious that considerable surgical risk may be justified if the mortality attending the first attack of subarachnoid hemorrhage (SAH) can be materially reduced (47).

Later in the same year, Norlén and Barnum presented a study of 24 surgically treated ACoA aneurysm patients with a 17% mortality: two operative deaths and two subsequent deaths from SAH ascribed to what the authors considered an inadequate surgical procedure. In their summary, the authors concluded that because of the poor outlook of conservative therapy, ACoA aneurysms are best handled by a direct surgical approach with occlusion of the aneurysm neck by clip or ligature (46).

Mid 1960s

In this decade (1955–1965), an increasing number of neurosurgeons learned that by delaying all aneurysm surgery until the cerebral circulatory dysfunction induced by the SAH had subsided, the operative results could be considerably improved. Some distinguished aneurysm surgeons, however, expressed their view that there was no proof that surgical treatment of ruptured aneurysms at any time had effectively lowered the management mortality (40) and neurologists tended to be more or less polarized toward conservative treatment for intracranial aneurysm.

Nevertheless, a few pioneers advocated operation as soon as possible during the acute stage after bleed. At the Society Meeting of British Neurological Surgeons in 1957, a group of Manchester neurosurgeons suggested that subarachnoid blood clot could maintain narrowing of cerebral vessels and cause serious ischemia and this might be an indication for early surgery in an attempt to free the main vessels quite apart from treatment of the aneurysm itself (23). A few years later Pool (53, 54) and Hunt (19) advocated operation in the acute phase in patients in good condition and in 1965 Norlén, a master of ligation of the aneurysm stalk, declared that he had become more and more convinced that patients in good condition should be operated upon in the first and second day after the bleed to prevent the disastrous effects of rebleeding (48).

In 1962, Tappura reported that 55% of patients who had survived their initial bleed eventually rebled with a 75% mortality rate (67). It was furthermore realized that besides rebleeds, a capricious dysregulation of the cerebral blood flow (CBF), which could be visualized on angiography at some time after the bleed in terms of arterial narrowing and sluggish circulation—cerebral vasospasm—took a further heavy toll during the first weeks after SAH (1, 31). The complexity of the problem of aneurysmal SAH and its consequences became better recognized and it was realized that such factors as the severity of the hemorrhage (expressed in the clinical condition of the patient), the presence of angiographic vasospasm, aneurysm location and local anatomy, the patient's age, and the presence of associated disease had to be considered in the total equation. The increasing awareness of a relationship between the severity of the initial hemorrhage, as expressed in the clinical condition of the patient and the prognosis, inspired several authors to design grading systems. The Hunt and Hess grading system, first reported in 1962, has well become known among most neurosurgeons and has proven useful and reliable (19, 20). More complicated multivariate prognostic equations have also been calculated for estimating the probability of deterioration and death within the first weeks after the hemorrhage.

Mid 1970s

During the period 1965–1975, neurologists learned that neurosurgeons with proper criteria for aneurysm operation were rather successful in their surgical treatment of cerebral aneurysms at all locations. With the techniques and surgical adjuncts of this era, renewed attempts were made to operate upon good condition patients during the acute phase after rupture. The difficulties encountered and the disastrous operative results obtained (10), however, led to the general advice that postponing surgery till the ill effects of the primary bleed had subsided ("late" surgery) also was preferable for patients in a good condition in the acute stage.

Nevertheless, Norlén in 1975 was able to confirm his hypothesis that surgery in the acute phase was possible, and, in his hands, had led to encouraging results. Despite the fact that he had not used the microscope, he could report a series of 45 individuals subjected to aneurysm surgery within a week after a SAH with only a 4% operative mortality; 70% of the survivors reported full working capacity 1 year after the SAH (49).

In this time period increased attention was focused on personality changes and psychosocial dysfunction in patients without gross neurological sequelae after aneurysmal SAH. Several authors reported a deterioration of cognitive faculties and disturbances in the emotional adjustment of their patients following a major bleed (32, 39, 59).

Mid 1980s

In the time period from 1975 until today, characterized by absolutely optimized neuroanaesthetical conditions, the general exploitation of microsurgical techniques and the utilization of specially designed microsurgical instruments, cerebrovascular surgery budded as a subspeciality from general neurosurgery. All possible aspects of operative techniques, microsurgical neuroanatomy, and most other aspects of the management of patients with ruptured intracranial aneurysms were covered in excellent reviews, book chapters, and a number of well-written and beautifully illustrated volumes (16, 22, 30, 50, 52, 62, 69). Great experiences were gained in aneurysm surgery and the operative mortality was brought down to almost zero in "late" aneurysm repair, including such technically difficult lesions as giant and basilar apex aneurysms. There was no longer any debate concerning the advantages of surgical treatment versus conservative management, whereas timing of the operative procedure remained controversial. Yet, during this period (21, 28, 29, 56, 57, 63) and especially in the last years (5, 25, 33, 41, 66, 68) increasing evidence indicated favorable results in a substantial series of patients subjected to "early" surgery, *i.e.*, within the first 48 or 72 hours after hemorrhage.

Distinguished neurosurgeons cautioned that most colleagues "only see the top of the iceberg," that is, are not confronted with the very many acutely devastated individuals who never reach the primary center. Thus, statistics from North America reported in 1982 showed that only approximately 36% of all individuals struck by aneurysmal SAH could be expected to become functional survivors (26). The opinion was increasingly expressed that results of different management regimes, especially with regard to timing of the operative procedure, should be expressed in terms of total outcome in well-defined populations or, although less preferable, in terms of overall management outcome, rather than as personal results in selected series of operated cases (37). A major impediment in assessing the overall efficacy of different treatment regimes is the lack of comparability in such clinical studies due to differences in the time interval from SAH to referral. Arguments were put forward that functional morbidity in terms of cognitive dysfunction and psychosocial disturbances should be incorporated in the final outcome assessment (4, 38, 55, 64).

TIMING OF THE OPERATIVE PROCEDURE

Eugene Flamm and Jack Fein in *"Cerebrovascular Surgery"* published in 1985 have put forward many arguments for delaying surgical intervention of the ruptured aneurysm (15). Comments regarding those arguments are provided in the following section.

Timing and Outcome

ARGUMENT

Much better results are obtained when surgery is delayed for 2 weeks (15).

COMMENT

In a consecutive series of patients with a ruptured aneurysm of the anterior part of the circle of Willis, referred to the neurosurgical clinic in Lund between June 1976 and August 1980, early intracranial operation (within 3 days post-SAH) was performed in 81 patients in neurological grades I–III according to the classification of Hunt and Hess (20). A comparison was made between the outcome for the patients receiving early operation and another group of patients who would have fulfilled our criteria for such an operation (grade I–III within 48 hours post-SAH) but who were not operated upon early (33). The comparison indicates that early operation that resulted in 74% good neurological recoveries, 10% morbidity, and 16% mortality was superior to delayed treatment, which resulted in 56% good neurological recoveries, 18% morbidity, and 26% mortality (Table 12.1). The latter outcome corresponds well with the report of Kassell and coauthors (24) for patients grades I–III on early admission (within 3 days), who were subjected to late surgery (no sooner than 12 days postictus) (Table 12.1). Early operations in 85 recent Grade I–III patients combined with continuous intravenous nimodipine resulted in

TABLE 12.1

Outcome for Grade I–III Patients with Early Operation for Ruptured Supratentorial Aneurysm versus Outcome for Comparable Patients Not Subjected to Early Surgery

	Early Surgery		Late Surgery	
			Fulfilled	Fulfilled
	Without	With	criteria for	criteria for
Outcome	nimodipine*	nimodipine	early operation*	early operation**
Good physical recovery (%)	74%	79%	56%	51%
Morbidity (%)	10%	15%	18%	22%
Mortality (%)	16%	6%	26%	27%
Total patients	81	85	55	190

* From: Ljunggren B, Brandt L, Kågström E, et al: Results of early operations for ruptured aneurysms. *J Neurosurg* 54:473–479, 1981.

** From: Kassell NF, Adams HP Jr, Torner JC, et al: Influence of timing of admission after aneurysmal subarachnoid hemorrhage on overall outcome: report of the cooperative aneurysm study. *Stroke* 12:620–623, 1981.

79% good neurological recoveries, 15% morbidity, and 6% mortality. In conclusion, these results (Table 12.1) favor the opinion that the overall outcome for grade I to III patients is improved by early operation as compared to delayed surgery. Concerning the important question of timing and total outcome, 41% of all our identified individuals struck by aneurysmal SAH made a good neurological recovery, while the total physical morbidity was 22%, and the total mortality was 37% (64). Comparable total outcome results have hitherto not been given in the literature supporting late surgery.

Timing and Cerebral Vasospasm

ARGUMENT

A strong argument can be made for delaying surgical intervention to reduce the morbidity and mortality associated with cerebral vasospasm (15). Vessel manipulation is required in early surgery to remove the blood undoubtedly contributing to vasoconstriction and may increase the risk of significant ischemic complications (15). Surgery during the acute stage after SAH may precipitate cerebral vasospasm and cerebral dysfunction of immediate or delayed onset (11).

COMMENT

Within a series of 100 consecutive individuals who were subjected to early aneurysm repair (64 patients were in preoperative Hunt and Hess neurological grades I–II, 21 were in grade III, and 15 subjects were in a poor condition, *i.e.*, equivalent to grades IV–V), the incidence of delayed ischemic dysfunction (DID) with permanent or fixed neurological damage (FND) was 5% (65). This low incidence of DID with FND certainly does not support the above concept that early surgery increases the risk of significant ischemic complications, but rather supports the opinion that clipping during the acute stage combined with evacuation of clots and blood-contaminated cerebrospinal fluid (CSF) containing a hell-broth of vasoconstrictive factors, combined with subsequent nimodipine administration, results in a significant reduction of delayed cerebral ischemic deterioration.

Timing and Treatment with Calcium Channel Blockers

ARGUMENT

The beneficial effects of calcium channel blockers in human vasospasm are still unproven (15).

COMMENT

This argument is indisputable. Nevertheless, during the last years, several studies have emerged indicating that treatment with the calcium channel blocker nimodipine significantly reduces the incidence of ischemic cerebral dysfunction associated with delayed SAH-induced reduction of CBF (vasospasm) (2, 3, 5, 35, 44, 51, 65). Furthermore, results of a multicenter, double-blind placebo-controlled study of patients with acute ischemic stroke showed a protective anti-ischemic cerebral effect of nimodipine with a significantly improved outcome (17). Assessment of the time course of cerebrovascular spasm with transcranial Doppler sonography has revealed that intravenous nimodipine treatment (2 mg per hour) in high risk patients with aneurysmal SAH (clinical grade III or worse and thick layers of cisternal blood on computerized tomography) reduces the severity of increased blood flow velocity (BFV) post-SAH; such increases of BFV in turn show a clear correlation to cerebral arterial constriction post-SAH (58). We found a markedly lowered incidence of DID with FND. In fact, in 61 recent ICA and MCA aneurysm patients (all grades) with early operation and intravenous nimodipine, none showed DID with FND (Table 12.2) (65). Early aneurysm operation furthermore permits a more aggressive anti-ischemic treatment of whatever type.

Timing and Surgical Trauma

ARGUMENT

The extravasated blood in the subarachnoid cisterns is more adherent to the vessels in the acute stage and tends to obscure the smaller perforating

TABLE 12.2

Early Aneurysm Operation without and with Nimodipine: Incidence of Delayed Ischemic Dysfunction (DID) with Fixed Neurological Deficit (FND) in Patients with Ruptured ICA and MCA Aneurysms in Relation to Preoperative Grade (Hunt & Hess Neurological Classification)

	Without Nimodipine		With Nimodipine	
	No. of Patients	DID with FND	No. of Patients	DID with FND
Grade I	23	1	9	0
Grade II	34	5	28	0
Grade III	19	6	13	0
Grades IV–V			11	0
Total	76	12 (16%)	61	0 (0%)

vessels (15). The brains are more swollen, soft, hyperemic, and prone to contusion and laceration during the acute stage when autoregulation is also impaired (27). The toll from the inevitable bruising of pial banks and injury to small vessels, particularly veins, that accompanies even the most gentle attempts to mechanically remove clot from the subarachnoid space must be considered (27).

COMMENT

Acute stage surgery usually permits evacuation of significant amounts of blood-contaminated CSF and with all probability facilitates and promotes a normalized CSF circulation and washout of vasoconstrictor material. Without doubt the surgical complications are higher with early (34) rather than with late aneurysm repair. Nevertheless, the decreased incidence of rebleeding and facilitation of the management of vasospasm is certainly worth this price and, apparently, early operation results in a lower overall unfavorable outcome. The expected outcome with delayed surgical intervention in our most recent series of 100 individuals, who were subjected to early operation and subsequent nimodipine infusion, would thus most certainly have been less favorable than the 7% management mortality and 22% management morbidity that was achieved (Table 12.3).

Timing and Intraoperative Aneurysm Rupture

ARGUMENT

The aneurysm is more friable and likely to rupture in acute stage operations (15).

TABLE 12.3

Site of Ruptured Aneurysm and Outcome in 100 Individuals (85 Grades I–III; 15 Grades IV–V) with Early Operation and Intravenous Nimodipine

| Outcome | Aneurysm Location | | | |
	Anterior Cerebral Artery Complex (ACA)	Internal Carotid Artery Complex (ICA)	Middle Cerebral Artery (MCA)	Total
Good recovery	24	23	24	71
Morbidity	10	5	7	22
Mortality	5	1	1	7
Total	39	29	32	100

COMMENT

In the above cited series of 100 individuals subjected to early operation the overall incidence of intraoperative aneurysm leak or bleed prior to occlusion was 25%. As shown in Table 12.4, MCA aneurysms were more prone to leak or rupture, while one out of four aneurysms originating from the ACoA or anterior cerebral arteries ruptured, and ICA aneurysms did not usually rupture. Intraoperative aneurysm bleeding during early operation certainly represents a complication, yet, as seen in Table 12.5, is not as a rule associated with an unfavorable outcome in any location.

Timing and Aneurysm Location and Preoperative Grade

ARGUMENT

It is possible that early surgery for relatively easy aneurysms of the carotid artery can be carried out without problems, but it is a different matter when dealing with ACoA, MCA, and basilar artery aneurysms (15).

TABLE 12.4

Incidence of Intraoperative Aneurysm Rupture or Leak in 100 Individuals with Early Operation and Intravenous Nimodipine

	Incidence	Percentage
Anterior cerebral artery complex (ACA)	11/39	28
Internal carotid artery complex (ICA)	1/29	3
Middle cerebral artery (MCA)	13/32	41
Total	25/100	25

TABLE 12.5

Incidence of Intraoperative Aneurysm Rupture and Relation to Outcome in 100 Consecutive Individuals with Early Aneurysm Operation and Intravenous Nimodipine

	Good Recovery No.	Unfavorable Outcome No.	Total No.
Anterior cerebral artery complex (39 cases) (ACA) — Nonrupture	18	10	28
— Intraoperative rupture	6	5	11 (28%)
Internal carotid artery complex (29 cases) (ICA) — Nonrupture	22	6	28
— Intraoperative rupture	1		1 (3%)
Middle cerebral artery (MCA) (32 cases) — Nonrupture	17	2	19
— Intraoperative rupture	7	6*	13 (41%)
Total	71	29	100 (25%) 25

* Of 6 MCAs with intraoperative rupture and unfavorable outcome, four individuals were preoperatively in poor condition (grades IV–V).

TABLE 12.6

Outcome in Relation to Preoperative Grade (Hunt & Hess) without (−) and with (+) Intraoperative Aneurysm Rupture

	Preoperative Grade							
	Grades I to II		Grade III		Grades IV to V		Total	
Outcome	−	+	−	+	−	+	−	+
ACA								
Good physical recovery	16	6	2	0	0	0	18	6
Unfavorable result	4	1	5	1	1	3	10	5
Total	20	7	7	1	1	3	28	11
ICA								
Good physical recovery	17	1	4	0	1	0	22	1
Unfavorable result	3	0	3	0	0	0	6	0
Total	20	1	7	0	1	0	28	1
MCA								
Good physical recovery	12	3	3	3	2	1	17	7
Unfavorable result	0	1	0	0	2	5	2	6
Total	12	4	3	3	4	6	19	13

Our series outcome with early surgery in relation to aneurysm location, intraoperative rupture, and preoperative grade is given in Table 12.6. Table 12.7 summarizes the final outcome in relation to the preoperative grade. From these results, we conclude that good-risk patients (grades I–II) with a ruptured supratentorial aneurysm should be operated on without unnecessary delay; grade III ICA and MCA aneurysm patients and younger individuals with such lesions who are in a poor condition (grades IV–V) may also benefit from this approach. It remains unproven whether grade III ACoA aneurysm patients should be subjected to early repair.

Timing and Functional Morbidity

ARGUMENT

The results of surgery must take into account long-range follow-up of neurological and psychological functioning, which is not discussed in the literature that advocates early surgery (15).

COMMENT

A recent study of all our patients during 1 year with a major aneurysmal SAH revealed that none of the survivors was left completely unaffected in terms of the remaining effects on psychosocial or cognitive status (64). When functional morbidity, in terms of persistent severe cognitive/psychosocial impairment, was included in the outcome assessment, the overall favorable outcome was decreased from 41 to 33% (64). It remains unproven whether early aneurysm operation precipitates later psychosocial and cognitive disturbances and results in an unacceptable functional morbidity. Results reported by Ropper and Zervas in patients not subjected to

TABLE 12.7

Preoperative Neurological Grade (Hunt & Hess) and Outcome in 100 Individuals with Early Operation and Nimodipine

| Preoperative Grade | Final Outcome | | | | | Success Rate |
	Good Recovery	Fair Result	Poor Result	Dead	Total	
Grade I	13		1		14	93%
Grade II	41	5	3	1	50	82%
Grade III	13	2	2	4	21	62%
Grades IV–V	4	4	5	2	15	27%
Total	71	11	11	7	100	71%

early surgery, however, indicated that psychosocial or emotional disturbances also were frequent in such patients (55). Thus, these authors found
a large proportion of individuals who were unable to resume their previous level of performance due to reported psychological or emotional
disturbances. These findings only point to the fact that aneurysmal SAH is
a catastrophic event from which few patients recover without sequelae
(4, 55).

Should younger, previously healthy individuals, who arrive in a moribund appearance, with a large intracerebral temporal hemorrhage (CT
finding) probably originating from a ruptured MCA aneurysm, be subjected
to surgery (evacuation of hematoma, cisternal washout, and clipping of
aneurysm) without preoperative angiography? Lives may be saved if such
patients are treated as top-priority surgical emergency cases in a fashion
similar to neurosurgeons who treat a rapidly deteriorating individual with
a suspected epidural hematoma after trauma. This interesting question has
so far not been discussed in the literature of aneurysm management.

Timing and Surgical Experience

It has been argued that a surgeon who performs relatively few aneurysm
operations but achieves excellent results with delayed surgery may have
considerably more difficulty in the acute situation. This certainly seems
true. In our opinion, however, aneurysm operations should always be carried out at centers with access to experienced aneurysm surgeons, *i.e.*, so
that shortage of experience does not become a factor that influences
timing of the operative procedure.

Timing and Hydrocephalus

In our opinion, early surgery with washout of clots and blood-contaminated CSF and sharp dissection of the arachnoid results in a lowered
incidence of hydrocephalus, or small likelihood in early operated grade I–
III cases (33, 34, 68).

Timing and Basilar Aneurysms

So far, no substantial series of patients subjected to early surgery for
ruptured basilar aneurysms have been reported in the literature. Favorable
results have, however, been reported with early surgical intervention in
occasional cases (5).

Timing and Giant Aneurysms

Favorable results following early surgery for ruptured giant MCA aneurysms have been reported (35, 36). It should be emphasized that temporary

clipping of the middle cerebral artery trunk, often a prerequisite in such surgery, appears to be well tolerated in early aneurysm operations (36).

Timing and Economy

Early surgery is accompanied by a markedly shortened hospital stay. Our patients with early surgery spent less than half the time in the hospital as compared to patients subjected to late surgery (33).

Timing and Medical Complications

Early surgery not only reduces bedrest but also results in significantly lowered incidence of medical complications.

EPICRISIS

Despite the marked differences in losses at the Battle of Jutland, it still remains controversial which side won the battle. There is, however, no doubt that a fateful failure to pass vital intelligence to Earl Beatty from the British Admiralty heavily contributed to the severe British losses. In our opinion, there is now vital information supporting the concept that early surgery in good risk patients (grades I–II) and in grade III patients with ruptured ICA or MCA aneurysms results in decreased losses compared to delaying the operation in such patients. Younger poor risk patients with ICA and MCA aneurysms also may benefit from early surgery. The neurosurgeon who remains an advocator of late surgery in such individuals may have reason to accuse himself in the words of Earl David Beatty: "There seems to be something wrong with my bloody aneurysm management today."

Regardless of the timing of aneurysm repair, aneurysmal SAH remains a most devastating disease. Despite the fact that early surgical intervention combined with anti-ischemic treatment with nimodipine has reduced the incidence of delayed ischemic deterioration with permanent deficit to only a few percent, not more than one out of three individuals struck by aneurysm rupture is prone to make a satisfactory physical and functional recovery. Future improvements in the outcome for patients harboring an intracranial aneurysm may depend upon improved devices to detect these most treacherous lesions before they rupture with all the severe consequences that are induced by the hemorrhage.

ACKNOWLEDGMENTS

Supported by grants from Thorsten and Elsa Segerfalk's Foundation for Medical Research and Education and from the Swedish Society of Medicine.

REFERENCES

1. Allcock, J. M., and Drake, C. G. Ruptured intracranial aneurysms. The role of arterial spasm. J. Neurosurg., *21:* 21–29, 1965.
2. Allen, G. S., Ahn, H. S., Preziosi, T. J., Battye, R., Boone, S. C., Chou, S. N., Kelly, D. L., Weir, B. K., Crabbe, R. A., Lavik, P. J., Rosenbloom, S. B., Dorsey, F. C., Ingram, C. R., Mellits, D. E., Bertsch, L. A., Boisvert, D. P. J., Hundley, M. B., Johnson, R. K., Strom, Jo. A., and Transou, C. R. Cerebral arterial spasm—a controlled trial of nimodipine in patients with subarachnoid hemorrhage. N. Engl. J. Med., *308:* 619–624, 1983.
3. Allen, G. S. Results of three dose multicenter randomized double blind nimodipine study. Presented at Subarachnoid hemorrhage investigator's meeting, Monterey, California, May 1985.
4. Artiola I Fortuny, L., Prieto-Valiente, L. Long-term prognosis in surgically treated intracranial aneurysms. Part 2: Morbidity. J. Neurosurg., *54:* 35–43, 1981.
5. Auer, L. M. Acute operation and preventive nimodipine improve outcome in patients with ruptured cerebral aneurysms. Neurosurgery, *15:* 57–66, 1985.
6. Ayer, W. D. So-called spontaneous subarachnoid hemorrhage. A resume with its medico-legal consideration. Am. J. Surg., *26:* 143–151, 1934.
7. Dandy, W. E. Intracranial aneurysm of internal carotid artery, cured by operation. Ann. Surg., *107:* 654–659, 1938.
8. Dandy, W. E. *Intracranial Arterial Aneurysms*, 147 pp. Comstock Publ. Co., New York/London, 1944.
9. Dott, N. M. Intracranial aneurysms: cerebral arterio-radiography: surgical treatment. Edin. Med. J., *40:* 219–240, 1933.
10. Drake, C. G. Discussion of Symon, L: Vasospasm in aneurysm. Presented at the 7th Princeton Conference, 1970; Grune & Stratton, New York, pp. 241–244, 1971.
11. Drake, C. G. On the surgical treatment of intracranial aneurysms. Ann. R. Coll. Phys. Surg. Can., *11:* 185–195, 1978.
12. Falconer, M. A. Surgical treatment of spontaneous subarachnoid haemorrhage. Preliminary report. Br. Med. J., *1:* 809–813, 1950.
13. Falconer, M. A. The surgical treatment of bleeding intracranial aneurysms. J. Neurol. Neurosurg. Psychiatr., *14:* 153–187, 1951.
14. Falconer, M. A. Surgical pathology of spontaneous intracranial haemorrhage due to aneurysms and arteriovenous malformations. Proc. Roy. Soc. Med., *47:* 693–700, 1954.
15. Fein, J., and Flamm, E. *Cerebrovascular Surgery*, Vol. I, 295 pp; Vol. II, 606 pp; Vol. III, 465 pp (pp 766–768; 779); Vol. IV, 251 pp. Springer Verlag, New York-Berlin-Heidelberg-Vienna-Tokyo, 1985.
16. Fox, J. L. *Intracranial Aneurysms*, Vol. I, 603 pp.; Vol. II, 498 pp.; Vol. III (appendices), 360 pp. Springer Verlag, Berlin-Heidelberg-New York-Tokyo, 1983.
17. Gelmers, H. J., Gorter, K., de Weerdt, C. J., and Wiezer, J. H. A. Effect of nimodipine on neurological deficits and outcome of patients with acute ischemic stroke: results of a multicenter double blind placebo controlled study. Presented at the XIIIth World Congress of Neurology, Hamburg, FR Germany, September 1985.
18. Hamby, W. B. *Intracranial Aneurysms*, 360 pp. Charles C. Thomas, Springfield, Illinois, 1952.
19. Hunt, W. E., Meagher, J. N., and Barnes, J. E. The management of intracranial aneurysm. J. Neurosurg., *19:* 34–40, 1962.
20. Hunt, W. E., and Hess, R. M. Surgical risk as related to time of intervention in the repair of intracranial aneurysms. J. Neurosurg., *28:* 14–20, 1968.

21. Hunt, W. E., and Miller, C. A. The results of early operation for aneurysm. Clin. Neurosurg., *24:* 208–215, 1977.
22. Ito, Z. *Atlas on Microsurgery of Cerebral Aneurysms,* 350 pp. Excerpta Medica, Amsterdam, the Netherlands, 1982.
23. Johnson, R. J., Potter, J. M., and Reid, R. G. Arterial spasm in subarachnoid haemorrhage: mechanical considerations. J. Neurol. Neurosurg. Psychiatr., *21:* 68, 1958.
24. Kassell, N. F., Adams, H. P. Jr., Torner, J. C., and Sahs, A. L. Influence of timing of admission after aneurysmal subarachnoid hemorrhage on overall outcome: report of the cooperative aneurysm study. Stroke, *12:* 620–623, 1981.
25. Kassell, N. F., Boarini, D. J., Adams, H. P., Sahs, A. L., Graf, C. J., Torner, J. C., and Gerk, M. K. Overall management of ruptured aneurysm: comparison of early and late operation. Neurosurgery, *9:* 120–128, 1981.
26. Kassell, N. F., and Drake, C. G. Timing of aneurysm surgery. Neurosurgery, *10:* 514–519, 1982.
27. Kassell, N. F. Discussion of Ljunggren, B., Säveland, H., and Brandt, L. Causes of unfavorable outcome after early aneurysm operation. Neurosurgery, *13:* 633, 1983.
28. Kikuchi, H., Furuse, S., and Karasawa, J. Microsurgery of cerebral aneurysm in acute phase (within 1 week after subarachnoid hemorrhage). *In Clinical Microneurosurgery,* edited by W. Th. Koos, F. W. Böck, and R. F. Spetzler, pp. 202–203. George Thieme Publ., Stuttgart, 1976.
29. Kobayashi, K., Okada, K., Tanimura, K., and Nakai, O. A follow-up study of the patients with ruptured aneurysms submitted to the microsurgery within one week. No Shinkey Geka (Japan), *7:* 661–668, 1979.
30. Koos, W. T., Spetzler, R. F., Pendl, G., Perneczky, A., and Lang, J. *Color Atlas of Microneurosurgery,* 420 pp. (pp. 302–352). Thieme-Stratton Inc, New York, 1985.
31. Kågström, E., Greitz, T., Hanson, J., et al. Changes in cerebral blood flow after subarachnoid hemorrhage. Presented at the 3rd International Congress of Neurological Surgery, Copenhagen, Denmark, 1965. In: Excerpta Medica Int. Congr. Series, Amsterdam, *110:* 629–633, 1966.
32. Lindqvist, G., and Norlén, G. Korsakoff's syndrome after operation on ruptured aneurysm of the anterior communicating artery. Acta Psychiatr. Scand., *42:* 24–34, 1966.
33. Ljunggren, B., Brandt, L., Kågström, E., and Sundbärg, G. Results of early operations for ruptured aneurysms. J. Neurosurg., *54:* 473–479, 1981.
34. Ljunggren, B., Säveland, H., and Brandt, L. Causes of unfavorable outcome after early aneurysm operation. Neurosurgery, *13:* 629–633, 1983.
35. Ljunggren, B., Brandt, L., Säveland, H., Nilsson, P-E., Cronqvist, S., Andersson, K-E., and Vinge, E. Outcome in 60 consecutive patients treated with early aneurysm operation and intravenous nimodipine. J. Neurosurg., *61:* 864–873, 1984.
36. Ljunggren, B., Säveland, H., and Brandt, L. Tolerance of temporary arterial occlusion in early aneurysm surgery. *In Cerebral Vascular Spasm,* edited by D. Voth and P. Glees, pp. 421–437. Walter de Gruyter, Berlin-New York, 1985.
37. Ljunggren, B., Säveland, H., Brandt, L., and Zygmunt, S. Early operation and overall outcome in aneurysmal subarachnoid hemorrhage. J. Neurosurg., *62:* 547–551, 1985.
38. Ljunggren, B., Sonesson, B., Säveland, H., and Brandt, L. Cognitive impairment and adjustment in patients without neurological deficits after aneurysmal SAH and early operation. J. Neurosurg., *62:* 673–679, 1985.
39. Logue, V., Durward, M., Pratt, R. T. C., et al: The quality of survival after rupture of an anterior cerebral aneurysm. Br. J. Psychiatr., *114:* 137–160, 1968.
40. McKissock, W., Paine, K. W. E., and Walsh, L. S. An analysis of the results of treatment of

174 CLINICAL NEUROSURGERY

ruptured intracranial aneurysms. Report of 772 consecutive cases. J. Neurosurg., *17:* 762–776, 1960.
41. Mizukami, M., Kawase, T., Usami, T., and Tazawa, T. Prevention of vasospasm by early operation with removal of subarachnoid blood. Neurosurgery, *10:* 301–307, 1982.
42. Moniz, E. Anevrysme intra-cranien de la carotide inferne droite rendu visible par l'arteriographie cerebrale. Rev. Oto-Neuro-Ophtal., *11:* 746–748, 1933.
43. Moniz, E. *Die Cerebrale Arteriographie und Phlebographie*, 413 pp. Springer Verlag, Berlin, 1940.
44. Neil-Dwyer, G. A controlled study of nimodipine in subarachnoid haemorrhage patients. Presented at the XIIIth World Congress of Neurology, Hamburg, FR Germany, September 1985.
45. Norlén, G. The pathology, diagnosis and treatment of intracranial saccular aneurysms. Proc. Soc. Royal Soc. Med. (London), *45:* 291–302, 1952.
46. Norlén, G., and Barnum, A. S. Surgical treatment of aneurysms of the anterior communicating artery. J. Neurosurg., *10:* 634–650, 1953.
47. Norlén, G., and Olivecrona, H. The treatment of aneurysms of the circle of Willis. J. Neurosurg., *10:* 404–415, 1953.
48. Norlén, G. Some aspects of the surgical treatment of intracranial aneurysms. Neurol. Med. Chir. (Tokyo), *7:* 14–27, 1965.
49. Norlén, G. Experiences with intracranial aneurysm surgery: results in early operations. Presented at XVI Congreso Latino-Americano de Neurocirurgia, Caracas, Venezuela, October 1975. In: Actas y Trabajos pp 235–245.
50. Ojemann, R. G., and Crowell, R. M. *Surgical Management of Cerebrovascular Disease*, 316 pp. (pp. 128–254). Williams & Wilkins, Baltimore-London, 1983.
51. Philippon, J. A., and Gross, R. A double blind trial of calcium entry blocker in the prevention of ischemic neurological deficits in subarachnoid haemorrhage patients. Presented at the XIIIth World Congress of Neurology, Hamburg, FR Germany, September 1985.
52. Poletti, C. E., and Ojemann, R. G. *Stereo Atlas of Operative Neurosurgery*, 350 pp. (pp. 16–39, 50–69, 106–119, 122–125, 146–151). C. V. Mosby, St. Louis-Toronto-Princeton, 1985.
53. Pool, J. L. Early treatment of ruptured intracranial aneurysms of the circle of Willis with special clip techniques. Bull. N.Y. Acad. Med., *35:* 357–369, 1959.
54. Pool, J. L. timing and techniques in the intracranial surgery of ruptured aneurysms of the anterior communicating artery. J. Neurosurg., *19:* 378–388, 1962.
55. Ropper, A. H., and Zervas, N. T. Outcome 1 year after SAH from cerebral aneurysm. Management morbidity, mortality, and functional status in 112 consecutive good-risk patients. J. Neurosurg., *60:* 909–915, 1984.
56. Samson, D. S., Hodosh, R. M., Reid, W. R., et al: Risk of intracranial aneurysm surgery in the good grade patient: early versus late operation. Neurosurgery, *5:* 422–426, 1979.
57. Sano, K., and Saito, I. Timing and indication of surgery for ruptured intracranial aneurysms with regard to cerebral vasospasm. Acta Neurochir., *41:* 49–60, 1978.
58. Seiler, R. W., Grolimund, P., Zurbrügg, H. R., and Reulen, H-J. Evaluation of the efficacy of nimodipine for the prevention of cerebral vasospasm following subarachnoid hemorrhage by transcranial Doppler sonography. Presented at the Satellite Symposium of the XIIIth World Congress of Neurology, Aachen, FR Germany, August 30–September 1, 1985.
59. Sengupta, R. P., Chiu, J. S., and Brierley, H. Quality of survival following direct surgery for anterior communicating artery aneurysms. J. Neurosurg., *43:* 58–64, 1975.

60. Sjöquist, O. Threat ligature of intracranial saccular aneurysms. Presented at the 5th Congress of Neurology, Lisboa, Portugal, *3:* 108–115, 1953.
61. Sosman, M. C., and Vogt, E. C. Aneurysms of the internal carotid artery and the circle of Willis, from a roentgenological viewpoint. *AJR, 15:* 122–134, 1926.
62. Sugita, K. *Microneurosurgical Atlas,* 274 pp. Springer Verlag, Berlin-Heidelberg-New York-Tokyo, 1985.
63. Suzuki, J., Yoshimoto, T., and Onuma, T. Early operations for ruptured intracranial aneurysms—a study of 31 cases operated on within the first four days after ruptured aneurysm. Neurol. Med. Chir. (Tokyo), *18:* 82–89, 1978.
64. Säveland, H., Sonesson, B., Ljunggren, B., Brandt, L., Uski, T., Zygmunt, S., and Hindfelt, B. Outcome evaluation of subarachnoid hemorrhage. J. Neurosurg., in press, 1985.
65. Säveland, H., Ljunggren, B., Brandt, L., and Messeter, K. Delayed ischemic deterioration in patients with early aneurysm operation and intravenous nimodipine. Neurosurgery, submitted 1985.
66. Taneda, M. Effect of early operation for ruptured aneurysms on prevention of delayed ischemic symptoms. J. Neurosurg., *57:* 622–628, 1982.
67. Tappura, M. Prognosis of subarachnoid haemorrhage. A study of 120 patients with unoperated intracranial arterial aneurysms and 267 patients without vascular lesions demonstrable in bilateral carotid angiograms. Acta Med. Scand. Suppl., *392:* 1–75, 1962.
68. Vapalahti, M., Ljunggren, B., Säveland, H., Hernesniemi, J., Brandt, L., and Tapaninaho, A. Early aneurysm operation and outcome in two remote Scandinavian populations. J. Neurosurg., *60:* 1160–1162, 1984.
69. Yasargil, M. G. *Microneurosurgery,* Vol. 1, pp. 1–371; Vol. 2, pp. 1–386. Thieme Stratton Inc., New York, 1984.

13

Management of Unruptured Cerebral Arteriovenous Malformations

MICHAEL J. AMINOFF, M.D., F.R.C.P.

INTRODUCTION

Cerebral arteriovenous malformations (AVMs) may become symptomatic in patients of any age and sex. AVMs are located supratentorially in at least 70% of cases, usually in the territory of the middle cerebral artery. Clinical presentation may be with subarachnoid or intracerebral hemorrhage, seizures, focal neurologic deficits, headache, or miscellaneous disturbances including hydrocephalus, increased intracranial pressure, and heart failure (Table 13.1). Differences between published series of cases in the proportion of patients presenting in these various ways must relate, at least in part, to differences in referral sources. A higher incidence of hemorrhage is to be expected among patients referred to neurosurgical units. Hemorrhage ultimately occurs in at least 50% of symptomatic cases, and once a hemorrhage has occurred, the risk of further bleeding is increased, although the extent and timing of subsequent bleeds cannot be predicted with any confidence. It is likely, nevertheless, that the true incidence of hemorrhage is underestimated since bleeding, as determined at operation, may be subclinical or produce only a minor exacerbation of a preexisting neurologic deficit.

With refinements in neuroimaging procedures, cerebral AVMs are being diagnosed earlier than before. Moreover, for many lesions previously deemed inoperable, surgical treatment has now become feasible with the use of microsurgical techniques. Thus, with the aid of the operating microscope, lesions beside or involving critical cerebral regions have been removed, as have small AVMs from the basal ganglia and other deeper structures.

There is little disagreement that in patients with a small, surgically accessible AVM not involving a critical region of the brain, operative treatment is indicated if hemorrhage has occurred. Controversy remains concerning the optimal management of patients with large lesions, with lesions having a complex blood supply, with lesions that are deep or located in critical areas of the brain, and with lesions that have never bled. Many

TABLE 13.1

*Initial or Presenting Symptoms of Patients with Cerebral AVMs
(Expressed as Percentages)*

Source (Ref no.)	Hemor-rhage	Epi-lepsy	Head-ache	Miscel-laneous*	Inci-dental
Olivecrona & Riives, 1948 (18)	40	40			
Mackenzie, 1953 (15)	30	32	24	14	
Paterson & McKissock, 1956 (20)	42	26	21	11	
Troupp, 1965 (25)	57	20	8	13	2
Henderson & Gomez, 1967 (6)	76	16		6	3
Kelly et al., 1969 (8)	51	37		12	—
Amacher et al., 1972 (2)	86	8	6		
Wilson et al., 1979 (28)	66	16	1	16	
Graf et al., 1983 (5)	63				
Fults & Kelly, 1984 (4)	52	27.5	6	14.5	

* Includes focal neurologic deficits.

neurosurgeons believe that all cerebral AVMs should be resected unless they are in surgically inaccessible sites, even if they have produced little (if any) clinical deficit, because of the risks of future rupture, with its associated morbidity and mortality. In order to justify this approach, however, it is necessary to show that the morbidity and mortality associated with AVMs (and especially of a first bleed) are not exceeded by that of surgery, especially since complications of surgery occur at or immediately following operation whereas clinical problems due to conservatively managed AVMs may not occur for many years after the diagnosis is first made. Such comparisons are complicated by the fact that the morbidity and mortality from rupture of untreated AVMs are higher in patients between 20 and 40 years of age than in older or younger patients. Clearly, some appreciation of the natural history of cerebral AVMs is essential before the issue can be resolved.

THE NATURAL HISTORY

Any study of the natural history of AVMs must take into account the age of patients, location of lesions, and modes of presentation. Troupp (26) has emphasized some of the difficulties that must be faced when the natural history of cerebral AVMs is to be evaluated. The mortality in unoperated cases cannot simply be compared to that in operated cases because this neglects any selection factors taken into account when determining whether or not operation should be undertaken. Again, a bias is introduced if surgical rejects are considered as unoperated cases for the purposes of determining natural history. It may well be, for example, that precisely those AVMs that are inoperable because of their location are more likely to bleed, although Stein (22) found no difference in the incidence of hemorrhage between deep-seated AVMs and those closer to the surface of the brain. Similarly, the results of surgery will depend in part upon the available facilities, and not all series show the same low mortality rates reported by certain neurosurgeons in major medical centers. Thus, it is hard to obtain unprejudiced data.

Svien and McRae (24) found from their study of 95 patients with an AVM that the mortality rate was 6% among 50 who had experienced a hemorrhage. If the initial symptom of the malformation was intracranial hemorrhage, as in 20 of their patients, the chance of rebleeding was 34%, with a mortality rate of 6% from subsequent hemorrhages.

Drake (3) indicated that for AVMs that had never bled, the incidence of hemorrhage was about 1% per year, with a 10% mortality rate for the initial hemorrhage; after the first bleed the annual incidence of further hemorrhage was about 3.7%, with a mortality rate of 0.9% per year from that hemorrhage. These figures are based on data from the Cooperative Study (21). However, in a series of 137 untreated patients followed for a mean period in the order of 12 years, Troupp—cited by Drake (3) and Luessenhop (11)—reported that 27 were well, 14 had slight disability, and 28 were disabled more severely; 33 died, 23 from their AVM and 10 from other causes. Three patients died as a direct result of operation after they had been followed for many years (12), and the remaining 32 patients were lost to follow-up. From this series, an annual mortality rate of 1–2% was calculated, with a morbidity rate of 3.5%. These rates are somewhat higher than those cited earlier, and exceed those projected by Michelsen (16) who stated that after 20 years, 33% of all symptomatic patients will be well, 22% will have mild deficits, 29% will be disabled, and 10% will have died from their AVM.

Recent studies yield even more sinister figures. Thus, Graf *et al.* (5) found that among 191 patients with cerebral AVMs, 102 had one hemorrhage, 32 had recurrent hemorrhages, and 57 never bled. The average yearly risk for the first hemorrhage was 2–3%, bleeding occurring most frequently in patients between 11 and 35 years of age. Among 93 patients followed after the AVM had ruptured, the risk of rebleeding was 6% in the first year, after which the average rebleeding rate was about 2% per year up to 20 years. The cumulative risk of first hemorrhage among 66 patients with an initially unruptured AVM who were followed was 2% at the end of the first year, 14% in 5 years, 31% in 10 years, and 39% in 20 years. Small lesions were more likely to bleed than large ones, as reported previously by others, such as Henderson and Gomez (6), Waltimo (27), and Luessenhop (12). Thus, the risk of hemorrhage at 5 years was 52% in those with small AVMs and 10% among patients with large AVMs. Among 134 patients with a bleeding AVM, there were 17 (12.7%) deaths from the hemorrhage.

Fults and Kelly (4) found that among 26 patients presenting with seizures and followed for an average of 11 years, seven (26.9%) had a hemorrhage and three patients died, but one of these deaths was unrelated to the AVM; if this last patient is excluded, the mortality rate was 8% (two of 25 patients). By contrast, among patients presenting with hemorrhage, they reported a mortality rate of 13.6% for the first bleed, a 67.4% chance of rebleeding, and overall a 40.5% mortality rate from hemorrhage. They found the prognosis was more favorable in patients presenting with seizures, confirming an impression gained from earlier studies.

Clearly, then, there is a discrepancy between different series with regard to the risk of hemorrhage. The mortality rate from a first bleed varies between 6 and 14% in these different studies.

OUTCOME OF SURGICAL TREATMENT

The above data must be borne in mind when considering the outcome of surgical treatment for AVMs, regardless of whether or not they have bled. Parkinson and Bachers (19) reported a mortality of 11% and morbidity of 23% in their recent studies, in which 90 of 100 serially encountered cases were treated surgically. Similarly, Fults and Kelly (4) reported a perioperative mortality of 11% in their series. Wilson et al. (28) reported in 1979 their more favorable results with microsurgical treatment of intracranial AVMs. Nevertheless among a total of 65 AVMs that were excised, four patients (6%) died, and in 18 (28%) there was a new postoperative deficit. The preoperative deficit was unchanged by operation in 10 patients and improved postoperatively in 21. An even more favorable outcome to surgical treatment was reported by Stein and Wolpert (23), who found that among 55 AVMs resected surgically they had a surgical mortality of one (2%) and morbidity of three (5%); surgery was the sole treatment of the AVM in 34 of their patients. These results and those from several other recent series are summarized in Table 13.2. Differences in operative morbidity and mortality presumably relate, at least in part, to differences in the preoperative state, and criteria for recommending surgical treatment.

Luessenhop and Rosa (14) reported a very low operative risk for AVMs that were less than 4 cm in size at angiography, finding a morbidity of 4% and no mortality among 74 patients. Therefore, they suggested that in patients with angiographically small AVMs the indications for operation need not be as strict as for patients with larger AVMs. For patients with large AVMs, they did not believe that surgery was justified for seizures, but agreed that it should be considered when presentation was with hemorrhage. However, operative treatment of such large AVMs was associated

TABLE 13.2

Results of Surgical Treatment of Cerebral AVMs

Source	Total Number of Patients	Number of Operated Patients (%)	Number of Operated Patients (%) with AVMs Less Than 2 cm	Operative Results	
				Percent Mortality	Percent Morbidity
Wilson et al., 1979 (28)	83	65 (78)	32 (49)	6	28
Parkinson & Bachers, 1980 (19)	100	90 (90)		11	20
Stein & Wolpert, 1980 (23)	81	55 (68)		2	5
Abad et al., 1983 (1)	112	70 (63)	29 (87)	11	26
Fults & Kelly, 1984 (4)	131	48 (37)		11	
Luessenhop & Rosa, 1984 (14)	450	90 (20)	29 (32)	2	11

with a mortality of 10% and morbidity of 30%, and therefore, they believed that for patients who were 50 years of age or older the risks of surgery for large lesions exceeded the morbidity and mortality of the untreated lesion.

DECISION ANALYSIS

Iansek et al. (7) have recently considered the management of cerebral AVMs in terms of decision analysis. They used probability estimates derived from the literature, and assigned values to different outcomes of surgical or conservative treatment. Their analysis involved a number of arbitrary judgments concerning the value of given outcomes. For example, death at operation was held to be the worst of all outcomes, and survival without any deficit following corrective surgery was held to be the best of all possible outcomes. Death following a major bleed was also considered a bad outcome, although not as bad as when death followed surgery; several years may pass before death occurs following a major bleed in patients undergoing conservative management, whereas perioperative death generally occurs much sooner, i.e., shortly after the time of diagnosis. Similarly, patients who survive and are intact following conservative management were held to have had a favorable response, although this was not as good as being neurologically intact following corrective surgical treatment for the AVM, and so was assigned a lower value. This is because in the former instance the risk still remains that the lesion will bleed in the future. The authors only considered the outcome over a 20-year period of follow-up, rather than over any longer time span. Based on published reports, they assumed an annual bleeding rate of 1% (18% cumulative total over 20 years) for AVMs that had not yet bled, and attributed to any hemorrhage an immediate mortality of 14% (based on findings in different series) and major morbidity of 20% (17–24% depending on the series); they also assumed a 10% mortality and 27% major morbidity rate for surgical treatment of an AVM that had not bled, with corresponding figures of 8% and 23%, respectively, for AVMs that had bled, basing this on previously published data. Their analysis showed unequivocally that conservative (nonoperative) treatment was the appropriate way to manage an AVM that had not bled.

For convenience, this approach can be simplified by assigning the same value to similar outcomes, regardless of whether these occur at the time of surgery or subsequently. If a common numerical scale is adopted so that death (regardless of whether it occurs at operation or at anytime within a 20-year period from hemorrhage due to the AVM) is assigned a value of 0, the development of major morbidity following operation or a naturally occurring complication of the AVM is assigned an arbitrary value of 0.5, and survival without neurologic deficit (regardless of whether or not the patient was treated operatively) is assigned a numerical value of 1.0, it can be shown that conservative treatment is generally the preferred method of management of AVMs (Fig. 13.1). This remains the case unless the surgical mortality is in the order of 1% and the surgical morbidity approximates 7% or less, when the chance of bleeding is taken as about 1% per year (or 18% over 20 years). If data from the more recent study of Graf *et al.* (5) are used, suggesting that AVMs have an annual bleeding rate of 2–3% (2.4% per year), medical management still remains superior unless the surgical mortality is only 1% and surgical morbidity is 18% or less.

Such a conclusion can be put in another way. If one considers a group of 1000 patients, and assumes a 2% surgical mortality rate and 10% morbidity rate (*i.e.*, very favorable rates), 880 patients will be completely intact following operation. When one considers, in turn, 1000 patients treated conservatively and determines the complications due to hemorrhage, assuming a bleeding rate of 1% per year, there will be approximately 180 hemorrhages (18%) over 20 years, leading to 25 deaths (14% of 180 cases), and 36 strokes (20% of 180 cases). Thus, the overall outcome from hemorrhage in the untreated group is that 939 patients remain intact over 20 years (820 who do not experience hemorrhage and 119 who do experience a hemorrhage but are left with no residual deficit). Utilizing the somewhat higher figures for bleeding published by Graf *et al.* (5), 390 hemorrhages would be predicted over 20 years, leading to 55 deaths (assuming a 14% mortality rate) and to residual deficits in 78 patients; 867 patients would then remain intact over a 20-year period. Thus, if one takes the best surgical and worst nonsurgical figures for mortality or significant morbidity, no clear advantage to surgery over nonoperative conservative treatment can

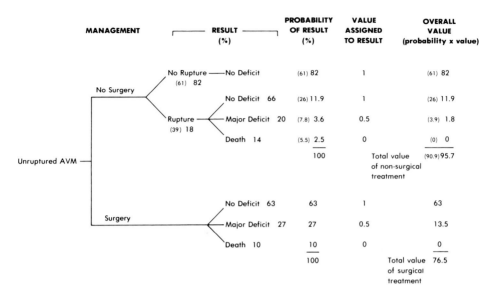

MANAGEMENT	RESULT (%)		PROBABILITY OF RESULT (%)	VALUE ASSIGNED TO RESULT	OVERALL VALUE (probability x value)
No Surgery	No Rupture (61) 82	No Deficit	(61) 82	1	(61) 82
	Rupture (39) 18	No Deficit 66	(26) 11.9	1	(26) 11.9
		Major Deficit 20	(7.8) 3.6	0.5	(3.9) 1.8
		Death 14	(5.5) 2.5	0	(0) 0
			100	Total value of non-surgical treatment	(90.9) 95.7
Surgery		No Deficit 63	63	1	63
		Major Deficit 27	27	0.5	13.5
		Death 10	10	0	0
			100	Total value of surgical treatment	76.5

Unruptured AVM

FIG. 13.1 Comparison of surgical and nonsurgical management of unruptured cerebral AVMs, using decision analysis, as described in the text. A higher total value indicates a more favorable outcome. The percent of conservatively managed AVMs that rupture is based on the findings in the Cooperative Study (3, 21). The more recent and more sinister figures of Graf *et al.* (5) are given in smaller numerals in parentheses. Outcome has been determined using both sets of figures. Postoperative morbidity and mortality rates, and those following spontaneous rupture, are based on data published in several different series described in the text, as also is the manner in which numerical values for each outcome have been arbitrarily assigned.

be shown from this analysis. Nevertheless, employing the most favorable estimates for surgery in this way implies that all the AVMs to be treated are small, superficial, and in clinically silent areas of the brain, that patients are young and otherwise well, and that the surgeons responsible for treatment are especially experienced in the management of AVMs.

CONCLUSION

It is generally not this author's policy to advise surgical excision for unruptured cerebral AVMs. As shown above, even with estimates of outcome that are most favorable to surgery and would only be obtained under optimal conditions, no clear advantage to surgical excision can be demonstrated. When more realistic figures for surgical mortality and morbidity are used, conservative treatment is clearly the best approach.

The management of unruptured cerebral AVMs should usually consist of symptomatic measures. The two most common symptoms not due to hemorrhage are seizures and headache (Table 13.1). Both of these are best managed pharmacologically, and usually respond well to this approach. In a recent study (17), no substantial improvement in seizure control occurred after resection of the AVM. Some surgeons feel obliged to operate when patients with unruptured AVMs are unable to come to terms with the presence within them of a potentially lethal lesion. Such patients are unable to make a rational decision based on judicious appreciation of the risks involved, however, and surgeons should therefore take especial care to avoid surgical treatment unless it is otherwise indicated. Firm reassurance may need to be accompanied by psychiatric treatment in such instances. Operative intervention can be justified in patients with unruptured AVMs when intracranial pressure is increased, cardiac decompensation occurs in children, or a focal neurologic deficit is progressing and leads to increasing disability. However, at least when progressive neurologic deterioration (not due to hemorrhage) is the reason for surgical referral, direct operative intervention may be unnecessary because the deficit often stabilizes or reverses with partial embolic obliteration of the AVM (10, 13). Long-term research is necessary to establish whether proton beam therapy (9) confers any benefit in the management of unruptured AVMs, and this form of treatment will not be considered further here.

REFERENCES

1. Abad, J. M., Alvarez, F., Manrique, M., and Garcia-Blazquez, M. Cerebral arteriovenous malformations: comparative results of surgical vs. conservative treatment in 112 cases. J. Neurosurg. Sci., 27: 203–210, 1983.
2. Amacher, A. L., Allcock, J. M., and Drake, C. G. Cerebral angiomas: the sequelae of surgical treatment. J. Neurosurg., 37: 571–575, 1972.
3. Drake, C. G. Cerebral arteriovenous malformations: considerations for and experience with surgical treatment in 166 cases. Clin. Neurosurg., 26: 145–208, 1979.
4. Fults, D., and Kelly, D. L. Natural history of arteriovenous malformations of the brain: a clinical study. Neurosurgery, 15: 658–662, 1984.
5. Graf, C. J., Perret, G. E., and Torner, J. C. Bleeding from cerebral arteriovenous malformations as part of their natural history. J. Neurosurg., 58: 331–337, 1983.
6. Henderson, W. R., and Gomez, R. de R. L. Natural history of cerebral angiomas. Br. Med. J., 4: 571–574, 1967.
7. Iansek, R., Elstein, A. S., and Balla, J. I. Application of decision analysis to management of cerebral arteriovenous malformation. Lancet, 1: 1132–1135, 1983.
8. Kelly, D. L., Alexander, E., Davis, C. H., and Maynard, D. C. Intracranial arteriovenous malformations: clinical review and evaluation of brain scans. J. Neurosurg., 31: 422–428, 1969.
9. Kjellberg, R. N., Hanamura, T., Davis, K. R., Lyons, S. L., and Adams R. D. Bragg-peak proton-beam therapy for arteriovenous malformations of the brain. N. Engl. J. Med., 309: 269–274, 1983.
10. Kusske, J. A., and Kelly, W. A. Embolization and reduction of the 'steal' syndrome in cerebral arteriovenous malformations. J. Neurosurg., 40: 313–321, 1974.

11. Luessenhop, A. J. Natural history of cerebral arteriovenous malformations. *In: Intracranial Arteriovenous Malformations*, edited by C. B. Wilson, and B. M. Stein. Williams & Wilkins, Baltimore, 1984, pp. 12–23.

12. Luessenhop, A. J. Operative treatment of arteriovenous malformations of the brain. *In: Current Controversies in Neurosurgery*, edited by T. P. Morley, W. B. Saunders, Philadelphia, 1976, pp. 203–209.

13. Luessenhop, A. J., and Presper, J. H. Surgical embolization of cerebral arteriovenous malformations through internal carotid and vertebral arteries. Long-term results. J. Neurosurg., *42:* 443–451, 1975.

14. Luessenhop, A. J., and Rosa, L. Cerebral arteriovenous malformations: indications for and results of surgery, and the role of intravascular techniques. J. Neurosurg., *60:* 14–22, 1984.

15. Mackenzie, I. The clinical presentation of the cerebral angioma. A review of 50 cases. Brain, *78:* 184–214, 1953.

16. Michelsen, W. J. Natural history and pathophysiology of arteriovenous malformations. Clin. Neurosurg., *26:* 307–313, 1979.

17. Murphy, M. J. Long-term follow-up of seizures associated with cerebral arteriovenous malformations: results of therapy. Arch. Neurol., *42:* 477–479, 1985.

18. Olivecrona, H., and Riives, J. Arteriovenous aneurysms of the brain. Their diagnosis and treatment. Arch. Neurol. Psychiatr. *59:* 567–602, 1948.

19. Parkinson, D., and Bachers, G. Arteriovenous malformations: summary of 100 consecutive supratentorial cases. J. Neurosurg., *53:* 285–299, 1980.

20. Paterson, J. H., and McKissock, W. A clinical survey of intracranial angiomas with special reference to their mode of progression and surgical treatment: a report of 110 cases. Brain, *79:* 233–266, 1956.

21. Perret, G., and Nishioka, H. Report on the cooperative study of intracranial aneurysms and subarachnoid hemorrhage. Section VI. Arteriovenous malformations. J. Neurosurg., *25:* 467–490, 1966.

22. Stein, B. Arteriovenous malformations of the brain and spinal cord. *In: Goldsmith's Practice of Surgery, Neurosurgery Volume*, edited by J. Hoff. Chap. 17. Harper & Row, Hagerstown, 1979, pp. 1–40.

23. Stein, B. M., and Wolpert, S. M. Arteriovenous malformations of the brain. II. Current concepts and treatment. Arch. Neurol., *37:* 69–75, 1980.

24. Svien, H. J., and McRae, J. A. Arteriovenous anomalies of the brain: fate of patients not having definitive surgery. J. Neurosurg., *23:* 23–28, 1965.

25. Troupp, H. Arteriovenous malformations of the brain: prognosis without operation. Acta Neurol. Scand., *41:* 39–42, 1965.

26. Troupp, H. Arteriovenous malformations of the brain: What are the indications for operation? In: *Current Controversies in Neurology*, edited by T. P. Morley. W. B. Saunders, Philadelphia, 1976, pp. 210–216.

27. Waltimo, O. The relationship of size, density and localization of intracranial arteriovenous malformations to the type of initial symptoms. J. Neurol. Sci., *19:* 13–19, 1973.

28. Wilson, C. B., U, S. H., and Domingue, J. Microsurgical treatment of intracranial vascular malformations. J. Neurosurg., *51:* 446–454, 1979.

14

Unruptured Arteriovenous Malformations: A Dilemma in Surgical Decision Making

ROBERTO C. HEROS, M.D., and YONG-KWANG TU, M.D.

INTRODUCTION

Neurosurgeons and neurologists frequently use the term "unruptured" arteriovenous malformation (AVM) to refer to an AVM diagnosed in a patient with no history of intracranial hemorrhage referable to the lesion. The diagnosis is usually made in these patients because of epilepsy, headaches, or a progressive neurologic deficit. Since the advent of computed tomography (CT), more and more AVMs have been diagnosed while they are completely asymptomatic in patients who had CT scans for a variety of unrelated reasons. In general, whether a patient with an AVM should be advised to have it surgically excised or not has, to this date, depended very heavily on whether the lesion is thought to be unruptured or whether it has bled either recently or in the past. Analysis of our personal experience and a review of the recent literature leads us to question the importance of this fact as a determining factor in the surgical decision making process when facing patients with AVMs. Table 14.1 lists some traditional concepts that we would like to challenge individually.

The morbidity and mortality of AVM surgery is very high. It is true that earlier reports indicated a relatively high risk for operations on AVMs (42, 43, 44). However, these reports represent early efforts, frequently in patients with serious neurologic deficits from acute intracerebral hematomas. Modern surgical techniques as well as refinements of criteria for surgical resection have brought combined surgical morbidity and mortality to about 15% when all lesions are considered (Table 14.2).

There is a definite, ascertainable "morbidity and mortality" in AVM surgery. In spite of the above statements about modern results, it must be clear to the experienced surgeon that the risk of surgery varies from practically no risk in small polar lesions to a 100% risk of neurologic devastation in large intrinsic lesions of the brain stem. Even so, one is very frequently asked by referring physicians and patients alike: "What is the risk of AVM surgery?" or "What are your morbidity and mortality rates with AVMs?" A perusal through Table 14.2 will indicate that, even in recent

TABLE 14.1

AVMs—Traditional Concepts

Morbidity and mortality of AVM surgery is very high

There is a definite, ascertainable "morbidity and mortality" in AVM surgery

If the patient has no neurologic deficit and is not incapacitated by seizures or headaches, he is "asymptomatic"

Whether the patient has bled in the past from his AVM is a clear-cut, ascertainable clinical fact

Risk of bleeding in a patient with an "unruptured" AVM is low

Risk of hemorrhage in patients that have never bled is much less than in patients who have bled in the past

First hemorrhage from an AVM is usually "benign"

Surgery is more dangerous in "unruptured" AVMs

---

series, the overall morbidity of AVM surgery ranges between 2% and 25.3% and surgical mortality ranges between 1.1% and 18.8%. Almost certainly these ranges reflect differences in patient population and thoroughness of assessment as to what represents morbidity; it is doubtful that differences

TABLE 14.2

AVMs—Modern Surgical Results

Year	Authors (Ref.)	No. of Cases	Morbidity (%)	Mortality (%)
1978	Cophignon (3)	45	?	4(8.5%)
1978	Mingrino (31)	98	2(2%)	4(4.1%)
1979	Drake* (8)	106	5(4.8%)	6(5.7%)
1979	Nornes (37)	63	2(3.2%)	3(4.7%)
1979	Wilson (59)	83	21(25.3%)	4(4.8%)
1980	Pellettiere (39)	116	18(15.5%)	6(5.2%)
1980	Stein (48)	55	3(10%)	1(2%)
1980	Guidetti* (13)	92	6(6.3%)	3(3.2%)
1980	Parkinson (38)	90	18(20%)	10(11%)
1982	Albert* (2)	140	?	10(7%)
1982	Suzuki (50)	173	8(4.6%)	8(4.6%)
1984	Luessenhop (26)	90	10(11%)	2(2.2%)
1984	Fults and Kelly (10)	48	3(6.2%)	9(18.8%)
1985	Adelt (1)	43	3(7%)	3(7%)
1985	Davis and Symon (5)	69	6(8.7%)	1(1.5%)
1985	Jomin (20)	128	6(8.5%)	16(12.5%)
1985	Heros	90	11(12.2%)	1(1.1%)
Total		1529	122/1344(9.1%)	91/1529(6.0%)

* In these series, the patients who were drowsy or comatose before surgery were excluded.

in surgical techniques account for much of the variance in these results. Within surgical series, for example, one finds that combined morbidity and mortality for lesions of less than 4 cm is 4%, for lesions more than 4 cm in diameter is 56.5% (26), and between "good risk" patients and "poor risk" patients is 10.5% and 62%, respectively (8).

If the patient has no neurologic deficit and is not incapacitated by seizures or headaches he is "asymptomatic." This is a grave misconception. Many a patient is psychologically devastated by the knowledge of having a potentially lethal lesion that could "explode" at any time. Within our modest series of 40 patients operated upon for unruptured AVMs (*vide infra*), we have two patients who were on disability pension because of the anxiety produced by this knowledge. Two other patients were under psychiatric treatment for the same reason. Several of the patients had traveled widely at considerable loss of time and money, seeking different, frequently contradictory opinions as to whether they should be operated on or not. Another patient tried to commit suicide because he could not live with the knowledge that the "time bomb" in his head, which was called "inoperable" by several physicians, could go off at any time. This last patient, incidentally, brought home to us the fact that we do a tremendous disservice to these patients by using phrases such as time bomb, "cocked pistol," "powder keg," etc., to refer to their AVM, particularly if the lesion is truly inoperable and the patient must live with it!

Whether the patient has bled in the past from his AVM is a clear-cut ascertainable clinical fact. This is frequently not so. In our small series we found two patients who presented with the sudden onset of a neurologic deficit accompanied by a severe headache in one; both patients were felt to have suffered an intracranial hemorrhage, but neither had evidence of hemorrhage by CT scan or at surgery. Conversely, in four patients with no history suggestive of a hemorrhage, we found evidence of old gross hemorrhage at surgery. This parallels the experience of Stein, who found evidence of previous hemorrhage at surgery in 10–15% of his patients with unruptured AVMs (47). Malis has had a similar experience (28) and MacKenzie quotes a 30% incidence of previous hemorrhage (27). It is also well-known that pathologically many unruptured AVMs are accompanied by signficant hemosiderosis in the adjacent brain, again indicating the presence of previous hemorrhage (28, 29).

The risk of bleeding in a patient with an unruptured AVM is low. Table 14.3 lists each reported series where the authors could clearly separate the results of no therapy in patients with unruptured AVMs. In an average follow-up of 12–20 years, there is a 25–39% risk of hemorrhage with a mortality, from AVM bleeding, of 11.5–18.2% and a morbidity about twice as high.

TABLE 14.3

Conservative Treatment of "Unruptured" AVMs

Author (Ref.)	No. of Cases	Bleeding (%)	Morbidity (%)	Mortality (%)	Average Years of Follow-up
Kelly (21)	26		34.5	11.5	12.5
Moody and Poppen (33)	6			17	3–10
Graf (12)	71	39			20
Fults and Kelly (10)	26	26.9	19.2	11.6	8.7
Forster (9)	46	25	20	17	15
Henderson (15)	11	36.4		18.2	5–20
Perret and Nishioka (42)	77	30			>20

The risk of hemorrhage in patients that have never bled is much less than in patients who have bled in the past. It is true that during the first few months after a hemorrhage a patient with an AVM has a slightly higher risk of rehemorrhage. This risk during the first year was estimated to be 6% in two different recent studies (12, 53). However, after the first year, the incidence of bleeding is almost identical in patients who have bled and in patients who have no history of hemorrhage. This yearly risk of bleeding has been estimated at 2–3% in the two studies quoted above (12, 53).

The first hemorrhage from an AVM is usually benign. This misconception has reassured us in the past when we have advised a patient with an unruptured AVM to wait and if he bleeds, from which he would almost certainly recover, then operate. Table 14.4 indicates that, in fact, a first hemorrhage from an AVM, though not as devastating as a first aneurysmal hemorrhage, is a very serious event with a mortality rate of 10% and a

TABLE 14.4

Severity of First Hemorrhage from AVM

Author (Ref.)	Morbidity (%)	Mortality (%)
Luessenhop (26)	30	10
Svien (51)	15	6
Forster (9)		30
Fults and Kelly (10)		13.6
Graf (12)	81.3	12.7
Kjellberg (22)	55	
Perret and Nishioka (42)	53	9.8
Perret (41)		11
Iansek (18)	20	14

morbidity rate of at least 30%. These figures are in agreement to those compiled by Luessenhop (25), Wilkins (58), and Michelsen (30).

Surgery is more dangerous in unruptured AVMs. There is no doubt about the fact that a large cavity from an old hemorrhage facilitates surgery. Obviously, if the patient has a severe pre-existing neurologic deficit from a hemorrhage it is more likely possible to remove the AVM without producing additional disability. However, a review of our material, as well as a review of two other series where the surgical results for ruptured and unruptured AVMs are separated, indicates that the overall surgical morbidity and mortality are very similar in these two groups of patients (see Table 14.5).

PRESENT SERIES

Ninety consecutive cases of cerebral AVMs operated by the senior author were reviewed in detail. Cases of dural AVMs, carotid-cavernous fistula, and small cryptic AVMs removed as part of an intracerebral blood clot were excluded. From this series, 40 patients had no history of hemorrhage and no CT scan evidence of previous bleeding from their AVM. In this group, four patients were found to have evidence of previous bleeding at surgery, but they were still left in the group and classified as unruptured. This group of 40 patients constitutes the present series. Table 14.6 give the age, sex, and type of surgical therapy for the group. The patient whose AVM was exposed only was an elderly lady who was operated because of an associated intracranial aneurysm that had bled. After the aneurysm was clipped, the incidental AVM of the left sylvian fissure was exposed. Because of the patient's age and the complexity of the lesion, determined at exposure, the decision was made to leave it alone. Another patient, treated with multiple embolizations, will be discussed later as a complication. Table 14.7 gives the presenting symptoms. Seven patients had AVMs de-

TABLE 14.5
Surgical Results in "Ruptured" vs "Unruptured" AVMs

Author (Ref.)	Ruptured			Unruptured		
	No. of Cases	Morbidity (%)	Mortality (%)	No. of Cases	Morbidity (%)	Mortality (%)
Perret and Nishioka (42)	148		12	28		14
Moody and Poppen (33)	40	2.5	10	57	7	14
Heros	50	12	2	40	12.5	0

TABLE 14.6
"Unruptured" AVMs

Age	
Range	12–75
Median	29
Sex	
Males	18
Females	22
Therapy	
Complete excision*	38
Exposure only	1
Multiple embolizations	1

* Confirmed in all cases by postoperative angiography.

tected as incidental lesions on a CT scan or an angiogram performed for unrelated symptoms. Of the three patients with "typical" migraine, two had occipital AVMs and one had a parietal lesion. Of interest is that all three had their headaches relieved by surgical excision of their AVM. Two patients presented with a fixed neurologic deficit of abrupt onset. The deficit was right leg weakness which eventually improved to a foot drop in a patient with a parasagittal AVM of the left parietal area and left partial hemianopsia associated with a severe generalized headache in a patient with a right occipital AVM. As discussed earlier, neither of these two patients had evidence of hemorrhage by CT scan or subsequently at surgery. The explanation for these deficits remains elusive since neither of the AVMs was large enough to postulate a "steal" phenomenon. Remarkably, the patient with the left parasagittal lesion regained almost all strength of her foot in the months following surgery. Of the 19 patients that presented with seizures, only two had poorly controlled seizures and the rest were

TABLE 14.7
"Unruptured" AVMs—
Presentation

Seizures	18
Headaches	
"Typical" migraine	3
Other	3
Progressive neuro deficit	4
Abrupt, fixed neuro deficit	2
Transient neuro deficit	3
Incidental	7

under acceptable control. In no case was the operation performed primarily to control the seizures. The main indication for surgery in each case was to prevent future hemorrhage although, in the patients with a progressive neurologic deficit and in the patients with poorly controlled seizures, it was hoped that the operation would result in some overall improvement.

Table 14.8 describes the size and general location of the lesions. The size given is a rough estimate of the diameter of the true nidus of the AVM based on the description in the record of the angiograms and the operative notes as well as, in some cases, the recollection of the surgeon. No effort was made to recall all the angiograms and carefully measure the lesion at the time of this review. As can be seen, most of the AVMs were of medium size and there was an unusually large number of deep temporal AVMs, perhaps due to a special interest of the surgeon in these lesions. Of the convexity lesions (presenting in the surface of a cerebral hemisphere), eight were located either in relation to the Rolandic fissure on either side or in the speech regions of the dominant hemisphere. Of the former lesions, most were parasagittal in location.

The results of surgery in this series of 40 patients have been rewarding. There have been no deaths. Only five patients required blood transfusion during surgery. All 38 patients from whom the AVM was excised had a postoperative arteriogram, usually just before discharge, 1–2 weeks from the time of surgery. In all, the angiograms confirmed that the lesion was completely excised. Several patients had a temporary neurologic deficit

TABLE 14.8
"Unruptured" AVMs—Size and Location

	Large >4 cm	Medium 2–4 cm	Small <2 cm	Total
Convexity				
Eloquent	3	3	2	8
Non-eloquent		3	1	4
Deep supratentorial				
Temporal		8	1	9
Parieto-occipital	2	3		5
Fronto-parietal	1	1		2
Callosal	1		1	2
Trigonal		1	1	2
Basal ganglia			1	1
Cerebellar				
Hemispheric		4		4
Deep	1	2		3
Total	8	25	7	40

after operation which cleared within a few weeks to months. This temporary deterioration after AVM surgery is frequent and can be quite striking with complete recovery within weeks of what appeared initially to be a serious deficit. The nature of this problem is multifactorial and includes postoperative swelling from retraction as well as complicated hemodynamic changes that have been eloquently addressed by others (8, 32, 35, 36, 45). Table 14.9 lists every case where there was permanent neurologic morbidity from the operation except for those patients who developed a partial visual field cut which was predicted before surgery and accepted by the patient. As noted, there were two additional patients who developed epilepsy after surgery; both are well controlled medically. The effect of the operation in seizure control was not specifically assessed, but it is our general impression that in most patients the frequency of seizures decreased. Of the two patients who had intractable seizures before surgery, one has been seizure-free for 2 years and the second one has had only one seizure in 3 years. Of the patients with a progressive or with a fixed neurologic deficit, one is unchanged, one is worse, and the rest are improved.

Figure 14.1 shows the pertinent x-rays in a patient with a deep cerebellar AVM that involved the cerebellar peduncles and at surgery was found to extend to the posterolateral aspect of the brain stem (see location of the clip in the postoperative CT scan—Fig. 14. 1D). Preoperatively, we had not predicted this deep extension and had not anticipated that the lesion was fed by small fragile perforating vessels coming right through the lateral medulla. This patient, who is our most serious complication, is home and independent, but is devastated by his severe ataxia and difficulty with swallowing which has required a tracheostomy and feeding gastrostomy. Obviously, this patient should not have been operated. Had we recognized,

TABLE 14.9

Permanent Morbidity*—5 Patients (12.5%)

Location of AVM	Complication
Deep cerebellar	Dysphagia, dysarthria, and severe ataxia
Parieto-occipital	Worsening of headaches and seizures
Temporoparietal	Hemianopsia
Frontoparietal	Worsening of preoperative hemiparesis
Frontoparietal	Foot drop

In addition, 2 patients developed de-novo seizures after surgery (well controlled). There were no deaths in this series of 40 patients.

* Predictable, incomplete visual field defects excluded.

from a more careful review of his preoperative angiograms, that the AVM extended into the medulla, we would have referred him for proton beam therapy (22).

Figure 14.2 illustrates the case of a teenager that presented with severe intractable headaches. She had a huge dominant temporoparietal-occipital lesion which also involved the thalamus. She has been treated over the last 3 years with multiple sessions of open and closed embolization. Her headaches were worse initially although recently, after embolization of some dural feeders, they have improved. She has a hemianopsia as a result of operative embolization and ligation of the posterior cerebral artery, she has developed epilepsy, and she has had probably at least two subarachnoid hemorrhages since the beginning of her treatment. She has been crippled psychologically by the effect of these therapies and she still has viable malformation left. She probably would have been better off if we never had undertaken any treatment at all since her only symptoms at presentation were headaches. The size of her malformation influenced us to attempt to reduce the flow by embolization. However, the literature suggests that, in fact, large malformations are less likely to bleed than smaller ones (8, 12, 34, 38, 57). This patient has influenced our present policy of not undertaking any form of embolization unless the AVM is estimated to be totally excisable by surgery or unless the embolization is reasonably expected to result in complete obliteration of the lesion. An exception to this policy is made in cases that present with a progressive neurologic deficit. In these patients even partial reduction of flow by embolization has frequently led to an improvement in the neurologic deficit. Also, occasionally a patient with intractable headaches and prominent scalp or dural feeders to the AVM can be improved by selective embolization of those feeders.

Figure 14.3 illustrates a patient with a high-flow AVM with large feeding arteries who developed massive brain swelling at surgery near the completion of her resection. Fortunately, we were able to excise the lesion completely and, with barbiturates and mannitol, were able control her brain swelling. Initially, she had a moderate hemiparesis and a nondominant parietal syndrome. Her deficit has resolved completely except for a complete hemianopsia which we did not predict preoperatively. This patient is one of the two patients in this series who was thought to have developed the syndrome of "perfusion-breakthrough" (45). This may been avoided by staging the procedure with pre-excision open or closed embolization as we have used in other cases where this problem was anticipated (6).

Figure 14.4 illustrates the pertinent angiograms of a dentist that presented with a progressive left hemiparesis probably due to a steal phenomenon. He also had seizures and had become unable to work because of inability to use his left hand. The lesion was completely resected after embolization, but his hemisparesis has been worse although he is ambulatory and presently working in an administrative capacity. He has never had a seizure since surgery and is very pleased with his decision to have the lesion resected; a decision he made in spite of the knowledge that resection would probably worsen his left hemiparesis.

Figure 14.5 illustrates the AVM of a young patient with seizures who developed significant leg weakness which eventually resolved into merely a foot drop for which she wears a short leg brace. This was a predictable deficit which she had accepted preoperatively. She has had no further seizures.

DISCUSSION

The traditional "indications" for resection in patients with AVMs have been a history of hemorrhage, intractable epilepsy, or a progressive neurologic deficit. The problem of what to do with a patient who has an unruptured AVM is one of increasing importance because more and more of these lesions are being detected by CT scan. Kumar *et al.* (24) have given

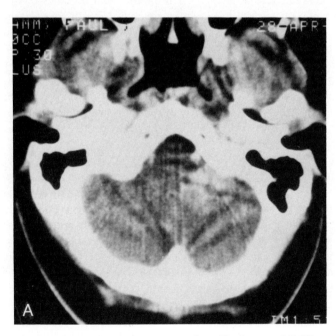

FIG. 14.1. Cerebellar AVM extending into posterolateral brain stem. (*A*) CT scan. (*B*) Left vertebral arteriogram, Towne's projection. (*C*) Left vertebral arteriogram, lateral projection. (*D*) Postoperative CT scan (note the deep position of the clip).

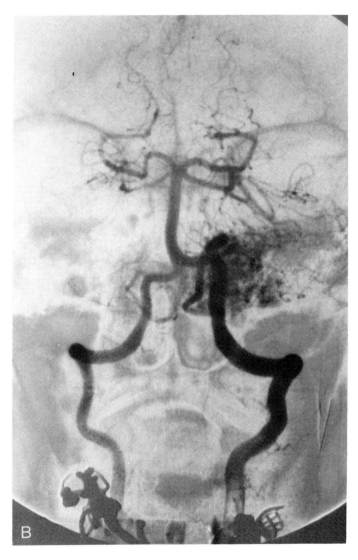

FIG. 14.1*B*

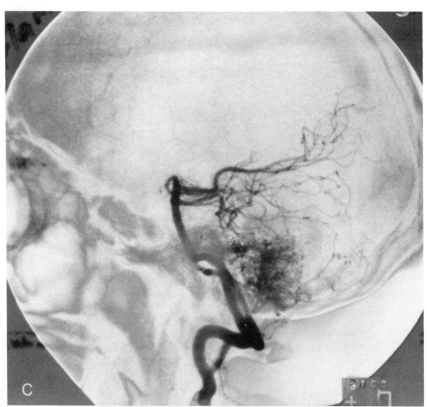

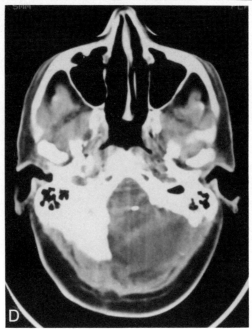

Fig. 14.1*C* and *D*

an excellent description of the CT scan appearance of unruptured AVMs. They analyzed a series of 60 patients and found evidence of mass effect in 33 of the 60. They also described the occurrence of extensive edema of the white matter surrounding the lesion, even though the patients had no history of hemorrhage. Many patients had lost the typical gray-white demarcation in areas around the lesion and several had hypodense lucencies within the lesion (24). These findings again raise the question of whether indeed these patients without a history of hemorrhage have had small hemorrhages in the past. The edema found around some of these lesions also indicates that they are probably not so "benign" hemodynamically.

Iansek and colleagues (18) addressed the question of whether unruptured AVMs should be treated and, through a complicated scheme of "decision

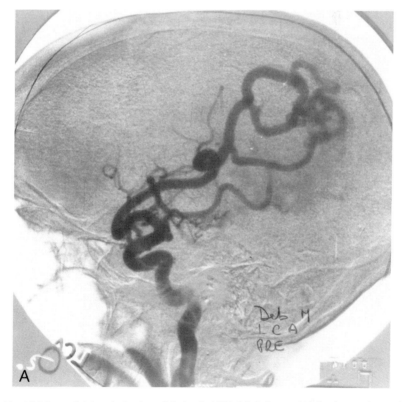

FIG. 14.2. Large left hemispheric and thalamic AVM. (A) Left carotid injection; early arterial phase showing very dilated middle cerebral feeders. (B) Right carotid injection showing pericallosal supply to the lesion. (C) Right vertebral injection (note the poorly defined margins of the lesion).

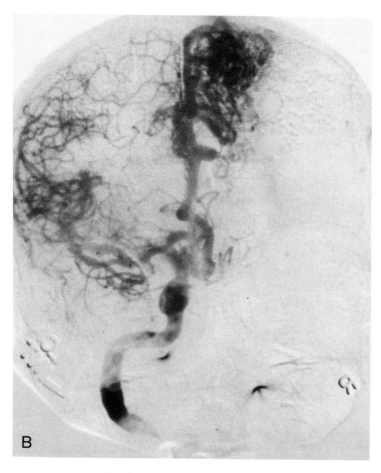

FIG. 14.2B

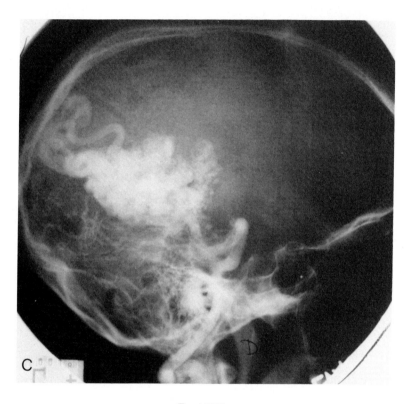

Fig. 14.2C

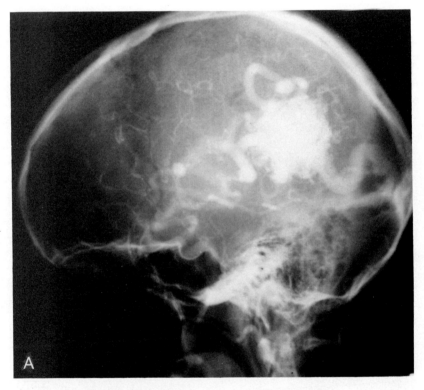

FIG. 14.3. Moderate size right parietal AVM. (A) Preoperative right carotid arteriogram showing large feeding vessels (note poor filling of rest of hemisphere). (B) Postoperative arteriogram (note residual dilatation and possible retrograde thrombosis [the vessels appear to be occluded proximally to the clips] of feeding vessels). Also note better arterial filling of the rest of the hemisphere (less "steal").

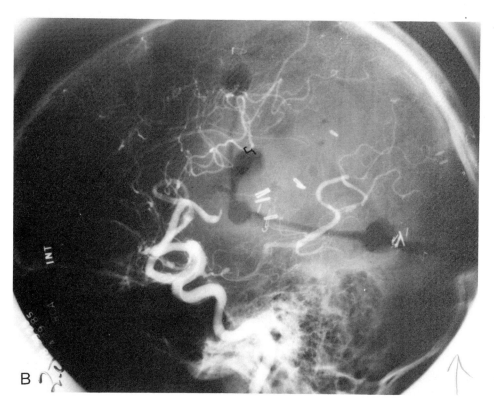

Fig. 14.3*B*

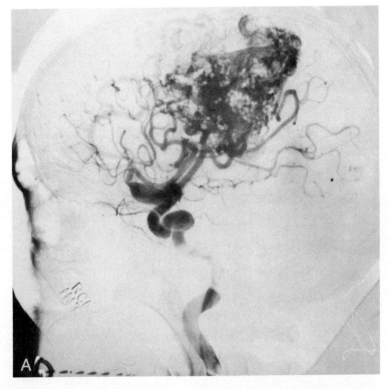

FIG. 14.4. Large right fronto-parietal AVM. (A) Right carotid injection (note pellets from preoperative embolization which effectively eliminated the upper [parasagittal] part of the malformation fed by pericallosal vessels). (B) Postoperative right carotid arteriogram (note better filling of the rest of the hemisphere).

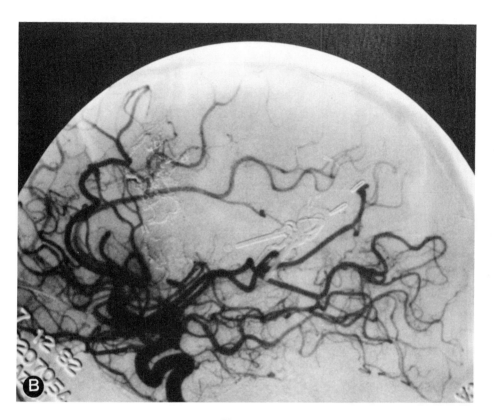

FIG. 14.4*B*

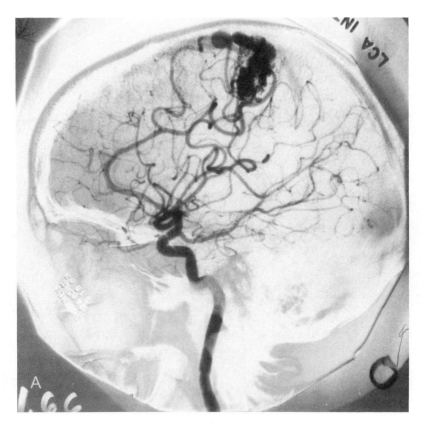

FIG. 14.5. Small rolandic parasagittal AVM. (*A*) Preoperative left carotid arteriogram. (*B*) Postoperative left carotid arteriogram.

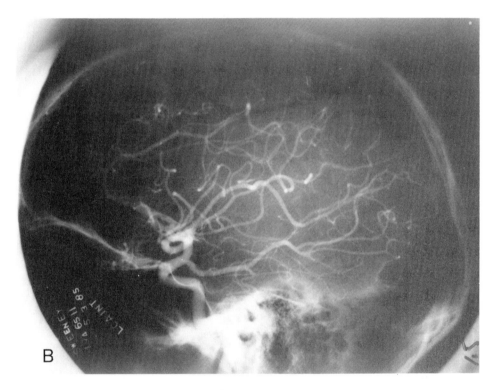

FIG. 14.5B

analysis," came to the conclusion that they should be left alone. However, as pointed out in subsequent letters to the editor in the same publication (4, 17), their analysis is a good example of how statistics coupled with inadequate data can lead to the wrong conclusion. They claim to have compiled a "summary of available data for use in decision analysis for cerebral AVM," however, their report contains only 12 references which are obviously selected references rather than "the data available." From these selected references, they estimate a surgical mortality of 10% and morbidity of 27%, clearly higher than the results presently obtainable as indicated in Table 14.2. They estimate the risk of bleeding of an unruptured AVM as 1% per year or about 18% in 20 years; an estimate clearly lower than the 2–3% per year risk estimated from larger patient pools by Graf and colleagues (12) and by Torner (53) or the 25% risk of hemorrhage in 15 years estimated by Forster (9).

A similarly conservative approach to AVMs in general was advocated by Svien and colleagues (51, 52) and later by Troupp and colleagues (54). Svien's conservative advice was, again, based on the generally poor, early surgical results with AVMs; still only 68% of their conservatively treated group were in good condition at follow-up, 16% had died as a result of their AVM, and an additional 10% were incapacitated (51). Troupp and colleagues treated 137 patients conservatively from 1942 to 1967. Fourteen died of their AVM, 33 were disabled, and only 55 were well at follow-up. Even so, they claimed that this represented a "cheerful outcome" as compared to early surgical results. Later, however, Drake quotes Troupp as reversing his position since, by 1977, of the same initial group of 137 patients, only 27 were well (8)—clearly a not-so-cheerful outcome.

More recently, neurosurgeons with considerable experience in AVM surgery have taken a more aggressive approach towards these lesions even when unruptured. Drake, after a comprehensive review of his own as well as the world's experience, concluded that "definitive treatment aimed at complete obliteration should be considered in every case, even those presenting with a convulsive disorder" (8). A similarly aggressive approach has been advocated by Stein (46, 47), Cophignon and his colleagues (3), Guidetti and Delitala (13), Mingrino (31), Malis (28), and Trumpy and Eldevick (55).

In view of the conflicting opinions, how then can a neurosurgeon decide whether or not to recommend surgical excision to a particular patient with an unruptured AVM? First, we want to re-emphasize our previously discussed thesis that it makes little difference whether the AVM is unruptured or there is a history of a remote hemorrhage. Second, we would like to emphasize our agreement with Pellettieri's opinion: "The problem cannot be resolved by comparing the overall results in different groups of oper-

TABLE 14.10

Surgery of AVMs—Helpful Hints

AVMs do not cross pial surfaces
Choroidal supply (as opposed to perforator supply) usually indicates resectability
Intraventricular hemorrhage without neurologic deficit is usually a good sign
Only the true "nidus" of the malformation as demonstrated in the very early arterial phase
   needs to be considered in determining resectability

ated and nonoperated patients" (39). Each patient is different and each AVM is different and, as discussed earlier, the risk of surgery in each patient is different and can only be estimated by the surgeon from previous personal or indirect experience with similar (though never identical) lesions.

Some clues that the senior author has found helpful in the decision-making process in "borderline" cases are given in Table 14.10. Figure 14.6 illustrates the case of a young man incapacitated by seizures and by progressive weakness of the left foot who had been told repeatedly that his AVM was inoperable because "it involved both sides of the brain." Indeed if his lesion had involved the medial basal portion of both frontal lobes, he could not have been operated without a resulting severe abulic syndrome as well as serious permanent affective changes. We felt that, in fact, his lesion was limited to the right hemisphere and that loops of the AVM protruded into the left frontal lobe but did not actually violate the pial interface of the interhemispheric fissure. At operation, which took nearly 24 hours, the latter was the case. He had an excellent result and is free of neurologic deficit. He is back to work and has had only one seizure in the 3 years since surgery.

Figure 14.7 illustrates a typical deep temporal AVM which had been called "inoperable" because of possible involvement of the basal ganglia or thalamus. The well-developed choroidal supply and the absence of lenticulostriate and thalamoperforating arterial supply indicated to us that the lesion was resectable. The only resulting deficit from surgery was a predictable partial visual field cut. Other clues of operability in these lesions of the medial temporal lobe have been emphasized in a previous publication (16).

Figure 14.8 illustrates a case in which the knowledge that the patient had had several purely intraventricular hemorrhages without ever developing neurologic deficit led us to suspect that the lesion was in the atrium of the ventricle and in the surface of the thalamus but did not involve the deep thalamic parenchyma. This lesion could be removed by a parasagittal, transparietal approach without a resulting neurologic or visual deficit.

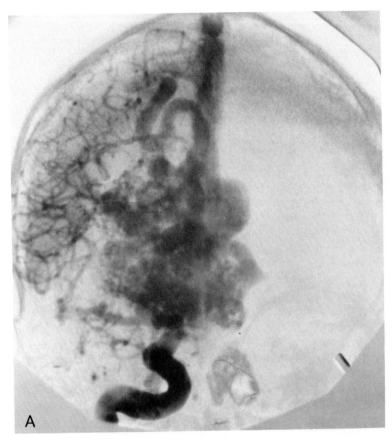

A

FIG. 14.6. Large right frontal AVM. (A) Right carotid injection, A-P projection (note how AVM loops protrude to the left side of the midline). (B) Right carotid injection, lateral projection. (C) Left carotid injection, A-P projection. (D) Postoperative right carotid injection. (E) Postoperative left carotid injection (note filling of both pericallosal arteries from the left.)

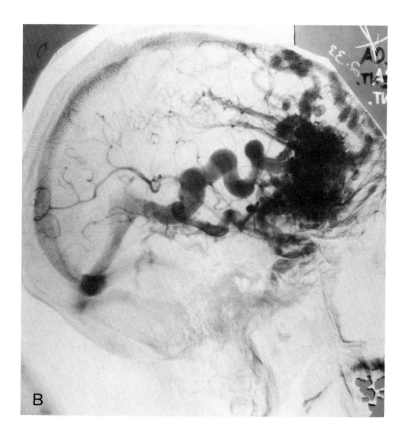

FIG. 14.6B

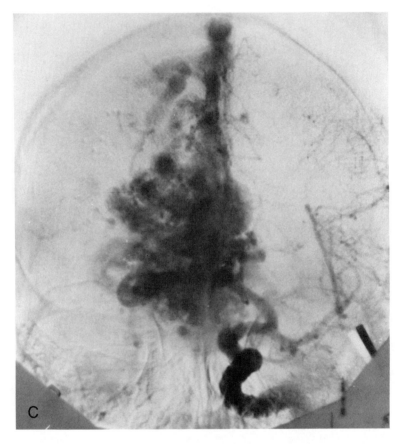

Fig. 14.6C

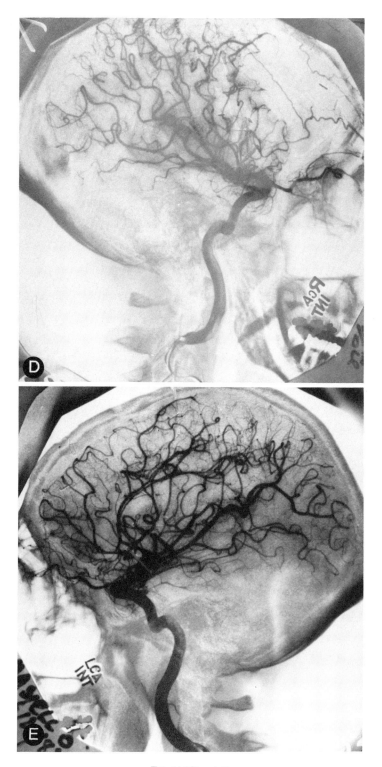

FIG. 14.6*D* and *E*

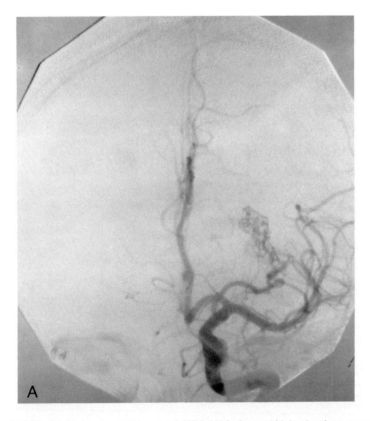

FIG. 14.7. Moderate size deep left temporal AVM. (A) Left carotid injection (note prominent anterior choroidal feeder and absence of lenticulostriate feeders). (B) Vertebral injection (note small posterolateral choroidal feeders and absence of thalamo-perforating feeders). (C) Postoperative left carotid arteriogram. (D) Postoperative vertebral arteriogram.

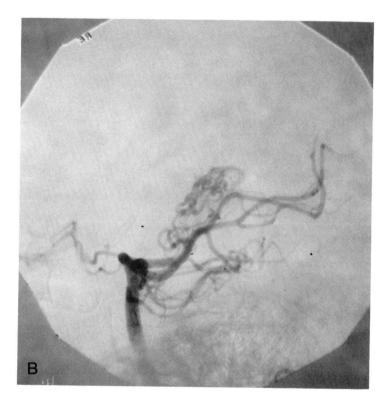

FIG. 14.7B

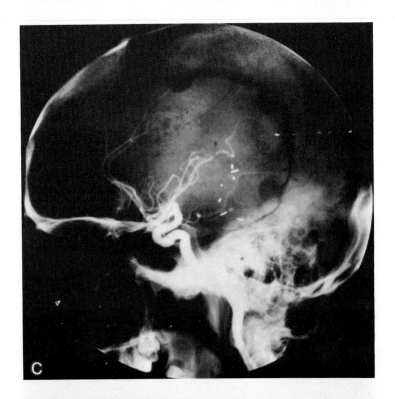

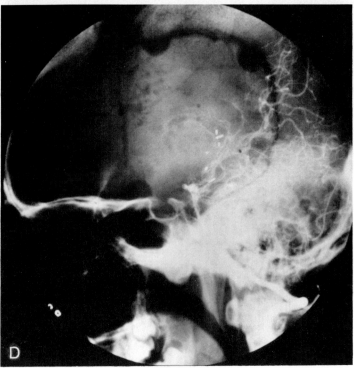

Fig. 14.7C and D

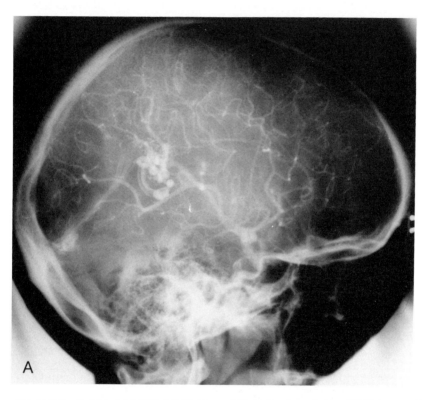

FIG. 14.8. Small right atrial AVM. (A) Right carotid injection, lateral view. (B) Right carotid injection, A-P view. (C) Postoperative arteriogram.

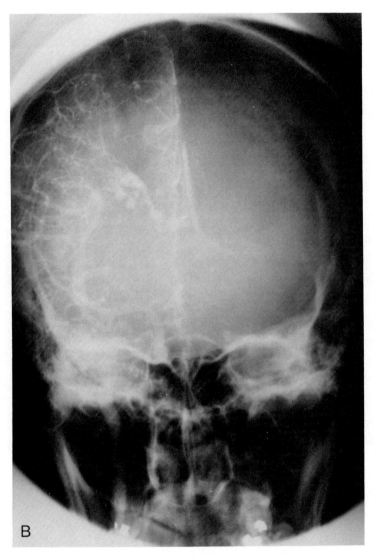

FIG. 14.8B

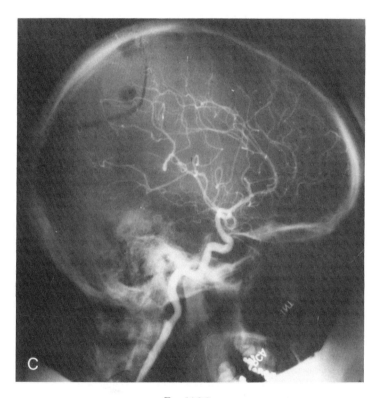

Fig. 14.8*C*

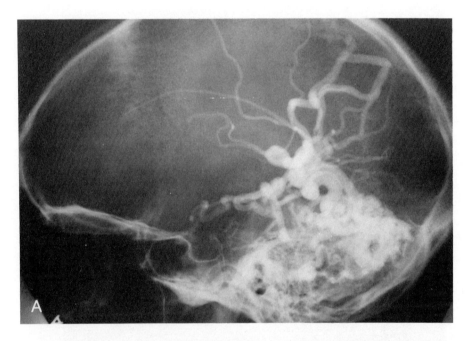

Fɪɢ. 14.9. Moderate size cerebellar AVM. (A) Vertebral injection, midarterial phase (note diffuse venous drainage which makes it difficult to delineate the extent of the lesion. (B) Vertebral injection, very early arterial phase (note good demarcation of the true nidus of the AVM). (C) Postoperative arteriogram.

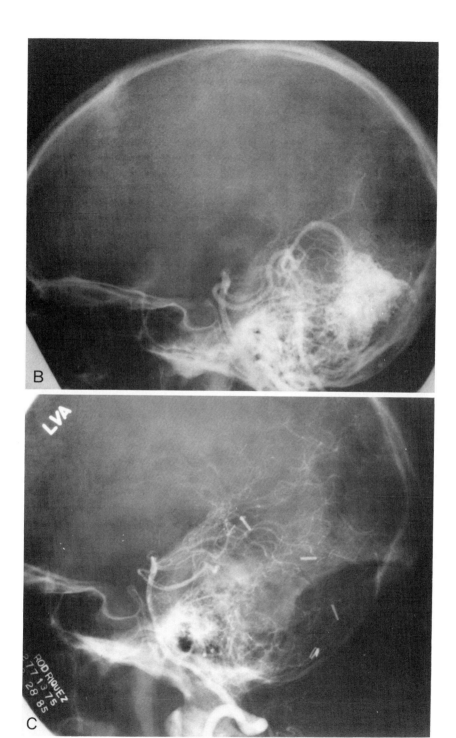

Fig. 14.9*B* and *C*

Fig. 14.9A illustrates that a lesion that appears formidable once the veins begin to fill can in fact be relatively circumscribed upon inspection of the early arterial phase of the arteriogram (Fig. 14.9B). This lesion was also removed without a resulting permanent neurologic deficit.

Some arteriographic clues that predict operative difficulty are listed in Table 14.11. Figure 14.10 illustrates a sylvian AVM with prominent lenticulostriate supply. Fortunately for this patient, all of the lesion was temporal and insular lateral to the internal capsule and, therefore, the minor hemiparesis that she had in the postoperative period cleared completely in time. However, this operation took many hours of very tedious dissection, sorting out which branches of the middle cerebral complex in the sylvian fissure went to AVM and which branches were simply "passing through" and going to normal brain. In addition, the deep lenticulostriate supply kept the lesion alive and bleeding until the very last hour of the operation. The fragility of these deep perforating vessels is well-known to surgeons and there is no access to them until the end of the resection. Also, when they bleed and retract, one must pursue them into the parenchyma of vital structures sometimes with catastrophic results.

The same applies to the small deep-feeding vessels that can be consistently predicted to exist when there is deep venous drainage. Figure 14.11, from a case previously illustrated and discussed in this chapter (Fig. 14.4), shows clearly one of these deep draining veins, in this case a very large ependymal vein. Even though no deep arteries are visualized in this case, there certainly was prominent deep supply from small arteries in relation to the deep vein. This added significantly to the difficulty of this case. The patient, who had a progressive hemiparesis preoperatively, was hemiplegic postoperatively, but fortunately his leg and proximal arm strength have improved considerably.

Another case previously discussed in this chapter (Fig. 14.2) is typical of the diffuse malformations with poorly defined margins and supply from all three major arterial territories. Most of these lesions are simply inoperable as was the lesion in point. Our attempts at partial treatment with repeated embolizations have only led to a worsening of her overall condition.

TABLE 14.11
Angiographic Clues of Operative Difficulty

Supply from perforating branches
Sylvian location
Deep venous drainage
Supply from three major arterial territories
Poorly defined margins
Large caliber feeding vessels

Lastly, Figure 14.12 illustrates the AVM of a patient who presented with a severe seizure disorder and failing intellect thought to be due to the large amounts of anticonvulsant medications he required. He had been unable to work for about 2 years. We excised the lesion without prior embolization. Again, as in the case discussed earlier under complications (Fig. 14.3), there was significant brain swelling at the time of craniotomy closure although there was no diffuse bleeding. He had a sluggish postoperative course with moderate left hemiparesis, drowsiness, and a marked right parietal syndrome. Fortunately, he responded to treatment for brain swelling and by about 3 months after surgery he was intact neurologically except for a partial visual field cut. Two years later, he is back to work and taking only a minimal amount of anticonvulsants. He has been seizure-free since the time of surgery. This is one of the two cases of probable "perfusion breakthrough" in our series of patients with unruptured AVMs. Both cases, fortunately, were not severe and postoperative bleeding did not occur in either. We feel that we would have seen this phenomenon more often if we had not embolized some of our other large lesions with high flow and large caliber feeding vessels prior to surgery.

In addition to the size and configuration (diffuse vs. compact), the location (deep vs. superficial; silent vs. eloquent brain), the number, caliber, and location of feeding vessels (superficial or choroidal vs. perforating), and the pattern of venous drainage (superficial vs. deep) what other factors have been important to us in the surgical decision making process when faced with a patient with an AVM? Table 14.12 lists some of these other factors. The importance of personal surgical experience with similar cases does not need to be elaborated. The patient's neurological condition is obviously a very important factor. The patient may already be so devastated that it would be unjustified to subject him to surgery to prevent death

TABLE 14.12
Surgical Decision Making in AVMs

Size and configuration of the lesion
Location of the lesion
Number, caliber, and location of feeding vessels
Pattern of venous drainage
Surgeon's experience with similar lesions
Patient's neurologic condition
Patient's age and general condition
Patient's psychological reaction to the lesion
Patient's occupation and hobbies
History of recent or multiple hemorrhages

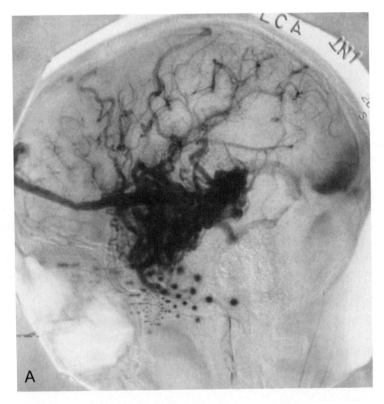

FIG. 14.10. Large left sylvian AVM. (*A*) Left carotid injection, lateral view. (*B*) Left carotid injection, A-P view (note prominence of lenticulostriate supply to the lesion). (*C*) Left carotid injection, very early arterial phase, lateral view (note the complexity of the mixture of normal branches and feeders to AVM in sylvian fissure). (*D*) Postoperative arteriogram.

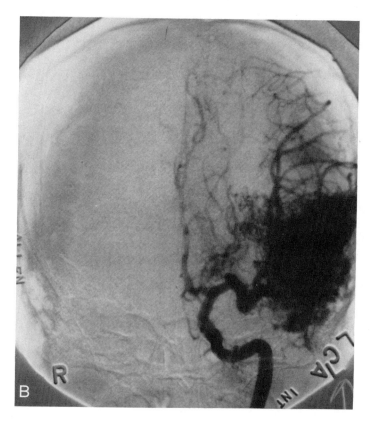

Fig. 14.10*B*

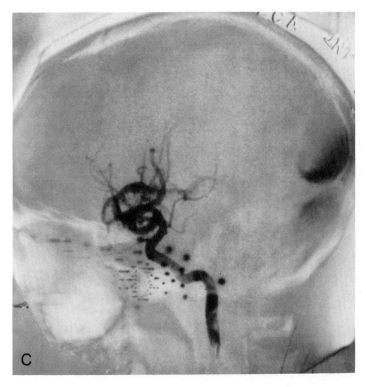

Fig. 14.10C

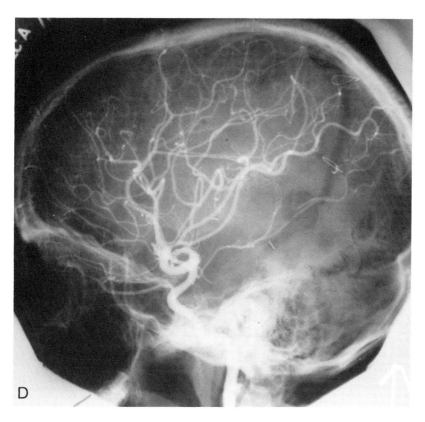

Fig. 14.10D

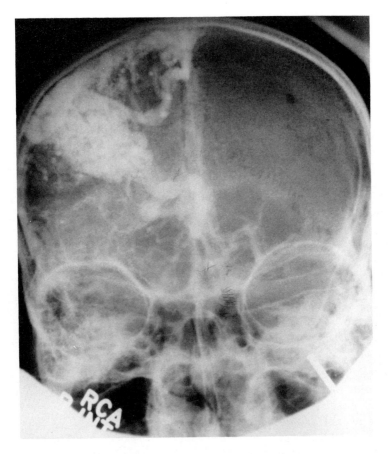

FIG. 14.11. Right midarterial phase carotid injection, A-P view from case previously illustrated in Figure 14.4 (note large deep draining vein).

from another hemorrhage which may be a blessing to the patient and his family. On the other hand, the patient may be functional and independent, but may already have the neurologic deficit that the operation would produce, in which case the AVM can be excised without additional disability. A word of caution should be given to the effect that, soon after a moderate hemorrhage, the patient may have a rather severe neurologic deficit which could well improve with time. It would be very wrong to excise his AVM and give him an irreversible deficit that, though not worse than the deficit he had at the time, could leave him permanently in that state from which he may have recovered significantly if left alone.

The patient's general condition and age are of obvious importance in assessing his ability to tolerate the operation. In addition, it is clear that once middle age is reached the risk of bleeding from an AVM decreases (26, 42). Also, whereas at younger ages AVMs more often than not tend to enlarge (7, 23, 26, 56), they seem to reach a stable size and occasionally decrease in size after middle age (26). Another important aspect of age is the well-known capacity of younger patients for neurologic recovery or adaptation to a neurologic deficit.

The patient's psychological reaction to his AVM is a factor commented upon earlier in this chapter. Some patients go on with their lives without giving it a second thought. Others are devastated by the thought that they could have a hemorrhage at any time; the latter group, as stated earlier, is far from being "asymptomatic" and sometimes they are quite willing to accept even a moderate neurologic deficit in exchange for being rid of their AVM. Garretson (11), in his very thoughtful recent review of AVMs, has emphasized the importance of not only the patient's age and condition, but also his occupation and hobbies. A mild hemiparesis has a very different meaning to a pianist than to a librarian, whereas a trial attorney whose hobby is to decipher hieroglyphics may be more amenable to accepting a moderate hemiparesis than any degree of aphasia.

Finally, although this chapter has emphasized the fact that the risk of hemorrhage is not very different in a patient with or without a history of a remote hemorrhage, there is no doubt that a patient is at a higher risk of rebleeding during the few months after a hemorrhage from an AVM (12, 53) and that patients with a history of multiple hemorrhages have a higher chance of rebleeding (9).

If, after all these factors are considered, the decision is made not to recommend surgical excision, what then should we do? First, and perhaps most importantly, we should never overemphasize the danger of a lesion that we cannot treat. Terms such as "a bomb in your head," "sitting on a powder keg," etc., should never be used under these circumstances. Perret (40) has found that hemorrhage from AVM occurs during sleep in 36% of the patients and during activities such as heavy lifting, defecation, coitus, urination, "emotional stress," etc., in less than 25% of the patients. Therefore, we recommend to our patients that they should continue their normal lifestyles and, save for such obviously dangerous activities as competitive weight lifting, they should continue to do whatever they enjoyed doing prior to diagnosis. An intelligent discussion of the relatively low risk of bleeding of such lesions (2–3% per year) is in order and will reassure most patients. Then the assessment can be made as to whether the lesion could possibly be completely obliterated by embolization even though it is in a surgically inaccessible location. This would indeed be a rare case since it

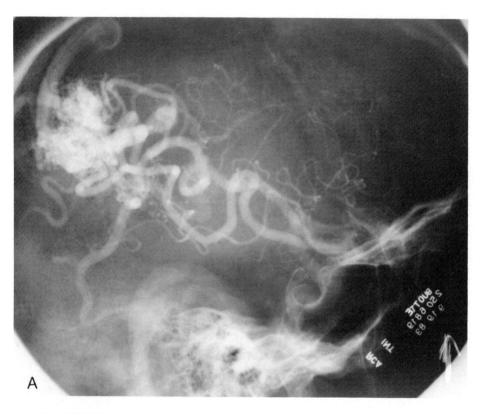

FIG. 14.12. Moderate size right parietal AVM. (A) Right carotid injection, lateral view (note large caliber feeding vessels). (B) Right carotid injection, A-P view. (C) Postoperative right carotid arteriogram.

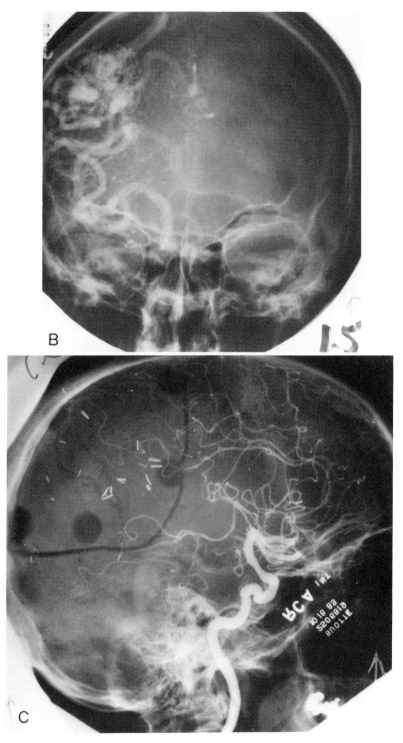

B

C

FIG. 14.12B and C

is usually the small superficial, surgically accessible lesions that can be completely obliterated by embolization (6). As stated earlier, we feel that partial embolization, if there is no hope of obliterating the lesion completely or surgically excising it after the embolization, is probably of no value and may be harmful. The possible exceptions, as discussed earlier, are in patients with progressive neurologic deficit and perhaps in patients with intractable headache who have prominent dural and scalp feeders to the AVM that are amenable to embolization. If the patient is not a candidate for complete surgical excision or embolization, other modalities such as proton beam therapy (22), stereotactic radiosurgery (49), conventional radiotherapy (19), or, more recently, electrothrombosis by stereotactic wire injections (14), can be considered. Each of these modalities have been shown to be of some value, but a thorough discussion of their pros and cons is beyond the scope of this chapter. They should not be considered definitive therapy and, as Drake (8) has discussed, they should not be thought of as an alternative to complete surgical excision of the lesion.

CONCLUSION

We have endeavored to show that the overall morbidity of AVM surgery with modern surgical techniques in experienced hands is acceptable and is similar in patients with ruptured or unruptured AVMs. We have also stressed that each AVM is different and, therefore, that overall morbidity figures are of little consequence when an individual case is analyzed. We have pointed out that simply because the patient has no neurologic deficit or seizures, he is not necessarily asymptomatic since the knowledge of having a potentially lethal lesion is psychologically devastating to many. We have emphasized the fact that whether or not a patient has bled in the past should not be the major factor influencing therapeutic decisions because, in the first place, it is sometimes difficult to determine whether or not a patient has bled in the past and, second, the risk of future hemorrhage is not very different in patients who have no history of hemorrhage than in patients who have bled in the past. We have also underlined the fact that the risk of bleeding in patients with unruptured AVMs is substantial (3% per year or 25% in 15 years) and that the morbidity of a first hemorrhage from an AVM is significant (at least 30%).

We have not solved the "dilemma" of whether or not to recommend surgery to a patient with an unruptured AVM or, for that matter, to any patient with an AVM. This dilemma will present itself to each surgeon with about one-half of the patients that come to him with an AVM, whether ruptured or unruptured. In the other one-half of the patients the decision will be straightforward; they either should be excised (small and moderately large AVMs of the "silent" cerebral convexities and cerebellar hemisphere) or should not be excised (intraparenchymal AVMs of the thalamus and brain stem and massive panhemispheric AVMs). We have argued that, in the roughly one-half of the cases where careful judgment must be exercised, the fact that the AVM is ruptured or unruptured is not the most important, or even a decisive factor. The most important factor is the size, location, configuration, blood supply, and drainage of the AVM itself. Other factors such as the surgeon's experience with similar lesions, the patient's age and his neurologic and medical condition, as well as his occupation and hobbies, and, importantly, his psychological reaction to the problem are at least as important as whether or not there has been a history of hemorrhage. We have presented a series of 40 consecutive patients with unruptured AVMs operated upon without mortality, but with a 12.5% morbidity. The cases in which morbidity occurred were illustrated. Of these, the only patient that is incapacitated is a man in whom we failed to recognize that his cerebellar AVM extended into the brain stem. Clues that we have found helpful in determining whether or not the lesion is operable and in predicting surgical difficulty, were discussed and illustrated.

ACKNOWLEDGMENTS

Dr. Robert Ojemann has referred several of the patients included in this series and has offered invaluable help to the senior author in preoperative decision-making as well as in operative planning and execution. Dr. Gerard Debrun has also referred several of the patients, has helped us greatly with neuroradiologic interpretations, and has carried out all of the embolization procedures in patients so treated.

REFERENCES

1. Adelt, D., Zeumer, H., and Wolters, J. Surgical treatment of cerebral arteriovenous malformations. Follow-up study of 43 cases. Acta. Neurochir. (Wien), 76: 45–49, 1985.
2. Albert, P. Personal experience in the treatment of 178 cases of arteriovenous malformations of the brain. Acta. Neurochir. (Wien), 61: 207–226, 1982.
3. Cophignon, J., Thurel, C., Djindjian, R., Rey, A., Visot, A., LeBesneraie, Y., and Houdart, R. Cerebral arteriovenous malformations. Modern aspects of investigations and treatment. Prog. Neurol. Surg., 9: 195–237, 1978.
4. Davis, C. Management of cerebral arteriovenous malformations. Letter to the editor. Lancet, June 18: 1391, 1983.
5. Davis, C., and Symon, L. The management of cerebral arteriovenous malformations. Act. Neurochir. (Wien), 74: 4–11, 1985.
6. Debrun, G., Vinuela, F., Fox, A., and Drake, C. G. Embolization of cerebral arteriovenous malformations with bucrylate. Experience in 46 cases. J. Neurosurg., 56: 615–627, 1982.
7. Delitala, A., Delfini, R., Vagnozzi, R., and Esposito, S. Increase in size of cerebral angiomas. Case report. J. Neurosurg., 57: 556–558, 1982.
8. Drake, C. G. Cerebral arteriovenous malformations: considerations for and experience with surgical treatment in 166 cases. Clin. Neurosurg. 26: 145–208, 1979.

9. Forster, D. M. C., Steiner, L., and Hakanson, S. Arteriovenous malformations of the brain. A long-term clinical study. J. Neurosurg., *37:* 562–570, 1972.

10. Fults, D., and Kelly, D. L. Natural history of arteriovenous malformations of the brain. A clinical study. Neurosurgery, *15:* 658–662, 1984.

11. Garretson, H. D. Intracranial arteriovenous malformations. In: *Neurosurgery*, edited by R. H. Wilkins and S. S. Rengachary. McGraw-Hill Book Co., New York, 1985, pp. 1448–1458.

12. Graf, C. J., Perret, G. E., and Torner, J. C. Bleeding from cerebral arteriovenous malformations as part of their natural history. J. Neurosurg., *58:* 331–337, 1983.

13. Guidetti, B., and Delitala, A. Intracranial arteriovenous malformations. Conservative and surgical treatment. J. Neurosurg., *53:* 149–152, 1980.

14. Handa, H., Yoneda, S., Matsuda, M., Shimizu, Y., and Goto, H. The surgical treatment of deep-seated or large arteriovenous malformations of the brain by means of electrically induced thrombosis. In: *Neurological Surgery (With Emphasis on Noninvasive Methods of Diagnosis and Treatment)*, Excerpta Medica, Amsterdam, 1978, pp. 143–148.

15. Henderson, W. R., Gomez, R. Natural history of cerebral angiomas. Br. Med. J., *4:* 571–577, 1967.

16. Heros, R. C. Arteriovenous malformations of the medial temporal lobe. J. Neurosurg., *56:* 44–52, 1982.

17. Hitchcock, E. R. Management of cerebral arteriovenous malformations. Letter to the editor. Lancet, June 18: 1391, 1983.

18. Iansek, R., Elstein, A. S., and Balla, J. I. Application of decision analysis to management of cerebral arteriovenous malformations. Lancet, *1:* 1132–1136, 1983.

19. Johnson, R. T. Radiotherapy of cerebral angiomas with a note on some problems in diagnosis. In: *Cerebral Angiomas: Advances in Diagnosis and Therapy*, edited by H. W. Pia, J. R. W. Gleave, E. Grote, and J. Zierski. Springer-Verlag, New York, 1975, pp. 256–259.

20. Jomin, M., Lesoin, F., and Lozes G. Prognosis for arteriovenous malformations of the brain in adults based on 150 cases. Surg. Neurol., *23:* 362–366, 1985.

21. Kelly, D. L., Jr., Alexander, E., Jr., Davis, C. H., Jr., and Maynard, D. C. Intracranial arteriovenous malformations: clinical review and evaluation of brain scans. J. Neurosurg., *31:* 422–428, 1969.

22. Kjellberg, R. N., Hanamura, T., Davis, K. R., Lyons, S. L., and Adams, R. D. Bragg-peak proton-beam therapy for arteriovenous malformations of the brain. N. Engl. J. Med., *309:* 269–274, 1983.

23. Krayenbühl, H. A. Angiographic contribution to the problem of enlargement of cerebral arteriovenous malformations. Acta. Neurochir., *36:* 215–242, 1977.

24. Kumar, A. J., Fox, A. J., Vinuela, F., and Rosenbaum, A. E. Revisited old and new CT findings in unruptured large arteriovenous malformations of the brain. J. Comput. Assist. Tomogr., *8:* 648–655, 1984.

25. Luessenhop, A. J. Natural history of cerebral arteriovenous malformations. In: *Intracranial Arteriovenous Malformations*, Edited by C. B. Wilson and B. M. Stein. Williams & Wilkins, Baltimore, 1984, pp. 12–23.

26. Luessenhop, A. J., and Rosa, L. Cerebral arteriovenous malformations. Indications for and results of surgery, and the role of intravascular techniques. J. Neurosurg. *60:* 14–22, 1984.

27. Mackenzie, I. The clinical presentation of the cerebral angioma: A review of 50 cases. Brain, *76:* 184–214, 1953.

28. Malis, L. I. Arteriovenous malformations of the brain. In: *Neurological Surgery*, Vol. 3, 2nd edition, edited by J. R. Youmans. W. B. Saunders Co., Philadelphia, 1982, pp. 1786–1806.

29. McCormick, W. F. The pathology of vascular ("arteriovenous") malformations. J. Neurosurg., *24:* 807–812, 1966.
30. Michelsen, W. J. Natural history and pathophysiology of arteriovenous malformations. Clin. Neurosurg., *26:* 307–313, 1979.
31. Mingrino, S. Supratentorial arteriovenous malformations of the brain. In: *Advances and Technical Standards in Neurosurgery,* Vol. 5, edited by H. Krayenbühl. Springer-Verlag, New York, 1978, pp. 93–123.
32. Mohr, J. P. Neurological manifestations and factors related to therapeutic decisions. In: *Intracranial Arteriovenous Malformations,* edited by C. B. Wilson and B. M. Stein. Williams & Wilkins, Baltimore, 1984, pp. 1–11.
33. Moody, R. A., and Poppen, J. L. Arteriovenous malformations. J. Neurosurg., *32:* 503–511, 1970.
34. Morello, G., and Broghi, G. P. Cerebral angiomas. A report of 154 personal cases and a comparison between the results of surgical excision and conservative management. Acta. Neurochir., *28:* 135–155, 1973.
35. Mullan, S., Brown, F. D., and Patronas, N. J. Hyperemic and ischemic problems of surgical treatment of arteriovenous malformations. J. Neurosurg. *51:* 757–764, 1979.
36. Nornes, H., and Grip, A. Hemodynamic aspects of cerebral arteriovenous malformations. J. Neurosurg., *53:* 456–464, 1980.
37. Nornes, H., Lundar, T., and Wikeby, P. Cerebral arteriovenous malformations: Results of microsurgical management. Acta. Neurochir. (Wien), *50:* 243–257, 1979.
38. Parkinson, D., and Bachers, G. Arteriovenous malformations. Summary of 100 consecutive supratentorial cases. J. Neurosurg., *53:* 285–299, 1980.
39. Pellettieri, L., Carlsson, A-A., Grevsten, S., Norlén, G., and Uhlemann, C. Surgical versus conservative treatment of intracranial arteriovenous malformations. A study in surgical decision-making. Acta. Neurochir. (Wien) (Suppl), *29:* 1–86, 1980.
40. Perret, G. E. Conservative management of inoperable arteriovenous malformations. In: *Cerebral Angiomas. Advances in Diagnosis and Therapy,* edited by H. W. Pia, J. R. W. Gleave, E. Grote, and J. Zierski. Springer-Verlag, New York, 1975, pp. 268–270.
41. Perret, G. The epidemiology and clinical course of arteriovenous malformations. In: *Cerebral Angiomas. Advances in Diagnosis and Therapy,* edited by H. W. Pia, J. R. W. Gleave, E. Grote, and J. Zierski. Springer-Verlag, New York, 1975, pp. 21–26.
42. Perret, G., and Nishioka, H. Report on cooperative study of intracranial aneurysms and subarachnoid hemorrhage. Section VI: Arteriovenous malformations. Analysis of 545 cases of cranio-cerebral arteriovenous malformations and fistulae reported to cooperative study. J. Neurosurg., *25:* 467–490, 1966.
43. Pool, J. L. Treatment of arteriovenous malformations of the cerebral hemispheres. J. Neurosurg., *19:* 136–141, 1962.
44. Pool, J. L. Excision of cerebral arteriovenous malformations. J. Neurosurg., *29:* 312–321, 1968.
45. Spetzler, R. F., Wilson, C. B., Weinstein, P., Mehdorn, M., Townsend, J., and Telles, D. Normal perfusion pressure breakthrough theory. Clin. Neurosurg., *25:* 651–672, 1978.
46. Stein, B. M. Arteriovenous malformations of the medial cerebral hemisphere and the limbic system. J. Neurosurg. *60:* 23–31, 1984.
47. Stein, B. M. General techniques for the surgical removal of arteriovenous malformations. In: *Intracranial Arteriovenous Malformations,* edited by C. B. Wilson and B. M. Stein. Williams & Wilkins, Baltimore, 1984, pp. 143–155.
48. Stein, B. M., and Wolpert, S. M. Arteriovenous malformations of the brain. II: Current concepts and treatment. Arch. Neurol., *37:* 69–75, 1980.
49. Steiner, L., Leksell, L., Forster, D. M. C., Greitz, T., and Backlund, E. O. Stereotactic

radiosurgery in intracranial arteriovenous malformations. Acta. Neurochir. (Suppl.), *21:* 195–209, 1974.

50. Suzuki, J., Onuma, T., and Kayama, T. Surgical treatment of intracranial arteriovenous malformations. Neurol. Res., *4:* 191–207, 1982.

51. Svien, H. J., and McRae, J. A. Arteriovenous anomalies of the brain. Fate of patients not having definitive surgery. J. Neurosurg., *23:* 23–28, 1965.

52. Svien, H. J., Olive, I., Angulo-Rivero, P. The fate of patients who have cerebral arteriovenous anomalies without definitive surgical treatments. J. Neurosurg., *8:* 381–387, 1956.

53. Torner, J. C. Natural history of arteriovenous malformations. Presented at a breakfast seminar at the 53rd annual meeting of the American Association of Neurological Surgeons. San Francisco, California, April 12, 1984.

54. Troupp, H., Marttila, I., and Halonen, V. Arteriovenous malformations of the brain. Prognosis without operation. Acta. Neurochir. *22:* 125–128, 1970.

55. Trumpy, J. H., and Eldevik, P. Intracranial arteriovenous malformations: Conservative or surgical treatment? Surg. Neurol., *8:* 171–175, 1977.

56. Walter, W. Conservative treatment of cerebral arteriovenous angiomas. In: *Cerebral Angiomas. Advances in Diagnosis and Therapy,* edited by H. W. Pia, J. R. W. Gleave, E. Grote, and J. Zierski. Springer-Verlag, New York, 1975, pp. 271–278.

57. Waltimo, O. The relationship of size, density and localization of intracranial arteriovenous malformations to the type of initial symptoms. J. Neurol. Sci., *19:* 13–19, 1973.

58. Wilkins, R. H. Natural history of intracranial vascular malformations: A review. Neurosurgery, *16:* 421–430, 1985.

59. Wilson, C. B., U, H. S., and Domingue, J. Microsurgical treatment of intracranial vascular malformations. J. Neurosurg., *51:* 446–454, 1979.

CHAPTER

15

Asymptomatic Carotid Disease

DONALD O. QUEST, M.D.

Patients with asymptomatic carotid disease may be divided into those patients with an asymptomatic carotid bruit, those with symptomatic cerebrovascular disease found to have contralateral carotid disease not causing symptoms, and those about to undergo other major noncarotid surgery who are found to have asymptomatic carotid disease. The aphorism: "It is difficult to make an asymptomatic patient better" sets an appropriate tone of caution in the approach to management of these patients.

THE ASYMPTOMATIC CAROTID BRUIT

Auscultation of a bruit in the neck leads to consternation for the physician, surgeon, and patient for several reasons: (*a*) There is increased awareness that stroke is a major cause of mortality (third most frequent cause of death in the United States in 1980—172,000 mortalities [18]) and morbidity (50% of victims requiring specialized care). (*b*) There is widespread understanding that lesions of the extracranial carotid artery are a major etiologic factor in stroke. (*c*) Carotid endarterectomy has been widely accepted as appropriate prophylaxis against stroke, though this procedure has yet to be proven conclusively better than the best medical treatment. (*d*) Carotid artery operations have become common with 85,000 cases done in 1982—a dramatic increase compared to 15,000 in 1971 (28).

Questions arise such as: What is the significance of a carotid bruit? What is the risk of stroke? Should surgery be performed? What is an appropriate plan of management? Some of the answers are clear-cut, others more problematical.

About 5% of people over age 65 have a cervical bruit, but the correlation of the bruit with carotid disease is poor (about 50%) (13). The overall risk of stroke in the patient found to have an asymptomatic bruit is about 2% per year and the risk of death 4% per year; however, the strokes are not always in the distribution of the carotid with the bruit (18).

With the advent of carotid endarterectomy and refinement of the operation, so that morbidity and mortality can be lessened to a small percentage, enthusiasm for surgery on the asymptomatic patient has increased. Two large studies in the past have advocated operation for such patients (6, 26).

Both studies followed nonoperated patients with asymptomatic bruits and reported higher rates of strokes (15–17%) over several years as compared to operated controls. These studies were retrospective in nature and neither documented the relationship of the neurological events to the territory of the carotid where the bruit was heard. It was also not reported whether these nonoperated patients suffered acute stroke or experienced warning transient ischemic attacks (TIA's) before the stroke (a warning TIA would have justified prophylactic endarterectomy in most cases).

There have been two large population studies, prospective and randomized, which have addressed the natural history of the patient with an asymptomatic bruit (14, 29). The Evans County Georgia Study identified carotid bruits in 72 of 1620 individuals, 10 of whom went on to develop strokes, but the strokes occurred in most cases in a different vascular territory from that of the asymptomatic bruit. The other study, from the Framingham population, confirmed that the patient with an asymptomatic bruit had an increased risk of stroke but the majority of these occurred in the opposite carotid or vertebral artery territory or were not related to the carotid at all—such as aneurysmal hemorrhage, lacunar infarcts, or embolic strokes related to cardiac sources. Both of these studies found that those patients with asymptomatic bruits are at increased risk for symptomatic cerebrovascular and cardiac disease but neither could provide justification for prophylactic surgery on the carotid artery for an asymptomatic bruit alone.

A recent study by Roederer et al. (24) addressed the issue of progression of carotid artery disease in patients with asymptomatic bruits followed with ultrasonography. A prior report of serial angiography in patients with carotid disease showed a progression of the disease in 20% of the patients over several years (16). Roederer et al. (24) followed patients with asymptomatic carotid bruits with ultrasound at 6-month intervals and found that there was indeed progression of the disease over a 3-year period. This progression did not always follow a linear fashion but sometimes occurred paroxysmally. It was found that those patients who had stenosis of the carotid artery greater than 80% were at 35% risk for stroke, TIAs, or occlusion of the carotid within a 6-month period. These authors recommended prophylactic surgery for the patient with 80% or greater stenosis of the carotid even if there are no symptoms.

The problem of the ulcerated but nonstenotic asymptomatic carotid lesion rarely has been addressed and is unsettled. One study found a 12% annual stroke rate in those with large or compound ulcers (22), whereas another found a rate of only 1% in several years (17). It is unclear from the available data whether or not surgery is indicated.

RECOMMENDED MANAGEMENT

In the asymptomatic patient in whom a cervical bruit is heard it is reasonable to proceed with noninvasive testing. Recommended is the duplex ultrasound study which includes Doppler imaging, showing velocity profile and degree of turbulence (Fig. 15.1 A-D), and B-mode scanning in sagittal and axial section which can outline the anatomy of the bifurcation relatively well (Fig. 15.2). It has been shown that duplex ultrasonography with pulsed Doppler and high resolution B-mode imaging is quite effective in delineating stenosis over 50% (9, 11). The correlation with angiographic documentation of stenosis is in the 80–90% range (1). Plaque morphology can be imaged but ulcerations may be missed (as they may be with angiography). An advantage of ultrasonography is that it is completely risk-free. A disadvantage is that the study depends significantly on the skill of the operator in order to detect stenosis. In experienced hands false-positives are quite rare; false-negatives range from 5–15% (15). Should there be evidence with either of these studies that there is significant stenosis (over 50%) an intravenous or intra-arterial digital subtraction angiogram should be performed.

Intravenous digital subtraction angiography has excellent sensitivity, specificity, and accuracy—about 94% compared to conventional angiography (10, 30) and it does not require intra-arterial catheterization or hospitalization. Problems include poor depiction of ulcerations and poor definition of the carotid siphon and intracranial vasculature (8). Technical difficulties include suboptimal resolution, patient motion causing artifacts, and superimposition of the vessels in the neck. In addition, there is a large contrast burden (more than with conventional angiography), which could cause problems with patients who have renal or cardiovascular disease. With an adequate study, stenosis can be readily detected.

Intra-arterial digital subtraction angiography has several advantages (Fig. 15.3A) (3). This study provides excellent detail with subtraction and magnification features. The ability to manipulate image contrast and brightness can help in depicting ulceration, and the intracranial vasculature is well seen (Fig. 15.3B-D). Less contrast agent is given than with either intravenous digital subtraction angiography or conventional angiography. In addition, a small catheter is used allowing the procedure to be performed on an outpatient basis in some instances.

If stenosis detected by ultrasonography is less than 50%, medical rather than surgical management is appropriate and should proceed with antiplatelet therapy (acetylsalicyclic acid) with attention directed toward the contributing risk factors of stroke, such as hypertention, diabetes, and

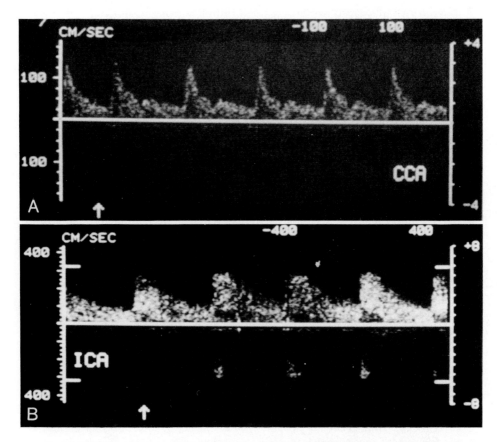

FIG. 15.1. Doppler ultrasound imaging showing velocity profile of a normal caliber common carotid artery with sharp peaks (A) and the velocity profile of a stenotic internal carotid artery with broad peaks (B). (C) shows the band width of velocities of a normal common carotid artery and (D) shows the band width of velocities of a stenotic internal carotid artery. Note the wide band width of velocities here, consistent with turbulent flow.

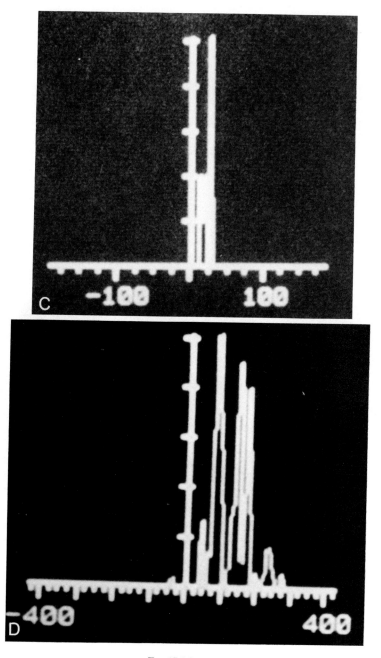

FIG. 15.1*C* and *D*

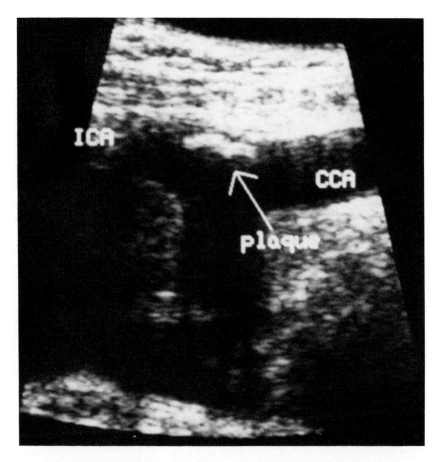

FIG. 15.2. B-mode ultrasound image in sagittal section of the carotid bifurcation plaque with moderate stenosis.

cigarette smoking. Follow-up ultrasonography at yearly intervals should be performed. A TIA would warn of an impending stroke in most patients; if a TIA occurs, surgery should be performed (5, 7, 9, 18, 20).

If stenosis greater than 50% is found on ultrasonography, either an intravenous or intraarterial digital subtraction angiogram should be performed. Those patients found to have progressing lesions on serial follow-up studies or who have stenosis greater than 80% are at high risk for TIA, stroke, or occlusion. They should be strongly considered for endarterectomy (15, 24, 31). If the digital studies do not show the intra- and extracranial vascular anatomy adequately, conventional angiography should be done. Surgical morbidity and mortality must be quite low, in the 3–5% range, in order to justify endarterectomy in these asymptomatic patients.

CONTRALATERAL CAROTID STENOSIS

A number of retrospective studies have been done in an attempt to define the risk of stroke in patients with contralateral carotid stenosis managed nonoperatively. Their aim was to determine what percentage of these patients progressed to a direct stroke in the appropriate carotid distribution without warning TIAs. In a number of reports no patients followed with contralateral asymptomatic lesions developed a stroke without a warning TIA (19, 21, 22). In two reports a few patients did develop strokes directly, but the incidence was less than 3% and thus less than the accepted risk of surgical morbidity and mortality in carotid disease (7). Some authors advocate surgery for such patients if there is angiographic documentation of stenosis in the 80–90% range as hemodynamic studies indicate that critical reduction of cerebral blood flow occurs with this degree of stenosis (2, 4, 23).

It seems best, in these patients, to follow a similar course as with those with asymptomatic bruits, operating only on symptomatic vessels and managing the contralateral asymptomatic carotid stenosis conservatively until such time as TIAs develop or greater than 80% stenosis or progression can be identified. It is reasonable to deduce that these patients with contralateral stenosis may be at the same risk as those with asymptomatic bruits found to have progressing lesions or 80% stenosis.

CAROTID RISK IN NON-CAROTID SURGICAL PATIENTS

Since the development of carotid artery surgery for occlusive disease, there has been interest in the proper management of those noncarotid preoperative patients who have auscultatory or radiographic evidence of otherwise asymptomatic carotid artery disease. It has been found that the incidence of asymptomatic bruit in random preoperative patients is about 15%. Although a perioperative stroke rate of about 1% has been identified in these patients there is no correlation between the presence or location of a carotid bruit and the risk of a perioperative stroke (12, 25, 27, 28). Recent investigations have prospectively studied operative patients with asymptomatic carotid bruits. These studies document higher perioperative mortality in patients with carotid bruits, but the mortality is primarily attributable to an increased risk of myocardial infarction. To date, there is no study analyzing the risk of stroke in preoperative patients with asymptomatic, but angiographically demonstrated carotid artery lesions.

Recommendations regarding this group of patients are similar to the asymptomatic bruit group and prophylactic surgery is not routinely recom-

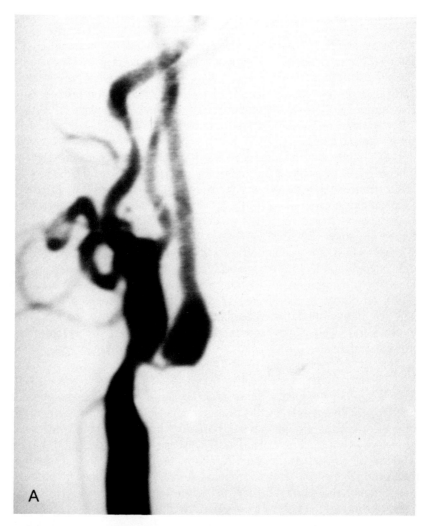

FIG. 15.3. Intra-arterial digital subtraction angiogram showing severe stenosis of the internal carotid artery (A) with acceptable visualization of the intra and extra-cranial vasculature (B-D).

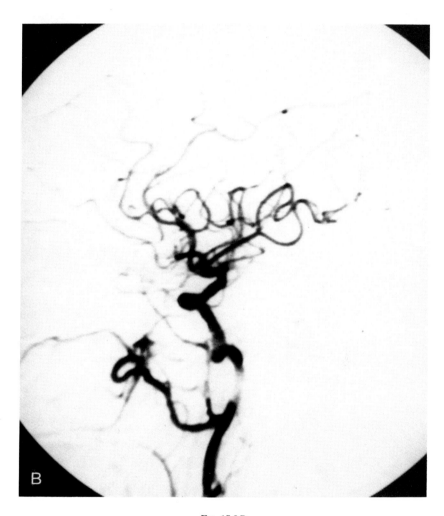

FIG. 15.3B

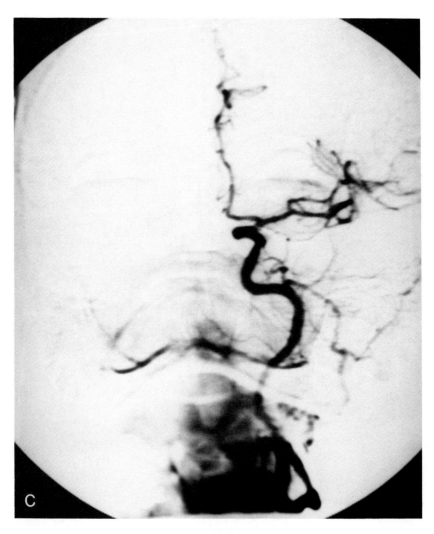

Fig. 15.3C

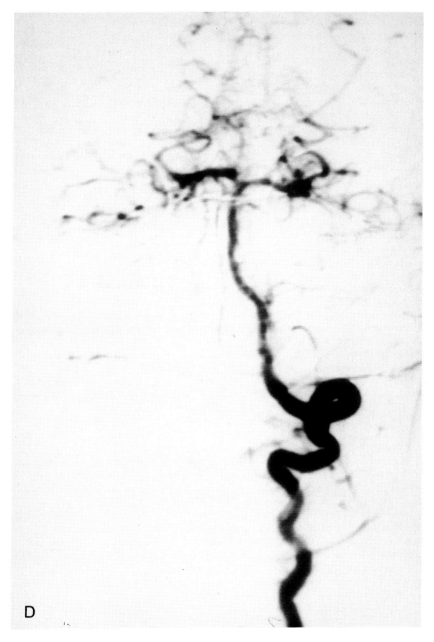

FIG. 15.3D

mended. If 80% stenosis of the carotid is demonstrated, surgery can be considered for the reasons previously discussed.

REFERENCES

1. Archer, C. W., Turnipseed, W. D., Sackett, J. F., Strother, M., Crummy, A., Mistretta, C. Digital subtraction angiography and continuous-wave doppler studies. Arch. Surg., *118:* 462–464, 1983.
2. Archie, J. P., Feldtman, R. W. Critical stenosis of the internal carotid artery. Surgery, *89:* 67–72, 1981.
3. Brant-Zawadski, M., Gould, R., Norman, D., Newton, T. H., Lane, B. Digital subtraction cerebral angiography by intrarterial injection: comparison with conventional angiography. Am. J. Radiol., *140:* 347–353, 1983.
4. Busuttil, R. W., Baker, J. D., Davidson, R. K., Machleder, H. I. Carotid artery stenosis— Hemodynamic significance and clinical course. J.A.M.A., *245:* 1438–1441, 1981.
5. Chambers, B. R., Norris, J. W.: The case against surgery for asymptomatic carotid stenosis. Stroke, *15:* 964–967, 1984.
6. Cooperman, M., Martin, Jr., E. W., Evans, W. E.: Significance of asymptomatic carotid bruits. Arch. Surg., *113:* 1339–1340, 1978.
7. Durward, Q. J., Ferguson, G. G., Barr, H. W. K. The natural history of asymptomatic carotid bifurcation plaques. Stroke, *13:* 459–464, 1982.
8. Earnest, IV, F., Houser, O. W., Forbes, G. S., Kispert, D. B., Folger, W. N., Sundt, Jr., T. M. The accuracy and limitations of intravenous digital subtraction angiography in the evaluation of atherosclerotic cerebrovascular disease: angiographic and surgical correlation. Mayo Clin. Proc., *58:* 735–746, 1983.
9. Flanigan, D. P., Schuler, J. J., Vogel, M., Borozan, P., Gray, B., Sobinsky, K. R. The role of carotid duplex scanning in surgical decision making. J. Vasc. Surg., *2:* 15–25, 1985.
10. Foley, W. D., Smith, D. F., Milde, M. W., Lawson, T. L., Towne, J. B., Bandyk, D. F. Intravenous DSA examination of patients with suspected cerebral ischemia. Radiology, *151:* 651–659, 1984.
11. Hames, T. K., Humphries, K. N., Powell, T. V., McLellan, D. L. Comparison of angiography with continuous wave Doppler ultrasound in the assessment of extracranial arterial disease. J. Neurol. Neurosurg. Psychiatr. *44:* 661–669.
12. Hart, R. G., Easton. Management of cervical bruits and carotid stenosis in preoperative patients. Stroke, *14:* 290–297, 1983.
13. Hennerici, M., Aulich, A., Sandmann, W., Freund, H. J. Incidence of asymptomatic extracranial arterial disease. Stroke, *12:* 750–758, 1981.
14. Heyman, A., Wilkinson, W. E., Heyden, S., Helms, M. J., Bartel, A. G., Karp, H. R., Tyroler, H. A., Hames, C. G. Risk of stroke in asymptomatic persons with cervical arterial bruits. A population study in Evans County, Georgia. N. Engl. J. Med., *302:* 838–841, 1980.
15. Jacobs, N. M., Grant, E. G., Schellinger, D., Cohan, S. L., Byrd, M. C. The role of duplex carotid sonography, digital subtraction angiography, and arteriography in the evaluation of transient ischemic attack and the asymptomatic carotid bruit. Med. Clin. North Am., *68:* 1423–1450, 1984.
16. Javid, H., Ostermiller, W. E., Jr., Hengesh, J. W., Dye, W. S., Hunter, J. A., Najafi, H., Julian, O. C. Natural history of carotid bifurcation atheroma. Surgery, *67:* 80–86, 1970.
17. Kroener, J. M., Dorn, P. L., Shoor, P. M., Wickbon, I. G., Bernstein, E. F. Prognosis of asymptomatic ulcerating carotid lesions. Arch. Surg., *115:* 1387–1392, 1980.
18. Kuller, L. H., Sutton, K. C. Carotid artery bruit: is it safe and effective to auscultate the neck? Stroke, *15:* 944–947, 1984.

19. Levin, S. M., Sondheimer, F. K., Levin, M. The contralateral diseased but asymptomatic carotid artery: to operate or not? Am. J. Surg. *140:* 203–205, 1980.
20. Loftus, C. M., Quest, D. O. Current status of carotid endarterectomy for atheromatous disease. Neurosurgery, *13:* 718–723, 1983.
21. Mohr, J. P. Asymptomatic carotid artery disease. Stroke, *13:* 431–433, 1982.
22. Moore, W. S., Boren, C., Malone, J. M., Roon, A. J., Eisenberg, R., Goldstone, J., Mani, R. Natural history of nonstenotic, asymptomatic lesions of the carotid artery. Arch. Surg., *113:* 1352–1359, 1978.
23. Ojemann, R., Crowell, R. M., Roberson, G. H., Fisher, C. M. Surgical treatment of extracranial carotid occlusive disease. Clin. Neurosurg., *22:* 214–263, 1975.
24. Roederer, G. O., Langlois, Y. E., Jager, K. A., Primozich, J. F., Beach, K. W., Phillips, D. J., Strandness, D. E. The natural history of carotid arterials disease in asymptomatic patients with cervical bruits. Stroke, *15:* 605–613, 1984.
25. Ropper, A. H., Wechsler, L. R., Wilson, L. S. Carotid bruit and risk of stroke in elective surgery. N. Engl. J. Med., *307:* 1388–1390, 1982.
26. Thompson, J. E., Patman, R. D., Talkington, C. M. Asymptomatic carotid bruit. Longterm outcome of patients having endarterectomy compared with unoperated controls. Ann. Surg., *188:* 308–315, 1978.
27. Turnipseed, W. D., Berkoff, H. A., Belzer, F. O. Postoperative stroke in cardiac and peripheral vascular disease. Ann. Surg., *192:* 365–368, 1980.
28. Warlow, C. Carotid endarterectomy: does it work? Stroke, *15:* 1068–1076, 1984.
29. Wolf, P. A., Kannel, W. B., Sorlie, P. Asymptomatic carotid bruit and risk of stroke. The Framingham Study. J.A.M.A., *245:* 1442–1445, 1981.
30. Wood, G. W., Lukin, R. R., Tomsick, T. A., Chambers, A. A. Digital subtraction angiography with intravenous injection: assessment of 1,000 carotid bifurcations. Am. J. Radiol., *140:* 855–859, 1983.
31. Yatsu, F. M., Hart, R. Asymptomatic carotid bruit and stenosis: a reappraisal. Stroke, *14:* 301–304, 1983.

16

Management of the Patient with Carotid Occlusion and a Single Ischemic Event

ROBERT L. GRUBB, Jr., M.D.

INTRODUCTION

The patient who experiences a single ischemic event referable to one cerebral hemisphere and is then discovered to have occlusion of the ipsilateral internal carotid artery (ICA) is a commonly encountered neurologic problem. A wide spectrum of clinical pictures is seen after occlusion of the ICA, ranging from an asymptomatic patient to a patient suffering a catastrophic, fatal cerebral infarction (26). Only 20% of patients who develop a severe neurological deficit with ICA occlusion will do this suddenly as the initial manifestation of this lesion. Sixty percent of patients with a severe stroke following ICA occlusion will have at least one prodromal transient ischemic attack (TIA), and 20% will develop a severe neurologic deficit after a fluctuating or step-wise course (48).

The management of patients presenting with a TIA, prolonged reversible ischemic neurologic deficit (PRIND), or no more than a mild neurologic deficit, remains controversial. In recent years many of these patients have been treated with an extracranial-intracranial (EC/IC) arterial bypass. It has, however, been difficult to demonstrate that the subsequent occurrence of stroke is less in patients undergoing EC/IC arterial bypass as compared to nonsurgical treatment (21, 78). The recently completed EC/IC Bypass Trial found the EC/IC arterial bypass did not improve the subsequent occurrence of stroke in patients with occlusion of the ICA, when compared to the best medical treatment (21). In spite of these studies, it is possible that a subset of patients may benefit from bypass surgery with a reduction in the risk of stroke. The existence of these patients is not proven at this time. Choosing the proper management for each individual patient is a complex process. Knowledge of the pathogenesis and prognosis for further ischemic events is critical for planning both immediate and long-term therapy of these patients.

PATHOPHYSIOLOGY OF ISCHEMIC EVENTS IN THE TERRITORY OF AN OCCLUDED
INTERNAL CAROTID ARTERY

Pathogenesis of Ischemic Events with Internal Carotid Artery Occlusion

Until recently, it was felt by many authors that ischemic events would cease once a stenosed carotid artery became completely occluded (25, 56). However, it is now recognized that further ischemic events can occur in the territory of an occluded carotid artery. Several pathogenic mechanisms can cause ischemic events in the territory of an already occluded ICA. Hemodynamic factors may play a role in some patients. Measurements of cerebral blood flow (CBF) and oxygen metabolism in patients with ICA occlusion have demonstrated that a number of these patients have a relative preservation of cerebral oxygen utilization ($CMRO_2$) in areas with reduced CBF and a resultant increased extraction of oxygen by the brain (6, 7, 8, 38, 62, 63). Following EC/IC arterial bypass, cerebral ischemic events stopped, CBF improved, and the oxygen extraction fraction (OEF) returned to normal levels.

In other patients with ischemic events following occlusion of the carotid artery, there has been evidence of embolization into the territory of the occluded artery. Stenotic or ulcerated plaques involving either the ipsilateral external carotid artery (ECA) or common carotid artery (CCA) may be a source of emboli through collateral circulation channels to the affected cerebral hemisphere (4, 9). Embolic material may also form in the "stump" of the occluded ICA and pass through collateral channels to the brain (4, 5, 16). A third source of emboli may be the distal end or "tail" of the thrombus occluding the ICA (28). The existing ICA thrombus may also propagate distally into the anterior and/or middle cerebral arteries, occluding collateral channels.

PROGNOSIS OF INTERNAL CAROTID ARTERY OCCLUSION

The long-term prognosis after symptomatic ICA occlusion has been studied by a number of investigators (Table 16.1). A potential problem in any investigation of the natural history of this lesion is knowing whether or not the carotid occlusion occurred before the ischemic event that brought the patient to medical attention. In all of these studies, many of the patients were treated medically with either antiplatelet agents or anticoagulants, and some also had a surgical procedure performed on the occluded carotid artery. Four of these studies list an overall stroke rate following carotid artery occlusion, but do not specify the exact vascular territory in which the strokes occurred. McDowell et al. (57) reported data on 38 patients who survived carotid artery occlusion. Nine of these 38 patients presented with a severe stroke, and 11 patients (29%) were treated

TABLE 16.1

Prognosis of Internal Carotid Artery Occlusion

Reference	Number of Patients	Mean Period of Follow-up	Patient Study	Type of Follow-up	Strokes during Follow-up	Stroke Rate per Year during Follow-up	Deaths during Follow-up
A. Overall Stroke Rate—Incomplete Reference to Vascular Territory Involved							
McDowell et al. (57), 1961	38	24 months	Includes major strokes	Retrospective	3(8%)	4%	5(13%)
Hardy et al. (40), 1962	121	48 months	Includes major strokes	Retrospective	30(23%)	6%	51(39%)
Dyken et al. (20), 1974	43	16.5 months	Includes major strokes	Prospective	3(7%)	5%	6(14%)
Fields et al. (24), 1976	359	44 months	Includes major strokes	Prospective	89(25%)	7%	155(43%)
B. Stroke Rate—Involved Vascular Territory Defined							
Grillo et al. (34), 1975	37	36 months	Majority with TIA or stroke	Retrospective	6(16%)*	5%*	10(27%)
Barnett (4), 1978	25	24 months	TIA or minor stroke	Prospective	7(28%)†	14%†	
Furlan et al. (30), 1980	138	60 months	TIA or minor stroke	Retrospective	11(8%)† 6(4%)*	2%† 1%*	30(21%)
Bogousslavsky et al. (9), 1981	23	27 months	Majority with TIA or minor stroke	Retrospective	0	0	0
Cote et al. (15), 1983	47	34 months	TIA or minor stroke	Prospective	7(15%)† 4(8.5%)*	5%† 3%*	4(8.5%)

* Stroke in other vascular distribution.
† Ipsilateral stroke.

with anticoagulant therapy. Over the next 2 years, 3 patients (8%) had a recurrent stroke, but the location of the infarction was not given. Hardy *et al.* (40) followed 133 patients who survived carotid artery occlusion. Many of these patients had a moderate to severe neurologic deficit. Twenty-three percent of these patients suffered a second stroke during the 4-year follow-up period. Again the location of the infarction was not given. More than 60% of these patients had some type of surgical procedure performed on the occluded carotid artery, but operative stroke morbidity and mortality was not discussed. Dyken and his associates (20) followed 43 patients with either common or ICA occlusion over an average follow-up period of 16.5 months. One-half of these patients had a moderate to severe neurologic deficit. During the relatively brief follow-up period three patients had a second stroke, but the location of these lesions was not discussed. The Joint Study of Extracranial Arterial Occlusion (24) followed 359 patients with unilateral carotid occlusion for an average of 14 months. Many of these patients had a severe initial stroke. Eighty-nine patients (25%) had a new stroke with 35 patients (10%) having a stroke ipsilateral to the occluded artery. However, the involved vascular territory was not described in 34 patients suffering a fatal stroke. All of these studies include a large number of patients who had a moderate to severe neurologic deficit following the carotid occlusion. The prognosis of these more severely affected patients may be different from that of patients with a minor or no neurologic deficit following carotid occlusion (40).

In a retrospective review of Grillo and Patterson (34) found that seven of 44 patients with ICA occlusion died from the initial stroke. The remaining 37 patients were followed for an average of 3 years. During this time, six patients suffered a second stroke. All of these strokes were in the cerebral hemisphere contralateral to the occluded carotid artery. Fourteen of these patients underwent endarterectomy of the carotid artery opposite to the occlusion. This study also included some patients with moderate to severe neurologic deficits.

Studies restricted to patients having either TIAs or a stroke with a minor neurologic deficit are more useful for the determination of the risk of further stroke following carotid artery occlusion. The chances of detecting new ischemic events in a vascular territory where a major infarction has occurred are probably limited. Four recent studies have included only patients having TIAs or minor fixed neurologic deficits following carotid artery occlusion. Two of these were retrospective studies. Furlan *et al.* (30) reported 138 patients with angiographically-proven carotid artery occlusion with either mild or no residual neurologic deficits with a mean follow-up period of 5 years. Seven percent of the patients were asymptomatic and the carotid occlusion was an incidental angiographic finding.

More than half the patients were treated with long-term anticoagulant therapy at some time following carotid occlusion and seven of these patients subsequently had a stroke. Among patients in good neurologic condition, 3% per year had strokes. Two-thirds, or 2% per year, were ipsilateral to the carotid artery occlusion. A few patients also continued to have ipsilateral TIAs but did not develop a cerebral infarction. Stroke rates were not significantly different for those who presented with TIAs only compared to presenting with cerebral infarction and residual neurologic deficits. The observed stroke rate for all patients 35 years old or over was eight times the expected rate for a normal population of a similar age and sex distribution. Bogousslavsky et al. (9) studied 23 patients retrospectively with a mean follow-up period of 27 months. Eight (34%) of the patients continued to have TIAs but none of the patients in the study developed a cerebral infarction during follow-up. Two other studies were prospective in design. Barnett (4) followed 25 patients for a 2-year follow-up period. Seven patients had strokes during this time ipsilateral to the occluded carotid artery. The stroke rate of 14% per year following carotid artery occlusion in this study is higher than that reported by most other studies. Cote et al. (15) followed 47 patients with occlusion of the carotid artery enrolled in the Canadian Cooperative Study on platelet inhibitory drugs in a prospective manner for an average follow-up of 34 months. Fifty-one percent of the patients continued to experience TIAs in the distribution of the occluded carotid artery. Over an approximately 3-year period the overall stroke rate was 23%, with 15% of the strokes occurring ipsilateral to the occluded carotid artery. The 5% annual ipsilateral stroke rate in this study is similar to the estimated long-term cerebral infarction 5–6% per year for most patients having TIAs (32, 77, 78).

The data from these studies indicate that patients with ICA occlusion with no or mild neurologic deficit have a risk of developing a subsequent infarction in the ipsilateral cerebral hemisphere of approximately 5% per year. This annual stroke rate is similar to the estimated long term annual rate of infarction for most patients having TIAs.

DIFFERENTIATION OF EMBOLIC AND HEMODYNAMIC ISCHEMIC EPISODES

Clinical Presentation

The differentation of embolic from hemodynamic factors in the pathogenesis of ischemic events in patients with ICA occlusion is critical. Unfortunately, there is no way to make this distinction with certainty since there is no way to absolutely prove or disprove either diagnosis. Some authors have felt that cerebral ischemia due to low blood flow can be differentiated from ischemic events due to emboli (47). Patients with transient low-flow, hemodynamic TIAs are said to describe their symptoms in a vague manner. A number of fleeting sensations such as "swelling" or "numbness" of an extremity or on one side of the face, brief losses of control or strength in an arm or leg, leg "buckling," or transient language problems may be described. Brief episodes of monocular blindness are sometimes described. Low blood flow leading to cerebral infarction may produce a progressive or "stuttering" type of neurologic deficit. In contrast, a single transient cortical or ocular event lasting an hour or longer is said to represent an embolic event (47). The size of the embolus determines the type of arterial branch that will be occluded, while the location of the occluded vessel and the adequacy of collateral circulation will determine the focal neurologic deficits produced by the embolus. However, in actual practice, the differentiation of hemodynamic from embolic factors on clinical grounds alone is difficult. Furthermore, we have observed a number of patients with well-described, discrete, sometimes prolonged, focal transient ischemic events in the territory of an occluded ICA who were found to have uncoupling of CBF and $CMRO_2$ in the affected cerebral hemisphere measured with positron emission tomography (PET) (62, 63). The depression of CBF with relative preservation of $CMRO_2$ was felt to be evidence of chronic ischemia due to hemodynamic factors in the symptomatic cerebral hemisphere. Recurrent attacks of focal neurologic deficits in association with assuming an upright posture are very suggestive of a hemodynamic cause. In patients with acute cerebral infarction, however, postural TIAs may be due to focal loss of autoregulation in the area surrounding the infarct and not secondary to hemodynamic compromise caused by the carotid occlusion. Thus, it is doubtful that hemodynamic causes can be reliably distinguished from embolic phenomenon by the clinical presentation in a given patient with ischemic events following occlusion of the internal carotid artery.

CT Scan Findings

Ringelstein and coauthors (66) felt that the location of a cerebral infarction on the CT scan, combined with angiographic and clinical data, was useful in differentiating infarction caused by hemodynamic factors from infarction due to emboli in patients with occlusion of the ICA. In an analysis of 107 patients with ICA occlusion, four patterns of cerebral infarction predominated. Infarctions felt to be of an embolic nature included cortical-subcortical infarctions in the territory of a pial artery and extended infarction of the lentiform nucleus. In contrast, infarctions felt to be secondary to hemodynamic factors included watershed or border zone infarctions of the cerebral convexities and infarctions in the subcortical terminal vascular supply. However, there were no measurements of cerebral hemodynamics and metabolism done in this group of patients to verify the interpretation and classification of the clinical and radiologic findings. The usefulness of this classification of cerebral infarction, as seen on CT scans, is unproven when applied to individual patients.

Measurements of Cerebral Hemodynamics and Metabolism

Quantitative measurements of cerebral hemodynamics and metabolism now give us the means to detect physiologic changes associated with decreased cerebral perfusion (7, 38, 62, 63). The ability to make the measurements is currently limited to a small number of medical centers. However, the presence of physiologic changes felt to represent chronic cerebral ischemia does not entirely exclude the possibility of the occurrence of emboli to a cerebral hemisphere with poor collateral circulation.

Clinical and experimental observations have demonstrated that the brain can tolerate a decrease in blood flow for a period without incurring permanent damage. Restoration of blood flow during this period of reversible ischemia can restore lost neurologic function and prevent the development of cerebral infarction. Because restoration of blood flow to irreversibly infarcted brain tissue is unlikely to be of benefit and can, in fact, be dangerous (81), a means to distinguish areas of the brain with reversible ischemia from those with irreversible infarction would be of great clinical value. Recent experimental studies have shown that measurements of regional CBF alone are inadequate for this purpose. The reversibility of cerebral ischemia depends both on the magnitude and duration of the decrease in blood flow and on other factors, including antecedent cerebral glucose stores and selective vulnerability of specific neurons (2, 45, 64). PET, with the capacity to make a variety of physiologic measurements in addition to regional CBF, has the potential to be of value for this discrimination and to identify patients with cerebral ischemia due to hemodynamic factors.

We have used PET to study the hemodynamic and metabolic changes that accompanied regional CBF reductions in ischemic but uninfarcted regions of the brain in seven carefully selected patients (62). These individuals, 47–70 years of age, all met the following criteria: (a) history of transient ischemic neurologic deficits referable to the territory supplied by one middle cerebral artery; (b) normal neurologic examination findings at the time of the study; (c) normal x-ray CT scan of the brain; (d) occlusion of the ICA on the symptomatic side; and (e) decreased CBF (as measured by PET) to the symptomatic cerebral hemisphere. Two groups of normal patients were studied for comparison: a younger group consisting of six patients, aged 20–39 years, and an older group of four patients, aged 68–74 years. These seven symptomatic patients were chosen from a larger group of patients who had had TIAs and normal CT findings, specifically because their PET studies demonstrated decreased CBF to the symptomatic hemisphere. (The other patients with TIAs showed infarction on CT scans or symmetrical flow to the two hemispheres.) PET was used to measure regional CBF, regional $CMRO_2$, regional cerebral blood volume (CBV), regional OEF, and regional mean vascular transit time.

All seven patients studied had both clinical and PET evidence of compromised flow to one cerebral hemisphere, yet demonstrated preservation of both cerebral structure (normal x-ray CT scan) and cerebral function (normal neurologic examination findings). We believe that the information provided by these studies provides the best criteria, short of neuropathologic examination, for defining areas of ischemic, uninfarcted brain. These methods do not enable us, however, to rule out the possibility that there has been some diffuse or patchy loss of a small number of neurons.

Concomitant with a decrease in regional CBF to the symptomatic hemisphere, these seven patients demonstrated a slight decrease in regional $CMRO_2$ and an increase in regional CBV, regional OEF, and regional mean vascular transient time. An increase in CBV in response to a reduction in cerebral perfusion pressure has been a consistent finding in experimental studies (35, 36). Although this increase most likely reflects the dilatation of precapillary resistance vessels in an attempt at CBF autoregulation (49), certain observations suggest that changes at the capillary level may also take place. In patients with subarachnoid hemorrhage, an increase in regional CBV has been observed in association with arterial spasm, suggesting that there is a dilation of more distal vessels (37). Morphologic studies of cerebral capillaries in animals subjected to hypoxia have demonstrated a variety of changes, including recruitment, dilatation, and proliferation (18, 69, 80). Taken together, these data suggest that the decrease in tissue oxygen supply produced by focal cerebral ischemia may cause the local increase in regional CBV that we observed. These capillary changes would facilitate oxygen delivery to brain tissue by decreasing intercapillary distance and increasing capillary surface area. Observations of dilated retinal veins in patients with carotid artery occlusion suggest that there may also be a venous contribution to the local increase in regional CBV (68).

Previous measurements of arteriovenous oxygen differences have demonstrated the capacity of the brain to increase its OEF in response to a diminished oxygen supply (23, 29, 44). Although the mechanism of this increase undoubtedly involves changes in oxygen-hemoglobin affinity produced by high local concentrations of carbon dioxide (39), our findings suggest that other factors may also be at work. The observed increases in intravascular volume and vascular transit time, if they occur at the capillary level, would facilitate the transfer of oxygen to tissue by increasing both the surface area and the time available for diffusion.

In these seven patients, the ischemic hemisphere showed loss of the normal coupling between flow and metabolism (62, 65) (Fig. 16.1). Regional $CMRO_2$ was maintained by an increase in regional OEF, with progressively higher extraction needed as flow decreased. The limits of local autoregulation had been exceeded, as shown by the decline in regional CBF. The greatest declines in regional CBF occurred in those patients with the least evidence of vasodilatation (smallest increase in CBV), suggesting that autoregulatory capacity may vary from individual to individual. In those with poor capacity for vasodilatation, CBF would be more sensitive to decreases in cerebral perfusion pressure.

The minimal value for regional CBF observed in these subjects with normal cerebral function was 22.1 ml/(min · 100 gm). This finding is consistent with the threshold value for regional CBF, defined in animal experiments, of approximately 20 ml/(min · 100 gm), below which neuronal function is impaired (2, 41, 45). Values above this threshold do not necessarily indicate viable tissue, because they may be measured during the period of luxury perfusion following infarction (53). The lowest value for regional $CMRO_2$ we observed was 1.43 ml/(min · 100 gm). In another recent PET study of 25 patients with acute ischemic stroke, those areas of the brain that later showed CT evidence of infarction had values for regional $CMRO_2$ below 1.5 ml/(min · 100 gm) (7). The slightly lower value found by us may be explained by the consistent overestimation of regional $CMRO_2$ by the technique used in this recent PET study (7, 51, 52).

An understanding of the local physiologic responses to decreased cerebral perfusion pressure is essential if PET is to be used clinically for differentiating reversible ischemia from irreversible infarction. This limited study provides helpful information in this regard but by no means offers a final answer. When compared with the findings in patients with ischemic stroke, our results suggest that a value for regional $CMRO_2$ greater than 1.4 ml/(min · 100 gm) is a good indicator of tissue viability in the face of decreased regional CBF. Regional CBV and regional OEF will also be increased, but these findings may not be specific for areas of reversible ischemia. The degree of ischemia in these patients was mild, however, and not associated with a clinical deficit. The hemodynamic and metabolic results of superficial temporal artery-middle cerebral artery anastomosis in five of seven of these patients were determined (63). Following bypass, CBF to the operated hemisphere increased to the point that OEF returned to normal. CBV and $CMRO_2$ did not change following surgery. Fig. 16.2 illustrates the PET scan findings in one of these patients before and after EC/IC anastomosis surgery. Although re-establishing

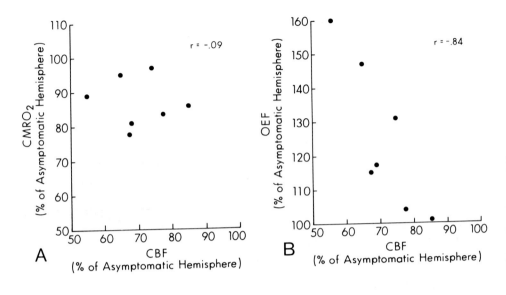

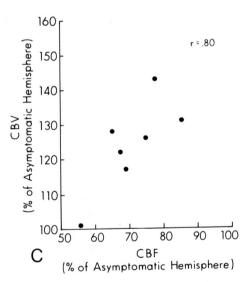

FIG. 16.1. Relationship of cerebral blood flow (CBF) to: (A) cerebral oxygen utilization (CMRO₂), (B) oxygen extraction fraction (OEF), and (C) cerebral blood volume (CBV) in the distribution of the middle cerebral artery of the symptomatic cerebral hemisphere in seven patients with local cerebral ischemia. The mean regional value for each patient is expressed as a percentage of the value of the opposite, asymptomatic cerebral hemisphere. (From W. J. Powers, R. L. Grubb, Jr., M. E. Raichle: Physiological responses to focal cerebral ischemia in humans. Ann. Neurol. 16: 546–554, 1984).

blood flow may reduce the risk of subsequent stroke in these patients, the real challenge remains in patients with clinical deficits in whom re-establishment of blood flow may reverse the disability.

MANAGEMENT OF PATIENTS WITH OCCLUDED INTERNAL CAROTID ARTERY

Once the diagnosis of an occluded ICA is made following a cerebral ischemic event, the clinician must decide whether or not any further diagnostic and therapeutic measures should be undertaken. The natural history of this lesion should be kept in mind while weighing various therapeutic options. It is essential that all patients being considered for further treatment have complete and detailed cerebral angiography before any therapeutic decisions are made. This is necessary for several reasons: (*a*) to be certain that the ICA is totally occluded and a "pseudo-occlusion" has been excluded; (*b*) to define the collateral circulation to the affected hemisphere; (*c*) to identify possible sources of further emboli to the territory of the occluded carotid artery; and (*d*) to demonstrate possible etiologies of the carotid occlusion. Measurements of cerebral hemodynamics and metabolism, if available, may be useful in differentiating reversible cerebral ischemia from irreversible cerebral infarction and separating hemodynamic causes from embolic causes of cerebral ischemic events. Patients with severe neurologic deficits are not candidates for surgical revascularization procedures in most instances and further treatment of these patients should be medical.

MEDICAL MANAGEMENT

Medical Therapy

ICA occlusion is a general marker for atherosclerotic disease. Mortality in these patients is more often due to cardiac disease than the cerebrovascular lesion. Thus, in addition to treatment of the cerebrovascular pathology, it is important to treat the general atherosclerotic disease by controlling risk factors for atherosclerosis. These general measures include long-term control of hypertension, control of diabetes, treatment of ischemic cardiac disease, lowering of elevated serum lipids with diet and drugs, if necessary, adequate exercise, and weight loss in obese patients.

In a patient with a symptomatic ICA occlusion, blood flow should be maximized (12). Aggressive reduction of elevated blood pressure should be avoided unless the hypertension is severe. Hypotension in these patients should be corrected by reducing antihypertensive therapy. Congestive heart failure should be vigorously treated and cardiac arrhythmias should be corrected with antiarrhythmic drugs. The patients should be adequately hydrated and kept on bed rest initially.

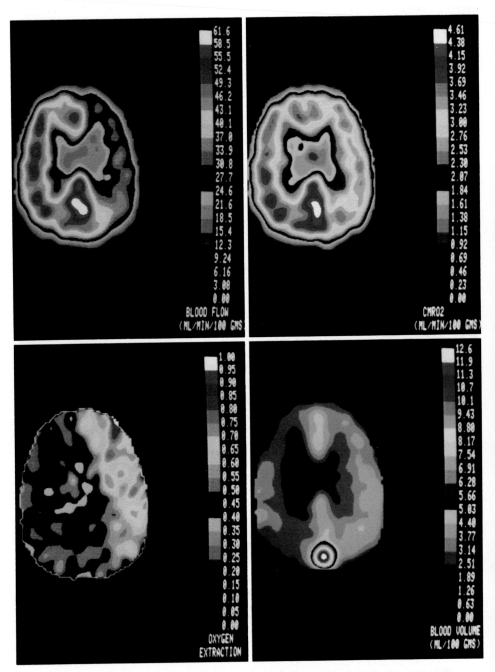

FIG. 16.2. Pre- and postoperative PET scans showing quantitative measurements of CBF (ml/(min · 100 gm)), CMRO$_2$ (ml/min · 100 gm) CBV (ml/100 gm), and OEF in one tomographic slice from a 69-year-old man who had a single right hemisphere TIA 6 weeks previously. Angiography showed total occlusion of the right internal carotid artery (ICA). Prior to surgery, the right cerebral hemisphere showed a marked decrease in CBF (*A*), slight decrease in CMRO$_2$ (*B*), increased OEF (*C*), and increased CBV (*D*).

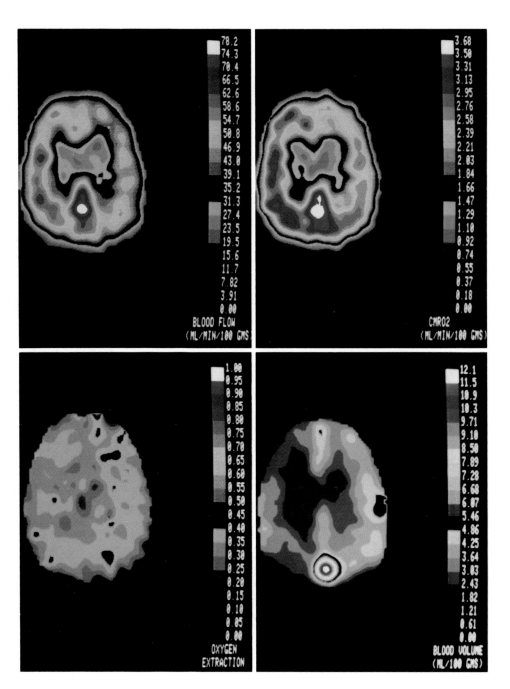

Following superficial temporal-middle cerebral arterial anastomosis, there was a relative increase in right cerebral hemisphere CBF (*E*), no change in $CMRO_2$ (*F*), and OEF became symmetric (*G*). There was little change in CBV (*H*). Each scan is accompanied by a 20-hue linear color scale showing 5% increments from zero to the maximum value for that slice. (From W. J. Powers, W. R. M. Martin, P. Herscovitch, M. E. Raichle, R. L. Grubb, Jr.: Extracranial-intracranial bypass surgery: hemodynamic and metabolic effects. Neurology *34:* 1168–1174, 1984).

Specific medical therapy for the cerebrovascular disease includes heparin anticoagulation, warfarin anticoagulation, and antiplatelet aggregation agents—aspirin, sulfinpyrazone, dipyridamole, indomethacin, and ibuprofen. Of these, the best data available to document effectiveness are for aspirin. Aspirin has been shown to be effective in preventing stroke secondary to carotid territory ischemic events presumed due to atherothrombosis (10, 11). Angiography was not done in many of the patients in these studies, and it is not known if aspirin is effective in the specific subgroup of patients with ICA occlusion. The effectiveness of other medical treatments specifically for occlusion of the ICA with a single ischemic event is also not known.

Spontaneous Dissection of the Internal Carotid Artery

A spontaneous carotid artery dissection has a number of typical, but variable, angiographic features including a "string sign," a "pouch" distal to the common carotid bifurcation in an otherwise normal-appearing artery, an aneurysmal pouch at the base of the skull, and a tapering complete occlusion of the internal carotid artery just distal to the bulb of the artery (Fig. 16.3) (27, 42, 55). The origin of the ICA is spared in nearly all of these typical angiographic pictures. If the ICA is not totally occluded, the dissection usually ends at the skull base and the artery returns to a normal caliber and appearance (27, 55). With time, the angiographic appearance of dissections usually improves and totally occluded vessels may become patent again (27, 42, 55, 58). In patients who do not present with a severe cerebral infarction the disease has a relatively benign natural history and good prognosis (22, 27, 42, 55, 58). Recurrent ischemic symptoms are thought to be the result of embolization (22, 55). Some patients have done well with no treatment. Because of the danger of embolization, however, anticoagulation for several weeks to months is usually employed (27, 55) and these patients usually do well. Angiography should be repeated at the end of the anticoagulation therapy. Surgical revascularization procedures in this condition should be reserved for recurrent ischemic symptoms occurring in spite of adequate anticoagulation and angiographic demonstration of severe stenosis or occlusion of the ICA.

SURGICAL MANAGEMENT

There is no current evidence that a surgical procedure should be performed in patients with a single ischemic event. While certain patients with a single ischemic event and carotid occlusion may benefit from a surgical revascularization procedure, the identification of such patients is not possible at this time. A variety of operations have been performed in patients with carotid occlusion, and surgery may play a role in some situations, especially if there are recurrent ischemic events.

Carotid Endarterectomy

Certain patients with ICA occlusion and cerebral ischemic events may have lesions that can be corrected by carotid endarterectomy. These lesions include: (*a*) ulcerated plaque and/or stenosis of the ipsilateral ECA and/or CCA where the ECA supplies collateral circulation to the symptomatic cerebral hemisphere; (*b*) persistent "stump" of the ICA where the ipsilateral ECA provides collateral channels to the cerebral hemisphere; (*c*) atheromatous pseudo-occlusion of the ICA; (*d*) complete occlusion of the ICA, and (*e*) contralateral ICA stenosis.

Ulcerative and/or stenotic plaques in the ipsilateral ECA and/or CCA and a persistent stump of the occluded ICA may be a source of emboli in the territory of an occluded ICA through collateral channels (Fig. 16.4). A significant ECA stenosis might also produce cerebral ischemic symptoms by hemodynamic mechanisms if this artery is the main source of collateral circulation to the cerebral hemisphere.

Endarterectomy of the ECA should be considered only when there is angiographic demonstration of blood supply to the symptomatic region by branches of the ipsilateral ECA. Operative techniques for external carotid endarterectomy are well described (14, 16, 43). In addition to removing the plaque completely from the ECA, it is essentially also to remove sufficient plaque from the ICA to ensure a smooth closure and obliteration of the ICA stump (42).

An occasional patient thought to have complete occlusion at the origin of the ICA in initial angiogram films will have a trickle of dye ascending the ICA in an anterograde fashion on the late angiogram films (17, 71) (Fig. 16.5). This type of lesion, the so-called pseudo-occlusion of the ICA, can be corrected by carotid endarterectomy with restoration of a normal caliber ICA and removal of a source of emboli. Careful, complete angiography is necessary to recognize this lesion.

In most instances, carotid endarterectomy will not restore patency of a chronically occluded ICA. In some patients, however, angiography will demonstrate patency of the internal carotid artery by retrograde filling of dye to the petrous canal or even more proximally (Fig. 16.6). Small branches of the ICA can develop anastomatic connections with ECA branches and keep the intracranial portion of the ICA patent. In this situation, carotid endarterectomy will often reestablish patency of the ICA (46, 50, 72). In many of these cases the obstruction of the ICA will be near the carotid bifurcation and the artery distally will be collapsed, containing a

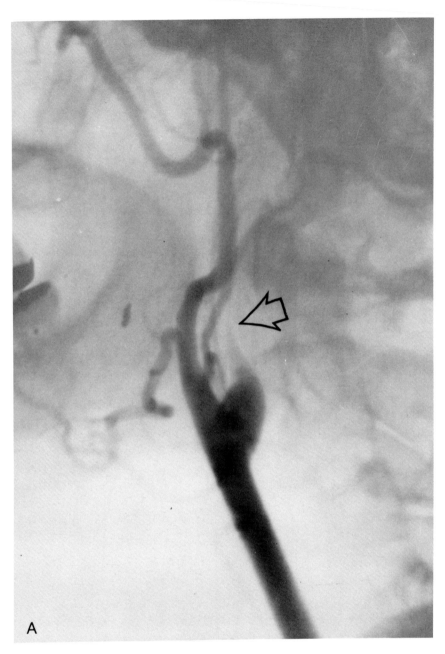

Fig. 16.3. (A) Angiogram in a 38-year-old female with a left cerebral hemisphere infarction showing a tapering, complete occlusion of the ICA just distal to the bulb of the artery (arrow), one of the typical appearances of a spontaneous dissection of the carotid artery. The patient was treated with warfarin anticoagulation. (B) Repeat angiogram 6 months later shows resolution of the occlusion and a patent ICA (arrow).

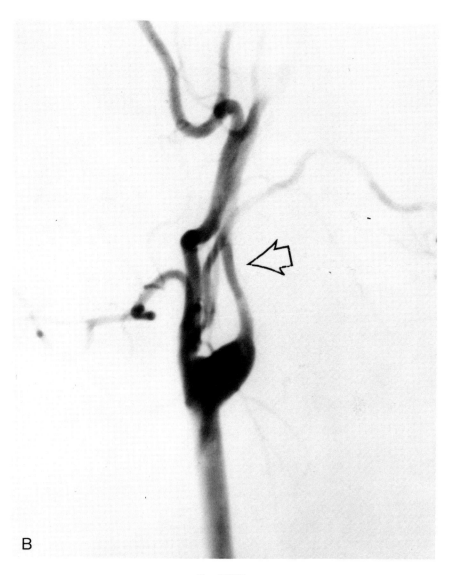

B

FIG. 16.3B

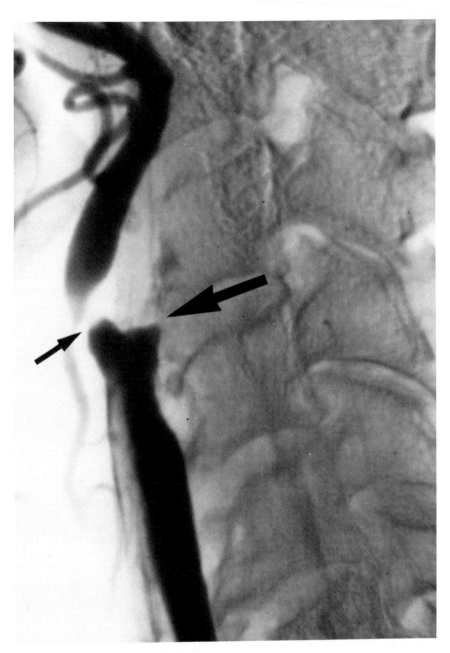

Fig. 16.4. Angiogram in a 75-year-old female patient with an occluded ICA and transient ischemic attacks in the territory of the occluded carotid artery. This cerebral hemisphere received its blood supply mainly from retrograde flow through ipsilateral external carotid artery (ECA) branches. There is severe stenosis of the proximal ECA (*small arrow*) and a persistent stump of the occluded ICA (*large arrow*).

thrombus that extends only to the skull base. This clot can usually be easily removed by suction or the careful use of a Fogarty catheter (42). Potential complications of carotid endarterectomy in this situation include dislodging distal thrombus with resultant embolism and the production of a carotid-cavernous fistula.

Some patients with cerebral ischemic symptoms in the territory of an occluded carotid artery have severe stenosis of the contralateral ICA. If there is good angiographic evidence that the main collateral circulation of the symptomatic cerebral hemisphere is from the opposite cerebral hemisphere vascular supply, endarterectomy of the contralateral stenotic carotid artery may be beneficial. There have been some reports that there is increased risk of performing a carotid endarterectomy when the opposite internal carotid artery is occluded (1, 24). However, other authors have reported an acceptable low rate of morbidity and mortality for carotid endarterectomy performed in this situation (31, 60, 61, 75). EC/IC arterial anastomosis can be considered if symptoms recur following successful carotid endarterectomy.

Extracranial-intracranial arterial anastomosis

In the late 1960s, Donaghy (19) and Yarsargil et al. (82) demonstrated that a microvascular anastomosis with long-term patency could be performed between the superficial temporal artery and a cortical branch of the middle cerebral artery, thus establishing blood flow between the extracranial and intracranial circulation and bypassing areas of occlusive disease not amenable to a direct surgical approach. The procedure can be done with high patency rate and low risk. Dilation of the donor and recipient vessels often occurs postoperatively (3, 13, 33, 59, 66, 69, 76). In situations where a suitable donor superficial temperal artery is not present, interposition vein grafts between the extracranial circulation and the middle cerebral artery have been successfully used (54, 59, 73, 75). The surgical techniques to perform EC/IC arterial anastomosis have been thoroughly described (19, 54, 59, 66, 73, 74, 82).

EC/IC arterial anastomosis has been performed with increasing frequency in recent years. Only two studies have compared the long-term results of patients undergoing EC/IC bypass with a comparable group of patients not treated surgically (21, 78). Whisnant et al. (78) compared 239 patients with TIAs, mild stroke, or transient monocular visual symptoms who had superficial temporal artery-middle cerebral artery (STA-MCA) bypass with 138 historical controls who had carotid artery occlusion, with either mild or no residual neurologic deficit, not treated with surgery. Both groups were followed for a mean period of 5 years. These authors found no difference in the risk of stroke comparing the STA-MCA bypass group of patients to the nonsurgical group. They felt that certain patients might

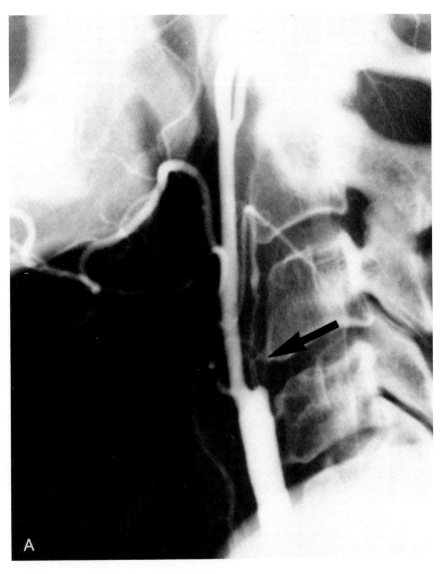

FIG. 16.5. (A)Angiogram in a 52-year-old female patient with transient ischemic attacks. An early film shows apparent complete occlusion of the ICA (*arrow*). (B) Late film shows the trickle of dye filling the ICA (*arrows*) in an anterograde fashion, indicating a "pseudo-occlusion" of the ICA.

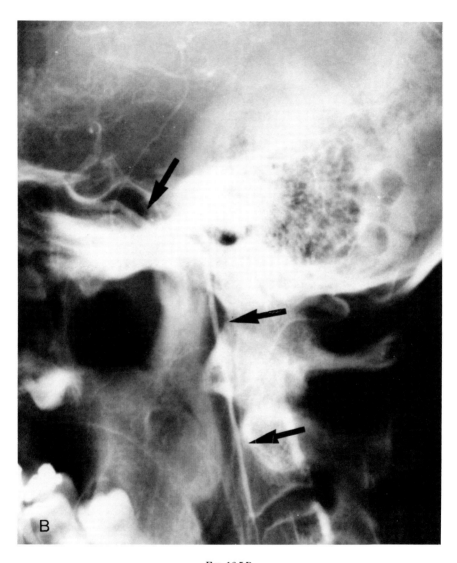

FIG. 16.5*B*

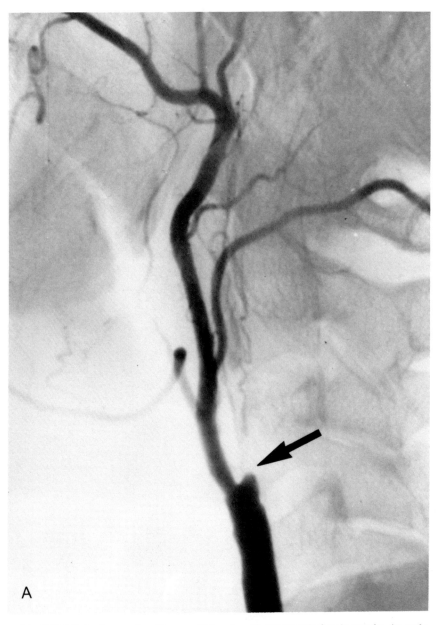

A

FIG. 16.6. (*A*) Angiogram in a 55-year-old female with transient ischemic attacks. An early film shows complete occlusion of the ICA (*arrow*). (*B*) Late film shows retrograde filling of the ICA (*arrows*) into the upper cervical region. Carotid endarterectomy restored patency of the ICA.

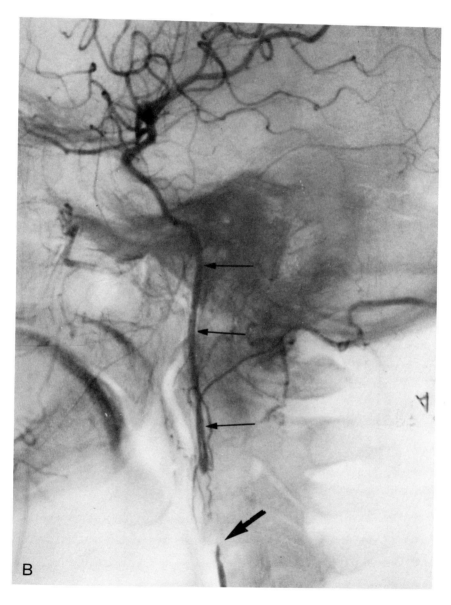

FIG. 16.6*B*

benefit from EC/IC arterial bypass surgery in regards to protection from stroke, but they were not able to identify them on the basis of their observations.

The EC/IC Bypass Trial (21) included 521 patients with ICA occlusion and no recurrent symptoms during this period of time between angiographic demonstration of ICA occlusion and randomization into a medical or surgical treatment group. Strokes, both fatal and nonfatal, in all locations were carefully recorded during the follow-up period. Two hundred and seventy-six patients were treated with the best available medical therapy, which included adequate blood pressure control and usually antiplatelet aggregation agents, with a few patients receiving warfarin for anticoagulation. In the medical group, 72 strokes were observed during follow-up. Two hundred and forty-five patients underwent EC/IC arterial bypass. Fifty-seven strokes in the perioperative and follow-up period occurred. There was no statistically significant difference in outcome between the medical and surgical group. In patients with ICA occlusion who had further symptoms during the time between angiographic demonstration of ICA occlusion and randomization into a treatment group, EC/ICA arterial bypass again was of no benefit in preventing stroke compared to the best available medical therapy. Thus EC/IC arterial bypass had no effect on the subsequent rate of stroke following ICA occlusion in this large cooperative study. Furthermore, EC/IC arterial bypass failed to reduce the incidence of stroke and TIA in the ipsilateral cerebral hemisphere compared to the best available medical therapy. Based on these studies there is no indication for EC/IC arterial bypass in the patient with an occluded ICA and a single ischemic event.

The natural history of patients with an occluded ICA is not, however, totally benign. If there is a role for EC/IC arterial bypass as a revascularization procedure in patients with this lesion, it would logically seem to be in the patients on medical therapy who develop further ischemic symptoms due to hemodynamic causes, i.e., inadequate perfusion of the cerebral hemisphere previously supplied by the occluded ICA. The challenge for neurosurgeons and neurologists is to learn how to identify such patients. We have observed a number of patients with an occluded ICA and ipsilateral cerebral hemisphere TIAs who seemed to have chronic cerebral ischemia in the symptomatic cerebral hemisphere based on PET measurements of cerebral hemodynamics and metabolism (62, 63). In these patients postoperative PET studies demonstrated that EC/IC arterial bypass improved cerebral hemodynamics and metabolism in the symptomatic cerebral hemisphere. However, patients who seem to have ipsilateral cerebral chronic ischemia following ICA occlusion are not common and, at this time, there is no proof that their natural history and prognosis is any worse then that of all patients as a group with ICA occlusion. This surgical procedure should not be entirely abandoned, but should be further investigated in centers with the means to study the pathophysiology of chronic cerebral ischemia and the effect of this operation on these patients.

CONCLUSIONS AND RECOMMENDATIONS

When the diagnosis of an occluded ICA has been made following a cerebral ischemic event, a decision must be made as to whether or not further diagnostic and therapeutic measures should be carried out. All patients with an occluded ICA should have appropriate supportive measures and control of atherosclerotic risk factors. Patients with a severe neurologic deficit following ICA occlusion are not candidates for surgical revascularization procedures and should be treated medically with antiplatelet aggregation agents. In patients with minor or no neurologic deficits there is no conclusive evidence that any surgical revascularization procedure reduces the long-term incidence of stroke ipsilateral to the occluded ICA following a single ischemic event compared to medical therapy. There is also no conclusive evidence that any medical therapy, including various anticoagulation and antiplatelet aggregation agents, improved upon the natural history of ICA occlusion with a single ischemic event, as this subgroup has not been specifically compared to a control group. Unfortunately, the natural history of this lesion is not totally benign. It has been difficult, however, to identify which patients are at further risk for cerebral ischemic events ipsilateral to the occluded ICA.

At the current time I would start a patient with ICA occlusion and a single cerebral ischemic event on aspirin and not do a surgical procedure. There is evidence that long-term anticoagulation with warfarin is effective in treating spontaneous dissection of the ICA. However, if further ipsilateral cerebral ischemic events occur while on medical therapy, a surgical procedure may be beneficial. Carotid endarterctomy can be considered in patients with recurrent symptoms if angiography demonstrates: (a) pseudo-occlusion of the ICA; (b) retrograde filling of the distal ICA to a point at or below the petrous canal; (c) severe stenosis and/or ulceration of an ECA, which is the main collateral blood supply to the ipsilateral cerebral hemisphere; (d) persistent stump of the ICA; (e) severe stenosis of the contralateral ICA with angiographic evidence that the main collateral circulation of the symptomatic cerebral hemisphere is from the opposite cerebral hemisphere. At this time, there is no evidence that EC/IC bypass reduces the incidence of stroke in the ipsilateral hemisphere following ICA occlusion. In patients with recurrent ipsilateral ischemic events where accurate quantitative measurements of cerebral hemodynamics and metabolism demonstrate changes of chronic cerebral ischemia in the symptomatic cerebral hemisphere, EC/IC arterial bypass might be of long-term benefit. Patients with recurrent TIAs associated with upright posture while on medical therapy may also benefit from bypass. There is no proof at this time, however, that such patients are helped by EC/IC arterial bypass. Further investigations of these problems would be helpful.

REFERENCES

1. Andersen, C. A., Rich, N. M., Collins, C. J., Jr., McDonald, P. T., Boone, S. C. Unilateral internal carotid arterial occlusion: special considerations. Stroke 8: 669–671, 1977.
2. Astrup, J. Energy-requiring cell functions in the ischemic brain. J. Neurosurg., 56: 482–497, 1982.
3. Ausman, J. I., Latchaw, R. E., Lee, M. C., Ramirez-Lassepas, M. Results of multiple angiographic studies on cerebral revascularization patients. In Microsurgery for Stroke, edited by P. Schmiedek, Springer-Verlag, New York, 1977, pp. 222–229.
4. Barnett, H. J. M. Delayed cerebral ischemic episodes distal to occlusion of major cerebral arteries. Neurology 28: 769–774, 1978.
5. Barnett, H. J. M., Peerless, S. J., Kaufman, J. C. E. "Stump" of internal carotid artery—a source for further cerebral embolic ischemia. Stroke 9: 448–456, 1978.
6. Baron, J. C., Bousser, M. G., Rey, A., Guillard, A., Comar, D., Castaigne, P. Reversal of focal "misery-perfusion syndrome" by extra-intracranial bypass in hemodynamic cerebral ischemia. Stroke 12: 454–459, 1981.
7. Baron, J. C., Rougemont, D., Bousser, M. G., Lebrun-Grandié, P., Iba-Zizen, M. T., Chiras, J. Local CBF, oxygen extraction fraction and $CMRO_2$: prognostic value in recent supratentorial infarction. J. Cereb. Blood Flow Metab. 3(Suppl. 1): S1–S2, 1983.
8. Baron, J. C., Steinling, M., Tanaka, T., Cavalheiro, E., Soussaline, F. Collard, P. Quantitative measurement of CBF, oxygen extraction fraction (OEF) and $CMRO_2$ with ^{15}O continuous inhalation techniques and positron emission tomography (PET): experimental evidence and normal values in man. J. Cereb. Blood Flow Metab. 1(Suppl. 1): S5–S6, 1981.
9. Bogousslavsky, J., Regli, F., Hungerbruhler, J.-P., Chrzanowski, R. Transient ischemic attacks and external carotid artery. A retrospective study of 23 patients with an occlusion of the internal carotid artery. Stroke, 12: 627–630, 1981.
10. Bousser, M. G., Eschwege, E., Haguenau, M., Lefaucconnier, J. M., Thibult, N., Touboul, D., Touboul, P. J. "AICLA" controlled trial of aspirin and dipyridamole in the secondary prevention of athero-thrombotic cerebral ischemia. Stroke, 14: 5–14, 1983.
11. Canadian Cooperative Study Group. A randomized trial of aspirin and sulfinpyrazone in threatened stroke. N. Engl. J. Med., 299: 53–59, 1978.
12. Caplan, L. R. Transient ischemic attacks. In Current Therapy in Neurologic Disease, 1985–1986, edited by RT Johnson. BC Decker, Philadelphia, Toronto, 1985, pp. 164–167.
13. Chater, N., Popp, J. Microsurgical vascular bypass for occlusive cerebrovascular disease: review of 100 cases. Surg. Neurol., 6: 115–118, 1976.
14. Clayson, K. K., Edwards, W. H. Importance of the external carotid artery in extracranial cerebrovascular occlusive disease. South Med. J., 70: 901–909, 1977.
15. Cote, R., Barnett, H. J. M., Taylor, D. W. Internal carotid occlusion: a prospective study. Stroke, 14: 898–902, 1983.

16. Countee, R. W., Vijayanathan, T. External carotid artery in internal carotid artery occlusion. Angiographic, therapeutic, and prognostic considerations. Stroke, *10:* 450–460, 1979.

17. Countee, R. W., Vijayanathan, T. Reconstruction of "totally" occluded internal carotid arteries. Angiographic and technical considerations. J. Neurosurg., *50:* 747–757, 1979.

18. Diemer, K. Capillarisation and oxygen supply of the brain. In *Oxygen Transport in Blood and Tissue,* edited by D. W. Lubbers, U. C. Luft, G. Thews, E. Witzleb, Thieme, Stuttgart, 1968, pp. 118–123.

19. Donaghy, R. M. P. Patch and by-pass in microangional surgery. In *Micro-Vascular Surgery,* edited by R. M. P. Donaghy and M. A. Yasargil, C. V. Mosby Co, St. Louis, 1967, pp. 75–86.

20. Dyken, M. L., Klatte, E., Kolar, O. J., Spurgeon, C. Complete occlusion of common or internal carotid arteries. Clinical significance. Arch. Neurol., *30:* 343–346, 1974.

21. EC/IC Bypass Study Group: Extracranial-intracranial arterial bypass surgery does not reduce the risk of ischemic stroke: Results of an international randomized trial (the EC/IC Bypass Trial). N. Engl. J. Med., *313,* 1985.

22. Ehrenfeld, W. K., Wylie, E. J. Spontaneous dissection of the internal carotid artery. Arch. Surg., *111:* 1294–1301, 1976.

23. Eklof, B., MacMillan, V., Siesjö, B. K. Cerebral energy state and cerebral venous PO_2 in experimental hypotension caused by bleeding. Acta Physiol. Scand., *86:* 515–527, 1972.

24. Fields, W. S., Lemak, N. A. Joint study of extracranial arterial occlusion: X. Internal carotid artery occlusion. J.A.M.A., *235:* 2734–2738, 1976.

25. Fisher, C. M. Concerning recurrent transient cerebral ischaemic attacks. Can. Med. Assoc. J., *86:* 1091–1099, 1962.

26. Fisher, C. M. Occlusion of the carotid artery. Arch. Neurol. Psych., *72:* 187–204, 1954.

27. Fisher, C. M., Ojemann, R. G., Roberson, G. H. Spontaneous dissection of cervico-cerebral arteries. Can. J. Neurol. Sci., *5:* 9–19, 1978.

28. Finklestein, S., Kleinman, G. M., Cuneo, R., Baringer, J. R. Delayed stroke following carotid occlusion. Neurology, *30:* 84–88, 1980.

29. Finnerty, F. A., Witkin, L., Fazekas, J. F. Cerebral hemodynamics during cerebral ischemia induced by acute hypotension. J. Clin. Invest., *33:* 1227–1232, 1954.

30. Furlan, A. J., Whisnant, J. P., Baker, H. L., Jr. Long term prognosis after carotid artery occlusion. Neurology, *30:* 986–988, 1980.

31. Gee, W., McDonald, K. M., Kaupp,. H. A., Celani, V. J., Bast, R. G. Carotid stenosis plus occlusion: endarterectomy or bypass. Arch. Surg., *115:* 183–187, 1980.

32. Genten, E., Barnett, H. J. M., Fields, W. S., Gent, M., Hoak, J. C. Cerebral ischemia: the role of thrombosis and antithrombotic therapy. Stroke, *8:* 150–175, 1977.

33. Gratzl, O., Schmiedek, P., Spetzler, R., Steinhoff, H., Marguth, F. Clinical experience with extra-intracranial arterial anastomosis in 65 cases. J. Neurosurg., *44:* 313–324, 1976.

34. Grillo, P., Patterson, R. H., Jr. Occlusion at the carotid artery: prognosis (natural history) and the possibilities of surgical revascularization. Stroke, *6:* 17–20, 1975.

35. Grubb, R. L., Jr., Phelps, M. E., Raichle, M. E. The effects of arterial blood pressure on the regional cerebral blood volume by x-ray fluorescence. Stroke, *4:* 390–399, 1973.

36. Grubb, R. L., Jr., Raichle, M. E., Phelps, M. E., Ratcheson, R. A. Effects of increased intracranial pressure on cerebral blood volume, blood flow and oxygen utilization in monkeys. J. Neurosurg., *43:* 385–398, 1975.

37. Grubb, R. L., Jr., Raichle, M. E., Eichling, J. O., Gado, M. H. Effects of subarachnoid hemorrhage on cerebral blood volume, blood flow and oxygen utilization in humans. J. Neurosurg., *46:* 446–453, 1977.

38. Grubb, R. L., Jr., Ratcheson, R. A., Raichle, M. E., Kliefoth, A. B., Gado, M. H. Regional cerebral blood flow and oxygen utilization in superficial temporal-middle cerebral artery anastomosis patients. J. Neurosurg., 50: 733–741, 1979.

39. Guyton, A. C.: Textbook of Medical Physiology. W. B. Saunders, Philadelphia, 1981, pp. 509–510.

40. Hardy, W. G., Lindner, D. W., Thomas, L. M., Gurdjian, E. S. Anticipated clinical course in carotid artery occlusion. Arch. Neurol., 6: 138–150, 1962.

41. Heiss, W.-D., Rosner, G. Functional recovery of cortical neurons as related to degree and duration of ischemia. Ann. Neurol., 14: 294–301, 1983.

42. Heros, R. C., Sekhar, L. N. Diagnostic and therapeutic alternatives in patients with symptomatic "carotid occlusion" referred for extracranial-intracranial bypass surgery. J. Neurosurg., 54: 790–796, 1981.

43. Jackson, B. B. The external carotid as a brain collateral. Am. J. Surg., 113: 375–378, 1967.

44. Jawad, K., Miller, J. D., Fitch, W., Barker, J. Measurement of jugular venous blood gases for prediction of brain ischemia following carotid ligation. Eur. Neurol., 14: 43–52, 1976.

45. Jones, T. H., Morawetz, R. B., Crowell, R. M., Marcoux, F. W., Fitzgibbon, S. I., DeGirotami, U., Ojemann, R. G. Thresholds of focal cerebral ischemia in awake monkeys. J. Neurosurg., 54: 773–782, 1981.

46. Kish, G. F., Adkins, P. C., Slovin, A. J. The totally occluded internal carotid artery: indications for surgery. Am. J. Surg., 134: 288–292, 1977.

47. Kistler, J. P., Ropper, A. H., Heros, R. C. Therapy of ischemic cerebral vascular disease due to atherothrombosis. N. Engl. J. Med., 311: 27–34, 1984.

48. Kistler, J. P. Personal communication, 1985.

49. Kontos, H. A. Regulation of the cerebral circulation. Ann. Rev. Physiol., 43: 397–407, 1981.

50. Kusunoki, T., Rowed, D. W., Tator, C. H., Lougheed, W. M. Thromboenarterectomy for total occlusion of the internal carotid artery: a reappraisal of risks, success rate and potential benefits. Stroke, 9: 34–38, 1978.

51. Lammertsma, A. A., Jones, T. Correction for the presence of intravascular oxygen-15 in the steady state technique for measuring regional oxygen extraction ratio in the brain. 1. Description of the method. J. Cereb. Blood Flow Metab., 3: 416–431, 1983.

52. Lammerstma, A. A., Wise, R. J. S., Heather, J. D., Gibbs, J. M., Leenders, K. L., Frackowiack, R. S. J., Rhodes, C. C., Jones, T. Correction for the presence of intravascular oxygen-15 in the steady-state technique for measuring regional oxygen extraction ratio in the brain. 2. Results in normal subjects and brain tumor and stroke patients. J. Cereb. Blood Flow Metab., 3: 425–431, 1983.

53. Lenzi, G. L., Frackowiak, R. S. J., Jones, T. Cerebral oxygen metabolism and blood flow in human cerebral infarction. J. Cereb. Blood Flow Metab., 2: 321–335, 1982.

54. Little, J. R., Furlan, A. J., Bryerton, B. Short vein grafts for cerebral revascularization. J. Neurosurg., 59: 384–388, 1983.

55. Luken, M. G., III, Ascherl, G. F., Jr., Correll, J. W., Hilal, S. K. Spontaneous dissecting aneurysms of the extracranial internal carotid artery. Clin. Neurosurg., 26: 353–375, 1979.

56. Marshall, J. The management of occlusion and stenosis of the internal carotid artery. Neurology (Minneap.), 16: 1087–1093, 1966.

57. McDowell, F. H., Potes, J., Groch, S. The natural history of internal carotid and vertebral-basilar artery occlusion. Neurology (Minneap.), 11: 153–157, 1961.

58. Mokri, B., Sundt, T. M. Jr., Houser, O. W. Spontaneous internal carotid dissection, hemicrania, and Horner's syndrome. Arch. Neurol., 36: 677–680, 1979.

59. Ojemann, R. G., Crowell, R. M. *Surgical Management of Cerebrovascular Disease*, Williams & Wilkins, Baltimore, 1983, pp. 71–92.
60. Ojemann, R. G., Crowell, R. M., Roberson, G. H., Fisher, C. M. Surgical treatment of extracranial carotid occlusive disease. Clin. Neurosurg., *22:* 214–263, 1975.
61. Patterson, R. H., Jr. Risk of carotid surgery with occlusion of the contralateral carotid artery. Arch. Neurol., *30:* 188–189, 1974.
62. Powers, W. J., Grubb, R. L., Jr., Raichle, M. E. Physiological responses to focal cerebral ischemia in humans. Ann. Neurol., *16:* 546–552, 1984.
63. Powers, W. J., Martin, W. R. W., Herscovitch, P., Raichle, M. E., Grubb, R. L., Jr. Extracranial-intracranial bypass surgery: hemodynamic and metabolic effects. Neurology, *34:* 1168–1174, 1984.
64. Raichle, M. E. The pathophysiology of brain ischemia. Ann. Neurol., *13:* 2–10, 1983.
65. Raichle, M. E., Grubb, R. L., Jr., Gado, M. H., Eichling, J. O., Ter-Pogossian, M. M. Correlation between regional cerebral blood flow and oxidative metabolism. Arch. Neurol., *33:* 523–526, 1976.
66. Reichman, O. H. Extracranial-intracranial arterial anastomosis. In *Cerebral Vascular Disease: Ninth Conference*, edited by J. P. Whisnant, B. A. Sandok. Grune and Stratton, New York, 1975, pp. 175–185.
67. Ringelstein, E. B., Zeumer, H., Angelou, D. The pathogenesis of strokes from internal carotid artery occlusion. Diagnostic and therapeutic implications. Stroke, *14:* 867–875, 1983.
68. Ross Russell, R. W., Page, N. G. R. Critical perfusion of brain and retina. Brain, *106:* 419–434, 1983.
69. Samson, D. S., Boone, S. Extracranial-intracranial (EC/IC) arterial bypass: past performance and current concepts. Neurosurgery, *3:* 79–86, 1978.
70. Scheich, H., Honnegger, H. W., Worrell, D. A., Kennedy, G. Capillary dilation in response to hypoxia in the brain of a gobiid fish. Respir. Physiol., *15:* 87–95, 1972.
71. Sekhar, L. N., Heros, R. C., Lotz, P. R., Rosenbaum, A. E. Atheromatous pseudo-occlusion of the internal carotid artery. J. Neurosurg., *52:* 782–789, 1980.
72. Shucart, W. A., Garrido, E. Reopening some occluded carotid arteries. Report of four cases. J. Neurosurg., *45:* 442–446, 1976.
73. Spetzler, R. F., Rhodes, R. S., Roski, R. A., Likavec, M. J. Subclavian to middle cerebral artery saphenous vein bypass graft. J. Neurosurg., *53:* 465–469, 1980.
74. Story, J. L., Brown, W. E., Jr., Eidelberg, E., Arom, K. V., Stewart, J. R. Cerebral revascularization: common carotid to distal middle cerebral artery bypass. Neurosurgery, *2:* 131–134, 1978.
75. Sundt, T. M., Jr., Sandok, B. A., Howser, O. W. The selection of patients for intracranial and extracranial surgery for cerebrovascular occlusive disease. Clin. Neurosurg., *22:* 185–198, 1975.
76. Sundt, T. M., Jr., Whisnant, J. P., Fode, N. C., Piepgras, D. G., Houser, O. W. Results, complications, and follow-up of 415 bypass operations for occlusive disease of the carotid system. Mayo Clin. Proc., *60:* 230–240, 1985.
77. Whisnant, J. P. A population study of stroke and TIA: Rochester, Minn. In *Stroke*, edited by F. J. Gillingham, L. Mawdsley, and A. E. Williams. Churchill, Livingstone, Edinburgh, 1976, pp. 21–39.
78. Whisnant, J. P., Sundt, T. M., Jr., Fode, N. C. Long-term mortality and stroke morbidity after superficial temporal-middle cerebral artery bypass operation. Mayo Clin. Proc., *60:* 241–246, 1985.
79. Wiebers, D. O., Whisnant, J. P., O'Fallon, W. M. Reversible ischemic neurologic deficit

(RIND) in a community: Rochester, Minnesota 1955–1974. Neurology (NY), *32:* 459–465, 1982.
80. Wiess, H. R., Buchweitz, E. L., Murtha, T. J., Auletta, M. Quantitative regional determination of morphometric indices of the total and perfused capillary network in the rat brain. Circ. Res., *51:* 494–503, 1982.
81. Wylie, E. J., Hein, M. F., Adams, J. E. Intracranial hemorrhage following surgical revascularization for treatment of acute stroke. J. Neurosurg., *21:* 212–215, 1964.
82. Yasargil, M. G., Krayenbuhl, H. A., Jacobson, J. H. II Microneurosurgical arterial reconstruction. Surgery, *67:* 221–223, 1970.

17

Emergency Cerebral Revascularization

ROBERT M. CROWELL, M.D.

Controversy reigns about emergency cerebral revascularization. On the one hand, there is a tantalizing rationale for the approach. Modern data indicate that focal cerebral ischemia may be fully reversible some hours after arterial occlusion (8). Medical measures have been developed which may prolong this "golden period" (22, 35, 36). Rapid revascularization may restore circulation to resuscitate nonfunctional ("paralyzed") but still viable neurons. Some clinical data exist to bolster this impression (14, 17, 25, 26, 31). On the other hand, some experimental and clinical data suggest the inadequacy or even deleterious effects of emergency revascularization (15, 32).

In the following chapter, we review the rationale, techniques, results, and complications of several forms of emergency brain revascularization. We offer an opinion as to current indications for this approach and possible future applications.

THRESHOLDS OF ISCHEMIA AND INFARCTION

Adequate perfusion is required to maintain the normal function and structure of the brain. Specific blood flow thresholds have been identified for a variety of reversible dysfunctions. Cerebral blood flow (CBF) determinations and electroencephalography (EEG) during carotid endarterectomy demonstrate EEG slowing when hemispheric blood flow falls to 16–20 ml per 100 gm per minute (29). Baboons lose somatosensory evoked potentials when regional CBF falls below 15 ml per 100 gm per minute (3). According to Heiss *et al.* (19), neuronal firing in anesthesized cats ceases when regional CBF falls below 18 ml per 100 gm per minute. In monkeys, average hemispheral CBF below 23 ml per 100 gm per minute causes a mild neurologic deficit (see Fig. 17.1) (21). CBF below 8 ml per 100 gm per minute causes flaccid hemiplegia.

The threshold for energy failure and loss of membrane function is a lethal threshold for cellular damage (2). Symon and Brierley found infarction in baboons corresponding to the zones with CBF less than 10 ml per 100 gm per minute. According to Morowitz *et al.* (25), infarction is a function of intensity and duration of ischemia. Monkeys with very brief

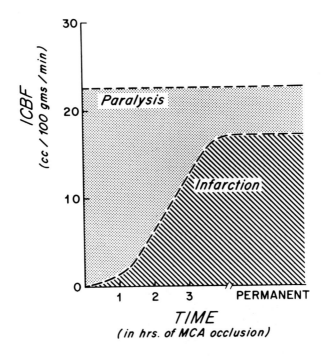

FIG. 17.1. *Thresholds of ischemia and infarction.* Correlation of CBF with deficient and infarction in awake monkeys with temporary MCA occlusion (see text). CBF below 23 ml per 100 gm per minute leads to reversible paralysis. Long-lasting ischemia below 17–18 ml per 100 gm per minute leads to permanent infarction. Note that elevation of CBF above 23 ml per 100 gm per minute may lead to full recovery unless CBF has gone below infarction threshold. (From Jones, T. H. *et al.*, J. Neurosurg., *53:* 773–782, 1981 with permission).

middle cerebral artery (MCA) occlusions tolerate marked ischemia without evidence of infarction. For permanent MCA occlusion, local CBF of 17–18 ml per 100 gm per minute causes infarction. Data from these studies suggest an infarction threshold, rising over 6–8 hours to a plateau.

Studies of local blood flow and metabolism indicate that following MCA occlusion there is a dense zone of ischemia below the threshold of infarction surrounded by a "penumbra" of moderate ischemia producing loss of synaptic transmission without necrosis. Restoration of flow to this penumbral zone, by either medical or surgical means, could restore useful function to stroke victims. Note that this strategy might hold even in chronic ischemia states, but the likelihood of useful recovery would obviously be greater in the acute stage before membrane destruction has occurred in the central zone.

The threshold and penumbra concepts are hopeful for the management of acute ischemic stroke. These ideas imply that some cases of fresh hemiplegia, with CBF in the penumbra range, might be improved by surgical revascularization. Recovery of animals and patients after restoration of MCA blood flow following occlusion of a few hours supports the approach. On the other hand, cases of acute hemiplegia with CBF in the infarction range for a sufficient interval will not be helped by restoration of flow. Rapid studies of local CBF and metabolism might help identify suitable cases for emergency cerebral revascularization.

Differential Diagnosis of Ischemia vs. Infarction

Once brain tissue is dead, brain revascularization cannot help. How can one identify infarction? Histopathologic changes can document infarction with certainty after several days, but this method has no clinical utility. Determination of extracellular potassium, which might indicate membrane irreversible failure, is not currently practical (2). Computed tomographic (CT) scanning can indicate by low proton attenuation an area of infarction, but only after 12–24 hours (12). Magnetic resonance imaging (MRI) seems more promising because experimental cerebral infarction may be demonstrated within 3 hours (13). Positron emission tomography (PET) scanning might also differentiate ischemia from infarction, but this instrument is likely to remain a research tool. Emergency determination of focal CBF might be useful to document transgression of the infarction threshold (21).

Angiographic studies are helpful in determining the mechanism of vascular insult. The angiographic anatomy may show distal embolus, occlusion of perforating branches, collateral circulation, and vessels for anastomosis. Carotid endarterectomy or distal bypass are unlikely to remedy ischemia resulting from multiple embolic occlusions or deep perforator obstruction.

Therapy to Extend Reversibility

Many treatments have been suggested to improve outcome after ischemia, but few are established. Barbiturate coma may under certain circumstances diminish infarct size (30, 31). Osmotic agents such as mannitol decrease cerebral edema and improve CBF (35). Hypervolemic hemodilution has been shown to increase CBF and decrease infarct size (36). Induced hypertension has been shown to be of some benefit (22), and perfluorochemicals may improve perfusion to the brain (35).

EMERGENCY CAROTID ENDARTERECTOMY

Since focal cerebral ischemia may be reversible in its early stages, there is a rationale for emergency carotid endarterectomy to restore flow through an occluded or stenotic internal carotid artery (ICA) This concept was applied in the 1960s but with discouraging results. Several reports appeared indicating that emergency endarterectomy led to cerebral hemorrhage and neurologic deterioration (4). Careful scrutiny of these reports, however, indicates that hemorrhage sometimes occurred on the opposite side from surgery and was almost always in conjunction with postoperative hypertension (6). Modern experience has suggested that in selected cases good results can be obtained with emergency endarterectomy if meticulous efforts at blood pressure control are applied in the postoperative period (27). Some patients have unstable neurologic syndromes of mild to moderate disability which may progress to severe disability without treatment. For such patients, we believe a diagnosis should be established as quickly as possible and then a rational program of treatment instituted. This same approach has been utilized in other centers with encouraging results in the surgical treatment of selected acute stroke patients (17, 33).

Evaluation for Emergency Surgery

A careful history and examination will lead to a correct diagnosis in a high percentage of patients. Almost every patient admitted with an acute stroke problem should have an electrocardiogram (EKG), and an immediate CT scan to differentiate between infarction and hemorrhage (5). Laboratory tests should include blood count, blood chemistries, and coagulation studies.

If the history, findings, or both, suggest carotid artery disease, then immediate angiography or digital subtraction angiography should be done (Fig. 17.2). This is especially important if the patient has had increasing transient ischemic attacks (TIAs) in preceding days, the sudden onset of a mild to moderate neurologic deficit, or a progressive or fluctuating deficit. TIAs which last more than 1 hour or TIAs involving face, arm, and leg are particularly worrisome and should be promptly investigated. If there is a severe ICA stenosis with delayed flow, thrombus in the distal lumen or stenosis, or occlusion with reflux to the intrapetrous segment of the ICA, surgery should be done to allow maximum blood flow to ischemic brain tissue, prevent extension of a thrombus, and remove a source of embolization. A stenosis with residual lumen diameter greater than 2.0 mm (not hemodynamically significant) or ulceration in the plaque at the common carotid artery bifurcation suggests embolus is the cause of the problem and the patient should be considered for anticoagulation. If an acute neurologic deficit occurs with loss of a previously documented carotid bruit, emergency endarterectomy should be undertaken without CT scan or angiography. Where there is sudden onset of severe neurologic deficit which

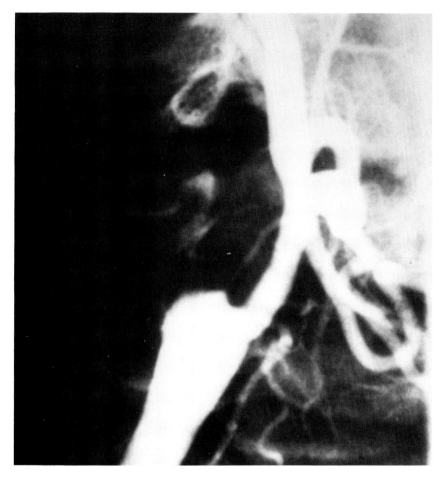

FIG. 17.2. *Emergency carotid endarterectomy.* (Case 1). Angiogram shows complete left internal carotid artery occlusion 8 hours after onset of moderate dysphasia and right hemiparesis.

persists, it is likely that significant infarction has occurred. This is almost certainly the case if there is a decreased level of consciousness. In this situation, restoration of blood flow either by emergency carotid endarterectomy or bypass graft has generally not been beneficial.

The technique of carotid endarterectomy is modified for emergency utilization (26). Every effort is made to expedite the procedure in order to minimize the progressive damage of acute ischemia. If there is a complete occlusion, then EEG monitoring may be omitted. While efforts to prepare for endarterectomy are underway, the blood pressure is elevated with volume administration, a dopamine infusion, or both to increase the mean arterial blood pressure (MABP) by 30%. A rapid exposure of the carotid bifurcation is achieved. In the case of complete or nearly complete occlusion, a shunt is ordinarily not required. Occasionally, in the presence of a large common to external carotid collateral circulation to the brain, we have used a common to external carotid intraluminal shunt during surgery.

When the angiogram indicates complete ICA occlusion, the majority of operations will disclose a thrombus at surgery. In many of these patients there will be good backflow, but in some there will be a further obstruction distally. If there is a longstanding occlusion, the artery may be a firm, fibrous cord. Hugenholtz and Elgie (19) noted that the angiogram correlates with the ability to obtain backflow. Of 35 patients with an occluded ICA, they were able to reopen the artery in 19 (53%). There was a clear-cut correlation between backflow and the collateral circulation to the distal ICA—six of 18 cases with modest retrograde filling of the ICA could be reopened (29%), whereas 13 of 15 patients with good retrograde filling of the intracranial ICA were reopened (87%).

Certain techniques may help in opening the completely occluded artery. If a thrombus is encountered in the ICA, an effort is made to withdraw it gradually using a hand-over-hand technique (Fig. 17.3). Thrombi as long as 20 cm have been removed. If this technique fails, a smooth-ended suction catheter is introduced into the ICA lumen, and suction is then applied to withdraw the thrombus. If this method fails, a Fogarty no. 3 catheter is passed gently as far as the base of the skull, inflated, and withdrawn. Care is required to avoid injuring the distal ICA with subsequent development of a carotid-cavernous fistula. Measurements on the angiogram from the ICA bifurcation to the base of the skull may help in determining the safe length of catheter which may be inserted. A single lateral intraoperative angiogram with 10 ml of Renografin through an Argyle shunt catheter is recommended to document restoration of flow without intimal flap or distal thrombus. If good backflow with satisfactory angiography cannot be achieved, the ICA is doubly ligated with 0 silk and its origin plicated with 3–0 Prolene to avoid a stump. In this setting, anticoagulation may be considered to avert propagation and embolization of clot when flow is reestablished, anticoagulation should be continued in the postoperative period to avoid recurrent thrombosis at the operative site. Heparin at 500 units per hour is recommended for 12 hours, then full heparinization to maintain a partial thromboplastin time of about 60 seconds. Heparinization may be continued for several days, and then a decision is made regarding Coumadin therapy. Where there has been carotid occlusion or in cases where recurrent thrombosis is particularly feared, we have favored Coumadin for a period of approximately 3 months.

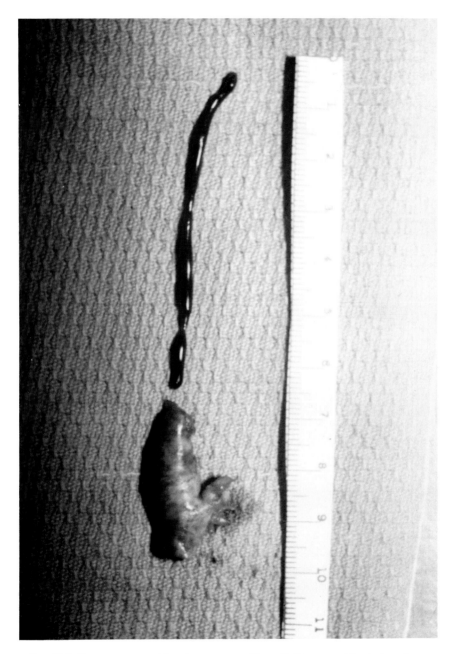

FIG. 17.3. *Emergency carotid endarterectomy.* (Case 1). Plaque and fresh thrombus removed at endarterectomy. Excellent backflow. Gradual complete recovery in a few hours.

Results of Emergency Endarterectomy

We base indications for treatment on experience with emergency carotid endarterectomy in 55 consecutive patients (2, 6). Table 17.1 correlates the outcome with preoperative status. Patients with crescendo TIAs had severe stenosis with either an intraluminal thrombus or marked reduction of flow in the distal ICA. Patients with mild to moderate neurologic deficits may be stable or have progressing or fluctuating deficits. In the series of 36 patients with worrisome TIAs, acute mild to moderate deficit, or fluctuating stroke, 29 enjoyed excellent or good outcome. In this group there was one death; the patient had complete neurologic recovery but then died of a cardiopulmonary complication. There were two occasions where the neurologic deficit was worse after the operation, but there were also several spectacular recoveries in the immediate postoperative period. In another study, 27 of 28 patients presenting with crescendo TIAs or stroke-in-evolution made a prompt recovery after emergency carotid endarterectomy (17). One patient died from a brain stem stroke.

Patients with sudden severe deficit do not benefit from endarterectomy (26). In 19 such cases, we noted seven deaths, six poor outcomes, and only one recovery to an excellent condition, a development that may be related to operating on this patient within one hour of the onset of difficulty. Five of the seven deaths were related to extensive cerebral damage and two were due to myocardial infarction. These cases were done early in our experience, and we no longer operate on such patients.

The correlation of surgical findings and outcome is striking, with 18 of 21 patients with total occlusion and restoration of internal carotid flow showing improvement (Table 17.2) (26). Only one of eight patients improved where occlusion could not be reopened. These findings strongly suggest that restoration of blood flow is the major factor in determining

TABLE 17.1
Results of Emergency Carotid Endarterectomy

Preoperative Neurologic Status	Outcome				
	Excellent	Good	Poor	Death	Total
TIAs	4				4
Mild deficit	2	2			4
Moderate deficit	7	14	6	1	28
Sudden severe deficit	1	5	6	7	19
Total	14	21	12	8	55

TABLE 17.2

Emergency Carotid Endarterectomy: Surgical Findings and Outcome

Findings	Outcome				
	Excellent	Good	Poor	Death	Total
Stenosis	8	11	4	3	26
Occluded (flow restored)	5	11	2	3	21
Occluded (flow not restored)		1	5	2	8
Total	13	23	11	8	55

neurologic improvement. The time elapsed from the onset of symptoms to revascularization in our study was usually under 24 hours, but an excellent result was reported as late as 36 hours after onset of symptoms. In other reports, it was possible to restore and maintain patency in patients who underwent surgery within 48 hours (33). Hugenholtz and Elgie (19) believe that an effort should be made to open all vessels seen within one week of occlusion.

EMERGENCY BYPASS

Laboratory results are mixed. Crowell and Olsen (9) in an experimental model of MCA occlusion in the dog found a favorable effect of superficial temporal-middle cerebral (STA-MCA) artery bypass, provided revascularization was completed within 6 hours. Levinthal *et al.* (23) report similar results. If blood brain barrier is damaged, however, revascularization may produce hemorrhage. Moreover, the STA may bring too little blood to overcome clinical ischemia. Experimental results in the dog reported by Diaz *et al.* (14) indicate STA-MCA bypass at 4 hours or 24 hours after cerebral vascular occlusion led to worse results regarding clinical deficit, infarct size, and incidence of hemorrhagic infarction.

Reports of clinical application of STA-MCA bypass grafting for acute stroke have been variable, but in general substantial benefit has been uncommon. Gratzl *et al.* (17) had five deaths in seven patients undergoing STA-MCA bypass for stroke-in-evolution. They concluded that emergency bypass was contraindicated. Crowell reported 11 bad results in 12 patients undergoing emergency STA-MCA bypass, but various factors including perforating artery occlusion and delay in surgery may have influenced outcome (7). Samson *et al.* (28) warned that STA-MCA bypass was not able to sustain adequate flow to a large segment of the cerebral hemisphere in the face of acute MCA occlusion. Sundt *et al.* (34) reported four good results in five cases with STA-MCA bypass for progressive stroke. Diaz and colleagues (14) performed STA-MCA bypass on 15 patients with crescendo TIAs, stroke-in-evolution, and completed stroke. Ten of the patients appeared to improve to some degree (Fig. 17.4), however, the five patients with fixed preoperative deficit showed no improvement. There were no deaths in this series. In a review of the literature, 67 cases of emergency bypass grafting were presented (Table 17.3) (14). If one considers delayed improvement as unrelated to bypass (Table 17.3), there were 27 instances of therapy-related improvement, 26 cases without improvement, and 11 deaths. It should be noted that this review contained a mixture of cases, some operated concomitant with intracranial occlusion, others operated several days after the onset of symptoms. The substantial majority of those that improved were operated on after a short interval of time (usually 6 hours). It should be noted that the Cooperative Study of Extracranial-Intracranial Bypass did not consider emergency cases.

More data are needed for firm indications, but rarely is bypass warranted for crescendo TIAs or moderate deficit less than 6 hours old with inaccessible ICA stenosis or occlusion.

MIDDLE CEREBRAL EMBOLECTOMY

The results of embolectomy (37) compared with the natural history of the disease remain inconclusive because of the paucity of case reports (Fig. 17.5). The natural history of MCA acute occlusion is not well-defined. Dr. C. M. Fisher believes that 90% of patients with MCA occlusion will sustain an unsatisfactory disabling deficit. Experimental results are encouraging provided operation is done within 4 hours (16).

Rapid evaluation of patients considered for MCA embolectomy is imperative if revascularization is to have a useful effect. In most cases the diagnosis can be strongly suggested from the clinical history and examination. The sudden onset of a substantial hemispheric deficit, particularly in the setting of known cardiac source of embolus, strongly suggests the

TABLE 17.3
Results of Emergency STA-MCA Bypass

Source	Outcome		
	Better	Same	Dead
Diaz *et al.* (13)	13	2	0
Literature	27	26	10
Total	40 (51%)	28 (36%)	10 (13%)

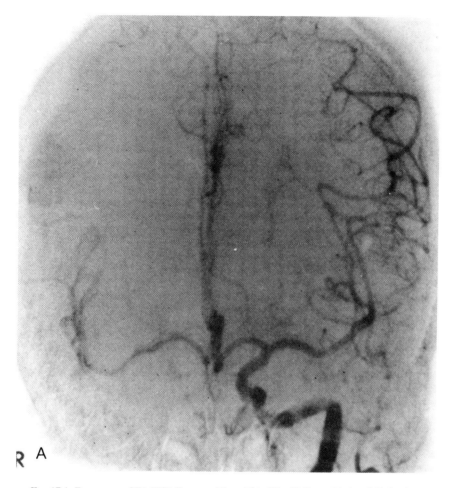

R A

FIG. 17.4. *Emergency STA-MCA Bypass.* (Case 13 in Diaz F. G. *et al.*) *A* and *B*: Angiogram shows right internal carotid occlusion with fair collateral circulation 6 hours after left hemiparesis in a 42 year old woman. *C*: Angiogram shows excellent MCA filling via STA-MCA bypass. Complete recovery. (From Diaz F. G. *et al.* J. Neurosurg., *63:* 200–209, 1985 with permission).

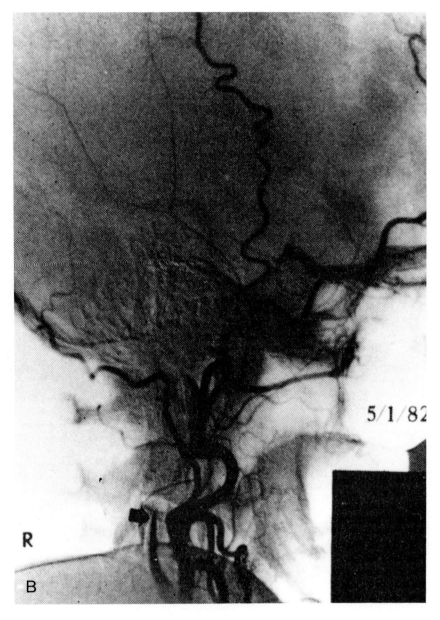

FIG. 17.4B

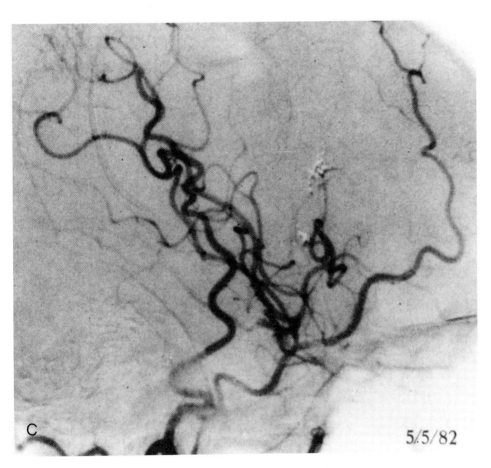

C   5/5/82

FIG. 17.4C

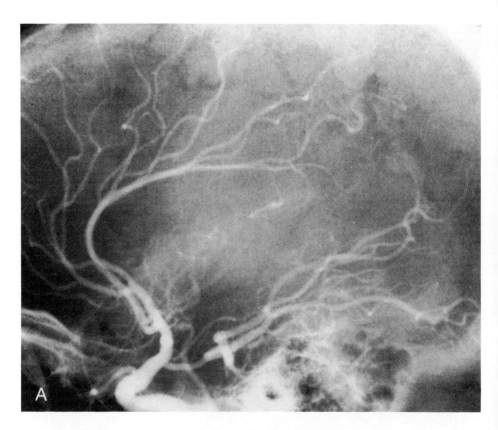

FIG. 17.5. *Emergency MCA embolectomy.* (Case 3). *A–C*: Angiogram shows complete left MCA occlusion with good collateral in a 42-year-old man 2 hours after onset of aphasia and hemiplegia. *D–F*: Good anterograde filling of left MCA after embolectomy. Gradual improvement with residual right brachial monoparesis and normal language. (From Ojemann R. G. and Crowell R. M.: *Surgical Management of Cerebrovascular Diseases.* Williams & Wilkins, Baltimore, 1983, with permission).

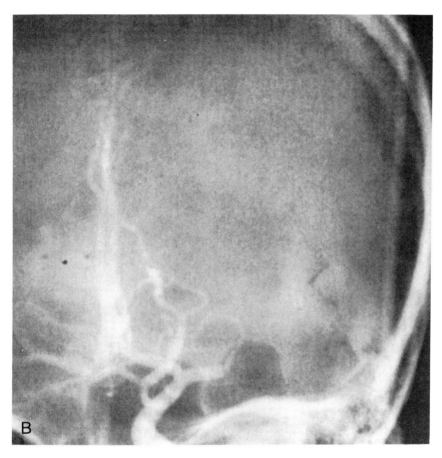

FIG. 17.5*B*

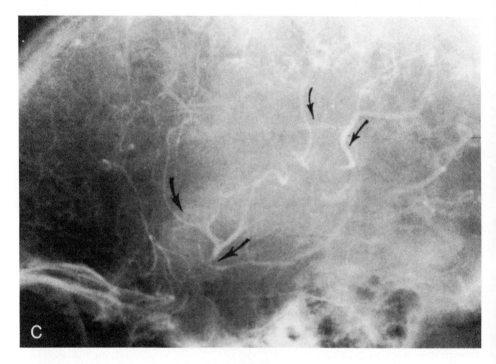

FIG. 17.5C

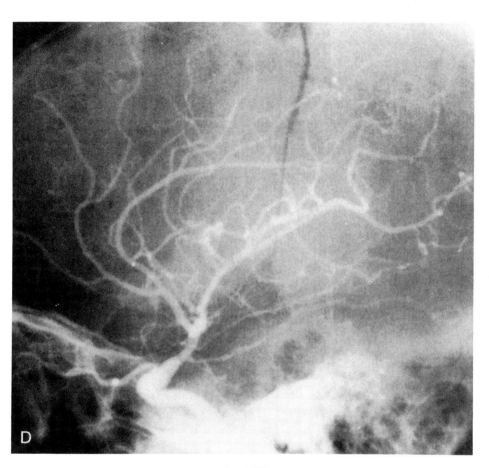

FIG. 17.5D

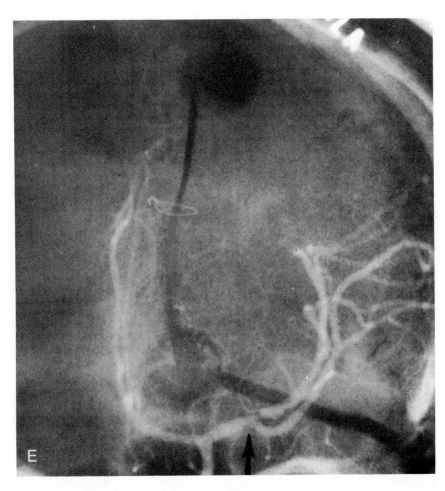

Fig. 17.5*E*

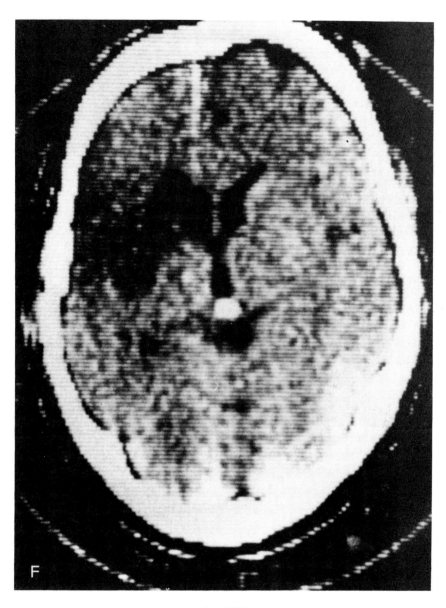

FIG. 17.5F

diagnosis. The diagnosis must be confirmed by cerebral angiography to pinpoint the site of occlusion, investigate possible multiple distal emboli, and evaluate collateral circulation. Emergency intubation with administration of barbiturate therapy or mannitol therapy together with the induction of hypertension and hypervolemic hemodilution may offer benefit during the evaluation phase.

Operative technique is aimed toward rapid exposure of the MCA-internal carotid artery complex (37). Ordinarily, this will involve opening the sylvian fissure. Occasionally, we have found it more expeditious to enter the fissure through a superior temporal gyrus cortisectomy if the fissure is difficult to open (26). Temporary aneurysm clips are placed on the M_1 segment and main divisions of the MCA distal to the embolus. The location of the embolus is identified by bluish discoloration of the nonpulsatile artery. Preferably, the arterotomy is made in one of the divisions although occasionally the main trunk of the MCA may be incised. The embolus is milked out by means of suction and forceps, with sequential use of antero-grade and retrograde flow to the MCA complex. After the embolus is removed, the arteriotomy is closed with 9–0 monofilament sutures. Patients may be given pentobarbital (4 mg per kg) at the start of the operation and MABP is elevated 30% to enhance collateral flow.

Results of MCA Embolectomy

The largest single series is that of Meyer *et al.* (24) from the Mayo Clinic (Table 17.4). They report 20 cases treated with emergency embolectomy. Flow was restored in 16 patients (75%). It was technically difficult to achieve patency with atherosclerotic emboli from the aorta. Two patients (10%) had an excellent result with no neurologic deficit, five (25%) were left with a minimal deficit but were employable, seven (35%) had a fair result but were still independent and employable, four (20%) did poorly, and two (10%) died. Patients with an associated ipsilateral carotid artery

TABLE 17.4
Results of MCA Embolectomy

	Outcome		
Source	Better	Same	Dead
Meyer *et al.* (24)	7	11	2
Literature	14	1	9
Total	21 (48%)	12 (27%)	11 (25%)

occlusion did poorly. Collateral flow, as judged from preoperative angiograms, was the best predictor of outcome.

Review of the literature disclosed 64 cases of MCA embolectomy (Table 17.4) (25). However, only 24 of these were performed within 24 hours of occlusion. In these cases, time for re-establishment of flow ranged from 40 minutes to 18 hours after occlusion. Among these 24 cases, 14 (58%) improved, one was unchanged, and nine (37.5%) died. Six of these deaths were either related to surgery or the actual ischemic event. There were two hemorrhagic infarctions, one resulting from use of anticoagulation therapy. Eighteen arteries were demonstrated to be patent. Seven of the eight patients with good preoperative collateral flow enjoyed improvement after surgery.

In the Mayo Clinic surgical group, at least seven patients (35%) did quite well, probably better than would have been expected without intervention (25). The seven patients with delayed improvement (35%) are probably a reflection of the natural history of the disease. Analysis of the preoperative cerebral angiograms in these cases suggests that collateral flow must have been sufficient to prevent irreversible cell damage in the majority of the compromised neurons maintaining them within the ischemic penumbra, thereby enhancing the salvaging effect of emergency embolectomy.

While more data are needed to establish indications, tentative guidelines for the procedure can be proposed: nonatheromatous debris should be the embolic source in that atheroma from aorta rarely can be removed with restoration of flow. Embolectomy after prolonged delay probably is unwarranted, and cases should be operated within 6 hours of onset. If there is an ipsilateral carotid occlusion, prognosis is poor and operation unwarranted. Good collateral flow to the MCA complex on the preoperative angiogram favors operative intervention. Younger patients probably are better candidates for surgery.

INTRAOPERATIVE OCCLUSION AND REVASCULARIZATION

Theoretically, the best opportunity for emergency bypass should be the occasional forced clipping of internal carotid or middle cerebral artery in the operating room. This situation would afford the opportunity for immediate (or even prophylactic) medical therapy (phenobarbital or mannitol with hypertension), followed by immediate revascularization. Samson et al. (28) found that immediate STA-MCA bypass in this setting may be inadequate to override infarction, suggesting that in some cases a long saphenous veins graft from the extracranial carotid artery to MCA is necessary to provide immediate high flow. Successful implementation by Spetzler et al. (31) bolster this concept. However, in the case of Lawner and Simeone (22), STA-MCA bypass was adequate to sustain an entire hemisphere after forced sacrifice of MCA. Consideration of the specific collateral circulation in individual cases might be helpful in selecting the appropriate revascularization procedure.

Suzuki and colleagues (35) performed STA-MCA bypasses within 10–20 hours in 10 patients with acute occlusion of ICA or MCA. For cerebral protection, the patients received mannitol and perfluorochemicals. All patients did well except for one who had a small hematoma and three with cerebral edema. Postoperatively, the blood pressure was maintained in the normal range. These observations suggest that preoperative therapy with cerebral protection, either in the form of mannitol, perfluorochemicals, or barbiturates with induced hypertension, may play a significant role in the resuscitation of brain neurons in preparation for revascularization.

CONCLUSIONS

There is a good rationale for emergency revascularization: surgery can supply blood flow needed by the ischemic brain. However, results indicate that in many cases, the required perfusion will come too late. Therefore, at present, emergency revascularization appears only occasionally warranted.

On the basis of present day experience, we recommend the following guidelines:

1. *Carotid endarterectomy* may be offered for patients with crescendo TIAs or mild to moderate deficit without drowsiness. Angiography should show occlusion or hemodynamically significant stenosis within 24 hours of onset (33). This will be the most commonly indicated emergency revascularizaton procedure.
2. *STA-MCA bypass* may be considered for patients with crescendo TIAs or mild to moderate deficit in whom infarction studies are negative. Angiography should show ICA occlusion with patent perforators. Patients should be ready for operation within 6 hours after onset. These cases will be very rare.
3. *MCA embolectomy* may be considered for patients with moderate to severe deficit seen within 6 hours where angiography discloses a single MCA occlusion, patent perforators, and good collateral circulation. These cases will be very rare.
4. *Immediate bypass* may be warranted for intraoperative ICA or MCA occlusion. Immediate institution of cerebral protection measures is clearly warranted. Saphenous vein bypass is probably advisable to achieve adequate flow.

Medical therapy is warranted in all such cases considered for emergency revascularization. Certainly hypotension is to be avoided and, in all cases where hemorrhage is not present, hypertension (MAPB increased by 30%) may be induced with volume loading. Hemodilution by colloid infusion (not whole blood) to achieve an optimum hematocrit (about 33%) for improved microcirculation is recommended (36). Mannitol therapy, though requiring further evaluation, is probably warranted for most cases during evaluation and surgery (35). Barbiturate therapy, because of its deleterious hemodynamic effect and effects on consciousness, is more difficult to recommend except in the case of intraoperative occlusion with revascularization (31). In this latter setting, encouraging results support measure.

Another critical variable is the surgical team. Emergency cerebral revascularization requires speed to be effective and carries high risk. Therefore, the approach can be recommended only for the experienced and prepared surgical team. Bad results with high-risk emergency surgery might well have an adverse effect on referrals for preventive cerebral vascular surgery.

Prevention of stroke is the best established goal for cerebral vascular surgery. *Reversal* of ischemia by emergency revascularization, despite the tantalizing rationale, is likely to remain a rarity. This therapy might become more practical with the development of public education for prompt referral, more effective therapy to extend reversibility, rapid differential diagnosis of ischemia versus infarction, and nonsuture techniques to accelerate revascularization.

REFERENCES

1. Astrup, J., Siesjö, B. K., and Symon, L. Thresholds in cerebral ischemia—the ischemic penumbra. Stroke, *12:* 723–725, 1981.
2. Astrup, J., Symon, L., Branston, N. M., *et al.* Cortical evoked potential and extracellular K^+ and H^+ at critical levels of brain ischemia. Stroke, *8:* 51–57, 1977.
3. Branston, N. M., Symon, L., Crockard, H. A., *et al.* Relationship between the cortical evoked potential and local cortical blood flow following acute middle cerebral artery occlusion in the baboon. Exp. Neurol., *45:* 195–208, 1974.
4. Bruetman, M. E., Fields, W. S., Crawford, E. S., *et al.* Cerebral hemorrhage in carotid artery surgery. Arch. Neurol. *9:* 458, 1963.
5. Buonanno, F., and Toole, J. F. Management of patients with established cerebral infarction. Stroke, *12:* 7–16, 1981.
6. Caplan, L. R., Skillman, J., Ojemann, R. G., and Fields, W. S. Intracerebral hemorrhage following carotid endarterectomy: a hypertensive complication? Stroke, *9:* 457–460, 1978.
7. Crowell, R. M. STA-MCA bypass for acute focal cerebral ischemia. In: *Microsurgery for Stroke,* edited by Schmiedek, P., Gratzl, O., Spetzler, R. F. Berlin, Springer-Verlag, 1977, pp. 244–250.
8. Crowell, R. M., Marcoux, F. W., and DeGirolami, U. Variability and reversibility of focal cerebral ischemia in unanesthetized monkeys. Neurology *31:* 1295–1302, 1981.
9. Crowell, R. M., and Olsson, Y. Effect of extracranial-intracranial vascular bypass graft on experimental acute stroke in dogs. J. Neurosurg., *38:* 26–31, 1973.

10. Crowell, R. M., Olsson, W., Klatzo, I., *et al.* Temporary occlusion of the middle cerebral artery in the monkey: clinical and pathological observation. Stroke, *2:* 439–448, 1970.

11. Davis, K. R., Ackerman, R. H., Kistler, J. P., and Mohr, J. P. Computed tomography of cerebral infarction: hemorrhage, contrast enhancement, and time of appearance. Comput. Tomogr., *1:* 71–86, 1977.

12. DeWitt, L. D., Buonnanno, F. S., Kistler, J. P., *et al.* Nuclear magnetic resonance imaging in evaluation of clinical stroke syndromes. Neurology, *16:* 535–545, 1984.

13. Diaz, F. G., Ausman, J. I., Mehta, B., Dujovny, M., *et al.* Acute cerebral revascularization. J. Neurosurg., *63:* 200–209, 1985.

14. Diaz, F. G., Mastri, A. R., Ausman, J. I., and Chou, S. N. Acute cerebral revascularization after regional cerebral ischemia in the dog. Part II: Clinical pathological correlation. J. Neurosurg., *51:* 644–653, 1979.

15. Dujovny, M., Osgood, C. P., Barrionuevo, P. J., *et al.* Middle cerebral artery microneurosurgical embolectomy. Surgery, *80:* 336–399, 1976.

16. Goldstone, J., and Moore, W. S. Emergency carotid artery surgery in neurologically unstable patients. Arch. Surg., *111:* 1284, 1976.

17. Gratzl, O., Schmiedek, P., Spetzler, R. *et al.* Clinical experience with extra-intracranial arterial anastomosis in sixty-five cases. J. Neurosurg., *44:* 313–324, 1976.

18. Heiss, W. D., Hayakawa, T., and Waltz, E. G. Cortical neuronal function during ischemia. Effects of occlusion of one MCA on single unit activity in cats. Arch. Neurol., *33:* 813–820, 1976.

19. Hugenholtz, H., and Elgie, R. G. Carotid thromboendarterectomy: a reappraisal. J. Neurosurg., *53:* 776–783, 1980.

20. Jones, T. H., Morawetz, R. B., Crowell, R. M., *et al.* Thresholds of focal cerebral ischemia in awake monkeys. J. Neurosurg., *53:* 773–782, 1981.

21. Kassell, N. F., Peerless, S. J., and Drake, C. G. Reversal of ischemic deficits by induced arterial hypertension. Stroke, *9:* 104–105, 1978.

22. Lawner, P. M., and Simeone, F. A. Treatment of intraoperative middle cerebral occlusion with phenobarbital and extracranial-intracranial bypass. Case Report. J. Neurosurg., *51:* 710–712, 1979.

23. Levinthal, R., Mosley, J. I., Brown, W. G., and Stern, W. E. Effect of STA-MCA anastomosis on the course of experimental acute MCA embolic occlusion. Stroke, *10:* 371–375, 1979.

24. Meyer, F. D., Piepgras, T. G., Sundt, T. M., Jr., and Yanagihara, T. Emergency embolectomy for acute occlusion of the middle cerebral artery. J. Neurosurg., *62:* 639–647, 1985.

25. Morowitz, R. B., DeGirolami, U., Ojemann, R. G., Marcoux, F. W., and Crowell, R. M. Cerebral blood flow determined by hydrogen clearance during middle cerebral artery occlusion in unanesthetized monkeys. Stroke, *9:* 143–149, 1978.

26. Ojemann, R. G., and Crowell, R. M. *Surgical Management of Cerebrovascular Disease.* Williams & Wilkins, Baltimore, 1983.

27. Ojemann, R. G., Crowell, R. M., Fisher, C. M., and Roberson, G. H. Surgical treatment of extracranial carotid occlusive disease. Clin. Neurosurg., *22:* 214, 1975.

28. Samson, D. S., Neuwelt, E. A., Beyer, C. W., and Ditmore, Q. M. Failure of extracranial-intracranial arterial bypass in acute middle cerebral artery occlusion: case report. Neurosurgery, *6:* 185–188, 1980.

29. Sharbrough, F. W., Messick, J. M., and Sundt, T. M., Jr. Correlation of continuous electroencephalograms with CBF measurements during carotid endarterectomy. Stroke, *4:* 674–683, 1973.

30. Smith, A. L., Hoff, J. T., Nielsen, S. L., *et al.* Barbiturate protection in acute focal cerebral ischemia. Stroke, *5:* 1–7, 1974.

31. Spetzler, R. F., Selman, W. R., Roski, R. A., et al. Cerebral revascularization during barbiturate coma in primates and humans. Surg. Neurol., *17:* 111–115, 1982.
32. Sundt, T. M., Jr., Grant, W. C., and Garcia, H. J. Restoration of middle cerebral artery flow in experimental infarction. J. Neurosurg., *31:* 311–322, 1969.
33. Sundt, T. M., Jr., Sandok, D. A., and Whisnant, J. P. Carotid endarterectomy: complications and preoperative assessment of risk. Mayo Clin. Proc., *50:* 301–306, 1975.
34. Sundt, T. M., Jr., Siekert, R. G., Piepgras, D. G., *et al.* Bypass surgery for vascular disease of the carotid system. Mayo Clin. Proc. **51:** 677–692, 1976.
35. Suzuki, J., Yoshimoto, T., Kodama, N., *et al.* A new therapeutic method for acute brain infarction: revascularization following the administration of mannitol and perfluorochemicals—a preliminary report. Surg. Neurol., *17:* 325–332, 1982.
36. Wood, J. H. Hypervolemic hemodilution: rheologic therapy for acute cerebral ischemia. Contemp. Neurosurg., *4:* 1–6, 1982.
37. Yasargil, M. G., Krayenbühl, H. A., and Jacobson, J. H. II. Microneurosurgical arterial reconstruction. Surgery, *67:* 221–233, 1970.

18

Indications for the Extracranial-Intracranial Arterial Bypass in Light of the EC-IC Bypass Study

SYDNEY J. PEERLESS, M.D., F.R.C.S.(C).

INTRODUCTION

The first human extracranial to intracranial (EC-IC) arterial microvascular anastomoses were performed by Yasargil and Donaghy in 1967 (33). This innovative surgical technique startled the neurosurgical world and soon became widely accepted and utilized for a variety of ischemic and potentially ischemic disorders of the brain. Perhaps more importantly, the EC-IC bypass became a symbol for modern neurosurgery utilizing the improved vision afforded by the operating microscope, elegantly designed instruments, ultra fine sutures and refined, precise surgical technique. Over the next decade, the technical limits of neurosurgery were rapidly expanded with microvascular anastomosis becoming the bench mark of this expansion.

A decade after the procedure was first done, it was estimated that more than 2000 EC-IC bypass operations were being performed each year. Although widely accepted and enthusiastically reported in the literature, concern was expressed that this was an elegant technique in search of an indication. At that time, the published indications for the EC-IC bypass were: (*a*) as a surgical collateral prior to major vessel occlusion in the treatment of aneurysms and tumors; (*b*) as a method of preventing stroke in patients with threatened stroke and cerebral vascular occlusive disease; (*c*) as a treatment to enhance the recovery from stroke; (*d*) for the treatment of dementia secondary to multiple extracranial vessel occlusion; (*e*) as a means of protecting asymptomatic patients with carotid occlusion against stroke when contemplating other major surgery; (*f*) in the treatment of ischemia in a remote territory such as the retina; (*g*) in the attempt to improve "abnormalities" in cerebral blood flow or metabolism studies in patients who had little or no clinical or even angiographic evidence of cerebral vascular occlusive disease; and (*h*) in Moya Moya disease (24, 28). Over the next decade, interest and enthusiasm for the EC-IC bypass procedure grew remarkably. Many small and several large series of case reports were published, monographs assembled, symposia and workshops eagerly attended, and variations and refinements in the instruments and technique were disseminated and debated. However, it was never certain just which patients should be selected for the operation and furthermore, although the procedure became accepted as standard therapy, the efficacy of providing a surgical collateral to the brain was unproven.

Of all the proposed indications for EC-IC bypass surgery, the one most frequently utilized was in the prevention of stroke. During the 1960s and 1970s, there was a parallel development and refinement of cerebral angiography and techniques to measure cerebral blood flow and cerebral metabolism. This emerging technology supported the notion of a hemodynamic cause for stroke and lent support to the idea that to add more collateral blood flow to the brain was biologically sound and always desirable. The logic of using the EC-IC bypass in patients with threatened stroke and inaccessible atherosclerotic cerebrovascular disease was compelling. Many reports of patients in uncontrolled series suggested that the EC-IC bypass reduced or stopped transient ischemic attacks (TIAs) and prevented stroke in otherwise stroke-prone individuals. Furthermore, several publications provided data derived from cerebral blood flow and metabolism studies, EEG analysis, and neuropsychological evaluations (4, 6, 7, 11, 12, 15–17, 20, 23, 25–27, 31, 34–36). These gave support to the premise that to add more blood to the brain via a surgical collateral was physiologically sound and worthwhile. It was shown that the perioperative morbidity and mortality rates were acceptably low and the ability to achieve a patent anastomosis remarkably high. Enthusiastic testimonials from patients who had undergone the procedure helped to stimulate the uncritical application of the bypass to an ever increasing number of patients.

In 1977, the International Cooperative Study of Extracranial-Intracranial Arterial Anastomosis (EC-IC Bypass Study) was organized to test, scientifically, for the first time, the value of this procedure among patients with symptomatic atherosclerotic lesions of the internal carotid and/or middle cerebral arteries. Although the EC-IC bypass was widely heralded as a significant therapy for stroke, the question remained—as compared to what?

THE EC-IC BYPASS STUDY

The EC-IC Bypass Study was a randomized clinical trial designed to determine whether anastomosis of the superficial temporal artery (STA) to the middle cerebral artery (MCA) could reduce, despite perioperative stroke and death, subsequent events of stroke and stroke-related death among patients with symptomatic, surgically inaccessible atherosclerotic stenosis or occlusion of the internal carotid or middle cerebral arteries.

The Study was administered clinically by the Central Office in the Department of Clinical Neurological Sciences at The University of Western Ontario in London, Ontario, and methodologically from the Methods Centre in the Department of Epidemiology and Biostatistics at McMaster University in Hamilton, Ontario. The day-to-day execution of the Study was supervised by a steering committee, made up of the principal investigators in the Central Office and the Methods Centre. Study policy and management were governed by an Executive Committee consisting of members of the steering committee and investigators from participating centers in North America, Europe, and Asia, and representatives from the National Institutes of Neurological Communicative Disease and Stroke (NINCDS). Seventy-one Study centers on three continents were accredited for participation in the trial. Each center was required to have specialists in neurosurgery, neurology, and neuroradiology. Every surgeon was required to document at least 80% microvascular graft patency, proven by angiography, on at least 10 consecutive patients. The principal investigators and participating clinicians were blinded to the result during the course of the Study. The conduct of the Study was reviewed twice yearly by a monitoring committee appointed by the Stroke and Trauma Program of the NINCDS. The participants in the trial are listed in the Appendix. The trial protocol and entry characteristics of the Study patients have been previously described (3, 13).

Between August 1977 and September 1982, a total of 1495 patients were entered into the trial. Of these, 118 (7.9%) were excluded from the analysis because they failed to meet the entry criteria in the opinion of a review conducted by the Central Office, the Methods Centre, and an independent evaluation by external adjudicators who were blinded to the treatment groups. All participating surgeons were asked to document all EC-IC bypass procedures done during the period of the trial including those patients that would have been eligible and those who underwent the bypass procedure for indications outside of the trial protocol. One hundred and seventy-eight (178) patients were reported by the participating centers including 115 eligible patients who refused to enter the trial, 52 patients whose physicians insisted that they undergo bypass surgery, and 11 patients with no reason given. All of the remaining patients were randomly allocated to two therapeutic arms. Those patients randomized to the surgical limb (663) underwent a microsurgical end-to-side anastomosis of the STA or occipital artery to a cortical branch of the MCA. The remaining patients (714) were assigned to the medical group. All patients (both medical and surgical) were given "best medical therapy," which included precise control of risk factors such as diabetes and hypertension; and acetylsalicylic acid (325 q.i.d.) unless contraindicated or not tolerated. The randomization process was effective in creating balanced treatment groups with respect to age, sex, clinical presentation, associated medical problems, medications taken at the time of entry into the trial, and angiographically demonstrated vascular pathology (Tables 18.1 and 18.2). At the time of entry, 93% of the patients had either minimal or no functional impairment, although 74% of the patients had detectable abnormalities on neurologic examination (Table 18.3).

During the follow-up period, no patients were lost and none were withdrawn. Each patient was examined by a Study neurologist every 3 months.

TABLE 18.1
Entry Characteristics

	Medical (N = 714)	Surgical (N = 663)
Age (mean years)	56	56
Sex male	82%	81%
Race		
White	77%	78%
Black	7%	6%
Asian	16%	16%
Associated disease		
Hypertension	48%	52%
Diabetes	18%	17%
Angina pectoris	8%	10%
Remote myocardial infarction	9%	11%
Claudification	11%	13%
Smoking history		
Never smoked	17%	19%
Former smoker	26%	22%
Current smoker	58%	57%
Employment status		
Employed	56%	53%
Unemployed due to cerebrovascular disease	15%	16%
Evidence of cerebrovascular disease		
Previous stroke	78%	78%
Previous TIA	62%	66%
Randomized for		
Stroke	66%	67%
TIA	34%	33%
Vascular exam		
BP at entry (mm Hg)		
systolic	144	145
diastolic	85	85
Carotid bruits		
Ipsilateral	4%	5%
Contralateral	7%	7%
Bilateral	7%	5%

TABLE 18.2

Site of Cerebrovascular Disease*

	Medical (N = 714)(%)	Surgical (N = 663)(%)
MCA stenosis	4	4
MCA occlusion	4	4
ICA stenosis (inaccessible)	17	15
ICA occlusion	59	58
Tandem lesion	17	19

* MCA = middle cerebral artery; ICA = internal carotid artery; tandem = more than one atherosclerotic lesion in the same vessel or sequence of vessels, i.e., ICA + MCA.

Of a potential total of 24,160 individual follow-up assessments, 21,428 were actually completed. The average duration of follow-up among surviving patients was 55.8 months, within a range of 28–90 months. The completeness of follow-up was similar in the smaller and larger centers. Nineteen centers entered fewer than 10 patients, but their pooled contribution was small, representing only 7% of the total.

Only nine patients randomized to the medical group (1.3%) crossed over and underwent EC-IC bypass on the same side for which they had been randomized. Six medical patients (0.8%) underwent bypass on the opposite side. Ninety-eight percent (652) of the patients randomized to the surgical group underwent surgery.

The technical performance of the many surgeons in the trial was exemplary. Angiographically proven graft patency rates were 95% in the smaller and 96% in the larger centers, and were high in all three regions: 98% in Asia, 97% in Europe, and 94% in North America. Ischemic complications of the postoperative angiograms were recognized in 0.5% of the studies.

TABLE 18.3

Neurologic and Functional Status at Entry

	Medical (N = 714)(%)	Surgical (N = 663)(%)
Neurologic examination normal	27	25
Neurologic examination abnormal		
No functional impairment	31	30
Minor functional impairment	36	36
Major functional impairment	6	8

SURGICAL PERFORMANCE

Although many surgeons participated in the trial, the perioperative morbidity and mortality were low, comparing favorably with those previously reported by the most experienced surgeons in the larger series (Table 18.4). During the perioperative period (defined as the time from randomization to 30 days after the surgery was completed), 81 surgical patients (12.2%) suffered cerebral and retinal ischemic events, ranging from minor to fatal strokes. Major stroke occurred in 30 patients (4.5%) and seven of these were fatal, resulting in a perioperative mortality of 1.1%. Major stroke occurred in 10 patients after randomization, but before surgery was performed and three of these resulted in death. During surgery and in the subsequent 30 days, there were 20 strokes—16 nonfatal and four fatal for a postoperative stroke morbidity or mortality of 2.5% and 0.6%, respectively. One hundred and twenty-five patients (19%) suffered 146 complications excluding stroke and death.

Because the average time between randomization and surgery was 9 days (range 0–44 days) and all events in that period between randomization and 30 days after the surgical procedure were counted against the surgical group, a similar analysis was made of the medical group in the 39 days following randomization. In this medically treated group, there were nine major strokes (1.3%) and 24 patients (3.4%) had a recognizable ischemic event involving the brain or retina. In the same period, one of the medical patients died of a myocardial infarction. Surgical patients had 3.2% more fatal or nonfatal strokes than the medical patients in the 39-day period following randomization.

RESULTS

The answer to the question, "Does the EC-IC bypass reduce the rate of stroke and stroke-related death in symptomatic patients with appropriate

TABLE 18.4
Stroke Morbidity and Mortality following EC-IC Bypass

		Stroke	
Author	No. of Patients	Morbidity (%)	Mortality (%)
EC-IC, 1985 (14)	652	2.5	0.6
Whisnant et al. 1985 (32)	239	3.3	0
Sundt et al. 1985 (30)	403	4	1.2
Chater, 1983 (7)	400	2.2	2.5
Yasargil and Yonekawa (1977)	84	2.3	3.5

atherosclerotic cerebral vascular occlusive disease?", is no (14). In this atherosclerotic population, there was no reduction in stroke risk (Fig. 18.1). Fatal and nonfatal strokes occurred both more frequently and earlier in the patients randomly allocated to surgery (Fig. 18.2). Thus, this primary analysis rejects with a statistical power greater than 99% the hypothesis of a surgical benefit of a one-third reduction in fatal and nonfatal stroke. Over the entire trial, there was a 14% increase in the relative risk of fatal and nonfatal stroke in the surgical group. The risk was much greater than 14% in the first 18 months after randomization and less toward the end of the trial. The average effect of surgery (90% confidence limits) ranged from a 34% increase to a 3% relative decrease. We can, therefore, reject ($p = 0.05$) a surgical benefit of 3% or more in the relative risk of fatal and nonfatal stroke.

Using the Cox proportional-hazards model, we have analyzed a number of base line and demographic factors including geographic region and size of the participating center, the type and site of angiographic lesion at the time of entry, the presence of a prior stroke or degree of functional impairment at entry, smoking history, comorbid conditions, age, sex, and employment status. None of these factors explain the negative result.

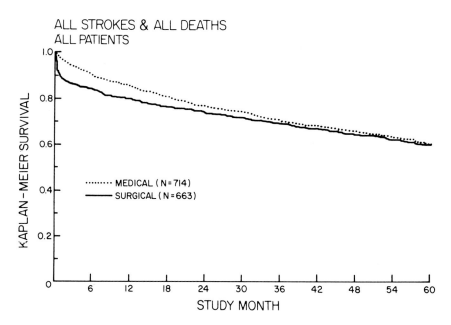

FIG. 18.1 There was no reduction in stroke risk in atherosclerotic patients who underwent EC-IC bypass surgery.

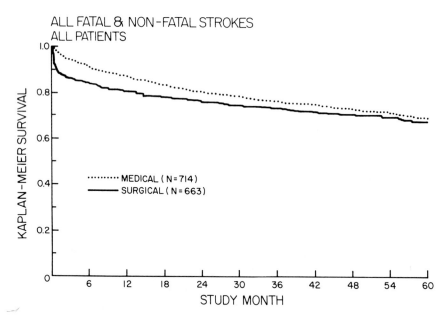

FIG. 18.2 Fatal and nonfatal strokes occurred more frequently and earlier in patients randomly allocated to EC-IC bypass surgery.

When minor and trivial ischemic events were excluded and the analysis restricted to strokes of sufficient severity to kill or seriously disable the patient (grades 5–11 on the Stroke Severity Scale), again no surgical benefit was observed. When the analysis was limited to only those major and minor events that occurred in the ipsilateral hemisphere (that is, the hemisphere operated upon), no surgical benefit was observed (Fig. 18.3). Again, this negative result could not be explained by the previously described base line factors.

Follow-up examination of the 118 ineligible patients excluded from the trial (67 surgical patients and 51 medical patients) revealed six fatal strokes (three surgical, three medical), 11 nonfatal strokes (five surgical, three medical) and 16 other causes of death (seven surgical, nine medical). When added to the eligible patients, these results did not alter the trial's conclusions.

A careful, systematic, functional status analysis of all of the Study patients at the time of their last evaluation and throughout the trial, demonstrated that identical numbers of medical and surgical patients achieved each level of function at the end of the trial and there was no difference found in the percentage of follow-up time spent in each functional level for

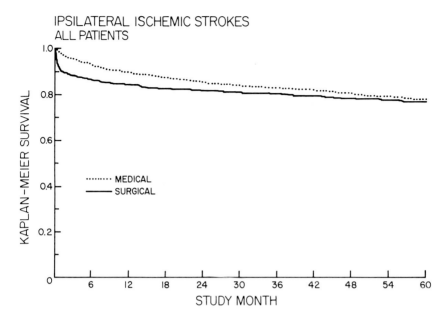

FIG. 18.3 When considering only those strokes that occurred in the hemisphere operated upon, no surgical benefit was observed.

the two treatment groups. Furthermore, in those patients who suffered a stroke following a surgical bypass, there was no enhancement of their recovery because the bypass was in place.

A number of clinically relevant subgroups were evaluated and analyzed. No statistically significant surgical benefit and indeed no trend toward a surgical advantage was found in the following patients: (*a*) those with internal carotid artery occlusion and no symptoms from the time the occlusion was identified; (*b*) those with internal carotid artery occlusion with continuing symptoms (Fig. 18.4); (*c*) those with frequent TIAs; (*d*) those from the various geographical regions, and (*e*) those entered from small centers (fewer than 25 patients entered) compared to large centers. Moreover, although patients who were entered into the trial with frequent, recent TIAs experienced a reduction in the number of TIAs, 80% of the patients were in the medical group and 77% in the surgical group. In this group of patients with frequent, recent (crescendo) TIAs, 13.8% of the medical patients and 20.3% of the surgical patients had suffered a stroke or death at 1 year.

It is important to note that two groups of surgical patients fared significantly worse than their medical counterparts. Patients who entered with

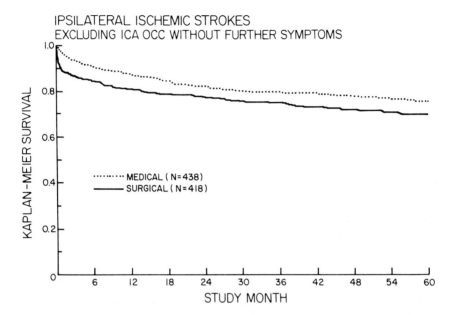

FIG. 18.4. Patients with internal carotid artery occlusion and continuing symptoms did not have significantly fewer strokes after bypass surgery.

either MCA artery stenosis or internal carotid artery occlusion with continuing symptoms experienced a significant increase in stroke with the operation than did the medically treated patients (chi square = 4.74 and 4.04, respectively). When the data were reanalyzed, excluding the 11 patients who were randomized into the surgery group but were not operated upon, we were still unable to generate evidence of a surgical benefit (14).

All of the postoperative angiograms were reviewed and classified on the degree of flow through the EC-IC bypass and rated on a perfusion index of 0 (no flow) to 12 (filling via the bypass of five cortical branches of the MCA, as well as the M1 segment and cross flow to the opposite hemisphere). The 200 patients with the least flow (0–4 rating) experienced fewer strokes and stroke deaths than the 225 patients with the most luxuriant flow (9–12 rating). These data would suggest that the simple expedient of providing increased cerebral blood flow via a surgical collateral to patients with atherosclerotic cerebral vascular occlusive disease, although apparently logical, offers no protection against subsequent ischemic events.

DISCUSSION

Despite repeated examination of the data, we have not been able to identify a group or subgroup of patients from the population studied that demonstrated any benefit or trend toward benefit from the EC-IC bypass. This result is disappointing and, to many, surprising. Understandably, enthusiastic practitioners of the EC-IC procedure and critics of the Study have voiced objections. These objections deserve comment.

It is our contention that the EC-IC Bypass Study was well done and is, indeed, a model of surgical studies. The randomization process was inviolate and produced precisely matched groups. The number of patients entered was impressively large and the objectivity, frequency, and consistency of follow-up admirable. The quality of the surgery was exemplary. The technical skills of the surgeons resulted in a patency rate of 96% and a combined surgical morbidity and mortality of 3.2%—a surgical performance exceeding that of contemporary published series (Table 18.4). All end-points (stroke, stroke-death, and death) were evaluated carefully and separately by the principal investigators in London and in Hamilton, Ontario, and independently adjudicated by neurologists and neurosurgeons who were not involved in the Study.

It has been suggested that the trial failed to show a benefit because a bias in the selection process resulted in the randomization of the wrong population of patients. We would suggest, however, that the patients in the EC-IC Bypass Study were similar, if not identical, in their entry characteristics to those previously reported and are highly representative of those patients being submitted to the operation in North America, Europe, and Asia during the time of the trial. It has furthermore been suggested that some centers participating in the trial were selecting patients for operation and leaving the remaining patients for randomization. It has also been implied that patients who "needed the operation" were indeed being operated upon and those not needing the operation (those at less risk for stroke) were by default left for the trial. It is unlikely that dilution of a clinically valuable effect has occurred because no subgroup analyzed can be shown to have benefited. Even those groups that theoretically should benefit most by the hemodynamic augmentation of cerebral blood flow (MCA stenosis, bilateral carotid stenosis, and occlusion) were not benefited by the procedure and, indeed, were more often injured by being taken to the operating room. It is incumbent upon those who criticize the Study's patient selection to identify those characteristics that allow for a better selection and to prove with scientific credibility that the operation does indeed reduce the rate of stroke and death.

In the same way, it has been intimated that patient selection could have been improved by the evaluation of collateral circulation on the angiogram, or by the consideration of evidence of impaired regional cerebral blood flow or altered oxygen delivery or metabolism based on positron emission tomography studies (21, 23). This contention may well prove to be correct and certainly has not been evaluated in the EC-IC Bypass Study. However, although a number of investigators have reported improvement in these laboratory evaluations following bypass in a very small number of patients, none has shown that the normalization of flow or increase in oxygen delivery is correlated with a clinical benefit (11).

It has been stated that the wrong operation was evaluated in the EC-IC Bypass Study. The suggestion has been made that an interposed vein bypass graft to a cortical or deep sylvian vessel or even to the intracranial carotid artery would provide even greater volumes of flow and, therefore, presumably even greater degrees of protection against stroke. Again, this speculation may be valid, but the comment is almost gratuitous in that the operation evaluated was the STA or occipital artery to MCA bypass and we do not preclude the possibility of surgical innovation resulting in new operations being designed with a putative benefit. A cautionary note must nonetheless be sounded. In reviewing the EC-IC Bypass Study data, one must be impressed by the fact that only 28% of the medically treated patients suffered a stroke over the average follow-up of almost 5 years. The disease in this population is clearly not as ominous as had been previously thought and any new or radical attempt at surgical revascularization must first be proven to be safe. It will be difficult, if not impossible, to show the benefit of a surgical procedure that carries with it a combined morbidity and mortality of greater than about 6%.

Finally, the concern about the validity of counting events into the surgical group that occurred following randomization, but before the surgery had been performed, is a particularly sensitive, even inflammatory, issue. Because there were more strokes in the 39-day perioperative interval in the surgical group compared with a similar 39-day period in the medical group, it has been implied that the groups must in some way be different and the outcomes cannot be considered equivalent. The data, however, are simple and the interpretation reasonable and rational. After randomization and before the EC-IC bypass was performed, 16 of the surgical patients had events, and 10 of these were major strokes. The time between the act of randomization and the bypass in these 16 patients ranged 0–44 days, with an average of 9 days. Three of the strokes were related to repeat angiography and two followed external carotid artery surgery done as a prelude to the bypass surgery. One patient suffered a stroke following a lumbar laminectomy carried out 4 days after randomization. Three other patients suffered their stroke the morning of, or the evening before, the contemplated surgical bypass. When the factors related to these ischemic events are evaluated, it is clear that the surgical group is faced with a greater risk from the preliminary surgery in preparation for the bypass, the additional angiography deemed necessary by the surgeon to plan his surgical approach, and the very real effect of the stress and possible dehydration that is part of the preparation for being taken to the operating room. It also must be reemphasized that even if all of these patients and events are excluded from the analysis (the best case scenario), a strategy that biases the results in favor of surgery, there is still no evidence of a surgical benefit.

A new and innovative procedure, often designed in the laboratory, will frequently be applied first to desperately ill patients in whom medical therapies have failed. With time, and if the procedure carries with it an acceptable morbidity and mortality, the technique will commonly be applied to progressively less ill patients, with an ever widening list of potential indications. The efficacy and scientific merit of new surgical technology as therapy may be evaluated in five different ways (19). The purpose of this evaluation is to let one draw a generalized conclusion which is reproducible and reliable for a group or class of patients. The five common methods of evaluating a new therapy include: (a) theoretical basis of the procedure; (b) personal experience; (c) historical control studies; (d) matched and alternate control studies; and (e) randomized control studies. The best of these techniques is relatively new to surgery and challenges the conventional wisdom, common practice, perceptions of ethical behavior, and even traditional surgical philosophy.

The theoretical basis for the EC-IC bypass was to prevent ischemic stroke by supplying extra blood to a part of the brain demonstrated to have a compromised blood flow. This theory was attractive and compelling. In the evolution of our thinking about cerebral revascularization, reports of improvement in regional cerebral blood flow, increased delivery of oxygen, enhanced metabolism after bypass, and improvement in cerebral function from computerized EEG records gave support to the notion that the theory was correct. These laboratory studies, although supportive of the theory, do not, however, provide data about the clinical benefit of the procedure. Although theories may be attractive clinically, they may be more attractive than real and imply but do not prove an understanding of the pathogenesis and natural history of the disease being treated. One need only recall the enthusiasm for bloodletting in the treatment of fever or irradiation of the thymus in the treatment of status thymicolymphaticus as examples of theoretical stands in medical therapy that have proved to be inappropriate if not calamitous (10).

Personal experience (one's last best or worst case) is perhaps the most common way physicians and surgeons evaluate their therapeutic endeavors. This method of evaluation though commonplace is hazardous. For some clinical events such as the use of penicillin in the treatment of pneumococcal pneumonia or insulin in diabetic coma or tracheostomy for a patient with upper airway obstruction, the individual experience or the published case report is all we need to know about the treatment. Unfortunately, there are few treatments which are as spectacularly successful as the above examples. Certainly with the EC-IC bypass, most surgeons were aware that we did not have a cure for stroke and that the benefits, if present, would be modest. Moreover, the experience, skill, and recall of one or a group of clinicians is usually too limited to detect minor differences between treatments or to be aware of the complexity of the clinical variables and end-points. Even the reports of the successful surgical treatment of a series of patients are possibly flawed when the outcomes are compared to those patients not operated upon; the selection of surgical patients involves a series of events and decisions that often excludes many patients and biases the result in favor of surgery (29, 30, 32, 37). Improvement attributed to our intervention may well be a spontaneous event unrelated to the surgery.

Historical controls suffer because of changing patterns of disease. The marked decline of stroke in the past two decades will cast doubt on any comparisons of therapy based on previous historical series.

Matched and alternate control studies provide a higher level of confidence than do anecdotes of personal experience. However, matching requires a very large pool of patients and implies that the investigator knows which characteristics to be matched are important to the outcome. Alternate control studies suffer because both the patient and the clinician may maneuver to allocate the patient to the treatment group of their choice and comparison of truly equal groups is thereby prevented (8).

The randomized control trial is, at this time, the gold standard of scientific evaluation of our therapeutic endeavors (18). Patients are assigned to treatment groups by chance to guarantee bias-free comparability. Neither the patient nor clinician can influence treatment assignment and, given adequate numbers, the matching of all significant variables will be assured and the therapy being tested will be the only certain difference between the two groups. Randomized clinical trials have in the past challenged theoretical wisdom and altered clinical practice. The gastric freeze technique for peptic ulcer disease, the internal mammary artery ligation for myocardial ischemia, and the failure of radical mastectomy to improve the outlook for patients with carcinoma of the breast are examples of surgical practice that has been abandoned or sharply modified after a randomized clinical trial showed no benefit (1, 5, 22).

In answer to the question posed by the title of this chapter, "What are the indications for the EC-IC bypass in the light of the EC-IC Bypass Study?", the answer is that there are no clear indications for this procedure. It should be understood, however, that the hypothesis that was tested in this Study was to determine whether or not the STA to MCA bypass would reduce the rate of stroke and stroke-related death among patients with symptomatic disease of the internal carotid arteries and MCAs. The Study has shown, with little doubt, that the operation failed to do this. We did not, however, test the other proposed indications for the procedure. It may well be that the bypass has value in the provision of surgical collateral prior to the intentional occlusion of intracranial vessels in the treatment of giant aneurysm or tumor, or that cerebral revascularization may be useful in patients with Moya Moya disease. These indications are relatively rare and it is unlikely that a randomized clinical trial could be mounted to test their value. Similarly, we did not evaluate the appreciation of the bypass in the treatment of multi-infarct dementia or its usefulness in providing new collateral flow to marginally ischemic brain to enhance the recovery from stroke. However, for the latter indication, there is indirect evidence from the trial that this will not be so. Two-thirds of the patients were entered into the trial after a nondisabling stroke. Although both groups showed some functional improvement in the first 3 months after randomization (the medical group significantly better than the surgical group) at 3 years, the functional status of both groups was identical. As well, 37 of the patients randomly assigned to surgery suffered a serious ipsilateral ischemic infarction despite the presence of a functioning bypass. This surgical group did not have a better functional recovery by the end of the trial than the 42 comparable patients in the medical group who suffered strokes in their ipsilateral hemisphere. It would seem that the addition of the surgical collateral was insufficient to protect any significant number of neurones in the penumbra (14).

Perhaps the two most important lessons that have been learned from the EC-IC Bypass Study are: (a) that the accepted theories of the pathogenesis of atherosclerotic cerebral ischemia have been challenged and need re-examination (2) and (b) the Study has shown that scientifically credible evaluation of surgical technology is possible. It is a credit to all surgeons involved in the study that they were prepared to put their intellectual curiosity and scientific credibility ahead of their personal beliefs, desires, and enthusiasm for a technically satisfying procedure. They recognized that it was preferable to offer their patients the opportunity to enter a randomized trial for, if the EC-IC bypass was not effective, then half of the patients, as controls, would be spared the very real, although small risk of the procedure and all future patients would be protected. We believe the neurosurgical and neurological community can look upon this Study with considerable pride. A unique and technically satisfying neurosurgical procedure has been found to be of little value, not because it is particularly hazardous or conceptually bad, but because a little aspirin every day is somewhat better.

APPENDIX

The EC-IC Bypass Study Group consisted of the following investigators, committees, and participating centers (members of the Executive Committee are indicated by an asterisk [*]): **Central Office** (University of Western Ontario), London, Ontario: principal investigator, H. J. M. Barnett; principal neurosurgical investigator, S. J. Peerless; principal neuroradiological investigator, A. J. Fox; senior staff, B. Valberg, J. Peacock. **Methods Center** (McMaster University), Hamilton, Ontario: principal epidemiologic investigator, D. L. Sackett; chief epidemiologist, R. B. Haynes; chief statistician, D. W. Taylor; senior staff, C. Collis, J. Mukherjee, P. Flanagan. Steering Committee: University of Western Ontario, H. J. M. Barnett (chairman), S. J. Peerless, A. J. Fox, B. Valberg, V. C. Hachinski; McMaster University, D. L. Sackett, D. W. Taylor, R. B. Haynes, J. Mukherjee. Monitoring Committee: M. Goldstein (chairman 1977–1982; National Institute of Neurological and Communicative Disorders and Stroke [NINCDS])*, M. D. Walker (chairman 1982–present; NINCDS)*, J. B. Benedict (NINCDS)*, W. Weiss (NINCDS), J. R. Marler (NINCDS), J. P. Whisnant (Mayo Clinic), H. G. Schwartz (Washington University), A. Heyman (Duke University Medical Center), W. H. Feindel (Montreal Neurological Institute).

Participating Centers (in order of number of eligible patients entered). University of Western Ontario, London, Ontario: H. J. M. Barnett*, C. W. McCormick, V. C. Hachinski, S. J. Peerless*, G. G. Ferguson; neuroradiologists, J. Allcock, A. J. Fox*; additional contributors, K. Meguro, R. Cote, D. Moulin, P. C. Gates, S. Lauzier. University of Toronto, Toronto, Ontario: R. Wilson, G. Sawa, H. Schultz, M. C. Chiu. University of Tennessee, Memphis: A. Heck, J. T. Robertson*, B. Gerald. National Institute of Neurosurgery, Budapest, Hungary: L. Ronai, E. Pasztor* (sponsoring neurosurgeon), J. Vajda, M. Horvath, I. Nyary, G. Deak. University of Essen, Essen, Federal Republic of Germany: A. Buch, H. M. Mehdorn, C. Nahser. Universita di Firenze, Florence, Italy: L. Amaducci*, D. Inzitari, S. Briani (deceased), R. Gagliardi, A. Nori. Neurochirurgia und Neurologica University Klinik Giessen, Giessen, Federal Republic of Germany: O. Busse, E. Grote, C. Hornig, R. Schonmayr. Kyoto University Medical School, Kyoto, Japan: M. Kameyama, I. Akiguchi, H. Shio, H. Handa (sponsoring neurosurgeon), Y. Yonekawa*. Hopital Pellegrin, Bordeaux, France: J. M. Orgogozo, J. J. Pere, J. P. Castel, J. M. Caille. New York University, New York: W. K. Hass*, E. S. Flamm*. University of Pecs, Pecs, Hungary: M. Bodosi, G. Gacs, F. T. Merei. Westeinde Ziekenhuis Den Haag, The Netherlands: J. Th. T. Tans, C. A. F. Tulleken*, P. Hoogland. University of Mississippi, Jackson: A. F. Haerer, R. R. Smith. Institute of Brain and Blood Vessels, Gunma, Japan: G. Araki, K. Nagata, M. Mizukami, C. Yunoki. Tokyo Medical and Dental University, Tokyo, Japan: H. Tsukagoshi, U. Ito, Y. Inaba (sponsoring neurosurgeon), T. Fujimoto, K. Komatsu. Neurochirurgische University Klinik Universitatsspital, Zurich, Switzerland: H. Zumstein, H. Keller, B. Zumstein, H. G. Imhof. Upstate Medical Center, Syracuse, NY: A. Culebras, C. J. Hodge. Case Western Reserve University, Cleveland, OH: D. L. Jackson, K. Chandar, R. Spetzler, R. B. Daroff, L. A. Hershey. University of Tokushima, Tokushima, Japan: S. Yasuoka, K. Matsumoto (sponsoring neurosurgeon), S. Ueda. Neurological Institute of Savannah, Savannah, GA: O. E. Ham, E. P. Downing, F. P. Wirth. University di Milano, Milan, Italy: P. Perrone, G. Cabrini. State University of New York at Buffalo, Buffalo, NY: E. J. Manning, D. Ehrenreich, L. N. Hopkins. University of Minnesota, Minneapolis, MN: M. C. Lee, D. Erickson. Royal Victoria Infirmary, Newcastle-upon-Tyne, England: D. A. Shaw, D. Bates, G. Venables, R. Sengupta. Veterans General Hospital, Taipei, Taiwan: Fu-Li Chu, Han-Hau Hu, W. Wen-Jang Wong, A. L. Shen*. Johns Hopkins University, Baltimore, MD: T. J. Preziozi, M. H. Epstein. University of Oregon, Portland, OR: B. Coull, F. Yatsu*, F. Waller, C. Tanabe. Sophia Hospital Zwolle, The Netherlands: W. G. M. Teunissen, P. W. Gelderman. Universita degli Studi, Naples, Italy: R. Cotrufo, P. Conforti, F. Tomasello, V. Albanese. Neurosurgical University Hospital, Belgrade, Yugoslavia: M. Panic, B. Milosavljevic, S. Domonji. Fujita-Gakuen University School of Medicine, Nagoya, Japan: M. Nomura, T. Kanno, H. Sano. Harvard Medical School, Boston, MA: P. Kistler, R. Crowell*. University of Pavia, Pavia, Italy: G. Brambilla, D. Locatelli, R. Rodriquez, P. Paoletti. University of North Carolina, Chapel Hill: J. N. Hayward, S. C. Boone, J. D. Mann. Emory University School of Medicine, Atlanta, GA: H. Karp, R. Schnapper, A. Fleischer. University of Iowa, Iowa City, IA: H. Adams, C. Gross. University of Texas, Dallas, TX: E. Ross, D. Samson. Legnano General Hospital, Legnano, Italy: G. Tonnarelli, I. Piazza. Tufts New England Medical Center, Boston, MA: M. Pessin, R. M. Scott. University of Missouri, Columbia, MO: J. Byer, C. Watts, M. Ditmore. University of Mainz, Mainz, Federal Republic of Germany: G. Kramer, G. Meinig. University of South Alabama, Mobile, AL: J. P. Mohr*, C. S. Kase, H. C. Mostellar. National Cardiovascular Center, Osaka, Japan: T. Yamaguchi, T. Sawada, H. Kikuchi. Mayfield Neurological Institute, Cincinnati, OH: R. Reed, J. Tew. Dalhousie University, Halifax, Nova Scotia: T. J. Murray, C. W. McCormick, W. J. Howes, M. Riding. Cleveland Clinic, Cleveland, OH: A.

Furlan, J. Little, D. Dohn. Institute of Brain Diseases, Tohoku University, Sendai, Japan: H. Saito. J. Suzuki (sponsoring neurosurgeon), N. Kodama, T. Yoshimoto. University of California, San Francisco, CA: M. S. Edwards. Hokkaido University Hospital, Sapporo, Japan: K. Tashiro, M. Tsuru (sponsoring neurosurgeon), Y. Nakagawa. North Manchester General Hospital, Manchester, England: D. Shepherd, G. M. Yuill, C. Bannister, I. W. Turnbull. Henry Ford Hospital, Detroit, MI: R. Teasdall, J. Ausman. Research Institute of Brain and Blood Vessels, Akita, Japan: T. Kutsuzawa, N. Nakajima, T. Kobayashi, N. Yasui, Z. Ito (deceased). University of Cincinnati, Cincinnati, OH: C. Olinger, R. Singh, G. Khodadad. Duke University Medical Center, Durham, NC: W. C. Olanow, R. H. Wilkins. Ciudad Sanitara v. del Rocio, Seville, Spain: R. Alberca-Serrano, F. Morales-Ramos. Barrow Neurological Institute, Phoenix, AZ: A. Yudell, R. Thompson, P. Carter. Mississippi Baptist Medical Center, Jackson, MI: W. Bowlus, L. Mahalak, D. Stringer. Neurological Institute, Tokyo Women's Medical College, Tokyo, Japan: S. Maruyama, K. Kitamura, M. Kagawa. University of Pittsburgh, Pittsburgh, PA: O. Reinmuth*, R. Heros. University of Nagasaki Medical School, Nagasaki, Japan: H. Matsumura, M. Takamori, K. Mori (sponsoring neurosurgeon), H. Ono. Osaka University Medical School, Osaka, Japan: M. Imaizumi, S. Yoneda, H. Mogami, T. Hayakawa. Nassau County Medical Center, East Meadow: NY: R. Carruthers, R. Decker. Naval Regional Medical Center, Oakland, CA: A. Chalmers, T. H. Rockel, R. Hodosh. University of Arizona, Tucson, AZ: J. Laguna, P. Weinstein. Tokyo University Medical School, Tokyo, Japan: T. Takasu, T. Eguchi, H. Sugiyama, N. Basugi, T. Asano. Queens University, Kingston, Ontario: H. B. Dinsdale, P. Murray. Albert Einstein College of Medicine, Bronx, NY: L. J. Thal. Hopital Neurologique, Lyon, France: D. Deruty. Daniel Freeman Memorial Hospital, Inglewood, CA: B. Dobkin. Scarborough General Hospital, Scarborough, Ontario: M. R. Goldman. Long Island-Jewish Hillside Medical Center, New Hyde Park, NY: M. Nathanson.

REFERENCES

1. Atkins, H., Hayward, J. L., Klugman, D. J., and Wayte, A. B. Treatment of early breast cancer: a report after ten years of a clinical trial. Br. Med., 2: 423–429, 1972.
2. Barnett, H. J. M. Pathogenesis of transient ischemic attacks. In: Cerebral Diseases, edited by P. Scheinberg. Raven Press, New York, 1976, pp. 1–21.
3. Barnett, H. J. M., and Peerless, S. J. Collaborative EC-IC Bypass Study: The rationale and a progress report. In: Cerebrovascular Diseases, edited by J. Moossy and O. M. Reinmuth. Raven Press, New York, 1981, pp. 271–288.
4. Baron, J. C., Bousser, M. G., Rey, A., et al. Reversal of focal "misery perfusion" syndrome by extra-intracranial arterial bypass in hemodynamic cerebral ischemia: a case study with ^{15}O positron emission tomography. Stroke, 12: 454–459, 1981.
5. Barsamian, E. M. The rise and fall of internal mammary ligation in the treatment of angina pectoris and the lessons learned. In: Costs, Risk and Benefits of Surgery, edited by J. P.

Bunker, B. A. Barnes, and F. Mosteller. Oxford University Press, New York, 1977, pp. 212–220.
6. Binder, L. M., Tanabe, C. T. Waller, F. T., and Wooster, N. E. Behavioral effects of superficial temporal artery to middle cerebral artery bypass surgery: preliminary report. Neurology (NY), *32:* 422–424, 1982.
7. Chater N. Neurosurgical extracranial-intracranial bypass for stroke: with 400 cases. Neurol. Res., *5*(2): 1–9, 1983.
8. Christie, D. Before and after comparisons: a cautionary tale. Br. Med. J., *2:* 1629–1630, 1979.
9. Conforti, P., Tomasello, F. and Albanese, V. Cerebral revascularization by microneurosurgical bypass. Piccin Nuova Libraria, Padua, Italy: 124–128, 1984.
10. Dawber, T. F. Annual discourse—unproved hypothesis. N. Engl. J. Med., *299:* 452–458, 1978.
11. de Weerd, A. W., Verring, M. M., Mosmans, P. C. M., *et al.* Effect of the extra-intracranial (STA-MCA) arterial anastomosis on EEG and cerebral blood flow: a controlled study of patients with unilateral cerebral ischemia. Stroke, *13:* 674–679, 1982.
12. Drinkwater, J. E., Thompson, S. K., and Lumley, J. S. P. Cerebral function before and after extra-intracranial carotid bypass. J. Neurol. Neurosurg. Psychiatr., *47:* 1041–1043, 1984.
13. EC/IC Bypass Study Group. The International Cooperative Study of Extracranial/Intracranial Arterial Anastomosis (EC/IC Bypass Study): methodology and entry characteristics. Stroke, *16:* 397–406, 1985.
14. EC/IC Bypass Study Group. Failure of extracranial-intracranial arterial bypass to reduce the risk of ischemic stroke. Results of an international randomized trial. N. Engl. J. Med., *313*(19): 1191–1200, 1985.
15. Gratzl, O., and Schmiedek, P. STA-MCA bypass: results 10 years postoperatively. Neurol. Res., *5*(2): 11–18, 1983.
16. Gibbs, J. M., Wise, R. J. S., Leenders, K. L., and Jones, T. Evaluation of cerebral perfusion reserve in patients with carotid artery occlusion. Lancet, *1:* 182–186, 1984.
17. Grubb, R. L. Jr., Ratcheson, R. A. Raichle, M. E., *et al.* Regional cerebral blood flow and oxygen utilization in superficial temporal-middle cerebral artery anastomosis patients: an exploratory definition of clinical problems. J. Neurosurg., *50:* 733–741, 1979.
18. Haines, S. J. Randomized clinical trials in the evaluation of surgical innovation. J. Neurosurg., *51:* 5–11, 1979.
19. Haynes, R. B., Sackett, D. L., and Taylor, D. W. The place of randomized control trials in the evaluation of new surgical treatments. In: *Cerebral Ischemia: Clinical and Experimental Approach,* edited by H. Handa, H. J. M. Barnett, M. Goldstein, and Y. Yonekawa. Igaku-Shoin, Tokyo, 1982, pp. 122–130.
20. Kletter, G. *The Extra-Intracranial Bypass Operation for Prevention and Treatment of Stroke.* Springer-Verlag, New York, 1979, pp. 117–128.
21. Laurent, J. P., Lawner, P. M., O'Connor, M. Reversal of intracerebral steal by STA-MCA anastomosis. J. Neurosurg., *57:* 629–632, 1982.
22. Miao, L. L. Gastric freezing: an example of the evaluation of medical therapy by randomized clinical trials. In: *Costs, Risk and Benefits of Surgery.* Oxford University Press, New York, 1977, pp. 198–211.
23. Norrving, B., Nilsson, B., and Risberg, J. rCBF in patients with carotid occlusion: resting and hypercapnic flow related to collateral pattern. Stroke, *13:* 155–162, 1982.
24. Peerless, S. J. Techniques of cerebral revascularization. Clin. Neursurg., *23:* 258–269, 1976.
25. Powers, W. J., Martin, W. R. W., Herscovitch, P., *et al.* Extracranial-intracranial bypass surgery: hemodynamic and metabolic effects. Neurology, *34:* 1168–1174, 1984.

26. Powers, W. J., and Raichle, M. E. Positron emission tomography and its application to the study of cerebrovascular disease in man. Stroke, *16:* 361–376, 1985.
27. Rhodes, R. S., Spetzler, R. F., and Roski, R. A. Improved neurologic function after cerebrovascular accident with extracranial-intracranial arterial bypass. Surgery, *90:* 433–438, 1981.
28. Samson, D. W., Boone, S. Extracranial-intracranial (EC-IC) arterial bypass: past performance and current concepts. Neurosurgery, *3:* 79–86, 1978.
29. Sundt, T. M. Jr., Siekert, R. G., Piepgras, D. G., *et al.* Bypass surgery for vascular disease of the carotid system. Mayo Clin. Proc., *51:* 677–692, 1976.
30. Sundt, T. M. Jr., Whisnant, J. P., Fode, N. C., *et al.* Results, complications, and follow-up of 415 bypass operations for occlusive disease of the carotid system. Mayo Clin. Proc., *60:* 230–240, 1985.
31. Tsuda, Y., Kimura, K., Iwata, Y., *et al.* Improvement of cerebral blood flow and/or CO_2 reactivity after superficial temporal artery-middle cerebral artery bypass in patients with transient ischemic attacks and watershed-zone infarctions. Surg. Neurol., *22:* 595–604, 1984.
32. Whisnant, J. P., Sundt, T. M. Jr., and Fode, N. C. Long-term mortality and stroke morbidity after superficial temporal artery-middle cerebral artery bypass operation. Mayo Clin. Proc., *60:* 241–246, 1985.
33. Yasargil, M. G. (ed.) *Microsurgery Applied to Neuro-Surgery.* Georg Thieme, Stuttgart, 1969, pp. 105–115.
34. Yonas, H., Gur, D., Good, B. C., *et al.* Stable xenon CT blood flow mapping for evaluation of patients with extracranial-intracranial bypass surgery. J. Neurosurg., *62:* 324–333, 1985.
35. Yonekawa, M., Austin, G., and Hayward, W. Long-term evaluation of cerebral blood flow, transient ischemic attacks, and stroke after STA-MCA anastomosis. Surg. Neurol., *18:* 123–130, 1982.
36. Younkin, D., Hungerbuhler, J. P., O'Connor, M., *et al.* Superficial temporal-middle cerebral artery anastomosis: effects on vascular neurologic, and neuropsychological functions. Neurology (NY), *35:* 462–469, 1985.
37. Zumstein, B., and Yasargil, M. G. Verbesserung der hirndurchblutung durch mikrochirurgische bypass-anastomosen. Schweiz Rundschau Med. (Praxis), *70:* 1866–1873, 1981.

19

Surgically Created Posterior Circulation Vascular Shunts

**JAMES I. AUSMAN, M.D., PH.D., LOUIS R. CAPLAN, M.D.,
FERNANDO G. DIAZ, M.D., PH.D.**

Vertebrobasilar territory ischemia can be caused by a heterogeneous variety of mechanisms (4). As in anterior circulation ischemic disease, the most important causes are:

1. Occlusive disease of the large proximal arteries and the vertebral and basilar arteries, with reduced distal flow.
2. Disease of small penetrating branch arteries.
3. Cardiogenic embolism.
4. Artery to artery embolism.
5. Functional constriction of arteries, *i.e.*, vasospasm or "migraine."

Selection of treatment should depend on stroke mechanism, the severity of neurological deficit, and the location, nature, and severity of the occlusive vascular lesion.

COMPARISON OF POSTERIOR CIRCULATION MECHANISMS WITH ANTERIOR CIRCULATION

The relative importance of these mechanisms differs in the two circulations. Collateral circulation, when there are no congenital anamolies, is even more plentiful in the posterior circulation. The nuchal vertebral artery has branches in contrast to the internal carotid artery (ICA), and there are two vertebral arteries, each able to help the other. Brain stem collateral circulation, especially to the tegmentum is also very rich. Because of the plentiful collaterals, unilateral vertebral or even basilar artery occlusion, may be well-tolerated. Posterior circulation vascular anomalies are more common; in patients with these anomalies, for example, hypoplasia of one vertebral artery, small posterior inferior cerebellar artery (PICA), atretic distal vertebral artery segment (vertebral artery ending in PICA), acquired occlusive disease can be disastrous.

The proportion of the posterior circulation fed by small penetrating arteries is much higher than in the anterior circulation, and so, lacunar infarcts and penetrating branch occlusion infarcts make up a larger portion of strokes than in the anterior circulation. Migraine, for unknown reasons, is predominantly a disorder of posterior circulation arteries; the most frequent symptoms of classic migraine are visual scintillations, paresthesiae, and vertigo, which all relate to constriction of the vertebral and posterior cerebral artery system. Adults do get basilar migraine.

About one in five cardiac-origin emboli lodge within the posterior circulation and usually cause an occipital lobe or cerebellar infarction. This fraction is about the proportion of the cranial circulation that goes to the vertebrobasilar system. The incidence of artery to artery emboli within the posterior circulation is not known. Occlusion of the vertebral artery can give rise to distal emboli (2, 8, 9). On the other hand, it has been said (although the data is very scanty) that ulceration within the vertebral artery is rare (10). There are too few necropsy or surgical studies of the vertebral artery to settle this point.

TREATMENT OF THESE MECHANISMS

On theoretical grounds, optimum treatment of cardiogenic embolism and artery to artery embolism of red clots would be standard anticoagulants-heparin, or warfarin. Migraine should respond to agents that diminish vasospasm. Artery to artery "white clots," that is, platelet aggregates, might respond to platelet antiaggregants such as aspirin. In patients with occlusion or stenosis of large arteries such as the vertebral or basilar arteries, warfarin is the first line of treatment. Only patients with large vessel occlusion and persistent or recurrent distal low flow would be candidates for surgically created posterior circulation shunts.

LARGE VESSEL POSTERIOR FOSSA DISEASE

Since only disease of large arteries seems relevant to bypass surgery, let us look briefly at the common loci and clinical picture of these occlusive lesions within the posterior circulation. More detailed accounts are available elsewhere (3, 5).

The most common location of atherosclerotic stenosis is at the proximal vertebral artery origin in the neck and the proximal subclavian arteries. Patients with disease at these sites are usually white and have a high incidence of associated angina, myocardial infarction, peripheral vascular disease with claudication, and accompanying ICA bifurcation disease. Blacks and patients of oriental origin rarely have vertebral artery or ICA origin disease. The most common symptoms are spells of dizziness, blurred vision, and arm ischemia if the lesion is subclavian. Transient ischemic attacks (TIAs) are more common than strokes, probably because of the great collateral potential. Even bilateral vertebral origin occlusions are usually well-tolerated (7). Since these patients have a relatively low incidence of stroke (11), and the TIAs disappear with time, we do not believe vertebral artery origin disease is an indication for shunting.

Disease of the distal extracranial vertebral artery is usually caused by neck motion or trauma. These vascular lesions develop precipitously. The most likely mechanism of stroke is embolism or propogation of clot from tears or dissections within the vessels, not "low flow." As in the anterior circulation these dissections usually heal well with time. It is unlikely that shunt therapy will prove useful for intrinsic distal extracranial vertebral artery disease. Some patients with intracranial vertebral artery occlusions have retrograde extension of clot into the neck just as ICA siphon occlusion can give rise to a tapered occlusion of the nuchal ICA. This circumstance should be considered as an intracranial occlusion.

Unilateral intracranial vertebral artery occlusion usually causes lateral medullary or cerebellar ischemia or infarction. Because of the usually adequate collateral circulation from the opposite vertebral artery and from the ICA/posterior communicating artery (PCA) system, chronic low-flow distally is very rare if the opposite vertebral artery is not hypoplastic or stenotic. Distal strokes are more often due to embolization of clot from an occluded vertebral artery. Shunts are seldom applicable.

Bilateral intracranial vertebral artery occlusion is a different matter. Once both distal vertebral arteries are severely compromised and the patient develops symptoms of ischemia, the course is often progressive and fatal in our experience (1). Cerebellar and pyramidal signs predominate. Posturally aggravated increases in symptoms are common (6). Ischemia is predominantly in the medulla, cerebellum, and caudal pons. Some of these patients will be saved by shunts and we vigorously support their use for this indication.

In basilar artery occlusion, the clot does not usually propagate beyond the next branch and cerebellar artery and ICA/PCA flow is often good. As a result, ischemia most often is to a local region, usually in the basis pontis. Most patients with basilar artery occlusion will either suffer a major stroke quickly or will be left with no or slight deficit (2). (3) Chronic recurrent low-flow symptoms are unusual, perhaps being more common in basilar stenosis than occlusion. Patients in this latter group might be candidates for shunting as would patients with acute basilar artery occlusions who do not respond to anticoagulants and have no evidence of severe infarction by magnetic resonance imaging scans (MRI) or newer generation computed tomographic scans (CT).

Another poorly studied group of candidates for shunting are those with so-called "basilarization" of the vertebral artery. Because of atresia, hypoplasia of the distal vertebral segment ("vertebral ending of PICA") or prior occlusion, the basilar artery is fed by the single vertebral artery. When this artery becomes stenosed or occluded, serious ischemia might occur and be prolonged.

Aneurysms of the posterior circulation vessels that are to be treated by ligation of the proximal large arteries might be another indication for posterior circulation vascular shunts.

In our opinion, candidates for posterior circulation shunts should meet all of the following criteria:

1. Have appropriate vascular lesion:
    a. Bilateral severe intracranial vertebral artery compromise (severe stenosis, hypoplasia, occlusion);
    b. Severe stenosis or occlusion of the proximal basilar artery or vertebral basilar junction;
    c. Aneurysm to be treated by ligation.
2. Excellent angiography that documents the site of disease and the available collaterals. The potential donor external carotid arteries and the available collaterals should be visualized.
3. Persistent ischemic symptoms, often with postural aggravation.
4. Failure to respond to therapeutic doses of anticoagulants or contraindication to their use.

REFERENCES

1. Caplan, L. R. Bilateral distal vertebral artery occlusion. Neurology, *33:* 552–558, 1983.
2. Caplan, L. R. Occlusion of the vertebral or basilar artery. Stroke, *10:* 277–282, 1979.
3. Caplan, L. R. Transient ischemic attacks and stroke in the distribution of the vertebral-basilar system: clinical manifestations. In: *Surgery for Cerebrovascular Disease*, edited by Moore, W. S. New York/Churchill Livingstone 1986 (In Press).
4. Caplan, L. R. Vertebrobasilar disease: time for a new strategy. Stroke, *12:* 111–114, 1981.
5. Caplan, L. R. Vertebrobasilar occlusive disease. In: *Stroke: Pathophysiology, Diagnosis and Management*, edited by Barnett, H. J., Mohr, J., Stein, B., Yatsu, F. New York/Churchill Livingstone, 1985 (In Press).
6. Caplan, L. R., Sergay, S. Positional cerebral ischemia. J. Neurol. Neurosurg. Psychiatr., *39:* 385–391, 1976.
7. Fisher, C. M. Occlusion of the vertebral arteries. Arch. Neurol., *22:* 1–19, 1970.
8. Fisher, C. M., Karnes, W. E. Local embolism. J. Neuropathol. Exp. Neurol., *24:* 174, 1965.
9. Koroshetz, W., Ropper, A. Local embolism as a cause of stroke in the posterior circulation. Neurology, *(Suppl. 1):* 214, 1985.
10. Moosy, J. Morphology, sites and epidemiology of cerebral atherosclerosis. Proc. Assoc. Res. New Ment. Dis., *51:* 1–22, 1966.
11. Moufarrij, N. A., Little, J. R., Furlan, A. J. *et al.* Vertebral artery stenosis: long-term follow-up. Stroke, *15(2):* 260–263, 1984.

CHAPTER
20
Posterior Circulation Revascularization

JAMES I. AUSMAN, M.D., PH.D., FERNANDO G. DIAZ, M.D., PH.D., AND
MANUEL DUJOVNY, M.D.

INTRODUCTION

Until the early 1960s, the only treatment available for cerebrovascular occlusive disease of the vertebrobasilar circulation was anticoagulation. Then, vertebral endarterectomy became a popular surgical procedure, but postoperative vessel patency was only 50%; because of these poor results, the operation fell into disfavor (11, 12, 17). Recently, the introduction of microsurgical procedures has permitted the application of reconstructive techniques to re-establish circulation to areas of the distal vertebrobasilar circulation previously considered inaccessible (1, 2, 3, 4, 6–10). Other operations have now been successfully performed for lesions in the extracranial vertebral artery (11). We will describe our experience with revascularization of the posterior circulation.

INDICATIONS

We consider candidates for revascularization of the posterior fossa all those patients who have ongoing symptoms of vertebrobasilar insufficiency (VBI) as described by Cartlidge et al. (16). The clinical syndromes may include any combination of two or more of the following symptoms: diplopia, dysarthria, bilateral visual loss, dysphagia, perioral numbness, crossed motor or sensory abnormalities, and vertigo. Dizziness alone is not considered a symptom of VBI. Other nonvascular causes of symptoms suggestive of VBI must be ruled out by a thorough medical evaluation. If this evaluation is negative, the patients may then undergo a computed tomographic (CT) scan and selective four-vessel angiography. We do not consider intravenous digital subtraction angiography a good substitute because it fails to provide sufficient detail of the vertebral and basilar arteries to make an adequate evaluation of the vertebrobasilar circulation (11).

With minimal risk, advances in cerebral angiography have permitted the complete evaluation of patients symptomatic for vertebrobasilar ischemia (11, 15). Since the episodes of VBI may be produced by structural lesions

located at any level of the vertebrobasilar system, we consider it mandatory to obtain a complete angiographic evaluation of the entire system,
including the origins of the vertebral arteries and their entire intracranial
course (13, 18). We will frequently obtain multiple intracranial projections
of the vertebrobasilar system because we have observed patients who
appeared to have normal vessels when evaluated only with single plane
angiograms. Oblique views and face views of the basilar artery combined
with good subtraction techniques are critical to the complete evaluation of
these patients.

The management of patients with VBI has been controversial. The natural history of VBI has not been fully documented; but 35% of patients who
presented with classical symptoms of VBI and did not undergo cerebral
angiography developed a cerebral infarction within 4 years (16). Anticoagulation has been accepted as the only effective treatment for these
patients (21). However, anticoagulation has never been proven to be valuable in preventing a cerebral infarction in patients symptomatic for VBI,
who have angiographically proven lesions (11). Although aspirin has reduced the incidence of cerebral hemispheric transient ischemic attacks
(TIAs) and infarction (14), there are no adequate studies regarding its
usefulness in patients with VBI (11).

SURGICAL PROCEDURES

The technical approach to the reconstruction of the vertebrobasilar
circulation presents several challenging problems. Since the syndrome of
VBI can be produced by lesions located at any level of the vertebrobasilar
circulation, the surgeon must be capable of approaching any segment of
the entire posterior circulation from beginning to end. In our opinion, the
best possible revascularization procedure is that which provides the wid-
est channel of flow to a point distal to the obstructive lesion (5). In general,
we would favor a direct reconstruction of the stenotic segment by an
endarterectomy, since this procedure would provide the optimum form of
restoration of the circulation to normal (8). When this is not possible, a
bypass can be performed.

Performing any of the anastomotic procedures for the posterior fossa
requires cerebral relaxation. This is obtained by the use of a lumbar subarachnoid drain, the intravenous administration of mannitol and furo-
semide, and by gentle retraction of the brain. The anastomoses are very
difficult to perform because of the depth at which they are done, they
require the use of very long instruments, and they are very taxing on the
surgeon. We use two teams of neurosurgeons who rotate during the 8–10
hour operation to perform the surgery in stages.

Vertebral Endarterectomy

Vertebral endarterectomies have been performed in patients with highly stenotic lesions in the third and fourth portions of the vertebral artery, usually associated with contralateral high-grade stenosis or vertebral artery occlusion (1, 8). The vertebral artery is approached through a suboccipital craniotomy performed with the patient lying in a three-quarter prone position. A midline approach is carried down and extended laterally until the vertebral artery is exposed, and the artery is dissected from its exit from the first transverse process to its entry into the dura through the atlanto-occipital membrane. The vertebral artery is surrounded by a venous plexus which must be carefully dissected, cauterized, and transected. When dissection is completed, the dura is opened over the vertebral artery. The perimedullary portion of the vertebral artery is dissected to expose the origin of the posterior inferior cerebellar artery (PICA). If a vertebral endarterectomy is required, the artery can be clipped proximally at C 1 and distally prior to PICA. A longitudinal arteriotomy is made, and the plaque is dissected under the microscope. After the plaque is removed, the arteriotomy is closed with running 6–0 or 7–0 polypropylene sutures (8). During the occlusion period, the patients receive an intravenous bolus of 250 mg of thiopental, 100 mg of xylocaine, and 5000 units of heparin.

Four of our patients underwent an endarterectomy in the distal portion of the vertebral artery. The plaque was completely removed in two with full anatomic reconstitution of the artery and both patients recovered from their previous symptoms. One had an immediate silent occlusion of the artery because of technical problems with the endarterectomy and, fortunately, his symptoms disappeared as well. The plaque was thought to be a source of emboli as a cause of the symptoms. We were unable to remove the plaque in the remaining patient because it had eroded through the outer vertebral artery wall and it was necessary to ligate the artery. This patient awoke with a lateral medullary syndrome.

Occipital Artery-PICA Anastomosis

For occlusive lesions of the vertebral artery proximal to PICA, the posterior circulation can be reconstructed by an anastomosis of the occipital artery to the PICA itself (3, 10, 19, 20, 22, 23). The patient is placed in a park bench or in a lateral position and the occipital artery is dissected by an incision placed directly over the occipital artery and then extended to the level of the mastoid process to obtain sufficient vessel length. After the incision has been carried down through the suboccipital musculature, a unilateral suboccipital craniectomy is completed from the foramen magnum to the transverse sinus and from the edge of the mastoid to the midline. Generally it is not necessary to remove the arch of Cl. After the dura is opened, the cerebellum falls away by its own weight once the cisterna magna has been drained of spinal fluid. When the perimedullary portion of PICA has been identified on the lateral medullary area and either the rostral or the caudal branches of PICA have been dissected, a section of PICA devoid of any branches to the brain stem is isolated and temporarily clipped with soft microvascular clips. A longitudinal arteriotomy is made on the lateral wall of the PICA branch and an end-to-side anastomosis is completed from the occipital artery to the perimedullary portion of PICA.

We have performed nine occipital artery-to-PICA anastomoses. Seven patients (78%) were asymptomatic or improved following the procedure. One patient developed a fixed neurologic deficit after surgery. One patient (11%) died as a result of the operation with pulmonary edema from transoperative fluid overload. Since that time, we have used Swan-Ganz catheters in all patients to monitor their fluid status. Postoperative angiography revealed a patent anastomosis in all surviving patients (Fig. 20.1).

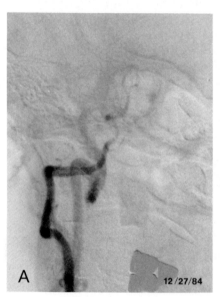
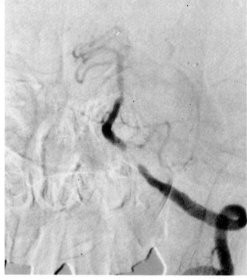

FIG. 20.1. A 65-year-old man who presented with repeated events of vertigo, ataxia and diplopia unresponsive to oral antiplatelet agents and anticoagulants. (*A*) Preoperative vertebral angiogram demonstrates an occlusion of the right vertebral artery distal to the origin of PICA. The left vertebral artery shows a severe stenosis just proximal to the origin of PICA. (*B*) Postoperative angiogram shows complete filling of the entire basilar tree through a patent anastomosis of the occipital artery to PICA.

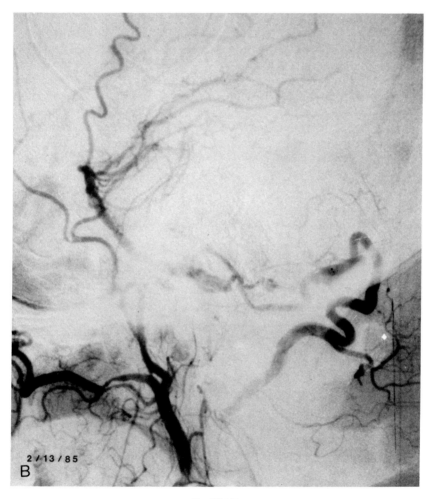

FIG. 20.1*B*

Occipital Artery-AICA Anastomosis

For occlusive disease of the vertebral arteries distal to PICA or at the vertebrobasilar junction, the EC-IC anastomosis must be completed to the anterior inferior cerebellar artery (AICA) (4). The exposure is essentially the same as that for the anastomosis to PICA, and the dissection of the occipital artery is completed in a similar manner. The cerebellum must be gently retracted laterally to expose the area of the seventh and eighth cranial nerves. AICA is identified as it extends from in front of the foramen of Luschka and is directed toward the anterior surface of the cerebellum. At this point, the vessel has already divided into its rostral and caudal branches. Choosing the anastomotic site, we prefer to use the branch without collateral branches to the brain stem. After the chosen branch is dissected carefully and isolated, an anastomosis is completed from the occipital artery to the AICA in a manner similar to that described above.

We have performed 18 occipital artery to-AICA anastomoses. Fifteen patients (83%) were asymptomatic or improved after surgery. One patient is unchanged and two are worse postoperatively. There have not been any deaths as a direct result of surgery. All anastomoses have been patent on postoperative angiography and have shown the best immediate filling of the vertebrobasilar circulation when the group is compared with the other procedures used to revascularize the posterior circulation (Fig. 20.2).

Superficial Temporal-Superior Cerebellar Anastomosis

In patients who have a stenosis or an occlusion of the proximal or midportion of the basilar artery without collaterals from the anterior circulation, any of the previously described procedures will not bypass the problem. These patients require an anastomosis to the superior cerebellar artery or to the posterior cerebral artery (6, 7, 9, 24) to connect to a vessel which will revascularize the distal basilar artery. In either case, the patient is positioned supine with the ipsilateral shoulder elevated and the head flat on the table. About 10 cm of the superficial temporal artery is dissected to gain as much length of the artery as possible. A subtemporal craniotomy is completed centered on the ear and flush with the middle cranial fossa. It is necessary to extend this craniotomy a minimum of 3 cm in front and 3 cm behind the external auditory meatus to have enough room to manipulate the instruments for the anastomosis and to reach the tentorial edge and superior cerebellar artery. After the dura has been opened, the temporal lobe is elevated. Care must be taken to preserve the temporal veins to prevent the development of postoperative swelling and cerebral contusions. To expose the superior cerebellar artery, we incise the tentorium by exposing first the fourth cranial nerve under the tentorial incisura and extending the incision toward the petrous apex. The two flaps of the tentorium are then retracted laterally and sutured back to the dura. This permits us to expose the perimesencephalic portion of the superior cerebellar artery, which at this point usually has no branches and divides into its rostral and caudal branches. The most available and largest of the two branches is carefully dissected and isolated. At this point, the distal end of the superficial temporal artery is transected, and a temporary clip is placed at the base. A fishmouth stoma is prepared ensuring that all of the length available for the superficial temporal artery is used, since, otherwise, the vessel is too short to use for the anastomosis. An end-to-side anastomosis is then completed from the STA to the SCA in a similar manner to that previously described.

We have performed 33 anastomoses of the superficial temporal to the superior cerebellar artery. These patients have been divided into those with stable symptoms and those with progressive ischemia refractory to intravenous anticoagulation. The patients we called stable had multiple ischemic events, but could still function and carry out some of their daily duties on antiplatelets or oral anticoagulants. The unstable patients required intravenous anticoagulants to control or modify their symptoms. No other medical causes of a cardiac or hypotensive nature existed in any of these patients to explain their symptomatology. In the stable group (16 patients), 12 (75%) had no further symptoms or were improved after surgery; one patient progressed to a brain stem infarction, and one patient died. Two were unchanged. In the unstable group (17 patients), ten (59%) became asymptomatic or were improved after surgery; one had persistence of symptoms, three developed brain infarction (two unrelated to the bypass), and three died in the immediate postoperative period. We believe that the group of patients classified in the unstable category were at higher risk for the surgical procedure. We must remember that these patients were failures of all medical therapy and would have most likely had a devastating infarct or death. Thus, our results represent salvage of a population for which there was no other treatment.

Previous neuroradiologic studies of patients with basilar artery occlusion suggest a dismal outcome with medical treatment only. Within 1 year 44–70% of the patients were dead in 3 months (21, 25).

Postoperative angiography has confirmed patency in 30 patients and occlusion of the anastomosis in two (Fig. 20.3). The degree of filling of the vertebrobasilar circulation has varied considerably in the first week after surgery. Sixty percent of the patients have only had filling of three or fewer major branches arising from the basilar artery opacified by the anastomoses. In Sundt's patients in whom a vein graft is used from the external carotid to the posterior cerebral artery, high volume flows can be achieved

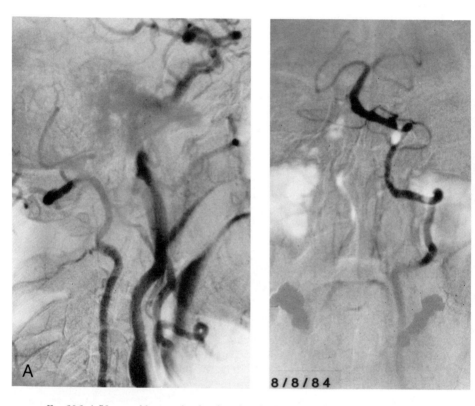

FIG. 20.2. A 56-year-old man who developed multiple events of ataxia, dysmetria, diplopia, and left body paresthesias unresponsive to anticoagulation. (A) Preoperative vertebral angiogram reveals a complete occlusion of the right vertebral artery distal to the origin of PICA. The left vertebral artery has a severe stenosis distal to the origin of PICA. (B) Postoperative angiogram demonstrates filling of the entire distai basilar artery through a patent anastomosis of the left occipital to the AICA.

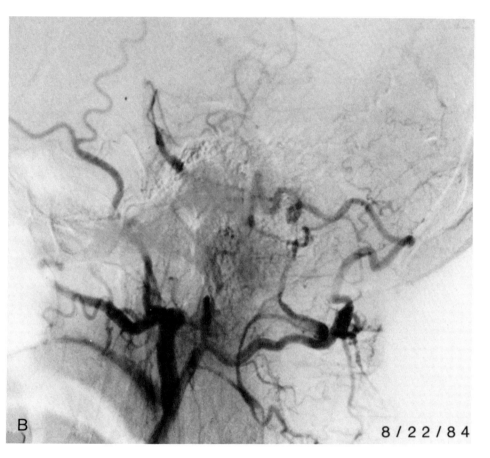

Fig. 20.2B

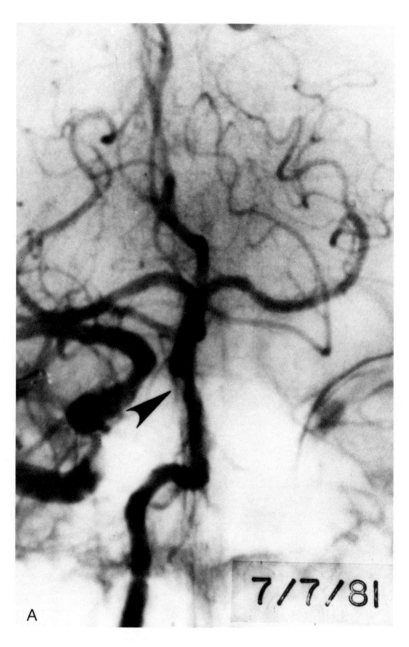

A

7/7/81

Fig. 20.3. A 60-year-old man who developed recurring events of dysarthria, diplopia, and left hemiparesis unresponsive to intravenous anticoagulation. (*A*) Preoperative angiogram shows a severe stenosis of the mid-basilar artery distal to AICA. (*B*) Postoperative angiogram demonstrates filling of the distal basilar artery system via a patent superficial temporal to superior cerebellar artery anastomosis.

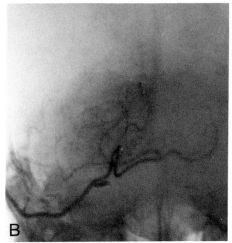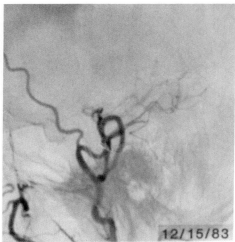

B

12/15/83

FIG. 20.3B

presumably early; but a higher incidence of graft failure and a more complicated surgical course is seen (24). Yet for extremely ill patients, this high volume immediate flow may be preferable.

The posterior cerebral artery may be used in patients with small or insufficient superior cerebellar arteries(24). We prefer not to use the posterior cerebral artery because its collateral circulation is not as extensive as the superior cerebellar artery and there is a risk of cortical blindness which we believe is a worse deficit than ataxia. The posterior cerebral artery is found in the perimesencephalic area just beneath the edge of the uncus of the hippocampus; the vessel is usually large and easy to isolate, although much more retraction is needed to identify and separate the posterior cerebral artery. The vessel has less mobility than the superior cerebellar artery, and the cortical perforators cannot be cauterized since they are usually large. Once the vessel has been isolated and temporarily clipped, an anastomosis is then completed with the superficial temporal artery or a saphenous vein graft to the posterior cerebral artery in a manner similar to that described previously. We have only performed two anastomoses to the posterior cerebral artery. Both patients had resolution of their symptoms and the anastomoses were patent immediately after surgery.

PATHOPHYSIOLOGIC CONSIDERATIONS

There are three possible pathophysiologic causes for the symptoms in these patients with vertebral basilar ischemia. First, ischemia of the vertebral or basilar segment distal to the stenosis or occlusion could produce the clinical syndrome (11). For this perfusion deficit, bypass surgery should be helpful. Second, for local disease or atheroma producing occlusion or stenosis of perforators, there is no treatment and bypass or anticoagulation are unlikely to help (11). For those with emboli as the third possible cause, anticoagulation should be helpful (11). In our patients, the unstable patients were anticoagulant failures. In our entire series, 50% of our patients were symptomatic on intravenous anticoagulants. Of these, surgical revascularization could help about 70%; so it would seem likely that a perfusion deficit would be a possible explanation for the symptoms in some of these patients. Embolization would not be reasonable as a cause in the face of failed anticoagulant therapy. Most likely, all of these factors are operant in producing symptoms but the perfusion deficit would seem a likely cause.

CONCLUSION

In conclusion, revascularization of the vertebrobasilar circulation appears a viable alternative in the management of patients with VBI. A variety of procedures have been developed for patients suffering from posterior circulation ischemia and who have vascular lesions previously considered surgically inaccessible. Any level of the cerebral circulation can now be revascularized with different and innovative procedures designed specifically for individual areas of the brain. These procedures can be completed in most cases with low morbidity and minimal mortality, but we have identified a subset of patients also described by Sundt who have progressed beyond the point where any reconstructive procedure may be of benefit. Our report represents another approach to the clinical problem. At this time there is no evidence that any form of therapy, medical, surgical, or no therapy, is superior to any other. Each case must, therefore, be evaluated and a therapeutic plan developed on an individual basis (11).

REFERENCES

1. Allen, G. S., Cohen, R. J., and Preziosi, T. J. Microsurgical endarterectomy of the intracranial vertebral artery for vertebrobasilar transient ischemic attacks. Neurosurgery, 8: 56–59, 1981.
2. Archer, C. R., and Hornstein, S. Basilar artery occlusion: clinical and radiological correlation. Stroke, 8: 383–390, 1977.
3. Ausman, J. I., Chou, S. N., Lee, M., et al. Occipital to cerebellar artery anastomosis for brain stem infarction from vertebral basilar occlusive disease. Stroke, 7: 13, 1976.
4. Ausman, J. I., Diaz, F. G., de los Reyes, R. A., et al. Anastomosis of occipital artery to anterior inferior cerebellar artery for vertebrobasilar junction stenosis. Surg. Neurol., 16: 99–102, 1981.
5. Ausman, J. I., Diaz, F. G., de los Reyes, R. A., et al. Microsurgery for athersclerosis in the

distal vertebral and basilar arteries. In *Microsurgery*, edited by R. W. Rand, 3rd ed., C. V. Mosby Co., St. Louis, 1984.

6. Ausman, J. I., Diaz, F. G., de los Reyes, R. A., *et al.* Posterior circulation revascularization. Superficial to superior cerebellar artery anastomosis. J. Neurosurg., *56:* 766–776, 1982.

7. Ausman, J. I., Diaz, F. G., de los Reyes, R. A., *et al.* Superficial temporal to proximal superior cerebellar artery anastomosis for basilar artery stenosis. Neurosurgery *9:* 56–60, 1981.

8. Ausman, J. I., Diaz, F. G., Pearce, J. E., *et al.* Endarterectomy of the vertebral artery from C2 to posterior inferior cerebellar artery intracranially. Surg. Neurol., *18:* 400–404, 1982.

9. Ausman, J. I., Lee, M. C., Chater, N., *et al.* Superficial temporal artery to superior cerebellar artery anastomosis for distal basilar artery stenosis. Surg. Neurol., *12:* 227–282, 1979.

10. Ausman, J. I., Nicoloff, D. M., and Chou, S. N. Posterior fossa revascularization. Anastomosis of vertebral artery to PICA with interposed radial artery graft. Surg. Neurol., *9:* 281–286, 1978.

11. Ausman, J. I., Shrontz, C. E., Pearce, J. E., *et al.* Vertebrobasilar insufficiency. A review. Arch. Neurol., *42:* 803–808, 1985.

12. Berguer, R., Bauer, R. B. Vertebral artery reconstruction: successful technique in selected patients. Ann. Surg., *193:* 441–447, 1981.

13. Boulos, R. S., Patel, S., Mehta, B., *et al.* Cerebral angiography in posterior revascularization. H. F. H. Med. J., *33:* 74–81, 1985.

14. Canadian Cooperative Study Group. A randomized trial of aspirin and sulfinpyrazone in threatened stroke. N. Engl. J. Med., *299:* 53–59, 1978.

15. Caplan, L. R., and Rosenbaum, A. E. Role of cerebral angiography in vertebrobasilar occlusive disease. J. Neurol. Neurosurg. Psychiatr., *38:* 601–612, 1975.

16. Cartlidge, N. E. F., Whisnant, J. P., and Elveback, L. R. Carotid and vertebral basilar transient cerebral ischemic attacks. Mayo Clin. Proc. *52:* 117–120, 1977.

17. DeBakey, M. E., Crawford, E. S., Morris, J. C., *et al.* Surgical consideration of occlusive disease of the innominate, carotid and vertebral arteries. Ann. Surg., *154:* 698–725, 1961.

18. Diaz, F. G., Ausman, J. I., de los Reyes, R. A., *et al.* Surgical reconstruction of the proximal vertebral artery. J. Neurosurg., *61:* 874–881, 1984.

19. Khodadad, G. Occipital artery—posterior inferior cerebellar artery anastomosis. Surg. Neurol., *5:* 225–227, 1976.

20. Khodadad, G. Short and long-term results of microvascular anastomosis in the vertebrobasilar system, critical analysis. Neurol. Res., *3:* 33–65, 1981.

21. Millikan, C. H., Siekert, R. G., and Schick, R. M. Studies in cerebrovascular disease. III. The use of anticoagulant drugs in the treatment of insufficiency or thrombosis within the basilar arterial system. Proc. Staff Meet. Mayo Clin., *30:* 116–126, 1955.

22. Spetzler, R. F., and Zabramski, J. Revascularization of anterior and posterior circulation ischemia. Clin. Neurosurg., *29:* 575–593, 1982.

23. Sundt, T. M., and Piepgras, D. G. Occipital to posterior inferior cerebellar artery bypass surgery. J. Neurosurg., *48:* 916–928, 1978.

24. Sundt, T. M., Piepgras, D. G., Houser, O. W., *et al.* Interposition saphenous vein grafts for advanced occlusive disease and large aneurysms in the posterior circulation. J. Neurosurg. *56:* 205–215, 1982.

25. Thompson, J. R., Simmons, C. R., Hasso, A. N., *et al.* Occlusion of the intradural vertebrobasilar artery. Neuroradiology, *14:* 219–229, 1978.

IV

Pediatric Neurosurgery

21

An Evaluation of the *In Utero* Neurosurgical Treatment of Ventriculomegaly

MICHAEL S. B. EDWARDS, M.D.

In 1963, Liley (10) reported the first instance of treatment of a fetus *in utero*. Despite his early success in the treatment of erythroblastosis fetalis, however, prenatal intervention for the treatment of neurologic disorders was not technically feasible until high-resolution obstetric ultrasound techniques became available. The vast majority of neural tube defects in fetuses are identified serendipitously during routine obstetric ultrasound examinations. In addition, ventriculomegaly can be identified readily on ultrasonograms during gestation. Ventriculomegaly is used here instead of hydrocephalus because sonograms cannot be used to differentiate active processes that cause obstruction of cerebrospinal fluid (CSF) flow from other causes of ventricular enlargement. In the discussion that follows, the rationale for prenatal treatment, the experimental and clinical evidence for the natural history of fetal ventriculomegaly and the methods of *in utero* treatment and clinical outcome will be reviewed.

RATIONALE

A prenatal diagnosis of ventriculomegaly may alter obstetric management in several ways. First, the mode of delivery may be altered. For cojoined twins or a fetus with either a large sacral-coccygeal teratoma or a large ruptured omphalocele, a caesarean section must be performed to protect both mother and fetus. Second, the prenatal diagnosis may alter the timing of delivery. Fetuses known to suffer bilateral hydronephrosis secondary to urethral obstruction, diaphragmatic hernia, or ventriculomegaly may suffer increased renal, pulmonary, or neurologic injury, respectively, if the condition is left untreated until term. It is generally assumed that documented ventricular enlargement occurs as an isolated phenomenon and not as the result of other central nervous system (CNS) or systemic abnormalities. Despite the fact that etologic factors cannot be differentiated, it has been assumed that ventricular enlargement *per se* can be diagnosed with a high degree of accuracy. Finally, it has been assumed that ventriculomegaly can be corrected *in utero* and the chances for a good outcome can be improved by a relatively simple, low-risk procedure.

To evaluate the validity of these assumptions and to provide a basis for the selection of appropriate treatment, the natural history of ventriculomegaly *in utero* must be known.

NATURAL HISTORY

In 1984, Chervenak *et al.* (2) reported the outcome for 50 fetuses with an *in utero* diagnosis of ventriculomegaly (Table 21.1). Only 14 (28%) survived; in 70% of fetuses, death was associated with severe congenital anomalies or intrapartum cephalocentesis. Two of the survivors had been treated by insertion of ventriculoamniotic (V-A) shunts at 28 and 29 weeks of gestation. The shunt functioned for 18 weeks in one fetus but migrated into the ventricular system in the other. Thirteen of the 14 survivors required shunting after delivery. Results of a neurologic examination in three infants showed no focal dysfunction, but in 11 infants a variety of neurologic disorders were identified. Bayley scores and/or Stanford-Binet testing showed that eight children had IQs of less than 80 (two patients with IQs of 65–80, six patients with IQs less than 65). Six infants had IQs of more than 80, however. Four of these children had myelomeningocele associated with ventricular enlargement, one had an arachnoid cyst, and the other had no associated malformations. The finding in this series of IQs greater than 80 in the majority of patients with myelomeningocele is not surprising because at least 70% of all children with myelomeningocele have IQs in this range (11).

In 1984, we (9) reported the outcome for 24 fetuses with a prenatal diagnosis of ventriculomegaly. Ventriculomegaly associated with other severe congenital abnormalities was detected early in gestation in 10 fetuses. After consultation with the Fetal Treatment Program at our institution, nine families decided to terminate the pregnancy. The tenth fetus died from severe nonCNS abnormalities 30 minutes after delivery. Ventriculomegaly was serendipitously diagnosed late in gestation in three fetuses. All

TABLE 21.1
Outcome in Chervenak's Series of 50 Fetuses

Outcome	Number	Percentage
Elective abortion	13	26
Antepartum death	0	0
Intrapartum death	7	14
Neonatal death		
Within 24 hours	11	22
24 hours to 28 days	3	6
After 28 days	14	28

were treated with cephalocentesis to permit vaginal delivery, and all died 30 minutes after delivery. The diagnosis was less well-defined in 11 fetuses, but we felt that they all suffered a form of isolated ventriculomegaly. The condition resolved in one fetus, remained stable in nine, and progressed slightly in one. Despite an increase of the size of ventricles in the fetus with slight progression, there was no evidence of increased intracranial pressure at birth. All 11 infants were viable at delivery, but one died from congenital heart failure shortly after birth. Three of the 10 infants required shunting at the time of birth, while two others required shunting within 5 months after birth.

In the hands of an expert ultrasonographer, high resolution obstetric sonograms can be used to detect anomalies associated with ventriculomegaly. In three of the fetuses with isolated ventriculomegaly in our series, agenesis of the corpus callosum, absence of the septum pellucidum, and septo-optic dysplasia were not recognized.

Ultrasonograms can be used to detect enlargement of the ventricles in fetuses by 15 to 18 weeks of gestation, and serial examinations can be used to determine the progression, stabilization, or resolution of the condition (6). As the results of both clinical series show, however, ultrasonography cannot always reliably define underlying anatomic and pathophysiologic abnormalities. With the resolution of the equipment currently available, it is not possible to differentiate ventricular enlargement that is the result of hydrocephalus from other CNS abnormalities such as septo-optic dysplasia and agenesis of the corpus callosum, conditions that have normal CSF dynamics. This limitation makes it difficult to select the appropriate patient for treatment.

RESEARCH

In an attempt to prove the assumption that ventriculomegaly will progress and cause cerebral damage if left untreated *in utero*, we developed a model of fetal hydrocephalus in sheep and monkeys (4, 9, 12). A 2% kaolin suspension is instilled through the intact uterus into the cisterna magna of the fetus at 90–100 days of gestation in lambs and at 96–130 days of gestation in rhesus monkeys. Fetal lambs are an excellent model because of the high incidence of twin pregnancies; one fetus can be treated and the other can serve as the age-matched control. In initial experiments, 12 fetal lambs and two fetal monkeys were instilled with kaolin. Massive hydrocephalus developed in six fetal lambs and both monkeys (Fig. 21.1). All treated animals had external signs of hydrocephalus with marked craniomegaly. On gross examination after sacrifice we found that the aqueduct of Sylvius and cisterna magna were filled with kaolin and that there was marked dilatation of the ventricles. The central canal of the spinal cord

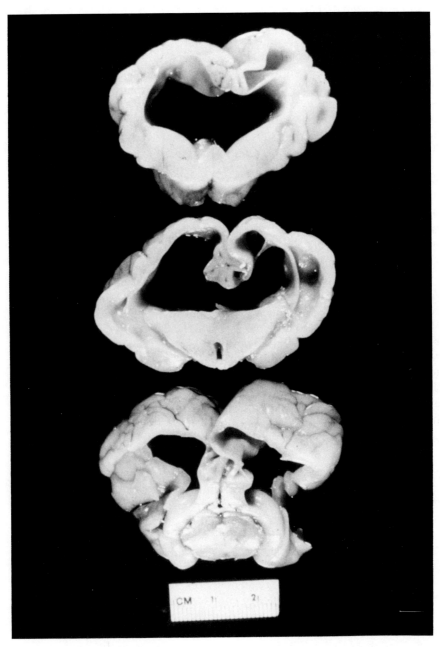

FIG. 21.1. Coronal section of formalin-fixed lamb brain at term; a 2% kaolin suspension was instilled into the cisterna magna during the third trimester. There is marked ventricular dilatation and compression of white matter with preservation of the cortex.

was not enlarged in any animal, but the basilar meninges were thickened secondary to the reaction with kaolin in all animals. On microscopic examination it was found that there was a moderate fibrotic reaction and inflammatory cell response along the basal meninges, which occluded the foramina of Luschka and Magendi in all animals and the aqueduct of Sylvius in some animals. Gray matter was relatively well-preserved, but white matter was extremely attenuated; the latter is often found in children with severe hydrocephalus.

This model was used to evaluate the effects of treatment by *in utero* placement of shunts in kaolin-treated animals. Hydrocephalus was induced in 28 fetal lambs and 17 fetal rhesus monkeys. At 21–25 days after instillation of kaolin, *in utero* ventricular decompression was performed by placement of a V-A shunt in 10 fetal lambs, a ventriculo-right atrial in nine, and a ventriculo-pleural shunt in one. Seven hydrocephalic lambs were used as controls. Intracranial pressure (ICP), measured in the ventricle at the time of shunt placement, was significantly elevated. The results are listed in Table 21.2.

Placement of the shunt significantly increased survival. Ten of 14 shunts were patent and functional at the time of delivery. Ventricular size was normal in eight of 14 shunted fetal lambs; ventricles were enlarged in all control lambs. Complications produced by the shunting procedure, including infection and subdural hematomas and hygromas, are listed in Table 21.3. The incidence of complication did not depend on the type of shunt used. Complications were present in six of 14 fetal lambs, which includes the improper placement of the catheter in two lambs. Despite these complications, most shunted lambs had decreased head circumference, over-

TABLE 21.2

Results of In Utero Shunting in Fetal Lambs with Kaolin-Induced Hydrocephalus

	Shunt Type			
	Ventriculo-amniotic	Ventriculo-right Atrial	Ventriculo-pleural	Control
Number in group	10	9	1	7
Viability*	6/10	7/9	1/1	1/7
Preshunt ICP (cm H$_2$O)	18.9 ± 8.6	23.0 ± 9.7	25.0	
Shunt patency	5/6	4/7	1/1	
Normal ventricular size**	3/6	4/7	1/1	0/1

* Viability of all shunted fetuses compared to unshunted, age-matched twin controls by a chi-square analysis, $p < 0.001$.

** Survivors only.

TABLE 21.3

Complications of In Utero Shunting in Fetal Lambs with Kaolin-Induced Hydrocephalus

	Shunt Type			
	Ventriculo-amniotic	Ventriculo-right Atrial	Ventriculo-pleural	Control
Number in group	10	9	1	7
Viability*	6/10	7/9	1/1	1/7
Shunt infection*	1/6	0/7	0/1	
Subdural hematoma*	1/6	0/7	0/1	0/1
Subdural hygroma*	2/6	1/7	0/1	0/1
Improper placement of shunt tip	1/6	1/7	0/1	

* Survivors only.

riding sutures, ventricles of normal size, and improved survival compared to untreated lambs. In a few lambs, however, marked destruction of white matter was found on histopathologic examination. Therefore, after instilling kaolin into the cisterna magnum we simultaneously monitored amniotic fluid pressure (AFP) and subdural ICP in fetal lambs *in utero* (Fig. 21.2). ICP and ICP minus AFP increased linearly, but AFP alone showed no trend. ICP reached a maximum value of 40 mm Hg by 40 days after injection, an ICP that is high enough to cause ischemic damage.

Eight fetal monkeys underwent V-A decompression 2 to 3 weeks after injection of kaolin. There was little or no improvement of ventriculomegaly in shunted monkeys. Brains from both shunted and untreated monkeys showed a severe inflammatory reaction and ventriculitis despite the finding that the size of the ventricles, monitored by ultrasonography *in utero*, was reduced after shunting. The size of the ventricles increased in several monkeys in which shunts failed to function. Even though these results are encouraging, they show clearly that additional research is necessary and that neither the ideal shunt nor the best technique for implantation have been found.

CLINICAL EXPERIENCE WITH V-A SHUNTING

In 1982, Clewell *et al.* (3) and Frigolleto *et al.* (7) reported the first use of a V-A shunt in a human fetus. Before 1982, only intermittent cephalocentesis had been used to treat progressive ventriculomegaly *in utero* (1). In the technique reported by Clewell *et al.* (3), at 24 weeks of gestation a V-A shunt was inserted transabdominally with sonographic guidance into a male fetus with a presumed X-linked aqueductal stenosis and hydrocephalus. The shunt appeared to function until 32 weeks of gestation. The fetus

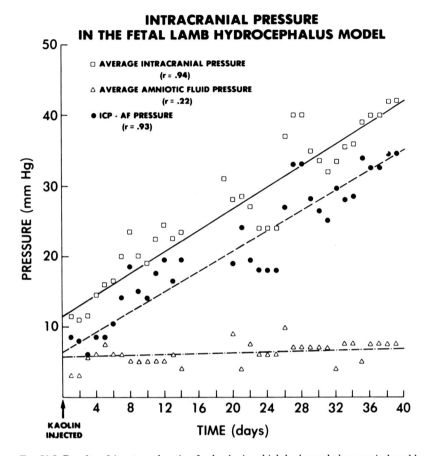

FIG. 21.2. Results of *in utero* shunting for lambs in which hydrocephalus was induced by kaolin instillation.

was delivered by cesarean section at 34 weeks of gestation and a ventriculopleural shunt was placed. Two major problems with *in utero* treatment are exemplified by this report. First, X-linked hydrocephalus is usually associated with mental retardation caused by associated CNS anomalies. Therefore, the selection of this fetus for *in utero* treatment seems inappropriate. Second, although the techniques are available to place the shunt, the appropriate shunt and the ability to keep it functioning for the entire gestation period are not.

On the basis of one case, obstetricians and ultrasonographers who presumably had no training in the procedure and who were undoubtedly much less technically capable, less thoughtful, and less talented than the members of the Denver group began placing V-A shunts in fetuses. It is not possible to estimate how many fetuses were treated or the number of complications that resulted from treatment. It is known that during this period neurosurgeons played a minor to negligible role in advising families and physicians of the propriety of this procedure. This disastrous experience emphasizes the point that personnel who are not thoroughly trained should never attempt a difficult procedure, and even if properly trained should never attempt a difficult procedure without the consultation and guidance of the appropriate specialists.

In June 1982, a conference was held under the auspices of the Kroc Foundation that brought together clinicians and researchers interested in treatment of fetuses *in utero*. The International Registry for *In Utero* Treatment of Fetal Obstructive Uropathy and Hydrocephalus was formed at this meeting. Case entry into the Registry is voluntary. Nineteen of 31 university centers have agreed to enter their patients. Eleven centers are in the United States, three are in Canada, two in Great Britain, and one each in Australia, Israel, and Chile. European centers are conspicuously absent.

As of June 1985, the cases of 39 fetuses treated *in utero* for hydrocephalus have been registered. Thirty-seven (95%) were treated with V-A shunting and two (5%) were treated with three to six serial ventricular taps. The mean gestational ages at diagnosis and treatment were 25 to 27 weeks, respectively. Thirty-two (82%) fetuses survived, but seven fetuses died during treatment or in the early prenatal period. Four of seven deaths were directly related to the treatment procedure (10% procedure-related death rate). The average follow-up for the 32 survivors is 8 ± 5 months. Eleven infants (34%) are developmentally normal, three (9%) are mildly to moderately handicapped, and 18 (56%) are severely handicapped (IQ less than 50). Five infants are cortically blind, two have severe seizure disorders, and two have spastic diplegia. Outcome does not correlate with the duration of function of the *in utero* shunt. The incidence of nonCNS abnormalities was 15%; if fetuses had been selected properly and if the natural history of the disease process were better understood, this incidence rate could be reduced significantly.

RECOMMENDED MANAGEMENT

Based on our experience and the initial results of the Registry program, we recommend the following approach to the *in utero* management of ventriculomegaly (Fig. 21.3) (5). After the initial diagnosis of ventriculomegaly is made, we perform a screening examination with high-resolution obstetric ultrasonography to rule out other associated anomalies. In practice, ultrasonography is performed at least twice at weekly intervals to help confirm the nature of the lesion and to document progression of

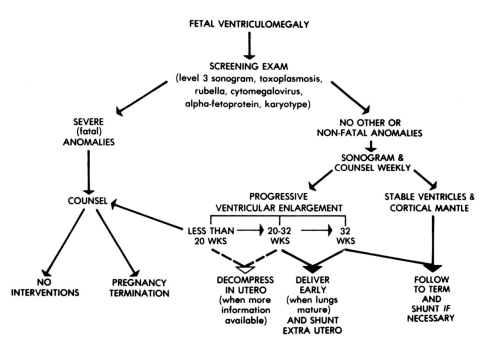

FIG. 21.3. Recommended approach to the *in utero* management of ventriculomegaly.

ventriculomegaly. Amniocentesis should be performed for karyotype, *alpha*-fetoprotein levels, and viral cultures in all pregnancies in which fetal ventriculomegaly is diagnosed in the second or early third trimester. If ventriculomegaly is severe, if other severe anomalies are identified, or if there is evidence of intrauterine toxoplasmosis, cytomegalovirus, or herpes infection, aggressive treatment may be inappropriate. If the prenatal evaluation is otherwise normal, however, we obtain serial weekly ultrasonograms. If the size of the ventricles remains relatively unchanged, the fetus is allowed to come to term, is delivered, and is followed closely for signs of hydrocephalus, which is treated by a shunting procedure if it develops. In some infants, hydrocephalus may not develop until many months after birth.

If ventriculomegaly is progressive, we determine the approach to treatment based on the period of gestation. Even though there is not sufficient information to evaluate our approach fully, we recommend preterm delivery and placement of a shunt in the immediate postnatal period for a fetus that is near-term (greater than 32 weeks of gestation) whose lungs appear to be mature. For fetuses with a gestation period of less than 32 weeks, the risks associated with pulmonary immaturity must be weighed against the potential damage that might be caused by progressive ventriculomegaly to determine the best time for delivery and postnatal shunting. We do not feel that the evidence currently available justifies *in utero* shunting. If new evidence should show that *in utero* shunting is effective, we would consider open surgical placement of an internalized shunt for the treatment of ventriculomegaly.

SUMMARY

Clinical results for *in utero* treatment of ventriculomegaly are not impressive; results may improve, however, with new techniques and more experience. Nonetheless, even in the best of hands, it is not always possible to identify associated and sometimes fatal congenital abnormalities on high resolution obstetric ultrasonograms, and not enough is known of the natural history of CNS congenital disease, in particular of ventriculomegaly, to select the appropriate fetus for *in utero* treatment. Results of animal studies are encouraging, but more work is needed to define the pathophysiology, knowledge of which might allow selection of the appropriate fetus and treatment modality.

REFERENCES

1. Birnholtz, J. C., Frigoletto, R. G. Antenatal treatment of hydrocephalus. N. Engl. J. Med. *304:* 1021–1023, 1981.
2. Chervenak, F. A., Duncan, C., Ment, L. R., Hobbins, J. C., McClure, M., Scott, D., and Berkowitz, R. L. Outcome of fetal ventriculomegaly. Lancet *ii:* 179–181, 1984.
3. Clewell, W. H., Johnson, M. L., Meier, P. R., Newkirk, J. B., Zide, S. L., Hendee, R. W., Rowes, W. A. Jr., Hecht, F., O'Keeffe, D., Henry, G. P., and Shikes, R. H. A surgical approach to the treatment of fetal hydrocephalus. N. Engl. J. Med. *306:* 1320–1325, 1982.
4. Edwards, M. S. B., and Filley, R. Diagnosis and management of fetal disorders of the central nervous system. In *Anomalies of the CNS*, edited by H. Hoffman and F. Epstein. Blackwells, Boston (in press).
5. Edwards, M. S. B., Harrison, M. R., Halks-Miller, M., Nakayama, D. K., Berger, M. S., Glick, P. L., and Chinn, D. H. Kaolin-induced congenital hydrocephalus in utero in fetal lambs and rhesus monkeys. J. Neurosurg. *60:* 115–122, 1984.
6. Fiske, C. E., and Filly, R. A. Ultrasound evaluation of the normal and abnormal fetal neural axis. Radiol. Clin. North Am. *20:* 285–296, 1982.
7. Frigolleto, F. D., Birnholtz, J. C., and Greene, M. F. Antenatal treatment of hydrocephalus by ventriculo-amniotic shunting. J.A.M.A. *248:* 2496–2497, 1982.
8. Glick, P. L., Harrison, M. R., Halks-Miller, M., Adzick, S., Nakayama, D. K., Anderson, J. H., Nyland, T. G., Villa, R., and Edwards, M. S. B. Correction of congenital hydrocephalus in utero II: efficacy of in utero shunting. J. Pediatr. Surg., *19:* 870–881, 1984.
9. Glick, P. L., Harrison, M. R., Nakayama, D. K., Edwards, M. S. B., Filly, R. A., Callen, P. W., Wilson, S. L., and Globus, M. S. Management of ventriculomegaly in the fetus. J. Pediatr. *105:* 97–105, 1984.

10. Harrison, M. R., Golbus, M. S., Filly, R. A. *The Unborn Patient: Prenatal Diagnosis and Treatment,* 445 pp. Grune & Stratton, Inc., Orlando, 1984.
11. McClone, D. G., Dias, L., Kaplan, W. E., and Sommers, M. W. Concepts in the management of spina bifida. *Concepts in Pediatric Neurosurgery,* Vol. 5. Karger, Basel, New York, 1985, pp. 97–106.
12. Nakayama, D. K., Harrison, M. R., Berger, M. S., Chinn, D. H., Halks-Miller, M., and Edwards, M. S. Correction of congenital hydrocephalus in utero I. The Model: intracisternal kaolin produces hydrocephalus in fetal lambs and Rhesus monkeys. J. Pediatr. Surg., *18:* 331–338, 1983.

22

Treatment of Myelomeningocele: Arguments against Selection

DAVID G. McLONE, M.D., PH.D.

In our pluralistic society it is difficult to gain agreement on purely moral or ethical grounds. It would be better to test whether the concept of selection can be supported on the basis of published evidence.

Let me first state that all children born with a myelomeningocele cannot be saved. To mandate either by law or standard of practice that all children born with a myelomeningocele must be operated upon is an absurdity.

In the neonatal period fetal development has ended and we have lost the legal option to terminate the child's life. It must be borne in mind that what and who we are talking about is a newborn child who is alive and who is not dying. This confronts us with serious moral and ethical issues. The situation is quite distinct from a child who is born dying or who has an irreparable defect which will initiate the dying process. A child born with anencephaly, severe irremediable cardiac anomalies, or absent kidneys is not the focus of this discussion. This unfortunate cannot be helped and must be made comfortable while dying. The child we are discussing has a problem which requires urgent medical attention if he or she is to survive. Moreover, if the problem is corrected and the child survives he or she is likely to have varying degrees of handicap. The significant question is not, "can the child survive?"; with surgery he can. Rather, the question is "what if the child survives?" The decision to treat the child has often been based on principally on what the likely outcome is or, more popularly, what will be the child's "quality of life."

To treat or not to treat has become a debatable issue presupposing several things to be true. In fact, each of these assumptions has a high degree of uncertainty. We need to ask some fundamental questions. Do valid medical criteria exist which accurately predict the outcome—the quality of life? What percentage of inaccuracy is acceptable for such criteria? How many children can we allow to die who would have done well in order to ensure that no severely handicapped child survives? Is the child assured expert opinion? Is there a universally accepted level of quality below which death is preferable? Can one person choose death for another? If one person can choose death for another, who should make the choice? The newborn is unable to choose for himself or herself. Can the parents choose? Whose interests are the parents serving? Is their choice informed? Is informed consent a realistic concept? Who should bear the initial and long-term cost for the decision? Has cost-benefit analysis been performed? Is this a subject that is properly studied in terms of cost-benefit analysis?

Spina bifida (myelomeningocele) serves very nicely as the test case for our discussion. Myelomeningocele is a disease that affects between 6000 and 11,000 newborns in the United States each year. The children are born alive but require urgent (not emergent) surgery to prevent exacerbation of their handicap or death. Paralysis, bladder and bowel incontinence, and hydrocephalus are all part of the child's future. Severe mental retardation requiring some form of custodial care is the likely fate of 10–15% of the children. Some 10–15% of the children will die prior to reaching the first grade, in spite of aggressive medical care. As you can see, the child with spina bifida confronts us with essentially all the problems faced by newborns with Down's syndrome, prematurity, cerebral palsy, or other severe diseases. I maintain that if we resolve the ethical issues surrounding spina bifida we will then have resolved these issues for nearly all handicapped newborns.

Now let us wrestle with the problem. For the sake of discussion, let us assume we are the parents facing this situation. If we withhold surgery our child has a high probability of dying within the first year of life. Can we morally and ethically choose to allow our child to acquire a lethal disease? Is this in his best interest? Do we have reliable information—facts—upon which to base our decision?

Some additional information must not be introduced. The ambiguous phrase *selective nontreatment* means in fact that (based on predetermined criteria) certain infants will be managed less aggressively. They will deliberately be managed so they will have a high probability of dying. In this plan, survival of the infant is considered a management failure. In Britain the children selected to die are heavily sedated and given food and water only "on demand." These children usually die within 3 months. Opinion in the United States is strongly opposed to withholding food and water from a child who can eat. Euthanasia is not acceptable in our country. Therefore, we must await death from an acquired illness, usually infection. This is passive euthanasia. Most available series indicate that if the child is given food and water and if antibiotics are withheld, about 40% of babies will survive. Most would agree that these survivors suffer from worse handicaps than do the infants treated surgically in the first days of life.

From a cost-benefit perspective, the cost of not treating some infants plus the cost of chronic institutional care for these unfortunate survivors of "benign neglect" far exceeds the cost of aggressive surgical care at the outset. The application of cost-benefit analysis to handicapped newborns, however, reminds me of the woman Oscar Wilde spoke of, "she knew the cost of everything and the value of nothing."

Between 1959 and 1984, 4 series of unselected newborns with a myelomeningocele were documented with a significant period of follow-up (1, 8, 13, 15). A review of this 25-year-period demonstrates a remarkable decrease in mortality and in the number of urinary diversions with an equally remarkable increase in urinary continence (13). This increase in continence is "social continence" with children staying dry for periods of 2–3 hours on clean intermittent catheterization (CIC). A gradual but significant improvement in ambulation and intelligence is also shown (Figs. 22.1 and 22.2). It is now rare for a child to die because of renal failure.

Lorber's 1971 (8) experience with an unselected population led to the initial set of criteria used to select children for nontreatment.

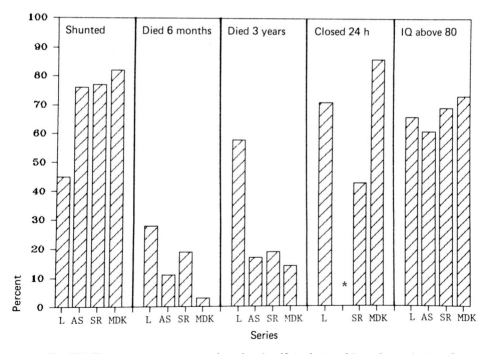

FIG. 22.1. Treatment outcome—unselected series. Note the trend in each area is toward preferred outcome and reflects progress. *L* = Lorber (8); *AS* = Ames and Schut (1); *SR* = Soare and Raimondi (15); *MDK* = McLone *et al.* (2).

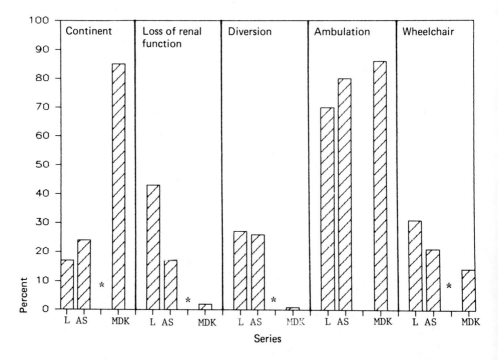

FIG. 22.2. Treatment outcome—unselected series. The remarkable increase in continence and decrease in renal function loss and urinary diversions is seen. Rate of community ambulation also shows improvement. * = Soare and Raimondi data not available.

In 1972, Ames and Schut (1) described the outcome of aggressive care of all newborns with a myelomeningocele. I feel that the results of this study remain the "gold standard" for care even today. They state, "Because no infallible criteria for determining potential at birth have evolved, all children are operated upon to close the defects and relieve the hydrocephalus."

Soare's (15) series was published in 1977 and was a nonsequential study. Therefore, the information is incomplete in some areas. McLone's 1985 study (12) is a sequential nonselected series of 100 children followed for at least 6 years.

One wonders why in the face of improved outcome for all children born with a myelomeningocele papers advocating selection continue to be published unless it can be shown that selected children fare better as a group in comparison to unselected children.

To return to selection criteria, let us discuss the criteria most frequently cited for selecting those children born with spina bifida who should not be treated. These criteria have, at one time or another, had international acceptance and are still in use in most English-speaking countries. An article this year in *Pediatrics* published these "adverse criteria" again without evidence of their validity (7). Lorber's 1971 criteria derive from his experience in the 1950s and 1960s in a large center in England. The criteria consist essentially of four items. Children will be selected for nontreatment if they have (*a*) severe hydrocephalus at birth, (*b*) total paraplegia, (*c*) angulation of their spine (kyphosis), or (*d*) any additional birth defect.

The reliability and "predictive value" of these four criteria can be considered for each criterion individually and then for the four criteria as a group. Criterion *a* (severe hydrocephalus) suggests that hydrocephalus is the principal cause of mental retardation in these individuals. This notion has been shown to be invalid by three studies performed in the United States. Simply, hydrocephalus is not the primary cause of mental retardation in patients with spina bifida. Rather, almost 80% of children with spina bifida born today should have normal intelligence. Lorber himself later questioned the impact of severe hydrocephalus on the function of the brain in a paper entitled "Is the Brain Important." The single most common cause of mental retardation in children with spina bifida is infection, either ventriculitis or meningoencephalitis (13). Such infection is most likely to appear in those infants from whom corrective surgery is withheld. The parents of Baby Jane Doe, a child born with spina bifida, were told she would inevitably be severely retarded. For that reason they decided not to allow a surgeon to treat her. Because she was not treated, she acquired ventriculitis, which means she is likely to be retarded. This becomes a self-fulfilling prophecy.

Regarding criterion *b* paraplegia has proved to be an unreliable criterion in our patients. In 37% of our children surgical closure of the back (10, 11) was followed by a significant motor recovery with development of active function of a previously nonfunctional joint (Fig. 22.3). This recovery is likely not the result of closure and has been noted in children without surgery. Thus, in 37% of our children the initial motor examination was an unreliable criterion for predicting outcome. The motor exam did not predict ultimate function. Beyond this inaccuracy in prediction one must ask further: What degree of motor function is necessary to compete in our culture? Even in the worse case, we do not feel that paraplegia is incompatible with meaningful participation in our society.

Criterion *c* is the presence of sharp angulation of the spine or kyphosis, such kyphosis is now in the majority of cases surgically correctable and, in our opinion is, again, not a valid criterion for predicting patient outcome. Although any curvature of the spine remains a difficult orthopaedic prob-

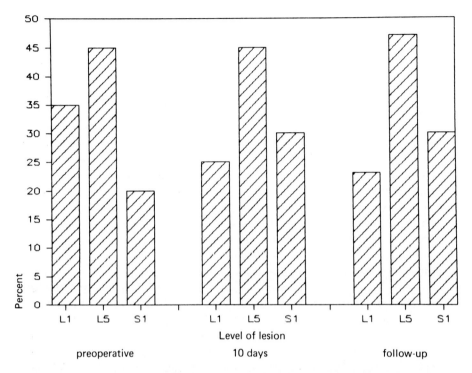

Fig. 22.3. Motor level in 100 consecutively treated patients. Percentage of children with L1 hip flexion or less, L5 knee extension or less, and S1 motor function in their feet. Preoperative, 10-day, and follow-up evaluation show sustained improvement.

lem for children with spina bifida, surgical correction at birth or a few years later provides a stable spine and maximum height in most cases.

Selection criterion d is the presence of any other birth defect. Additional congenital anomalies occur at a rate of 1% or less in patients with spina bifida. In our opinion, any concurrent defect must be considered individually to assess its own impact on the child. Significant defects like six fingers remain insignificant even in children with spina bifida. Obviously the child born with spina bifida and an additional lethal anomaly is a child born dying from the other defect and falls outside our discussion.

As to the validity of using all four criteria as a group, that approach also fails. Three studies have been published in the 1980s which utilized criteria to select children with a myelomeningocele for nonsurgical management (4, 7, 9). Lorber's long-term results in a highly selected population of "best" patients with myelomeningocele have recently become available (1981) (9). These may be compared with the results of treating an unselected population of all patients with myelomeningocele (12) (Fig. 22.4). The results of our treatment of all patients compare favorably with the results in the selected group of "best" patients. In the selected group, the overall mortality approaches 70%, because the selection process itself consigns a substantial number of children to death. The death rate in the remaining best, "selected" patients is not significantly different from the death rate we observe in the unselected group of all patients presenting to Children's Memorial Hospital. That is, the unselected, supposedly less viable children we treat at our hospital do not have any higher mortality than the best selected patients treated by Lorber. The selected group did better than the unselected group in IQ scores. Fifteen percent more children from the selected group had an IQ greater than 80. However, we must weigh a 70% mortality against a 15% increase in the number of children with an IQ greater than 80. Sixty percent of the selected children who died would have been considered competitive in our study.

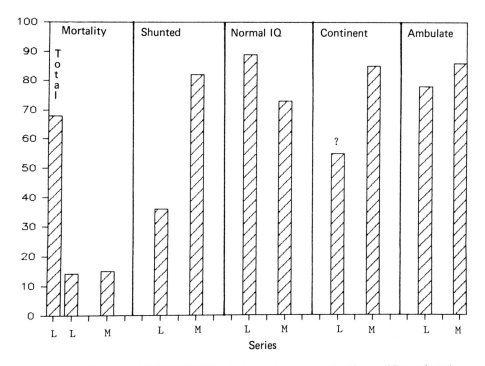

Fig. 22.4. Lorber and Salfield (9) (L) selected series compared with our (M) unselected series. L series indicates a 15% increase in number of children with an IQ greater than 80; but note increase in total mortality was greater than four times our total.

In 1984, a study was published from a university children's hospital in which children were selected for nontreatment based on the formula (7):

$$QL = NE \times (H + S)$$
$$NE = \text{Natural endowment}$$
$$H = \text{Home and family}$$
$$S = \text{Society}$$

This formula is thought to somehow predict the child's quality of life. Twenty-four of 69 babies were not operated upon and all died within 189 days. This paper evoked outrage in both the medical (19) and lay communities and led to threats of litigation from several groups representing handicapped individuals. This article contained no evidence that the children operated upon did any better than unselected children in other series published.

A thinly veiled selection paper emphasizing "Time for a Decision-Making Process," was published in 1985 (4). This paper purports to show that delay in surgical management allows time to inform the parents at no cost to the child and then offers no evidence that parents of children repaired in the perinatal period differ significantly from those where surgery was delayed. What it does show is a significant mortality (100%) occurred in the nonoperated group. Two children died during the first week of delay, 6 died in the first month, and a total of 14 died without surgery. Fifty-two were treated in the first 48 hours. Thus, 14 of 58 children with delay beyond the initial 48 hours died for a mortality rate of 24%. The mortality rate in the early group was 8%. The authors quote Fost as a supporter of this concept. I strongly recommend Fost's paper to anyone who is involved in the care of these children. Fost does state regarding the parents, "There is almost always an initial phase of severe shock, lasting days to months. During this time, the parents are typically incapable of assimilating information" (5). Our study, detailed later in this paper, would indicate that this period often extends for 6 months of the child's life.

Although selective nontreatment is not part of the title, it is the thrust of this paper. Adverse criteria, essentially the same as Lorber's, are listed, without evidence that they predict outcome for these infants. Children are treated at the request of the parents. Of the children operated upon in the first 48 hours, 10% had two or more of these adverse criteria, and of the children who were not operated upon, 86% had two or more of these criteria. Again, the authors quote Freeman (6) in the introduction. I prefer Freeman's quote in the same chapter: "Slow, natural death over weeks or months is not humane for the child, the family, or the staff." If nothing else, this paper suffers from prematurity due to a lack of long-term evidence that either the children or their parents are better because of this mode of management.

The weight of evidence would indicate that not only is each of the criteria invalid but the four criteria as a group do not ensure a significantly higher quality of life for the few patients treated.

In the Lorber (9), Gross (7), and Charney (4) articles, the child's life is weighed against the family's ability to cope. The deleterious effect of the handicapped child on the family is documented in the bleak results of series from the 1960s. Reports by Martin (1975) (14), Waisbren (1979) (18), and Vance et al. (1980) (16) in this country are ignored even though they demonstrate amazing family stability and ability to cope. It is important to note that the Spina Bifida Association of America, the national organization which represents individuals with spina bifida and their families, and the consumers themselves are very much protreatment and adamantly opposed to selection.

The issue of informed consent has several parts. The first involves the informant, usually a physician, and addresses the adequacy of the information provided to the parents. Is the information current and relevant to the problem? Objectivity on the part of the physician is beyond the scope of this paper. The only case in which we have documented sworn testimony of what the parents were told is the case of Baby Jane Doe (2). In the Baby Jane Doe case, the prognostic information provided to the parents, as testified in court by the managing "expert" physician, deviated substantially from the experience of other experts (3). From the information in the medical chart of Baby Jane's first 19 days and this "expert's" testimony, real questions exist about the quality of this informed consent. The parents may have acted in Baby Jane's best interest based on the information they were given. The reasons for this wide discrepancy between the testimony and medical literature remain speculative.

A second issue in informed consent, as pointed out earlier, is the individual's ability to assimilate sufficient knowledge to enable him or her to arrive at an informed consent within a reasonable period of time. As Charney has shown, prolonged delay in performing surgery increases the likelihood of the child's death. We have days, not weeks, in which to arrive at a decision.

I agree with Venes (17), "immediate operation is not indicated—but prolonged delay is (not) without hazard for increased rates of infection," and further, "certainly time is available for reasoned and considered discussion with at least one, and preferably both parents." It is essential that the parents participate in the decision-making process and feel that they have some control of the difficult situation thrust upon them.

In a review of 300 of the families followed at Children's Memorial Hospital in Chicago, 52% felt they had given informed consent at the time of the initial surgery. Almost half of those who felt they gave informed consent did not feel there was any other moral choice and information about outcome was irrelevant to their decision to treat. In reviewing the families' perception of their rate of acquisition of information, half the families indicated that it really took 6 months before they understood half of the information needed to be truly informed. The disease is complex and is difficult to comprehend quickly, even by medical professionals. Because we are a children's hospital we usually see only the father, however, we always send a team to talk to the mother about the significance of what has just occurred. All fathers seem to have equal ability to deal with this problem on the first few days of the child's life regardless of socioeconomic background. Realization that the child has been born with a significant handicap confounds the parents and reduces them all to equality. When parents were asked, "Do you regret your initial decision?" 13 of 300 answered "yes." It should be noted that nine of these 13 regretted that their initial decision was *not to treat* their child.

The manner in which the information is presented to the parents has a significant effect on how receptive the parent is to the physician's suggestions (overt or covert). The physician can introduce a significant bias at this point. You have heard some facts about spina bifida presented earlier in this paper. Although all true, they were selected because they emphasize the negative side of the quality of life. One could present equally true facts that produce a contrary perception of spina bifida. Primarily through medical progress we can now say that 85–90% of the children will survive; 70–80% will have normal intelligence; 80% will be socially continent of bladder and bowel; 89% of the survivors with normal intelligence will be able to ambulate in the community (walk with or without braces) by the first grade. This percentage of ambulation is likely to fall as the children reach their teen years. Although early to predict, it may be that 75% of the children will be independent and competitive as adults. True data presented positively and negatively provide different "informed consent" responses.

In my experience, in nearly every case the parents are acting in what they perceive to be the child's best interest. Armed with expert opinion presented positively, they almost invariably choose the recommendation of the expert.

Ideally at this difficult time for child and parent, consultation between caring parents and a truly informed physician, an expert, will permit a rational, best informed decision and the institution of the best possible care for the child. With this approach, the child and society have the best chance of success.

I would reiterate that proper decision making requires informed opinions. Any professional, physician, nurse, social worker, or other, who wanders into this process and out of ignorance misinforms a family, does a great disservice to the child, the parents, and us, the child's fellow citizens.

Neurosurgeons who treat children born with a myelomeningocele are, for better or worse, responsible for the child's survival. To walk away at that point is unacceptable. Participation, advocacy if you will, at all stages of the child's development is essential to the family's integrity and the child's potential for independence. A team approach utilizing social workers, psychologist, nurse specialists, and physicians is the method of choice. Education and support of family begun during the initial hospitalization will establish a relationship that will foster coping by the family and ensure optimal function on the part of the child. In the 10 years since I organized the myelomeningocele (MM) team at Children's Memorial Hospital, I have seen a small group of angry, confused families become a large group of optimistic informed advocates.

In conclusion, existing evidence casts doubt on the validity of the criteria advocated for selection. Also there is no evidence that children from selected populations are significantly more fit than unselected children. Those workers who use selection underestimate the ability of those families to rise to the challenge and to deal with both the short- and long-term problems of the handicapped child. They also significantly underestimate the advances in medical management and in society that now permit the handicapped to move freely and participate fully in the work day and recreational activities of our society.

REFERENCES

1. Ames, M., and Schut, L. Diagnosis and treatment. Results of treatment of 171 consecutive myelomeningoceles—1963 to 1968. Pediatrics (Springfield), 50: 466–470, 1972.
2. Baer, S. The half-told story of Baby Jane Doe. Columbia Journalism Review, November/December, pp. 35–38, 1984.
3. Butler, A. Personal Communication.
4. Charney, E. B., Weller, S. C., Sutton, L. N., Bruce, D. A., and Schut, L. B. Management of the newborn with myelomeningocele: time for a decision-making process. Pediatrics, 75(1): 58–64, 1985.
5. Fost, N. Counseling families who have a child with a severe congenital anomaly. Pediatrics, 67(3): 321–324, 1981.
6. Freeman, J. To treat or not to treat. In: Practical Management of Myelomeningocele. Baltimore, University Park Press, 1974.
7. Gross, R. H., Cox, A., Tatyrek, R., Pollay, M., and Barnes, W. A. Early management and decision making for the treatment of myelomeningocele. Pediatrics, 72: 450–457, 1983.

8. Lorber, J. Results of treatment of myelomeningocele. An analysis of 524 unselected cases, with special reference to possible selection for treatment. Devel. Med. Child Neur., *13:* 279–303, 1971.
9. Lorber, J., and Salfield, S. Results of selective treatment of spina bifida cystica. Arch. Dis. Childh., *56:* 822–830, 1981.
10. McLone, D. G. Technique for closure of myelomeningocele. Child's Brain, *6:* 65–73, 1980.
11. McLone, D. G. Results of treatment of children born with a myelomeningocele. Clin. Neurosurg., *30:* 407–412, 1983.
12. McLone, D. G., Dias, L., Kaplan, W. E., and Sommers, M. W. Concepts in the Management of Spina Bifida. *Concepts in Pediatric Neurosurgery*, Vol. 5. Karger, Basel, 1985, pp. 97–106.
13. McLone, D. G., Czyzewsky, D., Raimondi, A. J., Sommers, R. C. Central nervous system infections as a limiting factor in the intelligence of children born with myelomeningocele. Pediatrics, *70:* 338–342, 1982.
14. Martin, P. Marital breakdown in families of patients with spina bifida cystica. Devel. Med. Child Neurol., *14:* 757–764, 1975.
15. Soare, P. L., and Raimondi, A. J. Intellectual and perceptual motor characteristics of treated myelomeningocele children. Am. J. Dis. Child., *131:* 199–204, 1977.
16. Vance, J. C., Fazan, L. E., Satterwhite, M. A., and Pless, I. B. Effects of nephrotic syndrome on the family: a controlled study. Pediatrics, *65:* 948–955, 1980.
17. Venes, J. L. Letters to the Editor. Pediatrics, *74:* 162–163, 1984.
18. Waisbren, S. Parents' reactions after the birth of a developmentally disabled child. Am. J. Ment. Def., *84:* 345, 1979.
19. Letters to the Editor. Pediatrics, *74*(1): 162–167, 1984.

CHAPTER

23

Myelomeningocele—The Question of Selection

LESLIE N. SUTTON, M.D., EDWARD B. CHARNEY, M.D., DEREK A. BRUCE, M.D.,
and LUIS SCHUT, M.D.

The issue of selection for early surgery for the newborn with myelodys-plasia is an emotional one. Recently, greater attention to this problem by the popular press, the legislature, and various interest groups has height-ened general awareness but not resolved the ethical dilemma involved.

In the recent past, decisions regarding the aggressiveness with which a handicapped newborn would be treated were made privately in the physi-cian's office, often by the attending physician himself. As recently as 10 years ago, our group surveyed parents of children with myelomeningocele about their recollection of their own decision making process and found that the newborn's mother made the decision for or against early surgery in 1.9% of cases, and the father in 21.2%. The obvious implication was that the remainder of the decisions (76.9%) were, in fact, made by the surgeon. Certainly, in recent years the decision-making process has become more complex, but a decision-making process nonetheless remains. Even if one believes that every child with spina bifida deserves the maximum in ag-gressive care despite his eventual outcome, this still represents a decision.

The real issue then is not so much will there be a process of selection, but rather: (*a*) who shall make the selection? (*b*) what management op-tions are there? (*c*) what criteria shall be applied to an individual child at birth to determine which of the options are pursued? (*d*) how much time is there for the decision to be made? (4)

On April 15, 1985, the Department of Health and Human Services issued a set of rules under the provisions of the Child Abuse and Neglect Preven-tion and Treatment Program (5). This regulation would seem to resolve the issue questions. The government will make the decision, and all infants, no matter how damaged, will be treated with all of the facilities that modern medicine can muster unless the infant is in the process of dying. The parents are removed from the decision-making process entirely. Despite the seeming finality of this edict, discussion on the issue of selection of treatment of children with spina bifida is likely to continue as court chal-lenges and interpretations of the regulation emerge. It would, therefore, perhaps be worthwhile to review the process by which newborns with myelodysplasia have been managed at the Children's Hospital of Philadelphia, and place it in historical perspective.

HISTORY OF TREATMENT

In ancient times, no treatment was available for infants with severe congenital anomalies and the luxury of ethical decisions did not exist. Deformed and unwanted babies were thrown off a cliff in ancient Rome and placed in the woods alone with a hand-carved wooden doll for comfort by the ancient Japanese. As more effective forms of treatment for spina bifida were developed, selection was practiced. Frazier's comments represented the opinion from 1920 to 1935: contraindications to operation included "hydrocephalus, irreparable deformities, paralysis of the sphincters, complete paraplegia" or any ulcerative process in the region of the spina bifida (6). Frazier goes on to quote Hildebrand: "such children (those with complete paraplegia) should be left alone and should be allowed to die; in fact, the sooner they die, the better." The introduction of antibiotics and cerebrospinal fluid (CSF) shunts allowed for spontaneous closure of myelomeningocele sacs without surgical intervention and allowed for survival of severely handicapped individuals (10). In 1963, the group at Shefield reported a decreased incidence of ventriculitis in patients operated within the first 48 hours of life and became the prime advocates for aggressive comprehensive care of these patients. By 1971, however, this same group became disillusioned with the eventual outcome of their patients as they became older, despite satisfactory control of hydrocephalus. Lorber recommended that children with extensive paralysis, severe hydrocephalus, kyphosis, and major associated anomalies at birth be selected for no treatment:

> "The survival of so many severely handicapped children gave rise to progressively greater anxiety among doctors, nurses, parents, teachers, and the general public. This became evident with the rising tide of comments on television, radio, in newspapers, and other media. The ethical validity of prolongation of profoundly handicapped lives, consisting of frequent operations, hospital admissions, and absence from home and school with no prospect of marriage or employment became less and less tenable. The cost of maintaining such a child is now £3000 a year" (11).

Controversy arose regarding the manner of treatment given to patients selected for nonoperative treatment. Despite Lorber's insistence that "those infants were looked after as normal babies, given normal nursing care, and were fed on demand. Analgesics were given as required" (11), his report that death occurred within 9 months in all 25 infants did not agree with the experiences of most other workers who found that a signifi-cant number of children selected for no treatment will survive. Criticism focused on what was perceived as allowing babies to starve to death, as well as possible permanent increased damage to intellectual function in those unoperated patients who survived. Freeman expressed a frequently voiced response, stating that because active euthanasia of these infants is not acceptable, treatment of all affected infants is the preferred course (7).

Recently, several reports have described experiences with selection pro-cedures less controversial than Lorber's (2, 8, 12). These centers have emphasized parental involvement in decision making, counseling by ex-pert multidisciplinary teams with experience in managing children and adults with spina bifida, and continued follow-up and concern for children initially nonoperated with the opportunity for delayed surgical interven-tion. Concerns about these proposals have been both ethical and legal. It has been pointed out that although it is appropriate that parents be in-formed of the ramifications of medical care of their offspring, "one must remember that when that decision is followed by the death of the infant protagonist, his or her views are never heard!" (9) The legal aspects of selection procedures have been brought to general attention both by a few malpractice suits, and most dramatically by the "Baby Doe Cases" in which parents of newborn infants severely affected with spina bifida ini-tially opted to withhold surgical treatment and were subsequently emeshed in court battles, subjected to investigations by various advocacy groups, and ultimately stripped of their privacy and forced to watch as their family tragedies were paraded before the nations' television screens (1).

As the medical community was gradually beginning to deal with such issues by the establishment of voluntary "Ethics Committees" the federal government reacted abruptly in March of 1983 with the so-called "Baby Doe" rule, which was invalidated on May 23, 1984, by a United States District Court. A new set of regulations was issued in the Federal Register of April 15, 1985 (5). Under the rules governing child abuse and neglect, this regulation seeks to protect the rights of infants with severe or multiple handicaps and is explicit in its requirements. It first defines "medical ne-glect" as a form of child abuse, and includes within this term the "with-holding of medically indicated treatment from a disabled infant with a life threatening condition." Life-saving measures may be withheld when, in reasonable judgment (a) the infant is chronically and irreversibly coma-tose, (b) the provision of such treatment would merely prolong dying, not be effective in ameliorating or correcting all of the infant's life-threatening conditions, or otherwise be futile in terms of survival of the infant (c) and the provision of such treatment would be virtually futile in terms of the survival of the infant, and the treatment itself under such circumstances would be inhumane.

Lest there be any misunderstanding of the regulations, a set of interpretations and definitions are appended. It is clear from these that the regulation "does not sanction decisions based on subjective opinions about the future "quality of life" of a retarded or disabled person." (P.L. 4889). It is also clear that the regulation does not apply only to directly life-saving measures, but also requires medical treatment to be instituted where "the condition significantly increases the risk of the onset of complications that may threaten the life of the infant," (P.L. 4889) which, for example, would cover the care of myelomeningocele closure. The "merely prolong dying" provision is not intended to allow nontreatment in situations where many years of life will result from the provision of treatment though eventual death is expected. Thus, treatment is required in cases where death is inevitable but may be years distant (how long exactly is not stated).

Despite the seeming clarity and lack of room for interpretation of the regulation an ironic disclaimer is made:

"We want to emphasize that it is not the CPS Agency or the ICRC or similar committee that makes the decision regarding the care of and treatment for the child. This is the parents' right and responsibility. Nor is the aim of the statute, regulations, and the child abuse program to regulate health care. The parents' role as decision maker must be respected and supported *unless they choose a course of action inconsistent with applicable standards* established by law (P.L. 4880)."

As in the previous Baby Doe regulation, anyone may report suspected violations. The means of enforcement are not detailed but generally involve initiation of court-ordered evaluation of the child and treatment in instances where violations are found to have occurred. What becomes of the child afterward is not addressed, nor is the question of financial liability for the mandated treatment.

MYELOMENINGOCELE NEWBORN MANAGEMENT: A TIME FOR PARENTAL DECISION

It has been our practice at the Children's Hospital of Philadelphia over the past several years to counsel the parents of a newborn with spina bifida using a multidiciplinary approach, and to impart to them as objectively as possible the prognosis for their particular child concerning ambulation, sphincter continence, hydrocephalus, and general survival with and without surgery (2). Information is delivered at an initial meeting which ideally includes both parents, a neurosurgeon, pediatrician (Medical Director of the Spina Bifida Program), and the nurse and social worker for this program. The parents are then given the option of early surgery or conservative medical management including sterile back dressings and oral feedings to be initiated in the hospital but with the view toward continuation of conservative management at home. In general, the options of chronic institutionalization or adoption are not presented at this initial meeting. The parents are assured that should they opt for nonsurgical management the child would continue to be followed in the Spina Bifida Clinic, and that they could decide for surgery at any time should the baby survive. The parents are encouraged to choose either aggressive management or conservative treatment as outlined; partial measures such as shunting without closure of the back are not offered. Additional conferences are scheduled as needed, and any alterations in the baby's prognosis is discussed. Only in cases of severe associated anomalies felt to be incompatible with life were the parents advised against surgery, and even in these cases surgical treatment was instituted if the family wished.

The hospital records of 110 consecutive newborns referred during the period of 1978–1982 were reviewed and data collected, including level of paralysis, associated adverse criteria (kyphoscoliosis, hydocephalus, birth trauma, associated anomalies), time of back closure/shunting procedures, use of antibiotics, and disposition at discharge (home or chronic-care facility). Outcome was assessed from clinic records and consisted of mortality, degree of paralysis, incidence of ventriculitis, and developmental delay (developmental quotient <80 on the fine motor and adaptive portion of the Gesell Development Test performed at one or more years of age).

Patient Population

Forty-nine patients, 45% of the entire group, had thoracolumbar lesions (L1 and above), 20 (18%) had midlumbar paralysis (L3–4), and 41 (37%) had lumbosacral defects (L4 to sacral) (Table 23.1). Twenty (18%) of the infants had congenital hydrocephalus, eight (7%) had congenital kyphosco-

TABLE 23.1
Surgical Management and Clinical Newborn Physical Examination

Adverse Criteria	Early ($n = 52$)	Delayed ($n = 32$)	Late ($n = 12$)	None ($n = 14$)	Total ($n = 110$)
Paralysis					
L-1 ↑	17%(9)	44%(14)	100%(12)	100%(14)	45%(49)
L-3	27%(14)	19%(6)			18%(20)
L-4 ↓	56%(29)	37%(12)			37%(41)
Hydrocephalus	10%(5)	9%(3)	42%(5)	50%(7)	18%(20)
≥1 Adverse criteria	21%(11)	44%(14)	100%(12)	100%(14)	46%(51)
≥2 Adverse criteria	10%(5)	16%(6)	50%(6)	86%(12)	26%(29)

liosis, five (4%) had other gross congenital anomalies, and three newborns (3%) had associated birth injuries. Thus, 54% had no adverse criteria, 46% had one or more, and 26% had two or more.

Fifty-two (47%) of the infants had "early surgical closure" at the parents' request. Early surgical closure is defined as operation on the back within the first 48 hours of life: 17% thoracolumbar, 27% midlumbar, and 56% lumbosacral (Table 23.1). Of this group, 41 (70%) had no adverse criteria and 11 (21%) had one or more. Forty-one percent of this group received perioperative broad spectrum antibiotics and 92% required CSF shunts within the first 2 weeks of life.

Thirty-two children (29%) had "delayed surgical closure," defined as operation between 3 and 7 days of life as parents gradually reached a decision for surgical intervention: 44% thoracolumbar, 19% midlumbar, and 37% lumbosacral. Of these, 18 (46%) had no adverse criteria, and 14 (44%) had one or more. Fifty-six percent received perioperative antibiotics and 91% required shunts.

Twelve infants (11%) had "late surgical closure," sometime after the first week of life, as it became evident that the child was likely to survive and families became emotionally attached to their offspring. All of these children had thoracolumbar lesions and one or more adverse criteria. Twenty-five percent of this group had received some period of antibiotic therapy during the first week of life. Within this group there was considerable variation in length of time before surgery was eventually performed. Two underwent closure of the back within 2 weeks of life, and a total of seven were operated within a month (Table 23.2). All patients in this group were operated or discharged from the hospital before 2 weeks of age.

Fourteen patients (13%) never had surgical intervention. All had thoracolumbar lesions and adverse criteria, and 86% had two or more, including three with other gross congenital defects. One received antibiotic therapy during the initial hospitilization. Ten were discharged from the hospital (mean age 6 days), six to home, and four to community hospitals. Four died in our hospital prior to discharge.

Survival

Ninety-two percent of the babies treated with early surgery, 94% of those with delayed surgery, and 100% of the late surgery group were alive at 10 months of age. Deaths were attributable to sepsis or respiratory failure associated with severe Arnold-Chiari malformation. No patients survived past 10 months without surgery. Two died within the first week and six more within the first month (Fig. 23.1). By 8 weeks, only three infants who did not have surgery were still alive. The cause of death in this group was

TABLE 23.2

"Late" Surgical Intervention

Patient No.	Adverse Criteria*	Age at Discharge without Surgery (days)	Time at Home without Surgery (days)	Age at Surgery (days) Back	Shunt
1	A			9	15
2	A, C			19	10
3	A, C			14	16
4	A, B, C			19	14
5	A	6	11	23	18
6	A, C	9	9	23	19
7	A	10	14	25	26
8	A	8	17	57	26
9	A, E			45	45
10	A, C	1	47		49
11	A	8	41	50	52
12	A	1	300	365	302

* A = paralysis L1 and above, B = kyphoscoliosis, C = congenital hydrocephalus, D = birth injury, E = other severe birth defect.

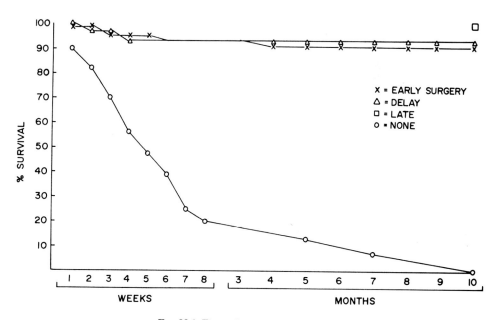

FIG. 23.1. Time of surgery and survival.

difficult to ascertain but appeared to be sepsis or complications of the Chiari malformation.

Ventriculitis

Of the 96 children who received surgical intervention, 10 (10.4%) developed ventriculitis: 5 of 52 (9.6%) of the group with early surgery, 4 of 32 (12.5%) of the group with delayed surgery, and 1 of 12 (8.3%) of those with late surgery. No association existed between time of surgery (early, delayed, or late) and incidence of ventriculitis at the .05 probability level by Fisher's exact test. Use of antibiotic coverage in the infants having surgery beyond 48 hours but within a week was associated with a decreased incidence of ventriculitis ($p < .03$).

Developmental Delay

Developmental delay, defined as developmental quotient (DQ) <80, was present in 37% of the children tested at one year of age or older. If the group is stratified by severity of the myelomeningocele and adverse criteria, we found that of 54 children tested without adverse criteria, 24% of those with early surgery and 31% of those with delayed surgery had developmental delay (Table 23.3). Of those with adverse criteria, 43% of those with early surgery, 55% of those with delayed surgery, and 67% of those with late surgery were retarded. A log linear analysis of these data revealed that although developmental delay was highly associated with severity of the lesion at birth, timing of surgery was not associated with developmental outcomes. Of five children without adverse criteria at birth who had delayed surgery and who were found to have developmental delay at 1 year or more of age, one had had fetal drug syndrome and one was quite premature. Only one child in this group had ventriculitis associ-

TABLE 23.3

Developmental Outcome in 84 Infants Who Had Surgery

Time of Surgery	No Adverse Criteria (n = 54)		>1 Adverse Criteria (n = 30)		
	Early	Delayed	Early	Delayed	Late
Developmental quotient <80	9(24%)	5(31%)	3(43%)	6(55%)	8(67%)
Developmental quotient >80	29	11	4	5	4
Total	38	16	7	11	12

ated with the poor developmental outcome. Of nine children without adverse criteria who had had early surgery but were found to have developmental delay, again, only one child had ventriculitis. Thus, developmental delay appeared to be largely determined at the time of birth and was not usually the result of ventriculitis acquired because of delay in surgery.

Paralysis

No infant appeared to gain lower extremity function as a result of surgery. Four children deteriorated one level following closure, but this was not associated with timing of surgery by Fisher's exact test.

DISCUSSION

The selective treatment of children with congenital anomalies depends upon the acceptance of the premise that it is possible to have a life so wretched that death is preferable. This is a point which is unclear both legally and ethically. Recently, the courts of three states (California, New Jersey, and Washington) have upheld the concept of suits for "wrongful life" by awarding damages on behalf of defective children in malpractice cases against obstetricians who did not counsel families to consider amniocentesis and presumably abortion (14). This would seem to suggest that the courts upheld the concept that a severely handicapped life was worse than no life at all, but the decisions were carefully worded in an attempt to avoid this issue. This is obviously dissonant when considered in light of the new federal regulations, which categorically forbid any consideration of "subjective opinions about the future 'quality of life' of a retarded or disabled person."

To be ethically defensible, a system of selection should ideally meet several tests:

1. As the infant cannot voice his or her own opinion, some person or group with the infant's interests foremost should make the ultimate decision, based on information conveyed by objective and knowledgeable sources. In the case of handicapped newborns, it is difficult to imagine people more caring for the child's well-being than the parents and physicians (1). Parental decision making does lead to an ethical dilemma in that two identical infants may be treated in different ways so that one may live and one may die simply because of parental "whim." However, the dilemma is resolved if one considers that the children cannot be considered in isolation, but rather in the context of the support and nurturing of the family milieu. Parents must be given information about prognosis of their individual infant by physicians who have extensive experience in management of spina bifida at all ages. All too often, parents of a newborn with a thoraic lesion are referred from a community hospital having been told

that "your baby has a lump in the back, but everything will be fine after he has surgery." We have found our multidisciplinary team approach to be satisfactory in that parents may be informed not only of their child's immediate perioperative outlook, but also the long-term prognosis to be expected as the child becomes older.

2. If active euthanasia is not to be employed, a group of infants will inevitably survive despite not being initially selected for surgical treatment. A selection procedure would be most acceptable if those children are not worsened by their nonoperative period of "conservative management." Our data suggest that those children who undergo delayed and late repair are intellectually worse off than the early group, not because of the timing of surgery or delayed ventriculitis, but because they were a worse group to start with. The brains of children with spina bifida are often dysmorphic, and this, more than ventriculitis, is the most likely cause of developmental delay in the majority of these children.

3. If any disagreement is present between the relevant parties, the decision should probably be surgical management. We have not encountered a situation where parents have refused surgery for a low lesion without adverse criteria, but if this were to occur, our institutional ethics committee might find a role. It should be emphasized, however, that the purpose of such committees should be education and consultation rather than actual decision making or usurping physician responsibilities (3). The ethics committee might also provide a forum for discussion when the patient's family appears incompetent.

4. For parents to make a truly informed decision, an atmosphere of "emergency decision" must be avoided (13). It is desirable that both parents engage in face-to-face exchange with the medical staff. The mother is often recovering from a cesarean section in a community hospital far removed from the center caring for the infant, and our data suggest that a period of time (a week with broad spectrum antibiotic coverage) is available for discussion without harm to the child.

In our series, the number of newborns who eventually died without surgical intervention is small (13%) in comparison with the Oklahoma group (35%) (8) and the Sheffield Group (68%) (11). Social change is perhaps part of the explanation for this, in that more recent series have shown an increased tendency for parents to ask for early surgical treatment despite a poor prognosis. This is true despite the fact that functional outcome in children has not materially changed in the past two decades (12). We feel, however, that even though the vast majority of our children with spina bifida eventually undergo surgical treatment, families are better able to cope with the result if they had some input into the decision-making process. Perhaps no group is in a better position to evaluate a selective approach to newborn management than are the parents who have been through the process themselves. We have interviewed the parents of older children with spina bifida about their feelings in this regard. When asked, "If you had the choice to make again for your child, would you still opt for surgery?", 96% of the parents responded that they would. However, when asked, "If you had another newborn with spina bifida would you withhold surgery?", 32.7% said yes. Finally, when asked, "Would you undergo amniocentesis (and presumably abortion) if you suspected a fetus with spina bifida?", 74.5% said that they would. It appears from this survey that this uniquely knowledgeable and sensitive group continues to perceive that there are judgments to be made and that they should have a role in making them.

REFERENCES

1. Angell, M. Handicapped children: Baby Doe and Uncle Sam. N. Engl. J. Med., *309(11):* 659–60, 1983.
2. Charney, E. B., Weller, S. C., Sutton, L. N., et al. Management of the newborn with myelomeningocele: time for a decision-making process. Pediatrics, *75(1):* 58–64, 1985.
3. Cranford, R. E., and Van Allen, E. J. The implications and applications of institutional ethics committees. Am. Coll. Surg. Bull. *79(6):* 19–24, 1985.
4. Delange, S. A. Selection for treatment of patients with spina bifida aperta. Devel. Med. Child Neurol., *16(32):* 27030, 1974.
5. Federal register part VI, Department of Health & Human Services, Vol. *50(72):* 14878–14901, April 15, 1985.
6. Frazier, C. H. *Surgery of the Spine and Spinal Cord,* pp. 303ff. Appleton & Co., NY and London, 1935.
7. Freeman, J. To treat or not to treat. In: *Practical Management of Myelomeningocele.* Baltimore, University Park Press, 1974. pp. 13–22.
8. Gross, R. H., Cox, A., Tatyrek, R., et al. Early management and decision making for the treatment of myelomeningocele. Pediatrics, *72(4):* 450–457, 1983.
9. Gutkelch, N. The indications and contraindications for early operation in myelomeningocele. In: *Current Controversies in Neurosurgery,* edited by T. Morley. Philadelphia, W.B. Saunders, 1976.
10. Ingraham, F. D., and Hamlin, H. Spina bifida and cranium bifidum. II. Surgical treatment. N. Engl. J. Med., *228(20):* 631–641, 1943.
11. Lorber, J. Early results of selective treatment of spina bifida cystica. Br. Med. J., *4:* 201–204, 1973.
12. McLaughlin, J. F., Shurtleff, D. B., Lamers, J. Y. et al. Influence of prognosis on decisions regarding the care of newborns with myelodysplasia. N. Engl. J. Med., *312(25):* 1589–1594, 1985.
13. Shurtleff, D. B., Hayden, P. W., Loeser, J. D., and Kronmal, R. A. Myelodysplasia: decision for death or disability. N. Engl. J. Med., *291(19):* 1005–1010, 1974.
14. Surgical Practice News, July 1985, p. 5.

V

Spinal Surgery

24

Chemonucleolysis versus Open Discectomy: The Case against Chymopapain

ARTHUR L. DAY, M.D., DOUGLAS F. SAVAGE, M.D.,
WILLIAM A. FRIEDMAN, M.D., and GEORGE W. SYPERT, M.D.

INTRODUCTION

Chemonucleolysis by injection of chymopapain is theoretically a very attractive method of treatment of lumbar disk herniation. Since its recent reintroduction into the United States, however, this technique continues to be surrounded by controversy regarding its safety and effectiveness. Our experience with this treatment modality has yielded a less than expected successful outcome rate, thus stimulating this retrospective analysis of our results in comparison to those achieved by standard or microsurgical open discectomy procedures.

MATERIALS AND METHODS

The last 151 consecutive cases of suspected lumbar disk disease, treated either by chymopapain injection (chemonucleolysis) or open surgical (standard or microsurgical) discectomy at the University of Florida, Department of Neurosurgery, were reviewed. Eleven patients were lost to follow-up, leaving 140 patients for analysis, including 70 patients who underwent the enzyme injection and 70 who had open disc procedures (17).

Historically, all patients in each group complained of unilateral leg pain (several subsequently complained of bilateral lower extremity symptoms) with or without low back pain; all were judged unresponsive to a minimum of 2 weeks of conservative therapy. Each patient's history was also classified according to duration of the sciatic component before consultation, and the presence of active workmen's compensation claims or previous lumbar spine surgery (including chymopapain injection in the open surgery group).

Physical examination findings were divided into three categories, depending on the number of signs pointing to a specific root lesion. A patient with a "classic" examination exhibited at least two of the following signs: (*a*) motor weakness of the quadriceps, dorsiflexors, or plantiflexors of the foot, (b) dermatomal sensory loss, (c) absent or asymmetrical knee or ankle reflexes, and (d) a positive crossed straight leg raise test. A patient's examination was judged "positive" when one of these signs was evident. The remaining patients did not exhibit any of these signs. All patients, however, had positive mechanical findings consisting of decreased lumbar range of motion and a positive straight leg raise test (Lasegue's maneuver).

Plain x-rays of the lumbar spine and sacrum were obtained in all patients to eliminate those with degenerative, neoplastic, or infectious etiologies. All patients underwent further radiologic assessment with lumbar metrizamide myelography and/or computed tomographic (CT) scanning. When findings were clear on clinical and CT examinations, myelography was often not performed.

If the radiologic assessment suggested a free-fragment herniation, patients were eliminated from chymopapain consideration. Initially, all other patients were then given a choice between an open surgical procedure (laminotomy and discectomy) or chemonucleolysis. More recently, after our chymopapain results were reviewed, only an open surgical procedure was offered (17).

Patients who chose chemonucleolysis were pretreated with diphenhydramine hydrochloride (50 mg po q6h) and cimetidine (300 mg po q6h) for 24–48 hours preoperatively. Routine laboratory screening included an erythrocyte sedimentation rate in all patients. Patients were also questioned about previous allergic reactions to meat tenderizer, beer, or papaya. The procedure was conducted in the operating room under flouroscopic control, using local anesthesia supplemented by intravenous sedation. Patients were placed in the prone position, and the surgeon approached the patient from the symptomatic side. For injection of the L3–4 or L4–5 interspaces, needle placement began 8 cm lateral to the appropriate intervertebral level and was aimed toward the axial plane at a 45° angle. For L5–S1 discs, the needle origination was identical to that for L4–5 discs, but was also directed 30° caudally to avoid the iliac crest. After the tip of the 18-gauge spinal needle was noted fluoroscopically to be in the center of the disc in both the anteroposterior (AP) and lateral planes, a discogram was usually performed. A test dose of 0.1–0.2 ml chymopapain was then administered, and if no allergic phenomena was observed after 15 minutes, the remainder of the enzyme was injected (3000 or 4000 units for single level patients, 6000 units for two levels). The majority of patients underwent a single level injection, and only five were treated at two levels.

Patients who elected an open surgical procedure were scheduled to receive either a traditional unilateral hemilaminotomy and discectomy under macroscopic visualization or a microsurgical discectomy with a more limited surgical exposure. In the former, the appropriate disc space was identified by counting upward from the sacrum, while the latter procedure was accompanied by intraoperative x-ray verification of spine level. In most instances, only one level was explored, and a discectomy was carried out only if pathology was surgically verified. The amount of bone removed was perhaps less in the microsurgical group, but an equivalent (and generous) discectomy was undertaken regardless of procedure type, after a window had been made in the anulus with a no. 15 surgical blade. Some patients received foraminotomy and/or hemilaminectomy in cases where bony encroachment on the root was identified.

All patients were hospitalized postoperatively at least overnight, and a decision regarding timing of discharge was thereafter made by a mutual discussion between the attending surgeon and patient. Patients were later seen in an outpatient clinic between 2 and 6 weeks after discharge, and as necessary thereafter. All 140 patients were later contacted by telephone in order to determine their final outcome. This interview was conducted by an individual other than the attending surgeon, and was performed at least 3 months after the treatment procedure.

Patients were questioned concerning activity level, pain, resumption of previous livelihood, use of analgesics, and overall satisfaction or dissatisfaction with the procedure. Based on the outcome of these interviews and the final examination findings, patients were classified into one of four groups: (a) excellent, (b) good, (c) fair, or (d) poor. Specifically, an excellent outcome was a patient who had no pain or limitation of activity. A good result was one in which the patient had occasional mild pain with only minimal limitation of activity. Patients in either of these two categories were not taking narcotic analgesics and had resumed their normal livelihood. A patient was judged to have a fair result if he was improved but still suffered moderate pain on a regular basis, had changed his activity level and/or job, and was still requiring analgesics. A poor result patient reported his pain to be unchanged or worsened after the procedure, was severely restricted in work and required frequent narcotics. For statistical and final clinical analysis, patients with excellent or good classifications were considered as satisfactory outcomes, while the other two groups (fair or poor) were considered as unsatisfactory results.

A subgroup of 19 patients subsequently underwent a second procedure because of continued pain or physical limitations. Seventeen patients received chymopapain as their initial procedure, and later underwent an open operation. The remaining two patients underwent two open procedures. In general, at least 6 weeks were allowed to elapse before consideration was given to the second procedure. Several other subpopulations with various different clinical factors were also analyzed, using both chisquare and Fisher's exact test methods, to determine their effect on outcome.

The clinical characteristics of the two large groups of patients (chymopapain vs open discectomy) are outlined in Table 24.1. There were no significant differences in age, sex distribution, workman's compensation claims incidence, duration or type of symptoms, examination findings, or duration of follow-up. Although the incidence of prior open lumbar surgery was similar in both groups, the open discectomy group also included 17 patients who had received prior chemonucleolysis, a population not matched in the chymopapain group.

Chymopapain Group (70 Patients)

Overall, 70 patients received chymopapain injections as their initial treatment for their symptomatic disc problem (17). Fifty-three patients underwent this procedure alone, while 17 (24.3%) subsequently required a second open procedure for persistent symptoms (Table 24.2). Approximately one-third of the patients suffered an increase in low back pain and/or spasm after the injection, resulting in a prolonged hospitalization in some cases. Six others (8.6%) developed complications that also could be attributable to enzyme injection, including three allergic reactions (1 major, 2 minor), one grand mal seizure, one increased deficit (foot drop), and one postoperative fever. There was no significant permanent morbidity from any of these events.

TABLE 24.1
Clinical Characteristics: All Patients*

	Chymopapain (70 pts)	Open Surgery (70 pts)
Age (years)	41.7	38.4
Sex (male/female)	49/21	43/27
Workman's compensation	20 (29%)	13 (19%)
Previous surgery (Y/N/Chym)	9/61/0	10/43/17
Duration of symptoms (% < 6 months)	9.5 (57%)	10.2 (56%)
Type of symptoms:		
Low back pain	65	60
Radiculopathy (U/B)	67/3	70/0
Physical examination findings:†		
Classic (2 signs)	32 (46%)	35 (50%)
Positive (1 sign)	22 (31%)	24 (34%)
Mechanical findings only	16 (23%)	11 (16%)
Duration of follow-up (months)	9.5	11.1

* (Y = yes; N = no; Chym = chymopapain; U = unilateral; B = bilateral).
† = all patients had (+) mechanical findings).

TABLE 24.2
Type of Treatment (All Procedures)

	No. of Patients	Ultimate Satisfactory Outcome (%)
1. Chymopapain	70	34 (49%)
2. Chymopapain and 2nd open procedure	17*	12 (71%)
Total	70*	46 (66%)
3. Microdiscectomy	43	35 (81%)
4. Standard discectomy	27	21 (78%)
5. 2nd open procedure	2	2 (100%)
Total	70	58 (83%)

* Two patients were lost to late follow-up after their second procedure.

Seventeen patients injected at our institution subsequently underwent an open procedure, and all had been screened radiographically to minimize enzyme injections into free-fragment situations. Fifteen patients underwent a hemilaminotomy and discectomy for continued nerve root compression; a free-fragment was identified in nine instances, and a bulging disc was found in 6 cases. Two of these 15 did not receive adequate follow-up and were discarded from analysis in the surgical series. Of the remaining two patients, one required a posterolateral fusion for bony instability at the previously injected level, and the other was found to have a swollen nerve root without any evidence of disc or bony compression. One of these two was also lost to late follow-up, while in the other, no disc was suspected preoperatively.

The treatment outcomes are recorded in Tables 24.2 and 24.3. Of the 70 patients injected with chymopapain, one patient had an excellent outcome and 33 had good outcomes, yielding an overall successful result in 34 (49%). Seven patients had a fair outcome, and 29 were judged as poor, providing an unsatisfactory result in 36 cases (51%). If the seventeen reoperation patients could have been screened and eliminated as having disease that would not benefit by chemonucleolysis, the success rate would be 64% (34 of 53 cases). Twelve patients with adequate follow-up in this reoperation subgroup later had successful surgery, and if their final outcomes were returned to the original group of 70 patients, 46 (66%) ultimately had a satisfactory result.

Two factors were associated with trends that favored poorer results, including a history of previous lumbar surgery and the presence of a workman's compensation claim. The only statistically significant indepen-

TABLE 24.3

Clinical Outcome: Chymopapain versus Open Discectomy†

Treatment Groups	Satisfactory E:G/S (%)	Unsatisfactory F:P/U (%)
All patients (one procedure only)*		
Chymopapain (N = 70)	1:33/34 (49%)	7:29/36 (51%)
Open discectomy (N = 70)	13:43/56 (80%)	11:3/14 (20%)
No previous surgery or WC**		
Chymopapain (N = 42)	1:20/21 (50%)	6:15/21 (50%)
Open discectomy (N = 38)	9:25/34 (89%)	4:0/4 (11%)
Classic examination, no previous surgery or WC:***		
Chymopapain (N = 21)	0:14/14 (67%)	2:5/7 (33%)
Open discectomy (N = 16)	2:12/14 (88%)	2:0/2 (12%)
No previous surgery or WC, and symptoms 6 < mo****		
Chymopapain (N = 24)	1:12/13 (54%)	3:8/11 (46%)
Discectomy (N = 23)	7:15/22 (96%)	1:0/1 (4%)

† Abbreviations: E = excellent; G – good; S = satisfactory outcome; F = fair; P = poor; U = unsatisfactory outcome; WC = workman's compensation.
 * p = 0.00009.
 ** p = 0.0001.
 *** p = 0.14.
 **** p = 0.003.

dent predictor of success was the presence of a classic clinical examination in which the success rate was 61%.

Multiple combinations of patient variables were then analyzed to try to identify a subpopulation of patients who might benefit most from enzyme injection (Table 24.3). In a subgroup from which patients with workman's compensation claims and a history of previous lumbar surgery were removed, only a 50% success rate was identified (21 of 42). The best success was found in a subgroup of patients who exhibited classic clinical features and had no prior history of surgery or workman's compensation claims in which 14 of 21 had satisfactory outcomes (67%).

The average length of hospitalization following chemonucleolysis was 3.3 days (Table 24.4). Nearly two-thirds of patients (64%) were discharged within 3 days of injection, and 90% were discharged within 1 week. The prime reason for any prolongation was worsened back pain or spasm. By adding the additional hospitalization experienced by those patients who underwent a second open surgical procedure, the average length of stay for a chymopapain patient was extended to 4.7 days.

TABLE 24.4

Length of Hospitalization (per Procedure)

Length of Post-treatment Hospitalization	Chymopapain (70 Patients)	Microdisc (43 Patients)	Standard Discectomy (27 Patients)
1–3 days	45 (64%)	25 (58%)	2 (7%)
3–5 days	13 (19%)	9 (21%)	12 (44%)
5–7 days	5 (7%)	7 (16%)	7 (26%)
7 days	7 (10%)	2 (5%)	6 (23%)
Mean:	3.3 days	3.9 days	6.6 days
	4.7 days*	4.9 days**	

* Mean hospitalization duration with additional stay required by 17 patients for second open procedure.
** Mean for all open procedures.

Open Discectomy Group (70 Patients)

Seventy patients received an open surgical discectomy (Table 24.1), including 43 patients who received a microsurgical discectomy and 27 who underwent a standard macroscopic discectomy (Table 24.2). There was no difference in clinical outcome regardless of the type of procedure performed. Complications consisted of increased root deficits in two cases, one brachial plexus stretch injury, four cases of urinary retention, three instances of fever, one dural laceration, and one wound infection. All of these problems resolved without sustained morbidity. Two patients who had initially received a standard discectomy later required a second open lumbar procedure during the interval of evaluation, and both had satisfactory results.

The open discectomy population differed from the chymopapain group by the presence of 17 failed chemonucleolysis patients thought to be harboring persistent disc herniations. This group included 13 of our original injected patients in whom follow-up was sufficient, and four others who had received their chemonucleolysis elsewhere. Eleven were subsequently found to have free-fragments, while the remaining six had herniations in continuity with the disc space. Fourteen (82%) had satisfactory outcomes, including all cases with free-fragments. Thus, the results for those patients who had undergone previous chemonucleolysis were similar to the remaining "virgin disc" patients.

The ultimate treatment outcomes are presented in Table 24.2. Initially, 56 of 70 patients (80%) achieved a satisfactory result from their original open procedure, including 13 classified as excellent and 43 as good. The two successful reoperations in this group yielded a final overall satisfactory result incidence of 83% (58 of 70 patients). Several individual clinical categories were statistically significant predictors of a successful outcome, including previous open lumbar surgery, a workman's compensation history, and a short symptom duration.

Several combinations of variables identified subgroups with significantly higher success rates (Table 24.3). If a subgroup of patients with no prior lumbar disc surgery (including chymopapain) or workman's compensation problems were excluded, 34 of 38 cases (89%) experienced a successful outcome. When patients with a classic examination were included in the patient subgroup that had no prior lumbar surgery or workman's compensation claims, 14 of 16 (88%) achieved a successful result. If all patients with prior surgery, workman's compensation claims, and symptom durations longer than 6 months were removed from analysis, the success rate reached 96% (21 of 22 cases).

The average length of hospitalization within the open discectomy group was 4.7 days post-treatment (Table 24.4). Microdiscectomy patients averaged 3.9 days, while standard discectomy patients stayed an average of 6.6 days.

DISCUSSION

Since its clinical introduction by Lyman Smith in 1965, chymopapain has been surrounded by controversy (20). While there is little doubt that the enzyme can dissolve the central portion of the nucleus pulposus, the effects on sequestered disc fragments (or even herniations in continuity) are less reliable and possibly are limited by failure of the substance to reach the area responsible for symptom production (22). In addition, the drug causes substantial allergic and/or toxic reactions (*i.e.*, paraplegia or subarachnoid hemorrhage) in approximately 1–2% of patients (21). Numerous reports in the literature have touted chemonucleolysis as the preferred initial treatment of all but the most obvious free-fragment herniations of discs in the lumbar region, with an average success rate of 70% (1, 4, 8, 12–15). A recent review of three randomized series confirms that chymopapain does have a statistically significant beneficial effect in the treatment of lumbar disc herniations when compared to placebo (6, 7, 9, 11, 18).

Using our strict grading system in defining success, however, our results and other retrospective series demonstrate a decisive advantage of open surgery to chymopapain in almost all patient subgroups, especially when those with prior workman's compensation and lumbar surgery are excluded (10, 23). Two similar prospective randomized studies comparing chymopapain to open discectomy have recently been published (3, 5). Both are limited by small numbers, but both support a clear superiority of an open procedure to that of enzyme injection.

When patients from all five randomized series are combined and reorganized according to our stricter criteria of success, the benefits of open surgery appear greater (Table 24.5). Even though the largest series does not differentiate which patients had fair results (and would thus be eliminated from the "successful" category) (9), the strictly defined success rate following chymopapain is only 53%, while open surgery achieved a 78% good outcome. These figures are nearly identical to our overall results herein.

The incidence of failure requiring a subsequent open procedure is also high (26%) in the combined randomized series, even though Javid *et al.*

TABLE 24.5

Prospective Series: Incidence of "Successful" Outcome†

Study	Placebo		Chymopapain		Open Surgery	
	S(%)	Re-op(%)	S(%)	Re-op(%)	S(%)	Re-op(%)
Schwetschenau	11/35	16/35	10/31	10/31		
Walter Reed	(31%)	(46%)	(29%)	(32%)		
(66 patients) 1976						
Fraser	9/30	11/30	17/30	5/30		
Australia	(30%)	(37%)	(57%)	(17%)		
(60 patients) 1982						
Javid	22/53	31/53*	40/55	6/55		
Smith Lab	(42%)	(58%)	(73%)	(11%)		
(55 patients) 1983**						
Ejeskar			5/15	8/15	9/14	0/14
Sweden			(33%)	(53%)	(64%)	(0%)
(29 patients) 1983						
Crawshaw			11/25	11/25	23/27	1/27
England			(44%)	(44%)	(85%)	(4%)
(52 patients) 1984						
Totals	42/118	58/118	83/156	40/156	32/41	1/41
	(36%)	(49%)	(53%)	(26%)	(78%)	(2%)

† S = satisfactory or successful outcome (excellent or good result); Re-op = received reoperation after failed initial procedure.

* All placebo failures later injected with chymopapain.

** Includes "fair" results as successes.

reported no laminectomies whatsoever in his placebo group and only six (11%) in his chemonucleolysis group (9). Our 24% incidence again nearly duplicated the composite series frequency (2, 24), and was substantially higher than the reoperation rate following an initial open procedure. Most explorations following chemonucleolysis revealed free-fragments which presumably could not be differentiated preoperatively by the best radiographic assessment. This high incidence of free-fragments implies that current radiologic techniques cannot accurately identify such lesions, or that the effects of enzyme injection may facilitate fragment extrusion. In addition, a disc "bulge" in continuity with the disc space was identified in approximately one-third of our patients, a situation that one would consider ideal for chemonucleolysis. Why were these "ideal" patients not cured by the enzyme therapy?

Included in our series is a subgroup of patients who underwent an open lumbar spine procedure for suspected disc herniation, but who had unexpected findings at time of surgery. Eight patients underwent decompressive procedures (laminectomies and/or foraminotomies) for concomitant lateral recess stenosis that closely resembled disc rupture radiographically, with a success rate of 75%. Presumably, these patients would have been unlikely to have benefited from chemonucleolysis, and it is quite possible that their bony compression would have been aggravated as the disc space collapsed following injection.

Who, then, is the ideal candidate for chemonucleolysis? Using multivarant analysis, we tried to identify which patients would be most suitable for this procedure, but were unable to isolate any subgroup that compared favorably with an open procedure. From our experience, if one takes an individual patient who has the clear-cut clinical and radiographic findings of a herniated lumbar disc (and no negative historical features such as workman's compensation or prior surgery), the success rate and ability to return to his or her former occupation is exceedingly high with an open procedure by an experienced surgeon (greater than 95%). The best possibilities offered to any subgroup in our chymopapain series did not exceed 70%, regardless of which factors were analyzed.

Furthermore, the "quality" of the successful outcome was also different between the two types of treatment. Only one of our patients receiving chymopapain alone could be categorized as an excellent result, defined as having no residual back discomfort or activity limitation whatsoever. In contrast, excellent outcomes were achieved in 13 open discectomy patients. Similar results have been reported in other nonrandomized series, and are confirmed by our data review from the prospective reports (10).

Can the shortened hospitalization and job-time loss provide justification of chemonucleolysis for economic reasons? In our series, while the initial hospital stay following the procedure was slightly less than for microsurgical discectomy, the subsequent readmissions for a second procedure quickly reversed this advantage in favor of the open procedure. In the preceding report by Shields (in this volume), this economic difference is further accentuated over longer follow-up. The average overall cost (including hospitalization and time lost from work) for the patient receiving chemonucleolysis was approximately $140,000, compared to $50,000 for that of open discectomy (19). Thus, in considering both economic and results end-points, our experience strongly favors an open microsurgical procedure as the treatment of choice for virgin lumbar disc herniations (10, 16, 19, 25).

CONCLUSIONS

Open surgical discectomy offers definite advantages over enzyme injection in the treatment of lumbar disc herniations, the greatest of which is that the compressive pathology can be directly visualized and removed. Although chemonucleolysis is quicker and avoids a skin incision (and perhaps general anesthesia), both the incidence and quality of successful outcomes are substantially less than for an open procedure. The higher failure rate, adverse tissue reactions, potentially severe neurologic catastrophes, and 1–2% anaphylaxis rates that accompany chymopapain administration do not justify its role as "the last step in conservative therapy." The severe muscle spasms and back pain lengthen the hospitalization in many patients, and combined with the high incidence of required reoperations, the drug enjoys no economic advantages. Furthermore, its ease of administration may lead to excessive number of patients receiving the treatment for inappropriate indications.

REFERENCES

1. Benoist, M., DeBurge, A., Heripret, G., *et al.* Treatment of lumbar disc herniation by chymopapain chemonucleolysis: a report on 120 patients. Spine, *7:* 613–617, 1982.
2. Carruthers, C., and Kousaie, K. Surgical treatment after chemonucleolysis failure. Clin. Orthop., *165:* 172–175, 1982.
3. Crawshaw, C., Frazer, A. M., Merriam, W. F., *et al.* A comparison of surgery and chemonucleolysis in the treatment of sciatica: a prospective randomized trial. Spine, *9:* 195–198, 1984.
4. Dabezies, E. J., and Brunet, M. Chemonucleolysis versus laminectomy. Orthopedics, *1:* 26–29, 1978.
5. Ejeskar, A., Nachemson, A., Herberts, P., *et al.* Surgery versus chemonucleolysis for herniated lumbar discs: a prospective study with random assignments. Clin. Orthop., *174:* 236–242, 1983.
6. Fraser, R. D. Chymopapain for the treatment of intervertebral disc herniation: a preliminary report of a double-blind study. Spine, *7:* 608–612, 1982.
7. Haines, S. J. The chymopapain clinical trials. Neurosurgery, *17:* 107–110, 1985.

8. Javid, M. J. Treatment of herniated lumbar disc syndrome with chymopapain. J.A.M.A., 243: 2043–2047, 1980.
9. Javid, M. J., Nordby, E. U., Ford, L. T., et al. Safety and efficacy of chymopapain (chymodiactin) in herniated nucleus pulposus with sciatica: results of a randomized, double-blind study. J.A.M.A., 249: 2489–2494, 1983.
10. Maroon, J. C., and Abla, A. Microdiscectomy versus chemonucleolysis. Neurosurgery, 16: 644–649, 1985.
11. Martins, A. N., Ramirez, A., Johnston, J., et al. Double-blind evaluation of chemonucleolysis for herniated lumbar discs: late results. J. Neurosurg., 49: 816–27, 1978.
12. McCulloch, J. A. Chemonucleolysis: experience with 2000 cases. Clin. Orthop., 146: 128–135, 1980.
13. Nordby, E. J., and Lucas, G. L. A comparative analysis of lumbar disk disease treated by laminectomy or chemonucleolysis. Clin. Orthop., 90: 119–129, 1973.
14. Onofrio, B. M. Injection of chymopapain into intervertebral discs. Preliminary report on 72 patients with symptoms of disc disease. J. Neurosurg., 42: 384–388, 1975.
15. Parkinson, D., and Shields, C. Treatment of protruded lumbar intervertebral disc with chymopapain. J. Neurosurg., 39: 203–208, 1973.
16. Ramirez, L. F., and Javid, M. J. Cost effectiveness of chemonucleolysis versus laminectomy in the treatment of herniated nucleus pulposus. Spine, 10: 363–367, 1985.
17. Savage, D. F., Friedman, W. A., and Sypert, G. W. Chemonucleolysis: The University of Florida Experience presented at the Annual Meeting of the Joint Section on Spinal Disorders, Grenelefe, Florida, 1985.
18. Schwetschenau, P. R., Ramirez, A., Johnston, J., et al. Double-blind evaluation of intradiscal chymopapain for herniated lumbar discs: early results. J. Neurosurg., 45: 622–627, 1976.
19. Shields, C. Current update of chymopapain. Clin. Neurosurg., 33: 1986.
20. Smith, L. Enzyme dissolution of the nucleus pulposus in humans. J.A.M.A., 187: 137–140, 1964.
21. Watts, C. Complications of chemonucleolysis for human disc disease. Neurosurgery, 1: 2–5, 1977.
22. Watts, C. Mechanisms of action of chymopapain in ruptured lumbar disc disease. Clin. Neurosurg., 30: 642–653, 1982.
23. Watts, C., Hutchison, G., Stern, J., et al. Comparison of intervertebral disc disease treatment by chymopapain and open surgery. J. Neurosurg., 42: 397–400, 1975.
24. Weir, B., and Jacobs, G. Reoperation rate following lumbar discectomy. Spine, 5: 366–370, 1980.
25. Wilson, D., and Harbaugh, R. Microsurgical and standard removal of the protruded lumbar disc: a comparative study. Neurosurgery, 8: 422–427, 1981.

25

In Defense of Chemonucleolysis

CHRISTOPHER B. SHIELDS, M.D., F.R.C.S. (C)

Much controversy has developed between the advocates and critics of chemonucleolysis with chymopapain. However, since the initial enthusiasm following its release by the Food and Drug Administration, there has been a reluctance by many neurosurgeons and orthopedic surgeons to continue using it for the treatment of lumbar disc disease. In a poll conducted by the American Association of Neurological Surgeons (AANS) and the Congress of Neurological Surgeons (CNS) in 1984 (36), it was noted that over half (52%) of the 858 neurosurgeons responding to the questionnaire had discontinued chemonucleolysis because the procedure was not efficacious (42%) or the risks were too great (33%). The poll also indicated that chemonucleolysis was believed by 60% of respondents to be less safe than surgery, by 36% to be equally safe, and by 4% to be safer than surgery. Furthermore, 87% of the surgeons believed that chemonucleolysis was less efficacious than surgery, 12% felt it was equally efficacious, and 1% believed it was more efficacious. This change in attitude had followed several reports of major neurologic complications consisting of paraplegia, strokes, and subarachnoid hemorrhage. However, the risks can be largely eliminated by (a) excluding patients allergic to chymopapain, (b) use of local anesthesia, (c) precise technique, and (d) careful postinjection care. Chemonucleolysis with chymopapain is not a panacea for the treatment for lumbar disc disease. Nonetheless, there is a small group of patients who may benefit by experiencing a shorter postoperative course, decreased morbidity, and cost savings.

BIOCHEMISTRY

The nucleus pulposus is a gel-like structure with few cells containing an amorphous ground substance with a high content of mucopolysaccharides (MPS) which binds to water. The annulus fibrosis is made up of both collagen I (40%) and collagen II (60%) in alternating sheets arranged in a criss-cross fashion (25). Chymopapain, a proteolytic enzyme, selectively disrupts the MPS-water-protein complex, the products of which all are soluble. The remaining products are keratosulfate and chondroitin sulfate, both soluble complex polysaccharides having a low molecular weight and viscosity. Urinary chondroitin-6-SO4 is increased for 3 days following chemonucleolysis. Chymopapain immunoreactive protein (CIP) is detected in serum within 30 minutes after injection and remains for 1 week (18). CIP is inhibited by α-2-macroglobulin (molecular weight 800,000), which is a general inhibitor of all proteolytic enzymes (31).

Toxicology studies demonstrate that chymopapain damages small blood vessels by acting on glycoaminoglycans. All vessels are vulnerable, but this effect is most significant in the central nervous system only when supratherapeutic doses are injected intrathecally since cerebrospinal fluid (CSF) contains a low concentration of α-2-macroglobulin (14, 31).

Chymopapain has no damaging effect on collagen of the annulus, dura, bone, or ligaments, and no injury to nerve roots is noted on electron microscopic studies after topical application of chymopapain (20). However, intrafascicular injection (19) produced widespread axonal damage and significant electrophysiologic changes. Topical application of chymopapain to the rabbit tibial nerve caused marked degeneration of nerve fibers as well as epidural and endoneurial fibrosis, presumably secondary to vascular changes (4, 5). Alternatively, Rydivik (28) and Watts (35) have suggested that pain relief occurs following direct neurolytic effect of small pain fibers located within the superficial layer of the annulus and nerve root.

Sequestered disc fragments have a high content of collagen (B protein) that resists dissolution by chymopapain, accounting for the poor results in patients harboring this condition (26, 27). Thus, the protruded disc with a fragment of nucleus impacted in the annulus may be the only type to obtain significant relief from chemonucleolysis to the extent that it contains protein-polysaccharides subject to hydrolysis. The development of the high resolution computed tomographic (CT) scan has facilitated the identification of such patients.

ANAPHYLAXIS

Chymopapain antigenicity is one-fortieth that of animal serum (23). Anaphylaxis is the most severe allergic complication of chymopapain. Use of local anesthesia with neuroleptic supplementation is associated with a 0.4% incidence of anaphylaxis, whereas use of general anesthesia has a 0.9% incidence (24). General anesthesia may act either as a secondary antigen causing further histamine release or by lowering the anaphylactic threshold to chymopapain. A 4:1 female preponderance to anaphylaxis has been reported (23), but is not widely supported. Prior sensitization to chymopapain in foods (meat tenderizer, papaya, beer), pharmaceuticals (toothpaste, digestive aids, cosmetics, contact lens wash solution), or environmental (leather treatment and laboratory reagents) is necessary to cause anaphylaxis. Persons living in the southern part of the United States, such as California (0.6%) or Texas (1.5%), have a higher incidence of anaphylaxis, while those in northern states have a much lower incidence (Minnesota, 0.09%) (2).

Anaphylaxis occurs through bridging of the chymopapain antigen to two adjacent IgE molecules situated on the basophil and mast cell membranes. Such binding precipitates a cascade of enzymatic reactions (both membranous and cytoplasmic), causing liberation of several chemical mediators. Adenylcyclase is activated, causing a rapid increase of cyclic adenosine monophosphate (cAMP) (15 seconds), methylation of membrane phospholipids (30 seconds), calcium ion flux (2 minutes), and histamine release 5 minutes after injection. Release of histamine causes tachycardia (<2 ng/ml), hypotension (<5 ng/ml), fibrillation (15 ng/ml), and cardiac arrest at concentrations greater than 50 ng/ml (23).

Several tests have been developed to identify the immunologically susceptible patient.

1. Direct antibody measurement (DAM). These tests quantitate the level of IgE antibodies against chymopapain, which are present in 2–3% of the population. Of patients suffering an anaphylactic reaction, 58% have chymopapain-specific IgE identified in their serum.

(a) The Radio Allergosorbent Test (RAST) exposes a paper impregnated with chymopapain to the patient's serum, allowing attachment of available IgE antibodies. A radioactive detector antibody (IgE) binds to IgE antibody on the paper, allowing the gamma activity to be quantitated. Patients demonstrating greater than 2% binding are classified as positive. If the RAST is negative, there is a 99% chance that an allergic response will not occur; if positive, an allergic reaction will occur in 14% of those undergoing injections (31).

(b) The Fluorescent Allergosorbent Test (FAST) is similar to the RAST test, but IgE antibody levels are quantitated by fluorescence rather than a radioactive technique (31).

2. Skin test (21). Although not FDA approved, this test is highly reliable, safe, and inexpensive in identifying a population allergic to chymopapain. McCulloch recommends that a solution consisting of 1 ml of Albay Buffered Saline and Phenol Diluent for Allergenic Extract (Holister-Stier, West Haven, CT), 1 ml of glycerol (99.5%), and 1 vial of chymopapain be used as the test solution. After sitting for 24 hours this solution loses its enzymatic activity but not its antigenicity, and 1 drop of this solution is used for a standard prick skin test. A positive reaction consists of a flare surrounding the test site (greater than control using a mixture without

chymopapain). A vial of the test solution is viable as an antigenic reagent for 3 months. McCulloch and Brock tested 970 patients, and they eliminated 26 skin test-positive patients. No case of anaphylaxis has occurred in a skin test-negative patient.

If any of the above tests are positive, the patient is rejected, even though 2–3% would have had only a minor allergic reaction. This is a small cost to protect the 0.5–1% population at risk for anaphylaxis.

Although the value of premedication is unproven, we administer 500 mg of hydrocortisone sodium succinate IV (Solu-Cortef-Upjohn Company, Kalamazoo, MI), and 50 mg of diphenhydramine (IV) (Benadryl-Parke Davis, Morris Plains, NJ) on call to the operating room and 300 mg of cimetidine every 8 hours for 24 hours (Tagamet-Smith, Kline and French, Philadelphia, PA) before injection (30). A test dose of 0.2 ml of chymopapain to identify the allergic patient is unnecessary because anaphylaxis is not dose dependent and a negative response often gives a false sense of security. Current experience based on phase IV drug monitoring has shown no clear difference between risk of anaphylaxis following injection of 0.2 ml or 2 ml of chymopapain. Indeed, 35 of 171 anaphylactic reactions occurred after a therapeutic dose, and 52 of 171 after a test dose. In the remainder (84 of 171) an anaphylactic reaction occurred after injection of a therapeutic dose despite the fact that a test dose had been administered at least 10 minutes earlier (23).

PATIENT SELECTION

Following a trial of complete bed rest for 10–14 days with continued intractable back and leg pain, a myelogram and/or CT scan demonstrating a protruded disc (bulging annulus with nuclear entrapment within the annular fibers) a patient may be offered the option of chemonucleolysis with chymopapain. Sequestered or extruded discs, in which larger nuclear fragments extend beyond the outer annular fibers, are unlikely to benefit from chemonucleolysis. Unfortunately, such a distinction is frequently impossible in clinical assessment, myelography, or CT scan, causing difficulty in deciding who may benefit. Absolute contraindications for chemonucleolysis are (a) allergy to chymopapain, (b) cauda equina syndrome (bladder or bowel paresis), and (c) pregnancy. Relative contraindications include patients harboring (a) diabetes with peripheral neuropathy, (b) spinal stenosis, (c) spondylolisthesis, (d) osteoarthritic spurs, (e) prior chemonucleolysis with chymopapain, (f) allergy to iodine-containing compounds, and (g) emotional or medical problems. If one excludes patients having sequestered or extruded fragments, or any of the above contraindications, perhaps only 15–20% of patients with a lumbar disc syndrome are candidates for chemonucleolysis.

DISCOGRAPHY

Discography performed in conjunction with chemonucleolysis is unnecessary and is associated with increased risk (17). Anteroposterior and lateral intraoperative radiograms adequately confirm correct needle tip position (26). Positive contrast agents used for discography may track into the subarachnoid space causing meningeal irritation, but no cases have been reported of cerebral subarachnoid hemorrhage, transverse myelitis, or cauda equina syndromes following discography (33). Some surgeons believe that abnormal discography is desirable to confirm the level to be injected. However, clinical assessment, myelography, CT scan, and magnetic resonance imaging are adequate enough to confirm the symptomatic disc level. Furthermore, the tract demonstrated by the contrast agent does not necessarily predict the flow direction of chymopapain since the latter is positively charged and immediately bound to the negatively charged nucleus pulposus. The potential relationship between major neurologic complications and use of positive contrast agents for discography has mitigated against discography in conjunction with chemonucleolysis. The leakage of both contrast agent and chymopapain into the subarachnoid space may increase the drug's neurotoxic effect in humans. Agre reported a high incidence of paraplegia in baboons receiving an intrathecal injection of chymopapain mixed with several radiopaque contrast agents, whereas none became paraplegic following intrathecal injection of chymopapain alone (1).

As chemonucleolysis avoids an incision, muscle stripping, bone removal, and nerve root retraction. Local wound pain is minimal. This usually results in a shortened hospital stay and earlier return to full activities (12).

FINANCIAL CONSIDERATIONS

The question of cost effectiveness of chemonucleolysis with chymopapain versus discography has been addressed by Ramirez and Javid (27), who noted an overall cost savings of 30% using chemonucleolysis as compared with laminectomy. This included a 77% savings in the professional fee and savings on the hospital charge of 51%. McCullough estimated a 20–30% failure with chemonucleolysis requiring reoperation, which would lessen the apparent financial savings of chemonucleolysis (21). Camp (7) has studied the total costs of various types of treatment for lumbar disc disease which included permanent partial disability, total temporary disability, closing award, and medical costs. The cost of microsurgical discectomy, "standard" discectomy, and chemonucleolysis is summarized in Table 25.1. The controversy concerning the cost of chemonucleolysis versus surgery remains unresolved and needs to be addressed from several points

TABLE 25.1

	Medical Costs (A)	Average Total Cost (B)	Total for Successful Outcome (C)
Microsurgical discectomy	$ 7,100	$17,100	$ 18,200
"Standard" laminectomy	$10,200	$28,900	$ 49,000
Chemonucleolysis	$17,300	$36,400	$143,197

of view, i.e., disability awards, duration of hospitalization, physician fees, and geographic region.

RESULTS

Surgical versus chemonucleolysis outcome is difficult to compare because series are not randomized, do not follow rules for clinical trials, have dissimilar patient groups, or represent series in which treatment modalities took place at different points in time (15).

Four double-blind studies have assessed the efficacy of chymopapain versus placebo (13, 16, 29). Three demonstrated the superiority of chemonucleolysis, and one showed no advantage. The first double-blind study, reported by Schwetschenau et al. (29), indicated a 58% efficacy rate using chymopapain compared to 49% with placebo (cysteine hydrochloride, disodium edetate, and sodium iothalamate—(CEI)). This study was criticized on the basis of a preponderance of veterans, use of a potentially pharmacologically active agent as placebo, inexperience of investigators, premature code breaks, and use of a low dose of chymopapain. Fraser (13) reported success in 80% of patients at 6 months, 73% at 2 years using chymopapain compared to 57% and 47% using saline, respectively. Javid et al. (16) reported the Illinois study in which chymopapain was successful in 72% of patients compared to 42% of patients using saline. Between 1979 and 1982 another U.S. study sponsored by the Travenol Corporation demonstrated a success rate of 71% using chymopapain and 45% using CEI 6 months following injection.

Ramirez and Javid (28) have summarized results from the literature of lumbar laminectomy for discogenic radiculopathy involving 13,212 patients; 77% had excellent-good results, 9% had a poor outcome, and 9% required reoperation. Published results of 14,438 patients undergoing chemonucleolysis demonstrated excellent-good results in 76% and a poor outcome in 15%, which was twice as frequent as following laminectomy. Chemonucleolysis failures were due to disc sequestrations and lateral canal stenosis in 50–80% of patients, most of whom subsequently had a good result following surgical discectomy.

COMPLICATIONS

Several major complications following lumbar discectomy and che-monucleolysis have been reported. Emotional and passionate descriptions of these complications have been cited as reasons to abolish use of chymo-papain (11, 32). Many patients described by Fager (11) as failures were inappropriate candidates for chemonucleolysis, most of whom presented with back pain, arthritic spurs, or spine instability. Nonetheless, well-docu-mented major complications have included anaphylaxis, paraplegia, and cerebrovascular accidents (1–3, 6, 8–10, 34).

1. Anaphylaxis has resulted in seven deaths, all occurring under general anesthesia. By excluding patients with a positive chymopapain sensitivity test and following a strict protocol in the treatment of anaphylaxis, this risk can be virtually eliminated.

2. Paraplegia has been documented in 35 patients both as acute trans-verse myelitis (8 patients) and cauda equina syndrome (27 patients). Acute transverse myelitis develops from 10–21 days following an uneventful postchemonucleolysis course. Once symptoms begin, a rapidly progress-ing thoracic transverse myelopathy develops, including sensory-motor and sphincter loss. Myelography has failed to disclose intraspinal mass lesions to explain the myelopathy. The neurologic deficits slowly improve over the course of several months. The etiology of acute transverse myelitis is unknown, but its delayed development has raised the possibility of an immune reaction. On the other hand, the cauda equina syndrome always follows a technically difficult procedure, with symptoms developing within 24 hours. Only infrequently has this syndrome shown any resolution (9). Myelography has demonstrated a large sequestered disc in three patients, but no abnormality to explain the cauda equina syndrome in the remain-der. Of the three patients demonstrating sequestered discs, two showed complete recovery and the other had a mild deficit following surgical removal of the disc. The pathogenesis of transverse myelitis and the cauda equina syndrome is unknown, but possibly an admixture of chymopapain and contrast agent (used for discography) extends intrathecally through a dural needle rent, creating a direct neurotoxic effect on spinal cord and/or nerve roots. Even though neurotoxic effects have followed the intrathecal injection of chymopapain in animals, virtually every patient suffering para-plegia had a combination of chymopapain and positive contrast agent (for discography) injected. If paraplegia in either form develops, the accepted management consists of thoracic and lumbar myelography if the CSF is not hemorrhagic. If a large intraspinal defect exists, the patient requires decompressive laminectomy and discectomy. If the CSF is bloody, barbo-tage with warm lactate Ringer's solution is performed, and systemic corti-costeroids are administered.

3. Cerebrovascular complications have caused eight deaths due to subarachnoid and intracerebral hemorrhages. The cause of the subarachnoid hemorrhage was unknown in four patients, was due to a cerebral aneurysm in one patient, and was caused by an arteriovenous malformation in three patients. Eight cerebrovascular accidents have been documented, consisting of three patients with transient ischemic attacks, and one each with a basal ganglia infarct, hemiparesis, and visual field defect.

Other complications have included discitis (aseptic and bacterial) in 51, seizures in four, Guillain-Barré syndrome in one, ocular nerve palsy in one, causalgia in four, and meningismus in one (34).

CONCLUSION

In spite of the potential risks, with careful patient selection, the use of local anesthesia, avoidance of discography, and single level injections, there is still a role for chemonucleolysis in the treatment of lumbar disc syndrome with radiculopathy. By using the proper techniques, risks are minimal and the hospital stay is shortened. Furthermore, there is less epidural, arachnoidal, intraneural, and muscular scarring compared to surgery. Surgery allows direct visualization of the pathology as well as providing superior results; however, this does require dissection of the lumbar spine with the potential attendant complications therein.

REFERENCES

1. Agre, K. Serious neurological adverse events associated with adverse events associated with administration of chymodiactin. In: *Chemonucleolysis*, edited by J. E. Brown, E. J. Nordby, and L. Smith, Chapter 15, pp. 203–216. Slack, Thorofare, NJ, 1985.
2. Agre, K., Wilson, R., Brim, *et al.* Chymodiactin post marketing surveillance. Demographic and adverse experience data in 29,075 patients. Spine, *9:* 479–485, 1984.
3. Bouilet, R. Complications of discal hernia therapy. Comparative study regarding surgical therapy and nucleolysis by chymopapain. Acta Orthorp. Belg. (Suppl. 1), 48–78, 1983.
4. Branemark, P. I. Tissue effects of chymopapain. J. Neurosurg., *42:* 488, 1975.
5. Branemark, P. I., Ekholdm, R., and Lundskog, M. L. Tissue response to chymopapain in different concentrations. Clin. Orthop., *67:* 52–67, 1969.
6. Buchman, A., Wright, R. B., Wichter, M. D., *et al.* Hemorrhage complications after the lumbar injection of chymopapain. Neurosurgery, *16:* 222–224, 1985.
7. Camp, P. Cost comparison: microsurgical discectomy, standard laminectomy, and chemonucleolysis. Presented at the Annual Meeting of the American Association of Neurological Surgeons, Denver, April, 1986.
8. Davis, R. J., North, R. B., Campbell, J. N., *et al.* Multiple cerebral hemorrhages following chymopapain chemonucleolysis. J. Neurosurg., *61:* 169–171, 1984.
9. Dyck, P. Paraplegia following chemonucleolysis: a case report and discussion of neurotoxicity. Spine, *10:* 359–362, 1985.
10. Equro, H. Transverse myelitis following chemonucleolysis. J. Bone Joint Surg. (Am), *65:* 1328–1330, 1983.
11. Fager, C. A., Freidberg, S. R., Tarlov, E., *et al.* The case against chymopapain, continued. Presented at the Annual Meeting of the American Association of Neurological Surgeons, Atlanta, 1985.

12. Farfan, H. F. The use of mechanical etiology to determine the efficacy of active intervention in single joint lumbar intervertebral joint problems. Surgery and chemonucleolysis compared: a prospective study. Spine, 10: 350–362, 1985.

13. Fraser, R. D. Chymopapain for the treatment of intervertebral disc herniation: a preliminary report of a double blind study. Spine, 7: 608–612, 1982.

14. Garvin, P. J., Jenings, R. B., Smith, L., et al. Chymopapain: a pharmacologic and toxicologic evaluation in experimental animals. Clin. Orthop., 41: 204–222, 1965.

15. Haines, S. J. The chymopapain clinical trials. Neurosurgery, 17: 107–110, 1985.

16. Javid, M. J., Nordby, E. J., Ford, L. T., et al. Safety and efficacy of chymopapain (Chymodiactin) in herniated nucleus pulposes with sciatica: results of a randomized double blind study. JAMA, 249: 2489–2494, 1983.

17. Junk, L., and Marshall, W. H. Neurotoxicity of radiological contrast agents. Ann. Neurol., 13: 469–484, 1983.

18. Kapsalis, A. A., Sterne, I. J., and Bornstein, I. The fate of chymopapain injected for therapy of intervertebral disc disease. J. Lab. Clin. Med., 83: 532–540, 1974.

19. Mackinnon, S. E., Hudson, A. R., Llamas, F., et al. Peripheral nerve injury by chymopapain injection. J. Neurosurg., 61: 1–8, 1984.

20. McCulloch, J. A. Chemonucleolysis: experience with 2000 cases. Clin. Orthop., 146: 128–135, 1980.

21. McCulloch, J. A. Thoughts on skin testing. Alternatives Spinal Surg., 2: 12–13, 1985.

22. Medical World News. Chymopapain: Help or hindrance? May 25, 1985.

23. Moneret-Vantrin, D. A., and Laxenaire, M. C. Anaphylaxis to purified chymopapain. In: Current concepts in chemonucleolysis, edited by J. C. Sutton, Series no. 72. Royal Society of Medicine International Congress Symposium, London, 1985.

24. Moss, J., McDermott, D. J., Thisted, R. A., et al. Anaphylactic/anaphylactoid reactions in response to Chymodiactin (chymopapain). Anesth. Analg., 63: 253, 1984.

25. Naylor, A. The biophysical and biochemical aspects of intervertebral disc herniation and degeneration. Ann. R. Coll. Surg. Engl., 31: 91–114, 1962.

26. Parkinson, D., and Shields, C. Treatment of protruded lumbar intervertebral discs with chymopapain (Discase). J. Neurosurg., 39: 203–208, 1973.

27. Ramirez, L. F., and Javid, M. J. Cost effectiveness of chemonucleolysis versus laminectomy in the treatment of herniated nucleus pulposus. Spine, 10: 363–367, 1985.

28. Rydevik, B., Branemark, P. I., Nordborg, C., et al. Effects of chymopapain on nerve tissue. Spine, 1: 137–148, 1976.

29. Schwetschenau, P. R., Archimedes, R., Johnston, J., et al. Double blind evaluation of intradiscal chymopapain for herniated lumbar discs: early results. J. Neurosurg., 45: 622–627, 1976.

30. Shields, C. B. Chemonucleolysis with chymopapain. Contemp. Neurosurg., 6: 1–7, 1984.

31. Sterne, I. J. The Biochemistry and Toxicology of Chymopapain in Chemonucleolysis, edited by J. E. Brown, E. J. Nordby, and L. Smith, pp. 11–28. Slack, Thorofare, NJ, 1985.

32. Sussman, B. J. Inadequacies and hazards of chymopapain injections as treatment for intervertebral disc disease. J. Neurosurg., 42: 389–396, 1975.

33. Taylor, W. K., and Pepe, R. G. Neurological complications related to contrast material. Alternatives Spinal Surg., 2: 6–9, 1985.

34. Watts, C. Complications of chemonucleolysis for lumbar disc disease. Neurosurgery, 1: 2–5, 1977.

35. Watts, C. Mechanism of action of chymopapain in ruptured lumbar disc disease. Clin. Neurosurg., 30: 642–653, 1983.

36. Watts, C. Chymopapain: is it safe and effective? Results of a 1985 AANS/CNS survey. AANS Newslett., 10: 1–2, 1985.

26

Microlumbar Discectomy

JOSEPH C. MAROON, M.D., and ADNAN A. ABLA, M.D.

The landmark paper by Mixter and Barr (23) in 1934 entitled, "Rupture of the Intervertebral Disc with Involvement of the Spinal Cord" established the degenerative or traumatic cause of lumbar disc herniation and its relationship to sciatica. Prior to that time, disc protrusions were considered neoplastic and were called enchodromas (13). Successful prior removal had been accomplished by Oppenheim and Krause (25), Stookey (34), Sashin (27), and Dandy (7), but they had not appreciated the true nature of these protrusions.

Initially, total laminectomy and transdural exploration was the procedure used to discover herniated discs, which were removed by separating the roots of the cauda equina. Love realized early that such aggressive procedures were not needed for disc removal (19). In 1939, he further improved upon this approach and recommended only an interlaminar fenestration of the ligamentum flavum as the procedure of choice for disc removal (20). Semmes (30) recognized that disc recurrences from the same interspace occurred and suggested curettement of the disc and cartilaginous endplates to avoid such recurrences.

In subsequent large surgical series, satisfactory results following lumbar disc operations have ranged 60–98% (2, 4, 9, 14, 24, 26). However, Sparup (32), in a review of 14 surgical series studied between 1942 and 1959 found 49% of the patients experiencing persistent back pain. In another review of operated patients, approximately 10% experienced reoperation at the same level (17, 28, 35). Postoperative perineural adhesions (16, 22), arachnoiditis, intraneural scarring, misdiagnosis, and performance of an incorrect operative procedure were cited as causes for failure (1, 3, 18, 21).

Fager (10), in an analysis of failures and poor results of lumbar spine surgery stated, "there remains a large if not increasing number of patients in whom results have been poor. Many of these patients have pain that is worse than that for which the procedure was undertaken." He considered inadequate surgical exposure to be a major technical problem in the failure to obtain good results in lumbar disc surgery. He advocated wide bone removal and even partial facetectomy to avoid nerve root damage and gain adequate exposure without excessive retraction of the nerve or dura. Using a wide operative exposure, Scoville reported in 1973 good to excellent results in 96% of his 779 patients (29). Despite admonitions of the need for meticulous surgical technique (5, 8, 11, 31, 33) and proper selection of patients, poor results still occur from disc surgery because of technical inadequacies. Undue retraction and trauma to the nerve root, the use of coagulation in the epidural space, and inadequate bone removal all contribute to the morbidity of the operation.

In an attempt to avoid such technical problems, Yasargil in 1967 advocated the use of the operating microscope and microsurgical techniques for lumbar disc removal (38). He cited the improved vision and illumination available, the ability to identify precisely structures in deep surgical wounds, the possibility of preserving epidural fat, the safe control of bleeding with bipolar coagulation, and the minimal trauma to paravertebral muscles when a small incision was used. In 1972, Williams published the results of his surgical experiences with microlumbar discectomy (36). Other authors including Goald (12), Hudgins (15), Casper (6), and Wilson (37) have subsequently published their surgical results and all indicated a 90%+ success rate. In addition, hospitalization time was reduced and earlier return to work was possible.

Four years ago we began using microsurgical techniques for disc removal and have been similarly impressed with reduced morbidity, earlier hospital discharge, and earlier return to work status. The purpose of this paper is to report our surgical technique and our preliminary results with this method.

METHODS

Selection of Patients

In this retrospective study, 120 patients were selected as candidates for microdiscectomy. All had symptoms of lumbar disc disease that included low back or radicular pain into one or both extremities that was not relieved after a strict conservative regimen, usually of a minimum of 4 weeks. Conservative treatment included bedrest, physical therapy, muscle relaxants, and analgesics. Positive physical findings consisted of one or more of the following: (a) a positive straight leg-raising test on the symptomatic side or a positive cross straight leg-raising test with pain referred to the symptomatic side; (b) weakness of the dorsal or plantar flexors of the foot; (c) an appropriate sensory loss; or (d) evidence of depressed or absent reflexes consistent with the clinical syndrome.

Diagnostic studies in all patients included the routine laboratory studies plus a myelogram and/or a CT scan that demonstrated an extradural defect consistent with a herniated lumbar disc and the clinical syndrome. Only "virgin" disc herniations were treated by microlumbar discectomy.

Patients were excluded from consideration if they exhibited a pending evaluation of or claim for compensation; or evidence of a narrow spinal canal syndrome as suggested by physical findings or myelography.

Microdiscectomy

The technique for microdiscectomy was patterned after that popularized by Williams (36), with a few modifications. All patients were placed in the lateral position with the affected side up, and the surgeon seated (Fig. 26.1). A midline 1-inch skin incision was made based on palpation of the spinous processes, the relationship of the L4–5 interspace to the iliac crest, and, when indicated, intraoperative roentgenograms. Although the incision is made directly over the interspinous space in the lateral position, it is approximately an inch from the midline. The skin and fascia are incised, and subperiosteal dissection is carried out. A Taylor or the Williams retractor is then inserted and fixed lateral to the facet.

At this point, the operating microscope is brought into use. A high speed air drill with a cutting bit is used to remove the inferior portion of the superior lamina, the medial portion of the facet if the interlaminar space is narrow, and the superior portion of the inferior lamina when the position of the herniation requires additional exposure (Fig. 26.2). Lateral exposure is essential to reduce nerve root retraction.

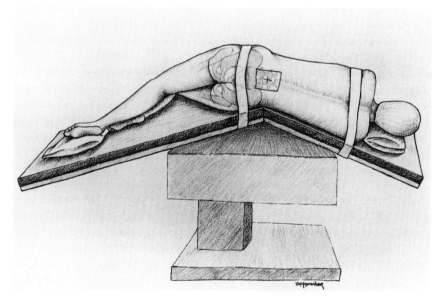

FOR POSITION ONLY

FIG. 26.1. Position of patient showing location of incision.

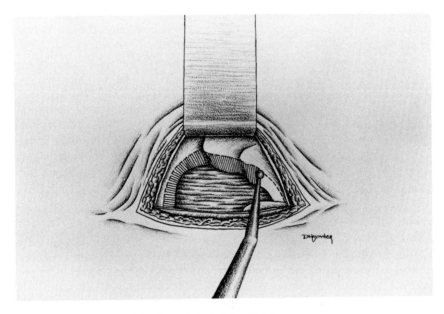

FIG. 26.2. Use of air drill for additional exposure.

The ligamentum flavum is incised with a no. 15 scalpel blade, and a cottonoid is inserted to protect the underlying dura matter and nerve root. A small curette is then inserted through the opening to detach the ligamentum flavum from its superior, lateral, and inferior points of fixation. That part of the ligament unremoved with this technique is grasped with a 45°, 1-mm rongeur. If the nerve root is immediately visualized and further lateral exposure is required, additional bone is removed with the angled Kerrison rongeur. The nerve root is protected during all dissection, particularly when introducing the angled rongeurs. In patients with large disc herniations, it may be necessary to approach the disc in an intraaxillary manner.

The epidural veins are identified and coagulated with bipolar coagulation on a low setting. Microscissors are used to transect the veins and also the epidural fat, which is separated with a blunt Penfield dissector. The nerve root and dural sac are displaced medially using a no. 5 suction tip or the Williams suction retractor (Fig. 26.3). Free-fragments of disc are mobilized using a 90° micronerve hook, or are grasped directly with the Williams disc forceps. If the disc remains under the posterior longitudinal ligament, the ligament is opened in a circular fashion with a knife. Removal of disc tissue is performed with variously sized rongeurs. An attempt is made to remove as much disc as possible consistent with safety.

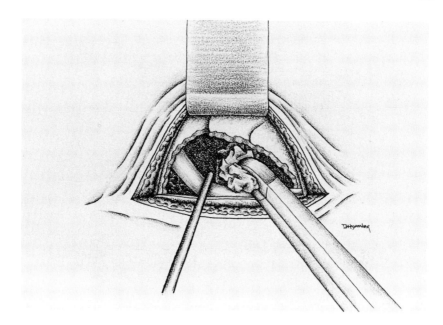

FIG. 26.3. Medial displacement of nerve root and dural sac.

After exploration superiorly, inferiorly, and medially with a Woodson-Adson dissector or a blunt nerve hook, a piece of fat from the subcutaneous tissue is placed over the dura mater. The fascia is closed with 2–0 absorbable suture, with no sutures placed in the paravertebral muscles. Generally, a subcuticular suture is used with an adhesive bandage dressing.

Postoperative Management

Patients are maintained in bed for 6–12 hours and then are allowed bathroom privileges. Ambulation is encouraged on the first postoperative day. Hospital discharge occurs whenever the patient feels comfortable enough to leave. All patients are instructed in an exercise regimen. Prolonged automobile travel in the sitting position is discouraged for 2–3 weeks.

RESULTS

The duration of symptoms was 1 month to 2.8 years in the 120 patients, with the median being 2.1 years (Table 26.1). The period of follow-up ranged 2–4 years.

Outcome was graded according to the following criteria: "Marked improvement" denoted progressive and sustained relief from radicular pain

TABLE 26.1

Patient Profile

Average age	40 years
Age range	10–75 years
Average hospital stay	6 days
Average time between operation and discharge	3 days
Median symptom duration	2.1 years
Follow-up period	2.4 years

or backache and diminution of clinical signs. This category included previous ratings of "good," "excellent," and "symptom-free." "Slight improvement" signified incomplete relief of radicular pain or backache with residuals of one or the other or both, but no incapacitating pain, and some improvement in the physical signs. "Unimproved" indicated no improvement. This included previous ratings of "no relief," "poor," and "no change." Marked improvement occurred in 112 (93%) (Table 26.2). The majority of patients awakened relieved of their radicular pain, but had persistent back pain for 2–6 weeks. All returned to their former occupations. Three patients (3%) experienced only slight improvement. In one of these, radicular pain was relieved, but back pain persisted and was aggravated by the operation. In the other two, despite the removal of herniated discs, radicular and back pain were relieved only partially.

Five patients (4%) were unimproved after 6 months of follow-up. One patient refused to undergo any further diagnostic studies. The second patient had a postoperative CT scan that was suggestive of a recurrent or possibly a missed herniated disc, but the patient refused surgical re-exploration. In the remaining three patients, a disc fragment was retrieved in a second operation. Two patients had disc herniation at another level. This

TABLE 26.2

Results of Microdiscectomy

	No.	Total No. of Reoperation
Surgical cure at first operation	112 (93%)	
Patients requiring reoperation	8 (7%)	
True recurrent herniated disc	4	4
Herniation same level opposite side	1	1
Herniation at different level	2	2
Persistent recurrent herniation	1	3

was verified by lumbar myelography and CT scan. One patient with hyperflexibility of all joints and suspected Ehlers-Danlos Syndrome had a recurrent disc fragment at the L5-S1 and required three operations.

Complications of Microdiscectomy

Four patients underwent exploration but not removal of the wrong disc. Intraoperative x-ray films showed the error, and the correct disc was then excised. Radiographic confirmation is now used routinely in all but patients with L5-S1 disc herniations. The dura matter under the nerve root was torn in one patient in an attempt to "fish out" a free disc fragment with a nerve hook. This was repaired and no subsequent complications occurred. One patient experienced dysesthesias that were not present before the operation and most likely occurred secondary to nerve root manipulation. The dysesthesias were moderate and did not prevent him from returning to his former occupation. One patient had increased weakness of the dorsiflexors of his foot which improved but not completely 6 months postoperatively. None required a transfusion. The average operating time was approximately 1 hour.

DISCUSSION

Although sciatica and low back pain were well known to ancient physicians, the surgical treatment of herniated lumbar discs is only 50 years old. Refined clinical judgment and innovative neurodiagnostic techniques such as the CT scan and metrizamide myelography now enable physicians to differentiate herniated lumbar discs from other entities such as spinal stenosis, lateral recess syndrome, foraminal stenosis, vascular and other conditions that mimic or contribute to this clinical syndrome. With the use of the operating microscope in spinal surgery for removal of arteriovenous malformations, intramedullary tumors, and cervical and thoracic discs, it was only a natural progression to adopt similar techniques for lumbar disc surgery.

The primary advantages of microsurgery include a smaller incision with less soft-tissue trauma and dissection, deep illumination and clear visualization of nerve roots and epidural contents, precise control of bleeding from epidural veins, microscopic dissection in the epidural space with protection of the epidural fat, direct visualization of the herniated disc or fragment, and the possibility of performing a simultaneous foraminotomy. There is no limitation to exploration of the paradiscal area and the same amount of disc material can easily be removed with this method as through a standard laminectomy. The micro technique has not been adopted by several investigators following Yasargil's early observations and results. Although Casper (6) has stated that removal of bone from the lamina and facet has no detrimental effect provided the joint facets are functionally preserved, Williams avoids excision of any bone from the lamina because of the apprehension of regenerative osteoblastic changes in the lamina which may produce focal thickening and entrap the nerve root by downgrowth. We also believe that adequate bone removal must be carried out to avoid undue nerve root retraction. This is particularly important in patients with narrow interlaminar spaces in whom removal of the medial third of the facet and a significant portion of the superior lamina can be routinely removed without consequences. The high speed drill accomplishes this expeditiously with complete safety, provided appropriate precautions are used.

Despite the refinement in surgical technique, the problem of recurrent discs remains most disconcerting. The question is still asked whether the removal of the protruded disc material alone is sufficient, as proposed by many microsurgeons, or if it is necessary to clean the intervertebral disc space of all accessible disc and cartilaginous material as advocated by Scoville and others. Comparison of published results indicate that the recurrence rate is higher if the intervertebral space has not been thoroughly cleaned of its contents.

Yasargil (38) and Casper (6) performed radical excision of disc material and curettage of the interspace, while Williams (36) advocates minimal evacuation of disc material without curettage to avoid macerating healthy disc material which may become a potential source for recurrence. Investigators who initially followed Williams' technique experienced a rate of recurrence approaching 9%. After they began to excise as much disc material as conveniently possible, the recurrence rate dropped to 4% (Table 26.3).

Our approach is to remove as much disc as possible at the site of herniation and then use various sized rongeurs to remove disc material

TABLE 26.3
Reported Recurrence Rate in Microlumbar Discectomy Series

	Goald (12)	Wilson (37)	Hudgins (15)	Williams (36)	Present
True recurrent disc	4.6%	2%	5%	5.6%	4.0%
Disc herniation at same level opposite side	1.0%		2%	1.4%	1.6%
Herniated at different level	2.0%	2%	1%	3.0%	0.8%
Total	7.6%	4%	8%	9.0%	6.4%

from the entire disc space where we are very careful to explore the potential space between the posterior longitudinal ligament and the posterior vertebral bodies since it is not uncommon to find disc fragments which have migrated out of the disc space lodged in this area causing symptoms. Despite complete removal of the disc contents, such hidden fragments may be the source of persistent pain or the subsequent diagnosis of "a recurrent disc."

Overall, the complications of microdiscectomy should be minimal. Wilson (37) encountered a 2–3% incidence of aseptic discitis. We have had one case of Staphylococcus epidermidis discitis. Postoperative nerve root complications are extremely uncommon but even with microsurgical techniques, hypalgesia and some additional weakness may occur when mobilization of the nerve root is necessary due to the configuration and location of a herniated disc fragment. Blood loss averages 30–60 ml.

A major economic advantage is the reduced hospital stay postoperatively. The average postoperative stay in our series is 3 days. We have instituted outpatient myelography and surgery on the day of admission with a further reduction of hospital days to a total average of approximately 3 inpatient days.

Even with conventional techniques, others including Fager and Scoville have reported discharging patients on an average of 1–3 days postoperatively. We feel that this further supports the imperativeness of using meticulous surgical technique and further bolsters the argument of using microsurgical techniques for this operation. Microsurgery permits the least possible violation of normal soft tissue and the least possible manipulation of sensitive nervous and vascular structures. These same factors, we believe, result in less morbidity in the removal of lumbar discs, particularly in the hands of those surgeons without the vast experience of the neurosurgical pioneers in this area.

When one realizes that over 200,000 disc operations are performed annually in the United States with an estimated cost of 7 billion dollars, reduction in postsurgical hospital stays can have an immense financial impact on health care financing. If microlumbar discectomy can assist in lowering the failure rate of surgical treatment and concurrently reducing the number of days required in the hospital to less than half, hundreds of millions of dollars could be saved annually. It is now the responsibility of physicians to effect greater efficiencies in health care. It appears that significant savings may be obtained safely with the above techniques.

REFERENCES

1. Abdullah, A. F., Ditto, E. W., Byrd, E. B., and Williams, S. R. Extreme lateral lumbar disc herniations: Clinical syndrome and special problems of diagnosis. J. Neurosurg., *41:* 229–234, 1974.

2. Aitken, A. P. Rupture of the intervertebral disc in industry: Further observation on the end results. Am. J. Surg., *84:* 261–267, 1952.
3. Armstrong, J. R. The causes of unsatisfactory results from the operative treatment of lumbar disc lesions. J. Bone Joint Surg. (Br), *33:* 31–35, 1951.
4. Barr, J. S., Kubik, C. S., Molly, M. K., McNeill, J. M., Riseborough, E. J., and White, J. C. Evaluation of end results in treatment of ruptured lumbar intervertebral discs with protrusion of nucleus polposus. Surg. Gynecol. Obstet., *125:* 250–256, 1967.
5. Balagura, S. Lumbar discectomy through a small incision. Neurosurgery, *11:* 784–785, 1982.
6. Casper, W. A new surgical procedure for lumbar disc herniation causing less tissue damage through microsurgical approach. Adv. Neurosurg., *4:* 74–79, 1977.
7. Dandy, W. E. Loose cartilage from inter-vertebral disk simulating tumor of the spinal cord. Arch. Surg. (Chicago), *19:* 660–672, 1929.
8. de Divititis, E., Spaziante, R., and Stella, L. Some technical modification of surgical treatment of lumbar disc lesions. Neuro. Chirurgia (Stuttg), *22:* 95–98, 1979.
9. Depalma, A. F., and Rothman, R. H. Surgery of the lumbar spine. Clin. Orthop. *63:* 162–170, 1969.
10. Fager, C. A., and Friedberg, S. R. Analysis of failures and poor results of lumbar spine surgery. Spine, *5:* 87–94, 1980.
11. Field, J. R., and McHenry, H. The lumbar shield: a preliminary report. Neurosurgery, *3:* 26–35, 1979.
12. Goald, H. Microlumbar discectomy: Follow-up of 477 patients. J. Microsurg., *2:* 95–100, 1980.
13. Goldthwaith, J. E. The lumbo-sacral articulation. An explanation of many cases of "lumbago," "sciatica," and paraplegia. Boston Med. Surg. J., *64:* 365–372, 1911.
14. Gurdjian, E. S., Ostrowski, A. Z., Hardy, W. G., Lindner, D. W., and Thomas, L. M. Results of operative treatment of protruded and ruptured lumbar discs. J. Neurosurg., *18:* 783–791, 1961.
15. Hudgins, R. W. The role of microdiscectomy. Orthop. Clin., North Am., *14:* 589–603, 1983.
16. LaRocca, M., and Macnab, I. The laminectomy membrane: studies in its evolution, characteristics, effects and prophylaxis in dogs. J. Bone Joint Surg. (Br), *56:* 545–550, 1974.
17. Law, J. D., Lehman, R. E. A. W., and Kirsch, W. M. Reoperation after lumbar intervertebral disc surgery. J. Neurosurg., *48:* 259–263, 1978.
18. Lindahl, O., and Rexed, B. Histologic changes in spinal nerve roots of operated cases of sciatica. Acta Orthop. Scand., *20:* 215–225, 1951.
19. Love, J. G. Root pain resulting from intraspinal protrusion of intervertebral discs. Diagnosis and surgical treatment. J. Bone Joint Surg., *19:* 776–804, 1937.
20. Love, J. G. Removal of protruded intervertebral disks without laminectomy. Proc. Staff Meet May. Clin., *14:* 800, 1939.
21. Macnab, I. Negative disc exploration. J. Bone Joint Surg. (Am), *53:* 891–903, 1971.
22. Mayfield, F. H., Keller, J. T., Dunsker, S. B., Ongkiko, C. M., and McWhorter, J. M. *Autogenous Fat for the Prevention of the Laminectomy Membrane.* Presented at the Forty-fifth Annual Meeting of the American Association of Neurological Surgeons, Toronto, Canada, April 28, 1977.
23. Mixter, W. S., and Barr, I. S. Rupture of the intervertebral disc without involvement of the spinal cord. Annual Meeting of the New England Surgical Society 1933. N. Eng. J. Med. *211:* 210–215, 1934.
24. O'Connell, J. E. A. Protrusions of the lumbar intervertebral discs: A clinical review based on five hundred cases treated by excision of the protrusion. J. Bone Joint Surg. (Br), *33:* 8–30, 1951.

25. Oppenheim, H., and Krause, F. Uber Einklemmung bzw. Strangulation der cauda equina. Dtsch. Med., *35:* 697–700, 1909.

26. Rosen, H. J. Lumbar intervertebral disc surgery: review of 300 cases. Can. Med. Assoc. J., *101:* 317–323, 1969.

27. Sashin, D. Intervertebral disk extensions into the vertebral bodies and the spinal canal. Arch. Surg., *22:* 527–547, 1931.

28. Schlarb, H., and Wenker, H. Reoperation performed on patients suffering from an intervertebral disc prolapse in the lumbar region. Adv. Neurosurg., *4:* 32–35, 1977.

29. Scoville, W. B., and Corkilig, G. Lumbar disc surgery: technique of radical removal and early mobilization. J. Neurosurg., *39:* 265–269, 1973.

30. Semmes, R. E. Ruptured lumbar intervertebral discs: Their recognition and surgical relief. Clin. Neurosurg., *8:* 78–92, 1960.

31. Shealy, C. N. Facet denervation in the management of back and sciatic pain. Clin. Orthop., *115:* 157–164, 1976.

32. Sparup, K. H. Late prognosis in lumbar disc herniation. Acta Rheum. Scand. (Suppl), *3:* 164, 1960.

33. Spengler, D. M. Lumbar discectomy: results with limited disc excision and selective foraminotomy. Spine, *7:* 604–607, 1982.

34. Stookey, B. Compression of spinal cord due to ventral extradural chondromas: Diagnosis and surgical treatment. Arch. Neurol. Psychiat. (Chicago), *20:* 275–291, 1928.

35. Torma, T. Post-operative recurrence of lumbar disc herniation. Acta Chir. Scand. *103:* 213–221, 1952.

36. Williams, R. W. Microlumbar discectomy; a surgical alternative for initial disc herniation. In Cauthen, J. (ed): *Lumbar Spine Surgery.* Baltimore, Williams & Wilkins, 1983, pp. 85–98.

37. Wilson, D. H., and Kenning, J. Microsurgical lumbar discectomy: preliminary report of 83 corrective cases. Neurosurgery, *4:* 137–140, 1979.

38. Yasargil, M. G. Microsurgical operations for herniated lumbar disc. Adv. Neurosurg. *4:* 81, 1977.

27

Lumbar Microdiscectomy: A Contrary Opinion

CHARLES A. FAGER, M.D.

Since the intervertebral disc has been recognized as a potential cause of some low-back problems, opinion among surgeons concerning treatment has seldom been uniform. Nevertheless, the most important consensus reached in the last 50 years is that most patients with a protruded disc and many others with a ruptured disc recover spontaneously. Their improvement occurs regardless of treatment and despite all forms of traction, intraspinal injections, many medications, chiropractic procedures, acupuncture, and several methods of intradiscal therapy. On the other hand, some patients whose back problems would have fared reasonably well without treatment are clearly worse as a result of ill-conceived therapy. Surgical treatment, therefore, must be reserved for the patient with unmistakable evidence of nerve root or cauda equina compression who has unremitting radicular pain or is in jeopardy of having a serious neurologic deficit.

It should be evident that an operation to remove or obliterate an intervertebral disc or to fuse a spinal segment is not curative but palliative since intervertebral disc disease is not curable even though a successful operation relieves neurogenic pain and may provide periods of freedom from back pain. The unsuccessful operation, which may result in persisting disability or additional neurologic deficit, is practically always the result of faulty patient selection or an operation inappropriate for the type of lesion (5).

Attempts at alternative procedures, such as injection of chymopapain and percutaneous discectomy, and modifications, such as microdiscectomy, seem to ignore the fact that surgical techniques have improved in this relatively new field. The patient of 35 years ago frequently endured great pain after disc surgery, had to be turned by "log rolling," often required catheterization and prolonged confinement in bed, and was in the hospital 10 days or more. Today, patients are ambulatory within hours of operation, are discharged from the hospital in 2 or 3 days, and return to work in 2–3 weeks. These changes preceded the needless introduction of 1-inch incisions, limited exposure, and superfluous magnification. Without denying the usefulness of microsurgery for many intracranial and spinal lesions, it remains doubtful whether microsurgery offers any advantage for the patient with a ruptured lumbar disc who requires operation; in fact, microsurgery is associated with several disadvantages and some additional risks.

DISCUSSION

Williams reported that lumbar microdiscectomy was a "conservative" surgical approach in which no lamina was removed, and reherniation was supposedly minimized by employing blunt perforation of the anulus rather than sharp incision (10). However, in his series of 661 operations performed on 530 patients over a 5½-year period, 37 patients required reoperation when results were unsatisfactory. Williams also referred to an "undulating" disc syndrome in 16 patients who required further operation for subligamentous deposits of extruded material. In his series, neither the average postoperative stay of 3.1 days nor return to work in 5 weeks (9 weeks in patients with work- or accident-related injuries) represents improvement when compared with results from neurosurgical centers having experience with conventional operations performed on large numbers of patients with ruptured disc. Williams' description of blunt surgical perforation of the anulus must be viewed with some skepticism because in most patients who require operation for ruptured disc, the anulus has already been perforated by a fragment of disc. Goald (6) surveyed his experience with microdiscectomy in 477 patients over a 4-year period and indicated a good result in 91% of patients after initial operation. Similar results were obtained in an additional 6% of patients who required a second operation. However, 21% of these patients had normal myelographic findings, and 18% had discs removed at two levels, raising serious questions about the indications for operation in this group as well.

Among the reported series of Williams (10), Goald (6), and Hudgins (7), the percentages of compensation cases were inordinately high—46%, 36%, and 40%, respectively—leading Hudgins (7) to suggest that these findings make the results of microdiscectomy seem even more favorable than believed previously. In my experience, less than 10% of patients with a severely ruptured disc requiring operation reported a history of work-related injury, suggesting that microsurgery may be a lesser operative procedure and more favorable for a number of patients after industrial accidents (often minor) in whom satisfactory recovery might be expected without any operation at all.

Furthermore, Hudgins (7) has been willing to operate on patients when 7 days of bed rest failed to provide "encouraging improvement" and apparently relied largely on history, physical examination, and computed tomography (CT) of the spine before operation. However, microdiscectomy was modified to include removal of lamina and the lateral shelf of ligamentum flavum as well as to permit curettage within the disc space. In addition, Hudgins (7) warned that because pieces of disc may appear larger when viewed microscopically, the tendency is to terminate surgery too soon!

After modifying Williams' technique, Wilson and colleagues (11, 12) compared results of microsurgery with those of standard removal of lumbar disc and reported a 93% rate of success for the standard operation. However, the two groups were not comparable so that the success rate of 97% in the microdiscectomy group and a slightly lower rate of recurrence may not be significant. Paradoxically, Wilson and associates (11, 12) described an excessive number of dural tears in the microsurgical group of patients. Merli et al. (8) also reported four dural tears and one footdrop in 120 patients. This high rate of complications occurred despite the authors' requirements of precise localization and limited operation to a single level. Bed rest was maintained for 24 hours, and patients were hospitalized for as long as 5 days. Oldenkott and Roost (9), while believing that microdiscectomy as an alternative treatment has some advantages, could not conclude that the long-term results using microdiscectomy were better than with other procedures. Ebeling and Reulen (1) thought the microsurgical techniques provided more favorable effects but no difference in either the frequency of poor results or repeat operations. Zeiger (13), reporting on a small number of patients, believed the technical improvements provided by the operating microscope made operation on the lumbar disc safer and more precise than other procedures, but these improvements did not reduce the incidence of recurrent disc or "failed disc syndrome."

REQUISITES OF SURGERY

Because the mechanics and pathologic status of ruptured discs are not uniform, patients obviously require different operative approaches for relief of nerve root or cauda equina compression. This fact constitutes the major flaw in the concept of microdiscectomy. When operation is necessary, the commonest finding is that a fragmented disc has thrust posterolaterally through the anulus fibrosus and distended the posterior longitudinal ligament overlying the disc space thus displacing nerve root and cauda equina (Fig. 27.1). A small portion of the disc is often found projecting through an opening at the apex of the thinned-out ligament. When the fragment is released, a conspicuous observation is that its larger mass in the spinal canal has often been propelled through a much smaller opening or tear in the anulus and remains incarcerated in a fixed position. From this basic trajectory, additional fragments of disc may erupt in any direction or occupy a less accessible area than the lateral epidural region overlying the disc space. Even in this common situation, the nerve root is

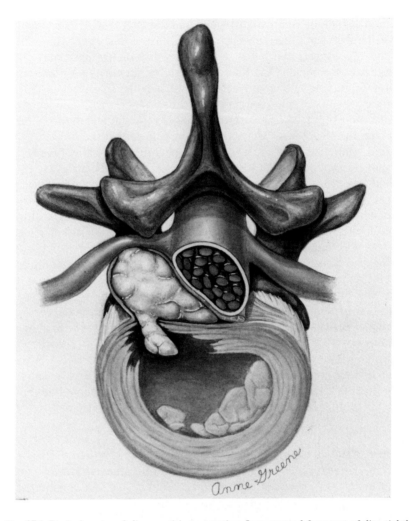

FIG. 27.1. Typical ruptured disc requiring operation. Incarcerated fragment of disc tightly compresses nerve root against posterolateral bony elements.

tightly compressed against posterolateral bony elements. An adequate exposure of bone above, below, and lateral to the lesion allows decompression for easy manipulation of nerve root and dura. This exposure provides the technical advantage of a conventional operation over that of the microsurgical approach.

The extruded fragment capable of even more severe compression may rupture through a small or larger opening in the anulus (Fig. 27.2) or

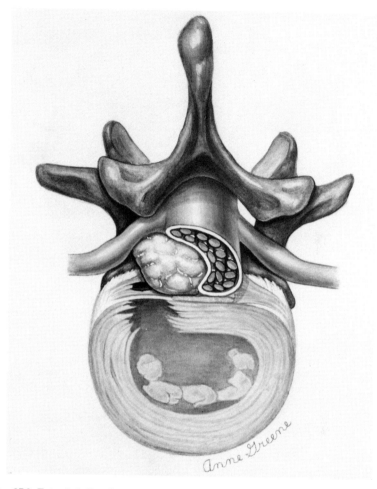

FIG. 27.2. Extruded disc. Severe compression of nerve root and cauda equina with little available space posteriorly.

through a marginal tear (Fig. 27.3). Once it is in the open spinal canal, the disc can extend medially, above, or below the disc space (Figs. 27.4–27.6). It may occupy a position close by or within a nerve root foramen or may straddle a nerve root at a considerable distance from the disc space itself. Whether incarcerated or extruded, fragments of discs vary tremendously in size. Yet, their impact on neural elements depends almost as much on the size of the spinal canal as on the size of the ruptured fragment. Thus, a small disc fragment may produce as much nerve root compression in a

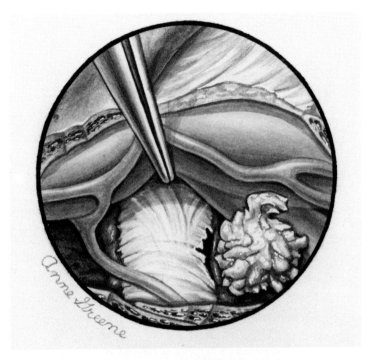

FIG. 27.3. Marginal tear through which fragment extends beyond the disc space. (From Fager, C. A. Surgery of the lumbar spine. In *Neurosurgery. Rob and Smith's Operative Surgery*, edited by Symon, L., Thomas, D. G. T., Clarke, K. London, Butterworths, 1986, ed 4, in press.)

spinal canal compromised by spondylosis and facet arthropathy (Figs. 27.7 and 27.8) or congenital stenosis (Fig. 27.9) as a large fragment in an otherwise normal canal.

Proponents of microdiscectomy advocate little or no removal of bone and less epidural dissection. While this microsurgical approach might be adequate for a protruded microdisc, it is difficult to imagine how it could be suitable for the large fragment of paramedian disc (Fig. 27.10), those fragments extrude beyond the disc space (Figs. 27.11 and 27.12), or calcified disc lesions (Fig. 27.13). All of these require more rather than less laminectomy to decompress neural elements for adequate access and less traumatic retraction. In my experience, a wider exposure and more lateral approach (Fig. 27.14) provide for less manipulation of the nerve root and cauda equina, better control of bleeding, much less chance of dural tear, and better postoperative recovery.

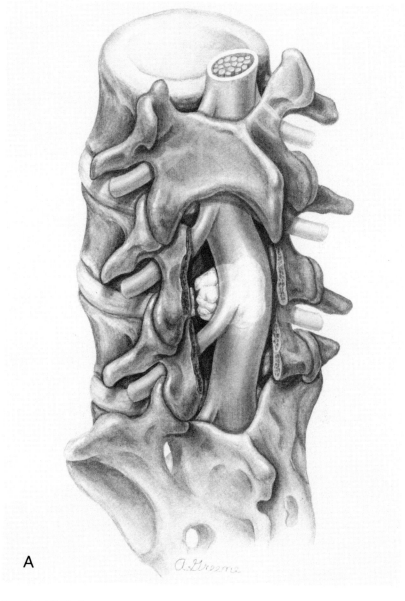

A

FIG. 27.4. (*A*) Median-paramedian fragment. (*B*) Laminectomy to decompress cauda equina before removal of disc. *Inset* shows limited exposure, *dashed line* indicates position of fragment. (From Fager, C. A. Facts and fallacies of spinal disorders: a neurosurgeon's viewpoint. In *Evaluation and Treatment of Chronic Pain,* edited by Aronoff, G. M., Baltimore, Urban & Schwarzenberg, 1985.)

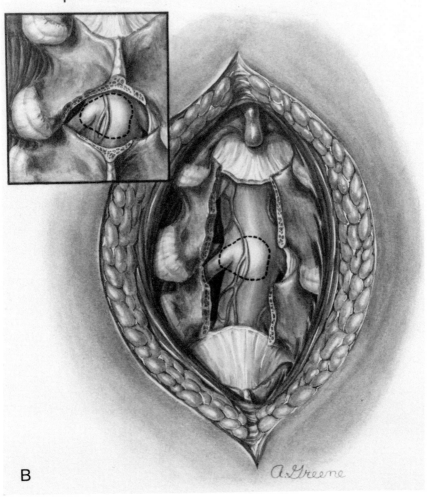

Limited
Exposure

B

a. Greene

FIG. 27.4*B*

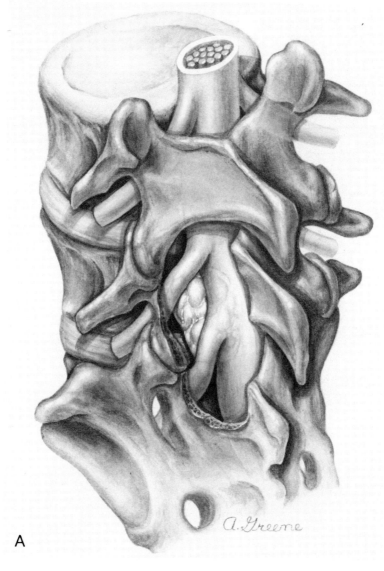

A

FIG. 27.5. (A) Fragment extruded laterally and above L5-S1 disc space compressing L5-S1 nerve roots. (B) Long and lateral hemilaminectomy required for adequate release of both nerve roots. *Inset* shows how inadequate exposure precludes satisfactory dissection of nerve roots and disc fragment (*dashed lines*). (From Fager, C. A. Surgery of the lumbar spine. In *Neurosurgery. Rob & Smith's Operative Surgery,* edited by Symon, L., Thomas, D. G. T., Clarke, K. London, Butterworths, 1986, ed 4, in press.)

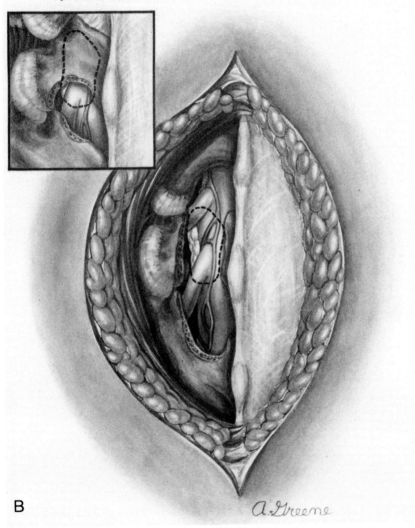

B

FIG. 27.5*B*

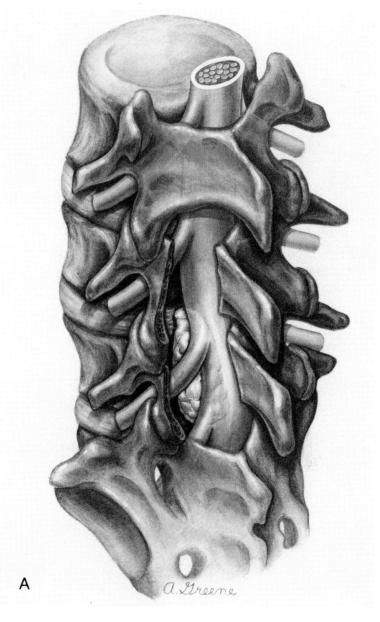

A

FIG. 27.6. (A) Fragment extending below L4–5 disc space. (B) Longitudinal release of nerve roots and cauda equina by complete hemilaminectomy of L4–5. Limited exposure fails to provide satisfactory decompression to remove disc easily. *Dashed line* shows position of fragment. (From Fager, C. A. Surgery of the lumbar spine. In *Neurosurgery. Rob & Smith's Operative Surgery,* edited by Symon, L., Thomas, D. G. T., Clarke, K. London, Butterworths, 1986, ed 4, in press.)

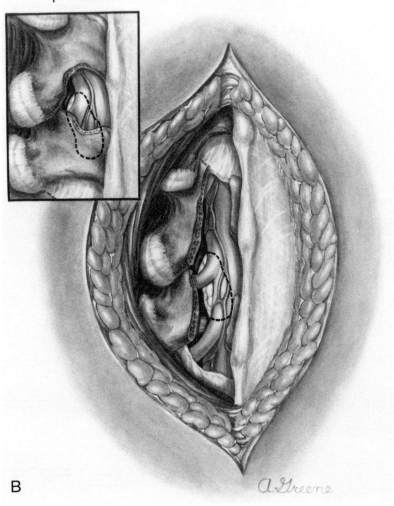

Limited
Exposure

B

FIG. 27.6B

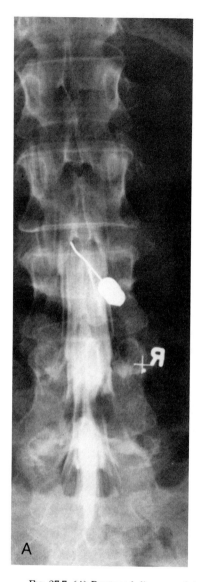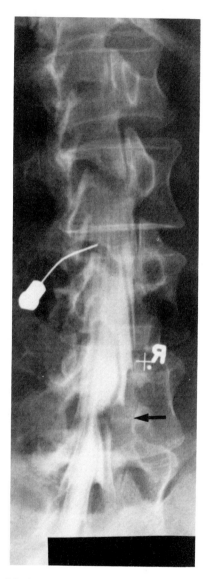

FIG. 27.7. (A) Ruptured disc associated with spondylosis. Facet arthropathy (*arrow*) produces additional compression of nerve root and cauda equina. (B) Facet arthropathy with ruptured disc.

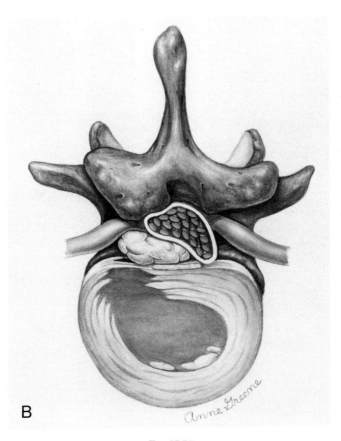

B

FIG. 27.7B

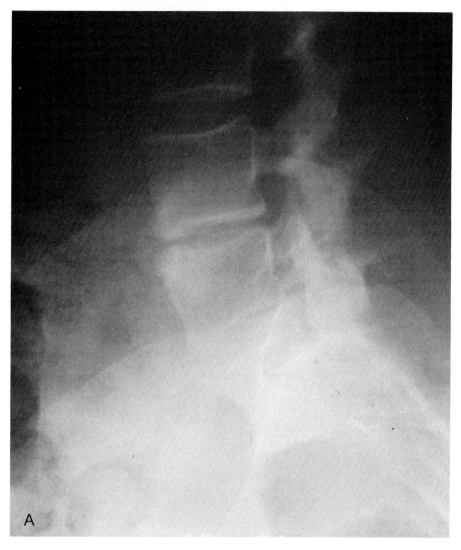

A

FIG. 27.8. Lateral radiograph (*A*) shows lumbar spondylosis with degenerative disc disease, and myelogram (*B*) of same patient discloses small ruptured disc fragment at L4–5 (*arrow*) associated with facet arthropathy.

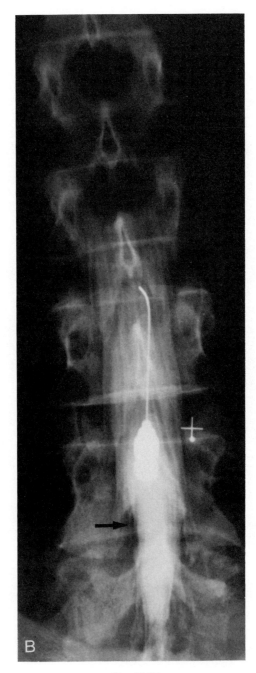

FIG. 27.8B

434

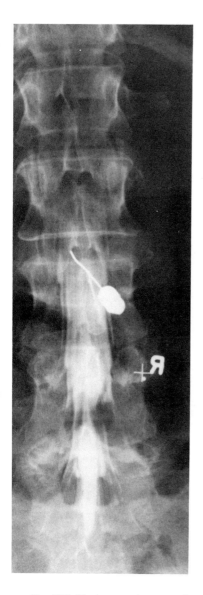 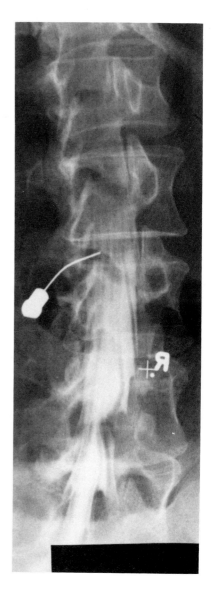

FIG. 27.9. Myelogram shows small ruptured disc at L4–5 (*right*) in patient with narrow lower lumbar canal.

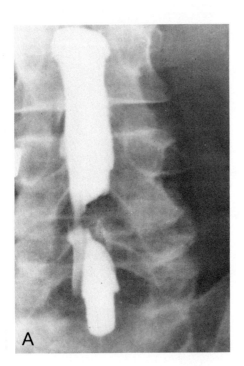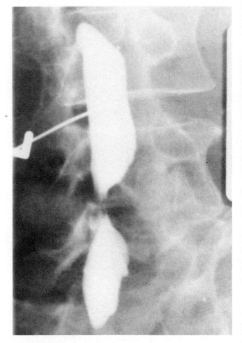

FIG. 27.10. Myelograms of two patients with right sciatica (A) and left sciatica (B) resulting from large paramedian ruptures at level of L4–5.

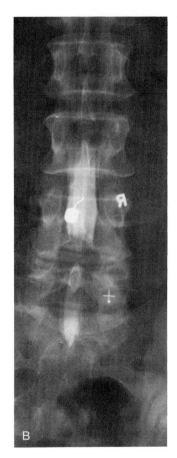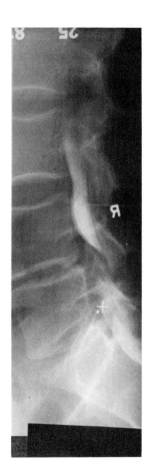

FIG. 27.10*B*

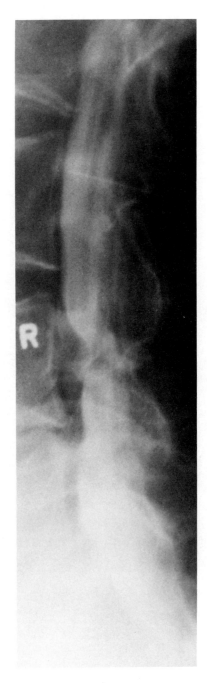

FIG. 27.11. Lateral myelogram showing disc fragment extruded from L3–4 disc lying against posterolateral body of L4.

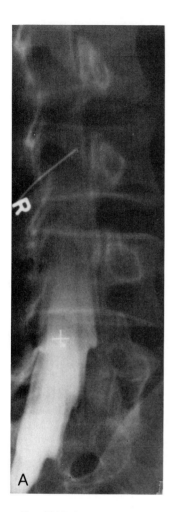
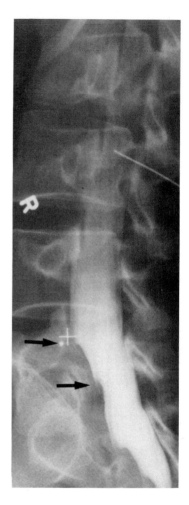

FIG. 27.12. Lumbar myelogram (A) and computed tomogram (B) showing fragment extruded upward and laterally from level of L5–S1 compressing right L5 nerve root at foramen. *Arrows* show extent and location of fragment.

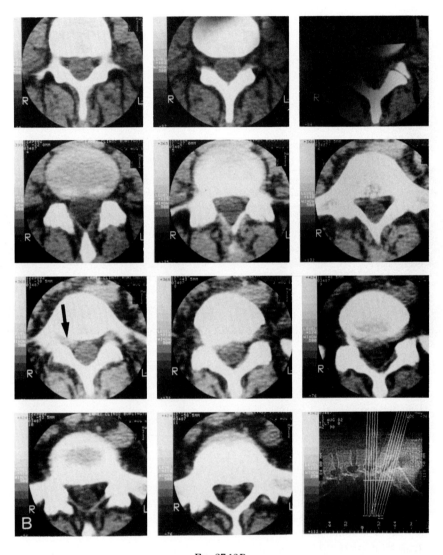

FIG. 27.12B

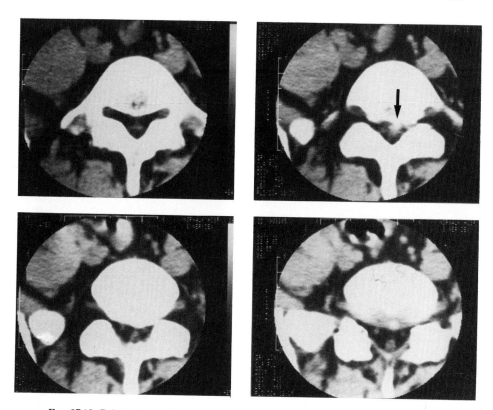

FIG. 27.13. Relatively small though partially calcified protruded disc shown by lumbar computed tomogram (*arrow*). (From Fager, C. A. Facts and fallacies of spinal disorders: a neurosurgeon's viewpoint. In *Evaluation and Treatment of Chronic Pain*, edited by Aronoff, G. M. Baltimore, Urban & Schwarzenberg, 1985.)

In performing subsequent myelography (Figs. 27.15 and 27.16) and surgical procedures for recurrent rupture, I have seldom encountered troublesome epidural fibrosis. Maintaining the principle of adequate exposure has virtually eliminated contusion, early nerve root edema, and later cohesion of nerve roots referred to as adhesive arachnoiditis. Furthermore, patients have had a relatively pain-free postoperative recovery after atraumatic dissection of muscles and adequate hemilaminectomy or laminectomy. Most patients at the Lahey Clinic, regardless of the size or location of the ruptured disc, are discharged from the hospital 2 days after operation and a smaller number of patients, within 3 days.

Adequate exposure requires the satisfactory release of paravertebral muscle over two interspaces enabling gentle muscle retraction to lateral

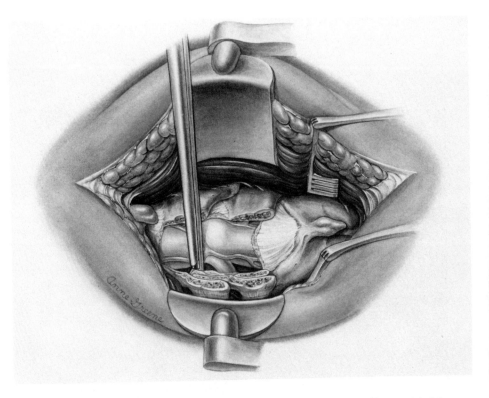

FIG. 27.14. Operative approach to large left paramedian disc rupture. Fragment bulging anterior to cauda equina. Laminae of L4–5 have been excised, and bone is removed beyond the lateral margin of dura on left. (From Fager, C. A. Ruptured median and paramedian lumbar disk: a review of 243 cases. Surg. Neurol., *23:* 309–323, 1985.)

facet margins at one or two levels. Adequate removal of bone for even ruptured disc at the disc space extending laterally, which is the most common presentation, necessitates hemilaminectomy above the superior margin of the ligamentum flavum and beyond the lateral margin of dura to remove a medial portion of facet and a portion of the lamina or sacrum below (Fig. 27.17), fully relaxing the nerve root (2, 4). For large fragments extending beyond the disc space, a complete hemilaminectomy may be essential, and, for better accessibility, a complete hemilaminectomy of two segments is often indicated. Median and paramedian disc rupture obstructing the spinal canal often requires complete lumbar laminectomy at two levels for their safe and effective extraction (Fig. 27.14) (3).

With more widespread use of a microsurgical approach for ruptured lumbar disc, more patients have required additional procedures because of

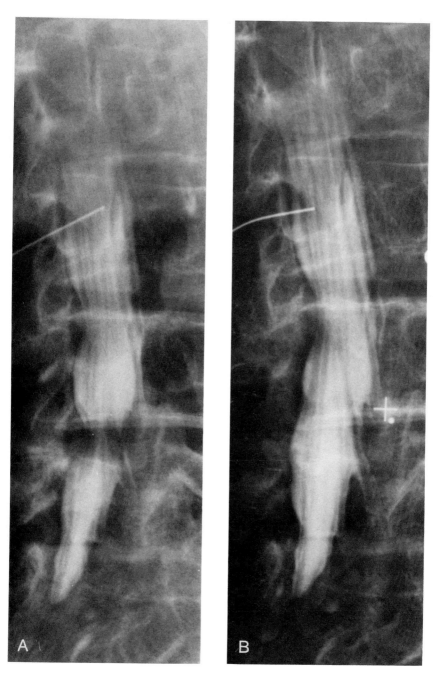

FIG. 27.15. (A) Oblique view. Myelogram shows ruptured disc in elderly man at L4–5 on right associated with spondylosis requiring full hemilaminectomy. (B) Postoperative appearance 9 months after operation; patient is free of sciatic pain.

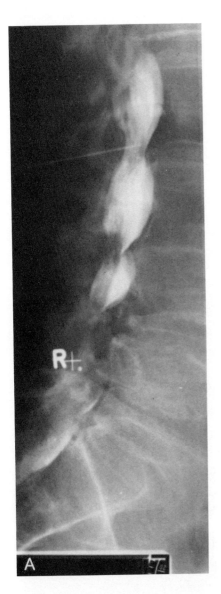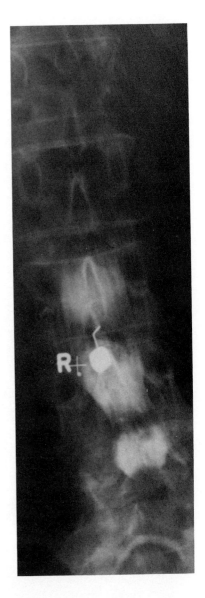

Fig. 27.16. (A) Preoperative myelogram showing lumbar spondylosis with associated chronic ruptured disc and partial block at L4–5. (B) Sketch of operation shows extensive decompressive laminectomy and excision of disc at L4–5. (From Fager, C. A. Surgery of the lumbar spine. In *Neurosurgery. Rob & Smith's Operative Surgery*, edited by Symon, L., Thomas, D. G. T., Clarke, K. London, Butterworths, 1986, ed 4, in press.) (C) Lumbar myelogram 2 years after extensive surgery shows no evidence of fibrosis or arachnoiditis.

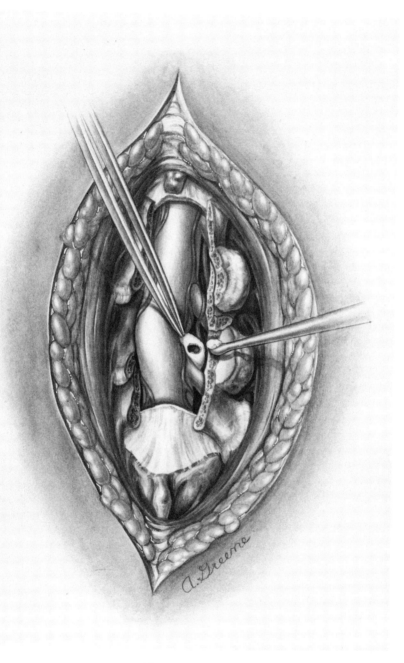

B

FIG. 27.16*B*

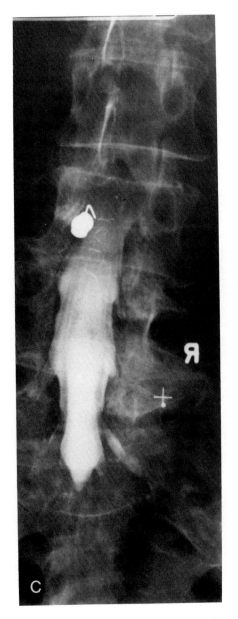
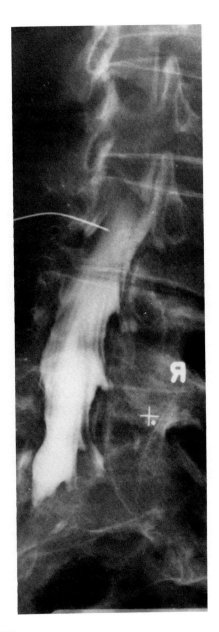

Fig. 27.16C

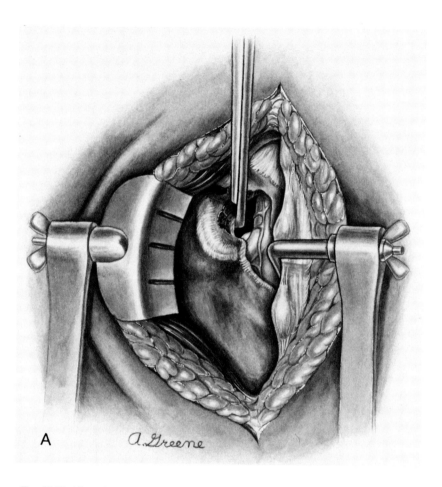

A

a. Greene

FIG. 27.17. (A) and (B) Surgical sketches show adequate bone removal for release of left first sacral nerve root and excision of lateral ruptured disc. (From Fager, C. A. Surgery of the lumbar spine. In *Neurosurgery. Rob & Smith's Operative Surgery*, edited by Symon, L., Thomas, D. G. T., Clarke, K. London, Butterworths, 1986, ed 4, in press.)

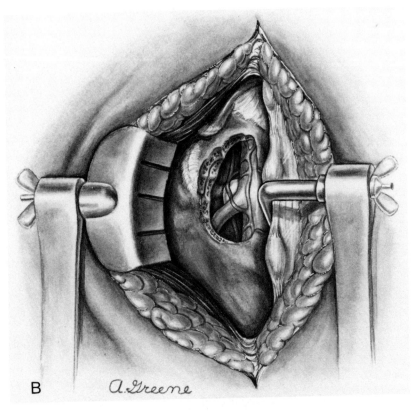

B

FIG. 27.17*B*

continued radicular pain and neurologic symptoms (Figs. 27.18 and 27.19). Many of these patients have had a retained fragment of disc either at the level of operation or at another level, usually one segment below the operative site (Fig. 27.20). Unfortunately, some of these patients had increased neurologic deficit after microsurgery (Fig. 27.21), presumably resulting from postoperative swelling of neural elements within a spinal canal already compromised by a mass lesion.

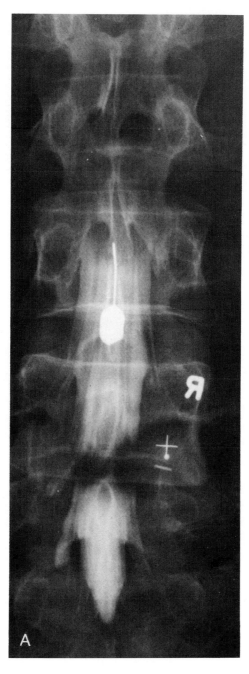

Fig. 27.18. Posteroanterior (*A*) and lateral (*B*) myelograms of patient with persistent right sciatic pain resulting from retained fragment of disc after microdiscectomy at L4–5 on right. Patient required further operation.

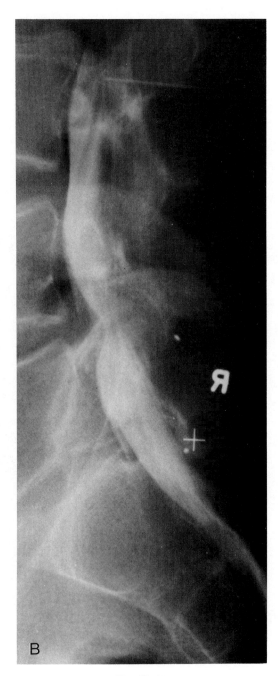

Fig. 27.18*B*

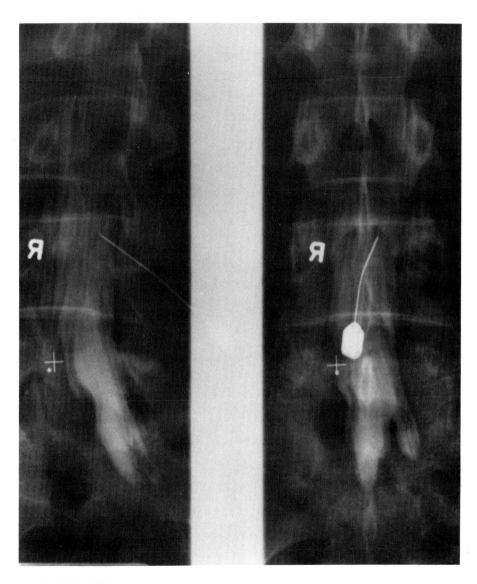

FIG. 27.19. Oblique and posteroanterior myelograms of patient with large retained disc fragment after microdiscectomy requiring further operation.

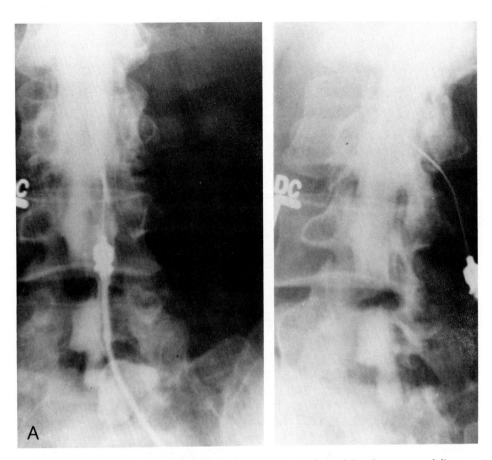

FIG. 27.20. (A) Preoperative myelogram of patient showing large defect from ruptured disc at L4–5 on left. Patient had left footdrop after operation and more severe left sciatic pain. (B) Myelogram 2 months later shows partial block resulting from large retained disc fragment. Initial microsurgery was thought to have been performed at L3–4.

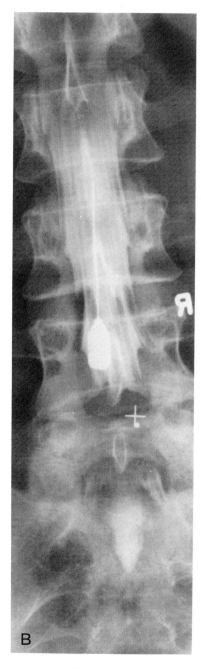

FIG. 27.20*B*

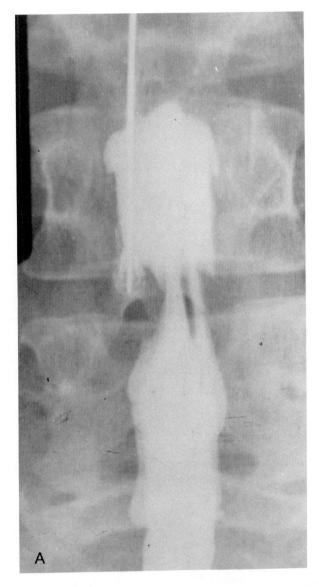

FIG. 27.21. (A) Myelogram of patient with large paramedian disc rupture at L4–5. Microdiscectomy was followed by partial cauda equina syndrome and more intense sciatic pain. (B) Myelogram 18 months after microdiscectomy shows large retained fragment. Surgical removal partially relieved pain but did not restore function.

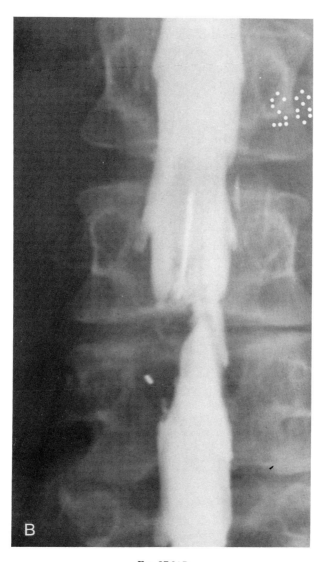

FIG. 27.21B

SUMMARY

Successful operation for ruptured lumbar disc is directly related to appropriate selection of patients and an operative approach designed for the particular size and location of the compressed fragment of disc. Lumbar microdiscectomy provides no advantage when operation is clearly indicated and adds the additional risks that have always accompanied inadequate exposure and incomplete decompression.

REFERENCES

1. Ebeling, U., and Reulen, H. J. Ergebnisse der mikrochirurgischen lumbalen Bandscheiben operation: Vorläufige Mitteilung. Neurochirurgia (Stuttgart), 26: 12–17, 1983 (Eng abstr).
2. Fager, C. A. Lumbar disc disease: surgical treatment. In Lumbar Disc Disease, edited by Hardy, R. W., Jr. New York, Raven Press, 1982, pp. 119–145.
3. Fager, C. A. Ruptured median and paramedian lumbar disk: a review of 243 cases. Surg. Neurol., 23: 309–323, 1985.
4. Fager, C. A. Surgical approaches to lumbar disk lesions and spondylosis. Surg. Clin. North Am., 60: 649–663, 1980.
5. Fager, C. A., and Freidberg, S. R. Analysis of failures and poor results of lumbar spine surgery. Spine, 5: 87–94, 1980.
6. Goald, H. J. Microlumbar discectomy: follow-up of 477 patients. J. Microsurg., 2: 95–100, 1980.
7. Hudgins, W. R. The role of microdiscectomy. Orthop. Clin. North Am., 14: 589–603, 1983.
8. Merli, G. A., Angiari, P., and Tonelli, L. Three years experience with microsurgical technique in treatment of protruded lumbar disc. J. Neurosurg. Sci., 28: 25–31, 1984.
9. Oldenkott, P., and Roost, D. V. Traitement microchirurgical de la hernie discale lombaire. Neurochirurgie, 26: 229–234, 1983 (Eng abstr).
10. Williams, R. W. Microlumbar discectomy: a conservative surgical approach to the virgin herniated lumbar disc. Spine, 3: 175–182, 1978.
11. Wilson, D. H., and Harbaugh R. Microsurgical and standard removal of the protruded lumbar disc: a comparative study. Neurosurgery, 8: 422–427, 1981.
12. Wilson, D. H., and Kenning, J. Microsurgical lumbar discectomy: preliminary report of 83 consecutive cases. Neurosurgery, 4: 137–140, 1979.
13. Zeiger, H. E. Microsurgical lumbar discectomy. Ala. Med. 58: 6–7, 1983.

CHAPTER

28

Low Back Pain Disorders: Lumbar Fusion?

GEORGE W. SYPERT, M.D.

INTRODUCTION

Lumbago (low back pain) and/or sciatica (radicular leg pain) is a major health problem in the United States, Canada, Australia, and Western Europe. Although accurate statistics are not available, various data suggest that approximately 75% of the population of adults over the age of 25 experience at least one incapacitating episode of lumbago and sciatica in their lifetime (25, 32, 39). The prevalence is about 20%, suggesting that at any one time, 20% of the adult population will complain about the back if asked (31). Moreover, approximately 10% of adults suffer disabling chronic low back pain syndromes and are either seeing a physician or seeking some form of treatment at any one time. The number of Americans currently suffering from chronic intractable low back pain disorders is greater than 18 million (5). In fact, lumbago and sciatica are the most common symptoms for which adults in these countries consult a physician. In most individuals suffering lumbago and/or sciatica, the exact cause of the pain cannot be accurately identified (28). Lumbago and sciatica of spinal origin are rarely related to disease processes that cause permanent loss of function or death. However, they achieve their importance because of reduction in the quality of life and disability resulting in inability to perform the normal activities of a given individual's life style. Given the magnitude of this health problem, it is not surprising that neurologic surgeons and orthopaedic surgeons have developed a variety of surgical strategies to treat chronic low back pain disorders, one of which is lumbar arthrodesis or fusion.

Despite a near half-century of application of lumbar spine fusion to low back pain disorders, this therapeutic modality remains a highly emotional and controversial subject among physicians treating these disorders. Such responses are appropriate given the absence of generally accepted operational definition(s) of mechanical lumbago/sciatica or so-called lumbar spinal instability. Careful review of the massive clinical literature regarding this subject fails to elicit scientifically interpretable data that may be used to determine the patient selection criteria that may ensure success of

457

lumbar arthrodesis in the treatment of low back pain disorders. Finally, there have been no well-designed prospective clinical studies that rigorously document the specific role of lumbar arthrodesis in the therapy of the low back pain disorders, particularly if one considers the role of primary lumbar fusion for spondylotic disease.

CLASSIFICATION OF LUMBAGO/SCIATICA OF SPINAL ORIGIN

The area of the body called the low back includes the lumbar spine, sacrum, sacroiliac articulations, coccyx, and associated joints, muscles, tendons, ligaments, and neural elements (cauda equina, individual nerve roots, and peripheral nerves innervating the low back structures). All of these structures are capable of contributing to low back pain syndromes. Lumbago and sciatica are merely descriptions of symptom complexes. Low back pain of spinal origin may result from numerous different pathologic conditions. Similarly, sciatica (radicular leg pain) may be caused by a variety of pathologic entities including lumbar radiculopathy, sciatic nerve entrapment syndromes, lumbosacral plexitis, and others. Lumbar radiculopathy itself is not only due to nerve root compression (*e.g.*, herniated lumbar disc, lateral recess stenosis, neoplasm, etc.) but may be caused by arachnoiditis, epidural scar formation, and intraneural pathologic changes, to mention a few. Finally, it should be recognized that a variety of pathologic conditions affecting low back structures can cause pain that is segmentally referred down the lower extremity. This latter form of pain is often misinterpreted by the inexperienced clinician as radiculopathic pain. Hence, lumbago and sciatica are often exceedingly complex pain syndromes caused by a variety of pathological conditions, some of which remain to be elucidated. The clinical investigation of low back pain disorders is further complicated in many cases by psychologic, social, and economic factors. Despite the development of numerous highly sophisticated diagnostic technologies (myelography, computed tomography, magnetic resonance imaging, etc.), which have contributed substantially to our understanding of low back disorders, it is frequently difficult for the neurologic surgeon experienced in the management of low back disorders to make an accurate diagnosis of the specific cause(s) of low back and leg pain in many patients. Furthermore, the natural histories of the low back pain disorders are poorly understood. It is well-known, however, that the vast majority of conditions producing lumbago/sciatica are benign and that they can generally be managed by conservative means.

The preceding discussion indicates that decision making regarding the surgical treatment of low back pain disorders is difficult and will remain so until further knowledge of the pathogenetic factors involved and their natural history is achieved. At present, surgical treatment of low back pain disorders is limited to one or more of four objectives: (*a*) decompression of compressed neural elements; (b) arthrodesis or fusion of a vertebral motion segment; (c) destruction of neural elements involved in the pathogenesis of pain; and (d) electrical stimulation of neural elements to reduce the perception of pain. The generally accepted primary indication for surgical treatment of low back pain disorders is the relief of persistent or recurrent "neural compression." Therefore, lumbar spine surgery is generally directed toward the restoration of nerve root or cauda equina function or the relief of intractable nerve root compression pain. It is the author's opinion that objectives c and d are investigational at this time, reserved largely for patients suffering the "failed back surgery syndrome." However, the author is also of the opinion that a lumbar spine stabilization-fusion procedure may be indicated for those infrequent patients with carefully documented intractable and incapacitating "mechanical" low back pain syndromes. In this respect, prior to contemplating any form of interventional therapy, the author has found it useful to make a rigorous attempt to classify a patient's principal complaint of pain of spinal origin into one or more of six general categories (Table 28.1). Although such a classification scheme appears somewhat simplistic, it is consistent with available knowledge regarding the pathogenesis of lumbago and sciatica. Moreover, this categorical scheme has been very helpful in the early education of neurologic surgery residents regarding diseases affecting the spine as well as substantially reducing the application of unnecessary diagnostic and interventional therapy.

DEFINITION: MECHANICAL SPINE PAIN SYNDROME

"Mechanical" pain syndrome of the lumbar spine is defined as low back and/or hip and/or segmental leg pain due to "instability" of a lumbar motion segment. Characteristically, such patients complain of low back pain syndromes that are aggravated by weight bearing, bending, twisting, lifting, or other activities that mechanically stress the lumbar spine. These patients typically obtain near complete relief of symptoms from recumbency. A clinical trial in an appropriate lumbar orthosis used to reduce forces acting on the lumbar spine may be an important adjunct to the sympto-

TABLE 28.1

Classification for Low Back Pain Disorders of Spinal Origin

1. Myofascial syndromes
2. Inflammatory syndromes
3. Neural compression syndromes
4. Mechanical (instability) syndromes
5. Neuropathic syndromes
6. Psycho-social-economic syndromes

matic determination of mechanical pain. It must be kept in mind that the only orthotic device that offers significant immobilization of the L4–5 and L5-S1 motion segments is a well-fitted "spica" that incorporates one thigh. In fact other orthotic devices designed for the lumbar region may actually aggravate motion or stress of the lower lumbar region in certain circumstances. Neurodiagnostic laboratory investigations (computed tomography, myelography) appear to be of limited usefulness (see below) unless they are carefully correlated with the patients symptoms. Table 28.2 lists some of the conditions that may contribute to mechanical pain syndromes of spinal origin. The present discussion will deal primarily with spondylotic (degenerative disc disease) aspects of lumbar spine disease, which may result in intractable and incapacitating mechanical pain syndromes.

INDICATIONS FOR SPONDYLOTIC LUMBAR FUSION

Although the circumstances which make lumbar fusion beneficial in the treatment of spondylotic low back pain disorders have yet to be clearly delineated, various indications for lumbar fusion have been suggested. These "so-called" indications may be classified as clinical, radiologic, and surgical.

Clinical Indications

Clinical indications include (a) intractable and incapacitating "mechanical" pain syndromes (see above): (b) high demand activity (sports, laborer, etc.); (c) relative youth; (d) extension lag (reversal of spinal rhythm); (e) temporary relief with repeated facette anesthetization; and (f) pain relief with trial in external orthosis.

Radiological Indications

Radiological indications include (a) positive stress radiograph (flexion-extension, lateral bending); (b) traction spur(s); (c) facet sublaxation

TABLE 28.2
*Mechanical Low Back Pain Syndromes:
Etiologic Factors*

Degenerative disease—spondylosis
Isthmic spondylolysis—spondylolisthesis
Congenital disease
Traumatic disease
   Postoperative disorders
Neoplastic disease
Inflammatory-infectious disease

and/or degeneration; (d) pseudospondylolisthesis; (e) disc abnormalities (severe degeneration-gas shadow, wide space, central prolapse, and bilateral displacement); and (f) diagnostic discography (abnormal discogram, reproduction of symptoms).

Surgical Indications

Surgical indications include (a) disc excision; (b) repeat disc excision at same level; (c) facetectomy-unilateral or bilateral; and (d) loose joint at surgery.

In order to apply treatments rationally, it is essential to determine the predictors of success or failure for the therapeutic modality, particularly if that modality is spinal arthrodesis. Lumbar fusion, whether posterolateral fusion (PLF), posterior interbody fusion (PLIF), or anterior interbody fusion (ALIF), is a major operative procedure associated with substantial risks and complications for the patient. This is especially true for lumbar mechanical pain syndromes which are benign in the sense that they are not generally associated with loss of neurologic function and death. Unfortunately, none of the above listed indications for lumbar arthrodesis has been subjected to well-designed clinical studies to determine the predictive value.

The author is of the opinion that some of these indications have not been shown to be of any predictive value in low back pain disorders; they are easily misinterpreted and should not be routinely used in the evaluation of patients suffering low back pain disorders. An example is diagnostic discography. Degenerative disc disease and, hence, abnormal discograms are a biologic consequence of the normal aging process. Moreover, one suggested indication, routine PLIF at time of excision of a herniated lumbar disc (3, 11, 12), is to be deplored. There is absolutely no evidence that lumbar fusion improves the results of a well-executed decompressive discectomy in an appropriately selected patient (16, 17, 33). Given currently available data, the only rational conclusion that can be reached is that the routine addition of a lumbar fusion can only add to the morbidity of the treatment.

The author can, in fact, produce numerous examples of patients with one or more of the above indications who were successfully treated with either a conservative (nonsurgical) program or appropriate surgical decompression (Fig. 28.1). Although the *only indication* for lumbar fusion in low back pain disorders is *intractable and incapacitating symptomatic segmental instability*, there are no generally accepted clinically useful operational definitions for a symptomatic mechanically unstable intervertebral joint. Therefore, rigorously designed prospective clinical studies are required if we hope to evolve patient selection factors and predictors that

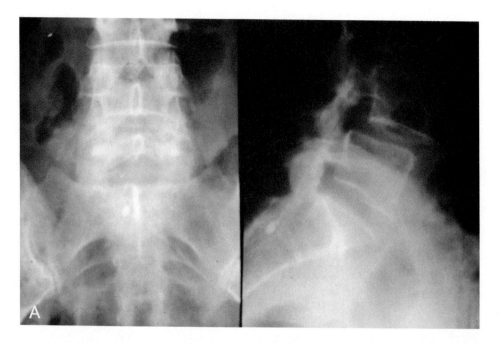

FIG. 28.1. Radiographic studies of a 58-year-old white female competitive square dancer who 2 years earlier developed progressively intractable and incapacitating low back and bilateral leg pain whenever weight-bearing. She was asymptomatic at bed rest. Her general and neurologic examination was within normal limits. (A) AP and lateral lumbosacral spine films which reveal Grade 1 spondylotic spondylolisthesis at L4–5. Stress flexion-extension x-rays revealed 5 mm of dynamic subluxation. (B) AP and lateral metrizimide lumbar myelogram which reveals central and lateral spinal stenosis at L4–5. (C) CT scan of L4–5 which reveals hypertrophic facets, vertebral subluxation, and spinal stenosis. A wide L4–5 decompressive laminectomy and bilateral L4–5 foraminotomies (undercutting of hypertrophic facets) was performed despite the multiple radiographic features consistent with so-called "instability". (D) Postoperative AP lumbosacral spine radiograph. Five years later, the patient remains completely free of back and leg pain and has resumed competitive square dancing.

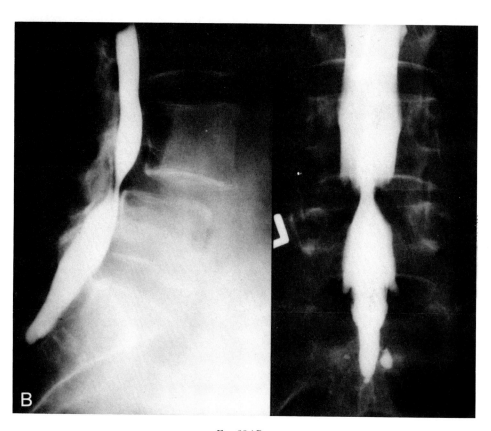

FIG. 28.1B

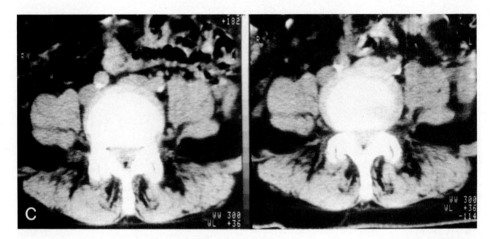

Fig. 28.1C

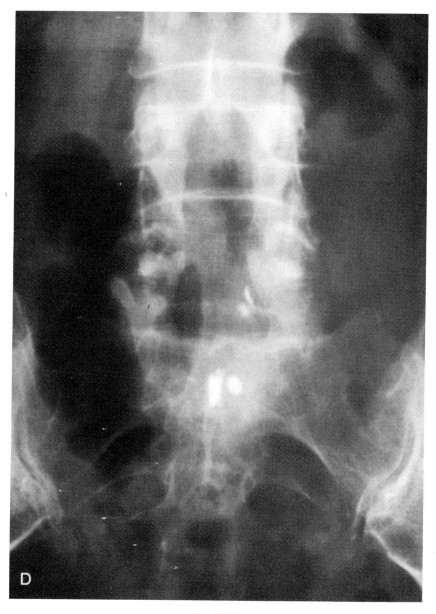

FIG. 28.1D

will be able to guide the choice of the most appropriate therapy for individual patients who suffer from intractable and incapacitating lumbago and sciatica.

Indications

The etiology of low back and leg pain of spinal origin in the vast majority of patients is unknown. Some clinicians assume that the basic problem is degeneration of the lumbar discs, but this is an unproved hypothesis. Most such patients complain of lumbago, often with diffuse nonspecific hip and leg radiation. Although the pain frequently follows the proximal course of the sciatic nerve, unlike true sciatica its termination and associated symptoms, such as numbness and paresthesias, are generally quite vague. Moreover, objective neurologic findings are typically absent. The symptoms are usually worsened by activity and improved by rest. Although a rare patient will reverse this complaint. Vigorous physical activities, particularly bending, twisting, and lifting, commonly exacerbate the symptoms, whereas restriction of pain-producing activities results in at least temporary improvement. Typical physical findings are nonspecific and include paravertebral muscle spasms, scoliosis, limited range of motion of the spine, muscular trigger points, tenderness, and aggravation of symptoms with the straight leg raising test. Objective reflex, motor, and sensory alterations are usually not present. Included in this group are patients who have been categorized by some spine specialists as lumbar facet syndrome and pyriformis syndrome. The author classifies these patients as predominantly "myofacial pain syndromes." They generally do quite well on a conservative back rehabilitation program if given sufficient reassurance, education, and encouragement by the treating physician. Furthermore, the concept cannot be overemphasized that such patients should be treated as a "human being with low back pain" and *not* turned into "a patient with a chronic pain syndrome" (low back cripple).

The patient with intractable and incapacitating "mechanical low back pain syndrome" is frequently difficult to differentiate from the patient suffering with a benign myofascial pain syndrome. These patients typically complain of low back and leg pain symptoms that are related to activities that mechanically stress the lumbar spine. Characteristically, these patients obtain almost complete relief of symptoms from recumbency or assuming a nonweight-bearing position. If the pain is relatively constant, being present even at bedrest, the clinician should be very cautious in considering the diagnosis of a mechanical pain syndrome. If the latter complaint is prominent, then psychosocial-economic pain syndrome (or neoplasia) should be given strong consideration, particularly when the patient requires larges doses of addicting drugs, requests antidepressants or tranquilizers, and must have medications for sleep. Hence, it is quite likely that the most important data for making the diagnosis of mechanical pain are historical in nature. Although a meticulous physical examination is essential, it may be unremarkable in some patients suffering intractable mechanical low back pain disorders.

The best results for fusion of the lumbosacral spine are achieved when a localized pathologic lesion is identified and definite indications of mechanical pain are determined (18). If an anatomic lesion firmly related to mechanical pain is not determined, a lumbar arthrodesis will not succeed (11, 40, 43). Essential data include a detailed history, a meticulous physical and neurologic examination, and appropriate laboratory investigation. An important component of this evaluation includes consideration of the emotional and personality characteristics (psychosocial-economic aspects) of the patient.

Since strong evidence is lacking regarding the specific role of lumbar fusion in patients suffering intractable low back pain syndromes, primary lumbar fusion has been rarely offered to our patients unless the patient is reasonably young with an exceedingly strong history of mechanical pain and overwhelming evidence of spinal instability (e.g., spondylolisthesis). Hence, we have limited lumbar fusion largely to highly motivated patients who failed appropriate decompressive surgery and appear to suffer chronic incapacitating mechanical low back pain syndromes (salvage spine surgery). Therefore, prior medical records, laboratory studies, operative reports and findings, and postoperative course(s) should be reviewed in detail. Moreover, the patients should be tried on an intensive conservative therapy program during which they are assessed by a surgeon on multiple occasions prior to consideration for a major lumbar reconstructive operative procedure. A 3 week trial of immobilization of lumbosacral spine in an appropriate orthotic device that incorporates one thigh (spica) appears to be beneficial in determining whether the patient's pain syndrome is mechanical in nature as well as in evaluating the patient's motivation.

Laboratory studies that appear to be helpful include: plain x-rays (lumbosacral spine and hips), water-soluble contrast lumbar myelography followed by computed tomography, and, occasionally, a radionuclide bone scan. These studies should verify the presence of a pathologic lesion consistent with spinal instability. However, the clinician must be very cautious because the presence of a pathologic lesion does not imply that it is symptomatic or causally related to the patient's complaints. The predictive values of lateral flexion and extension and anteroposterior right and left lateral bending films, electrodiagnostic testing, facet injections, diagnostic nerve blocks, differential spinal, and discography have not been rigorously or prospectively evaluated in any clinical study published to date despite their widespread use. Hence, we have not used these latter studies in the diagnostic work-up of our patients.

Posterolateral Fusion

Since we have largely restricted our prospective study of the role of lumbar fusion to patients suffering intractable and incapacitating mechanical low back pain disorders following previously performed low back surgery, we have elected to perform decompressive surgery when appropriate followed by a posterolateral (intertransverse) fusion in combination with a posterior element distraction-fixation device (Knodt rods). The rationale for this approach is founded on three separate concepts: (a) posterolateral fusion has proven to be highly reliable in achieving arthrodesis with minimal operative risk (23, 35); (b) internal fixation improves the probability of ensuring successful multilevel arthrodesis (4, 37, 42); and (c) posterior element distraction may relieve neural compression. Whether this surgical approach has any advantage over adequate neural decompression, adequate neural decompression plus posterolateral fusion without internal distraction-fixation, or posterior interbody fusion remains to be determined. Two case reports are presented to illustrate our approach to this problem.

CASE REPORT 1

An attractive, 38-year-old, white, female, physician's wife was referred to me with a past medical history of L4–5 laminotomies and discectomies two times 5 years earlier and a third L4–5 laminotomy and discectomy and L5-S1 exploration 2 years earlier. She sustained a low back injury 6 months earlier with a severe exacerbation of intractable and incapacitating low back and bilateral buttock and proximal leg pain related to weight bearing. Absolute bedrest temporarily and completely relieved her pain.

Physical examination revealed a well-developed, well-nourished, thin, white female with healed lumbar incisional scars and a marked limitation of motion of her lumbar spine. Straight leg raising and sciatic nerve stretch tests were positive for sciatica at 60° bilaterally. Patrick's maneuvers were negative. Her neurologic examination was within normal limits except for atrophy of her left extensor digitorum brevis (EDB) muscle.

A recently obtained CT scan and lumbar myelogram were interpreted to be consistent with epidural scarring at L5-S1 on the right (Fig. 28.2).

A 3 week trial in a University of Florida Lumbosacral Immobilizer

(UFLSI-polyform clam shell spica) completely relieved her pain. The pain immediately recurred with temporary discontinuation of the orthosis.

An exploration was performed at L5-S1 followed by internal distraction-fixation with Knodt instrumentation and posterior lateral fusion from L4-S1 (Fig. 28.2D). At surgery, epidural scar tissue was found at L5-S1.

The postoperative course was uncomplicated. During the next 3 months, the patient was required to wear the UFLSI whenever weight bearing. She is now some 4 years postoperative without back or leg pain. She has resumed all of her athletic activities (tennis, swimming, aerobic dancing, and jogging). In fact, at 2 years postoperative, she was able to complete a marathon run.

CASE REPORT 2

This 71-year-old white female was referred to me with a 2-year history of progressively intractable and incapacitating low back and left lower extremity sciatica when weight bearing. She was asymptomatic at bedrest. Her past medical history revealed that 5 years earlier she had undergone a decompressive laminectomy L4–5 for hypertrophic spondylotic spinal stenosis with an excellent result for 3 years.

Physical examination revealed a markedly obese, short, white female with a healed lumbar incision and limited range of motion of the lumbar spine. Straight leg raising, sciatic nerve stretch tests, and Patrick's maneuvers were negative. Her neurologic examination was within normal limits except for bilateral, decreased ankle tendon reflexes. Her radiographic studies are illustrated in Figure 28.3.

During a 3-week trial in a UFLSI, she obtained excellent relief from her pain. Upon temporary cessation of the othrosis, her pain rapidly recurred.

An L3 decompressive laminectomy and bilateral foraminotomies were performed followed by internal distraction-fixation with Knodt spinal instrumentation and posterior lateral fusion from L2-S1 (Fig. 28.3D). The postoperative course was uncomplicated. She was required to wear a UFLSI whenever weight bearing for the first 3 months following surgery. She was then begun on a course of low back rehabilitation walking 3 miles/day and extensor muscle stretching exercises.

The patient is now pain-free some 3 years postoperative and has resumed all of her normal activities, including bicycling 10 miles every day.

Preliminary Results

A preliminary analysis of the first 57 patients treated with posterolateral fusion techniques in a prospective study of the role of lumbosacral arthrodesis in mechanical low back pain syndromes at the University of Florida

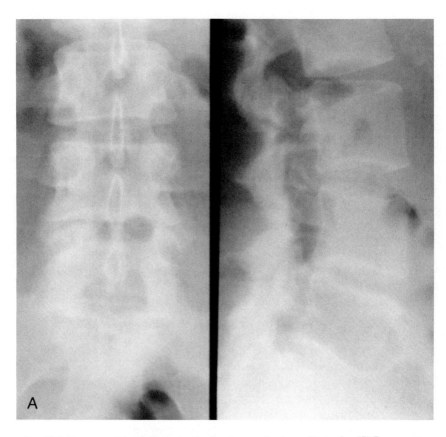

FIG. 28.2. Case report 1. (A) Preoperative lumbosacral spine radiographs. (B) Preoperative metrizimide myelogram. (C) Preoperative CT scan sections at L4–5. (D) One year postoperative lumbosacral spine radiographs. Note excellent posterolateral fusion mass L4-S1.

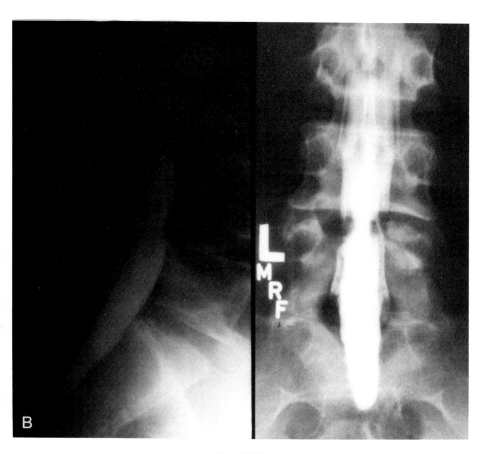

FIG. 28.2B

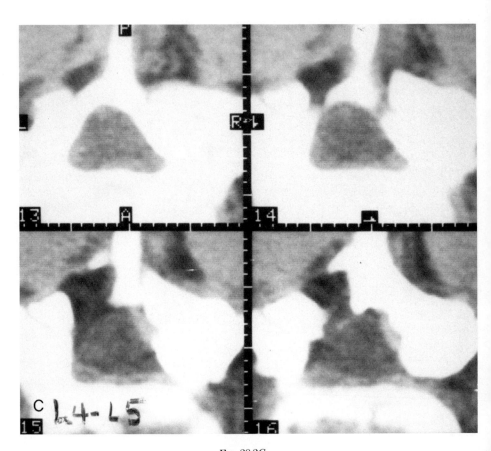

Fig. 28.2C

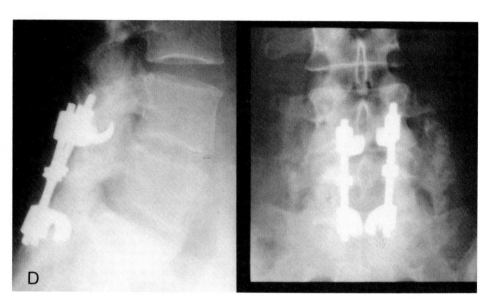

FIG. 28.2D

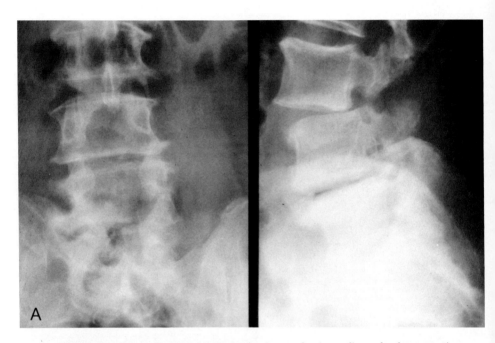

FIG. 28.3. Case report 2. (*A*) Preoperative lumbosacral spine radiographs demonstrating wide laminectomy L3–4, absent facets L3–4, and spondylotic spondylolisthesis L3–4. (*B*) Preoperative myelogram revealed no evidence of neural compression. (*C*) Preoperative CT scan L3–4 demonstrates severe spondylotic and surgical facet abnormalities. (*D*) One year postoperative lumbosacral spine radiographs demonstrating internal distraction-fixation with Knodt instrumentation and excellent posterolateral fusion mass extending from L2 to S1.

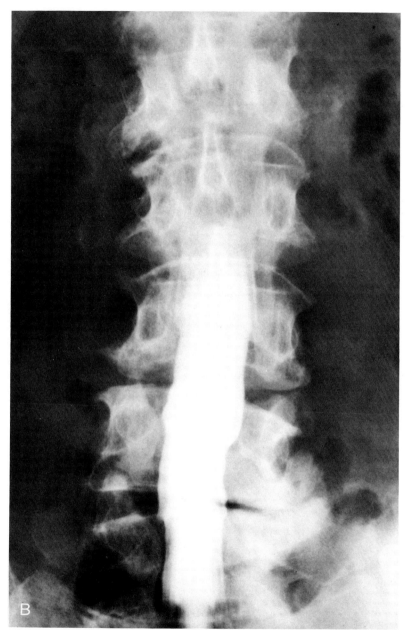

FIG. 28.3*B*

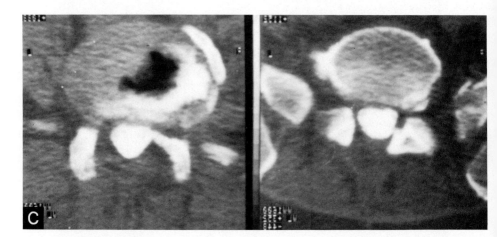

FIG. 28.3C

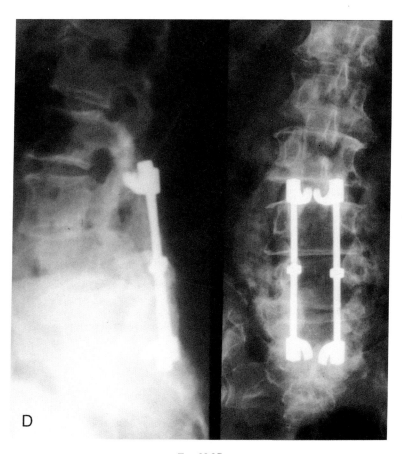

D

FIG. 28.3D

TABLE 28.3

Lumbosacral Arthrodesis for Low Back Pain Syndromes

U.F. Prospective Study—Preliminary Data Analysis

	N	
Patient Population		
Adults (mean age 42 yrs)	57	
Previous Surgery (1-3 ops)	41	(72%)
Compensation/Litigation	18	(32%)
Surgical Procedures*		
H-rods + PLF	30	(53%)
K-rods + PLF	11	(19%)
PLF (± wire fixation)	16	(28%)
Successful Results**		
Entire Population	37/57	(65%)
H-rods + PLF	18/30	(56%)
K-rods + PLF	10/11	(91%)
PLF (± wire fixation)	9/16	(56%)
H-rods (no complications)	14/16	(88%)
H-rods (with complications)	4/14	(29%)
Successful Fusion		
H-rods + K-rods	38/41	(93%)
PLF (± wire fixation)	13/16	(81%)
Complications		
H-rods	14/30	(47%)
K-rods and PLF	0/27	(0%)

* H-rods = Harrington distraction rods; K-rods = Knodt distraction rods; PLF = posterolateral fusion.

** Defined as an excellent (no pain or limitation) or good (occasional mild pain with minimal limitation of activity) outcome. All had resumed their normal livelihood and none were taking prescription medications.

was performed (Table 28.3). The patient population represented the most challenging segment of those patients with low back pain disorders evidenced by the percentage of patients with prior low back surgery (72%). Despite the difficulties involved in patient selection, the results are surprisingly good, with an overall success rate of 65%. Moreover, if one limits the analysis to that patient sample who underwent an uncomplicated operation which included the application of an internal distraction/fixation implant and posterolateral fusion, the results were dramatic with 24 of 27 patients classified as successful outcomes (89%) with a fusion rate of 96%. It should be noted that the subpopulation in which the internal distraction/fixation implant was Harrington distraction rod instrumentation had an unacceptably high incidence of complications (47%). These complications included seven cases of sacral nerve root injuries (23%) related to sacral canal compromise by the caudal hooks and seven cases of mechanical failure of the implant (loosening or displacement). The preliminary conclusions based on these data are as follows: (a) lumbosacral arthrodesis has a role in the treatment of certain rigorously selected patients suffering intractable and incapacitating low back pain disorders; (b) internal distraction-fixation implants appear to improve the probability of a successful clinical result; (c) internal distraction-fixation implants improve the incidence of bony fusion; (d) operative complications decrease the probability of a successful clinical result; and (e) Harrington distraction rod instrumentation should not be used in the operative treatment of low back pain disorders.

LUMBAR FUSION TECHNIQUES

Fusion of the lumbosacral spine is one of the original surgical methods used to treat low back pain disorders. Its historical foundation began in 1911 when Hibbs proposed spine fusion for treatment of progressive, deforming spinal disease (21). Its use was extended to degenerative spinal diseases soon thereafter. The first spinal fusions utilized the posteromedial spinal elements. Hibbs layered the spinous processes over the lamina. Albee (2) subsequently added a tibial cortical graft in an attempt to achieve arthrodesis. Distraction used in conjunction with fusion was first reported by Breck and Basom in 1943 (7). This concept was popularized in 1945 with the "H" graft of Bosworth (6). McBride developed another distraction technique that required no internal fixation (30). Cleveland et al. (10) published the first major series of posteromedial lumbosacral fusions. That series demonstrated that autogenous iliac bone grafting improved the fusion rate and that multilevel fusions have a higher incidence of pseudoarthrosis. Unfortunately, posteromedial fusions have proven to have an unacceptably high incidence of complications: high pseudoarthrosis rate and risk of iatrogenic spinal stenosis related to overgrowth of the fusion mass. Hence, a modified "posterior fusion," utilizing corticocancellous and cancellous strip grafts (matchstick size) harvested from the posterior iliac crest applied to the decorticated laminae and spinous processes combined with packing of the denuded facets with small chips of cancellous bone, is reserved for special circumstances. An example would be when the patient's condition does not permit prolonging the operative procedure.

A major advance in lumbosacral fusion occurred with the evolution of arthrodesis of the posterolateral spinal elements. The first clinical series was published by Cleveland et al. in 1948 (10). Autogenous matchstick iliac grafts were shown to be the optimal material for induction of fusion (23, 35, 38, 40, 41). Utilizing this approach, one can anticipate a 7% nonunion rate following a single-segment fusion and a 15% pseudoarthrosis rate for a two-segment posterolateral fusion (18). Because of the low rate of pseudoarthrosis and complications, posterolateral (intertransverse) fusion (PLF) has become the technique of choice for lumbosacral arthrodesis by the majority of orthopaedists.

Interbody fusions were recognized by Burns (8) and Capener (9) as early as 1932 as being the most mechanically advantageous. Anterior interbody fusion (ALIF) was attempted both transperitoneally (26) and retroperitoneally (20). Despite improvements in techniques over the years, ALIF continues to have a high rate of pseudoarthrosis and complications (1, 19, 22, 34). Posterior lumbar interbody fusion (PLIF) was introduced by Cloward in 1945 (11). Its initial acceptance was less than enthusiastic due to its technical difficulty, potential complications, and the understandable controversy as to the place of lumbosacral fusion in the low back pain disorders. However, the technique of PLIF has improved over the years, and interest in this technique has increased (12, 13, 24, 27, 29).

At present, the three generally accepted techniques for arthrodesing the lumbosacral spine for lumbosacral pain syndromes include PLF, PLIF, and ALIF. The role of internal fixation devices in the treatment of low back pain disorders is currently being evaluated prospectively at a number of institutions. Despite any lack of consensus regarding the role of lumbosacral arthrodesis in low back pain disorders and an absence of a useful clinical definition of lumbosacral "instability," a brief summary of the hypothetical advantages and disadvantages of these three operative approaches is attempted.

Posterolateral (Intertransverse) Fusion

Advantages: High fusion rate (90% single level, 80% two levels)
Neural elements need not be exposed
No bone overgrowth leading to spinal stenosis
No risk of neural injury from graft extrusion
Conventional posterior midline incision may be used
Excellent biomechanical support for resistance to torsional forces which appear to be highly detrimental to degenerating intervertebral joints

Disadvantages: Blood loss from donor site and recipient bone
Absence of contact compressive forces
Absence of distraction-decompression of spinal canal and foramina

Posterior Lumbar Interbody Fusion

Advantages: Distraction-decompression of spinal canal/foramina
Total discectomy prevents recurrent disc herniation
Relatively immediate mechanical stability
Alloimplant bone may be used
Contact compressive forces present

Disadvantages: Technically difficult
Pseudoarthrosis rate high (15–30%)
Excessive retraction of neural elements with risk of neurological and CSF complications
Graft migration (6–15%) with risk of neural injury
Constrictive epidural scar may form
Risk of great vessel and intra-abdominal injury

Anterior Lumbar Interbody Fusion

Advantages: No need to work in area of previous spinal surgery
Avoidance of intraspinal neural injury and scarring
Distraction-decompression of spinal canal/foramina
Relatively immediate mechanical stability
Alloimplant bone may be used
Contact compressive forces present

Disadvantages: Inability to surgically decompress neural elements
Lack of familiarity with anterior approaches
High pseudoarthrosis rate (20–30%)
Risk of gastrointestinal, genitourinary, and great vessel injury
High incidence of thromboembolic disease (5–8%)
Risk of retrograde ejaculation

SUMMARY

The role of lumbar spine arthrodesis in the treatment of low back pain disorders remains a highly disputed and controversial subject. There are no clear-cut indications for lumbar spine fusion in lumbar degenerative disc disease. In fact, lumbosacral fusion when added to appropriate decompressive surgery has failed on careful statistical analysis to significantly improve the results over decompressive surgery alone (14). Moreover, in several large series in the literature of lumbosacral fusion in conjunction with discectomy, the results in patients who developed a pseudoarthrosis did as well as matched cases who obtained an excellent arthrodesis (14–16, 36). These results should not be surprising since there does not appear to exist a generally accepted operational definition of mechanical (lumbar instability) pain. The author, however, is of the opinion that lumbosacral arthrodesis will prove to have a definite, albeit small, role in the management of the intractable and incapacitating low back pain disorders. This is based on personal clinical experience and the belief that the phenomenon of intractable and incapacitating mechanical low back pain syndromes do exist. Carefully performed prospective clinical studies are requisite to define the mechancial low back pain syndrome and the role of lumbar arthrodesis in the treatment of the low back pain disorders.

Given our present limitations, the author suggests that lumbosacral arthrodesis be reserved for patients suffering spondylotic low back pain syndromes who have the following characteristics: (*a*) intractable and disabling pain; (*b*) primary complaint of segmental *mechanical pain;* (*c*) radiologic evidence consistent with "instability"; (*d*) minimal or no segmental disease above proposed site of arthrodesis; and (*e*) minimal or absent psychosocial-economic pain.

REFERENCES

1. Adkins, E. W. O. Lumbosacral fusion after laminectomy. J. Bone Joint Surg., *37B:* 208–223, 1955.
2. Albee, F. H. Transplantation of a portion of the tibia into the spine for Pott's disease: a preliminary report. J.A.M.A. *57:* 885–886, 1911.
3. Barr, J. S., Kubik, C. S., Molloy, M. K., McNeill, J. M., Riseborough, E. J., and White, J. C. Evaluation of end results in treatment of ruptured lumbar intervertebral discs with protrusion of nucleus pulposus. Surg. Gynecol. Obstet., *125:* 250–256, 1967.
4. Beattie, F. C. Distraction rod fusion. Clin. Orthop., *62:* 218–222, 1969.
5. Bonica, J. J. *Pain.* Raven Press, New York, 1980.
6. Bosworth, D. M. Clothespin graft of the spine for spondylolisthesis and laminal defects. Am. J. Surg., *67:* 61–67, 1945.
7. Breck, L. W., and Basom, W. L. The flexion treatment of low back pain. J. Bone Joint Surg., *25:* 58–64, 1943.
8. Burns, B. H. An operation for spondylolisthesis. Lancet, *224:* 1233, 1933.
9. Capener, N. Spondylolisthesis. Br. J. Surg., *24:* 50–58, 1936.
10. Cleveland, M., Bosworth, D. M., and Thompson, F. R. Pseudoarthrosis in the lumbosacral spine. J. Bone Joint Surg., *30A:* 302–311, 1948.
11. Cloward, R. B. The treatment of ruptured intervertebral discs by vertebral body fusion. J. Neurosurg., *10:* 151–168, 1953.
12. Cloward, R. B. Posterior lumbar interbody fusion updated. Clin. Orthop., *193:* 16–19, 1985.
13. Collis, J. S. Total disc replacement: a modified posterior lumbar interbody fusion. Clin. Orthop., *193:* 64–67, 1985.
14. DePalma, A., and Rothman, R. The nature of pseudoarthrosis. Clin. Orthop., *59:* 113–118, 1968.
15. Flynn, J. C. Anterior fusion of the lumbar spine. J. Bone Joint Surg., *61A:* 1143, 1979.
16. Frymoyer, J. W., Hanley, E., Howe, J., Kuhlman, D., and Matteri, P. Disc excision and spine fusion in the management of lumbar disc disease: a minimum ten-year followup. Spine, *3:* 1–6, 1978.
17. Frymoyer, J. W., Matteri, R. E., Hanley, E. N., Kuhlmann, D., and Howe, J. Failed lumbar

disc surgery requiring second operation: a long-term followup study. Spine, *3:* 7–11, 1985.

18. Goldner, J. L. The role of spine fusion. Spine, *6:* 293–303, 1981.
19. Goldner, J. L., Wood, K. E., and Urbaniak, J. R. Anterior lumbar discectomy and interbody fusion: Indications and technique. In: *Operative Neurosurgical Techniques: Indications, Methods, and Results,* edited by H.H. Schmidek and W. H. Sweet, pp. 1373–1397. Grune Stratton, New York, 1982.
20. Harmon, P. Anterior extraperitoneal disc excision and vertebral body fusion. Clin. Orthop., *18:* 169, 1961.
21. Hibbs, R. A. An operation for progressive spinal deformities. NY Med. J., *93:* 1013–1016, 1911.
22. Hodgson, A. R. A description of a technique and evaluation of results in anterior spinal fusion for deranged intervertebral disc and spondylolisthesis. Clin. Orthop., *56:* 133, 1968.
23. Hoover, N. W. Methods of lumbar fusion. (AAOS Instr. Course Lect.), J. Bone Joint Surg., *50A*(1), 1968.
24. Hutter, C. G. Posterior intervertebral body fusion: A 25-year study. Clin. Orthop., *179:* 86, 1983.
25. Kelsey, T. L., and White, A. Epidemiology and impact of low back pain. Spine, *5:* 133–142, 1980.
26. Lane, J. D., and Moore, D. S. Transperitoneal approach to the intervertebral disc in the lumbar area. Ann. Surg., *127:* 537, 1948.
27. Lin, P. M. Posterior lumbar interbody fusion technique: Complications and pitfalls. Clin. Orthop., *193:* 90–102, 1985.
28. Loeser, J. D. Low back pain. In: *Pain,* ed. J. J. Bonica, pp. 363–377. Raven Press, New York, 1980.
29. Ma, G. W. C. Posterior lumbar interbody fusion with specialized instruments. Clin. Orthop., *193:* 57–63, 1985.
30. McBride, E. A mortissed transfacet bone block for lumbosacral fusion. J. bone Joint Surg., *31A*, 1949.
31. Nagi, S. Z., Riley, L. E., Newby, L. G. A social epidemiology of back pain in a general population. J. Chron. Dis., *26:* 769–779, 1973.
32. Poussaint, A. F. Psychological and psychiatric factors in the low back pain patient. In: *AAOS Symposium on Idiopathic Low Back Pain,* ed. A. A. White and S. L. Gordon, pp. 39–46. C. V. Mosby Company, St. Louis, 1982.

29

Management of Cervical Radiculopathy

WILLIAM E. HUNT, M.D. AND CAROLE A. MILLER, M.D.

PATHOPHYSIOLOGY

Acute cervical radiculopathy is usually due to herniated nucleus pulposus whereas chronic cervical radiculopathy is often the result of osteophyte formation. Acute herniation of soft disc material is but one facet of the larger process of chronic disc degeneration, (20, 40, 41). With aging, a series of biochemical changes occurs in which the nucleus polposus loses its normal gel consistency and its ability to distribute stress evenly. As the nucleus shrinks, the anulus must bear weight instead of providing circumferential restraint of the nucleus. Concomitantly, certain pathologic changes occur with loss of structural integrity which may, but only rarely does, allow herniation of dessicated nuclear material. More often, the space narrows, motion is limited, and osteophytes develop. The relationship between biochemical changes and structural stress is not entirely clear, but upright posture and the aging process are both operative (2, 8, 15–17, 21, 23, 26).

The morphology of the articulations between the cervical vertebrae are different from the lumbar segments. The latter are joined by three joints (the intervertebral disc anteriorly and two zygapophyseal joints posteriorly), the lower five cervical vertebrae are connected by five joints (the intervertebral disc anteriorly, the two zygapophyseal joints posteriorly, and the neural central joints of Luschka).

Cervical spondylosis is related to cervical disc degeneration, a complex process. Degeneration implies a mechanical breakdown of the integrity of the disc, initially producing symptoms because of mechanical instability, and only in the later stages causing root or cord compression due to the development of osteophytic overgrowths (3, 9, 12). This is a universal process with age first affecting the lower cervical and lumbar discs. It is a prerequisite to anular rupture and nuclear prolapse, events which are actually rare in view of the ubiquity of the degenerative process. If there is prolapse of nuclear material, symptoms are produced by pressure on the dura, posterior longitudinal ligament, root or spinal cord.

In the early stages of cervical disc degeneration, reflex pain syndromes may develop (11, 13). Acute trauma, however, does not appear to be the primary factor for most of the cervical radiculopathies under discussion, although it certainly can aggravate the pre-existing condition in the disc substance. Some persons are more susceptible than others and degenerative changes in the disc are frequently seen in patients without symptoms. The fact that the lesions more frequently occur at the interspaces (94% at the sixth and seventh) which are subjected to everyday stress and strain may be used as an argument in favor of chronic trauma as a primary or a secondary factor (27, 29).

Spurs and ridges are another result of degenerative changes in the cervical disc and may represent teleologically an attempt of the body to stabilize the degenerating interspace. These "osteophytes" may not be symptomatic.

Acute cervical monoradiculopathy is a common neurologic lesion in the cervical spine (1, 10, 13, 21, 39). Specific neck trauma is relatively uncommon, many patients awaken with neck pain and/or brachialgia as the first symptom. The pain is aggravated by movements such as coughing, breathing, sneezing, and Valsalva's maneuver. Hyperextension and turning the neck away from the side of the lesion with compression (Spurling's sign) characteristically produces a poorly localized but radicular type of pain. It may also cause tingling in the distal dermatome. Sensory deficit, motor and reflex changes more accurately define the level of the radiculopathy. By contrast, chronic monoradicular syndromes are a poorly defined entity, usually without clear monoradicular deficit. The attribution of root pain and vague numbness to osteophytes is difficult to prove, since spurs are so common, and insidious chronic pain can arise from joint capsules or ligament without root compression. Trauma often precipitates symptoms in the arthritic spine. Osteophytic spurs per se rarely cause chronic progressive monoradicular syndromes, although a soft protrusion superimposed on an osteophytic spur may cause the acute syndrome.

Stookey (41) was the first to define typical syndromes, referring to group I as compression of the spinal cord, group 2 as mixed lateral cord and root compression, and group 3 as the monoradicular syndrome, the subject of this essay.

Scoville and Whitcomb (34–38) described five distinct categories of cervical disc lesions. They believe such categorization is mandatory if one is to approach the management of cervical spine lesions rationally. The five categories are as follows: (a) the lateral "soft" disc; (b) the lateral arthritic "hard" or osteophytic disc; (c) the central "bar" or ridge disc; (d) the rare central "soft" disc; and (e) fracture dislocation with disc injury. In almost 95% of the cases culled from the literature, the disc lesions are lateral with the majority of those producing the classic acute monoradicular syndrome soft discs. Miller (25) has pointed out the role of congenital narrowing as a predisposing factor to pain or deficit as degenerative changes occur.

Acute cervical nerve root compression produces a characteristic clinical picture which is consistent in its pattern and is not difficult to diagnose; but the diagnosis is seldom made when the patient first presents (13, 18, 19). Bursitis, arthritis, neuritis, "myositis", and other painful conditions may be simulated by nerve root compression since pain referral is largely to the suprascapular region, shoulder, or arm. It may also present as occipital headache, interscapular pain, pain into the chest and down the arm, and even retro-ocular pain.

There are several factors involved here. First, the pain is of C-fiber origin due to inflammation and stretching of ligament or root, probably caused by ischemia plus recurrent trauma. Pressure on the nerve without inflammation, as in sleep and tourniquet palsies, is not painful. It blocks axonal conduction, beginning with the largest A-fibers producing the weakness, distal numbness, and reflex changes that accurately identify the root. The deep, aching, predominantly proximal pain is too diffuse for accurate localization. It is the A-fiber deficit that identifies the root. In addition to pain and deficit there may be a third phenomenon, the congeries of diffuse reflex phenomena that can obscure the origin of the nociceptive input. There may be headache, suboccipital "neuralgia," blurred vision, light headedness, and other complaints sometimes labeled the "cervical tension syndrome." All clinicians are familiar with this; none, to our knowledge, can explain it with any precision.

Since the interpretation of symptoms affects the choice of treatment and even the surgical approach, the history is essential (19). Seven major points deserve inquiry:

1. *Onset.* In nuclear extrusion, the onset is usually acute and rarely due to an episode of trauma. The patient may awaken with a severe pain radiating to one shoulder and arm. Numbness may be delayed, and focal weakness may be masked by pain inhibition. If the cervical radiculopathy is of insidious onset and steady progression, symptoms may be difficult to distinguish from tumor.

2. *Progression.* Progression of the pain syndrome is often irregular, with recurrent attacks of varying severity. The patient has ordinarily been through several bouts of stiff neck and brachalgia before he or she finally presents with a full-blown root syndrome.

3. *Character.* The character of the pain is more visceral than somatic. That is to say it is "deep" and poorly localized, tends to be aching, and

tends to be felt more proximally than distally. The numbness is a different matter, best appreciated in the distal part of the dermatome. As noted, because of the acute onset and diffuse referral the character and location of pain can simulate that of myocardial infarction or bursitis.

4. *Location.* As noted, the pain is of little value in identifying the involved nerve root, although the slightest numbness or tingling is quite reliable in identifying the dermatome.

5. *Remissions and exacerbations.* The familiar aggravation of pain with cough, sneeze, straining at stool, or specific moments of the spine are indications of inflamed tissue (root and/or ligament) affected by movement or by pressure fluctuations in the dural sac. In the cervical region, if the patient recovers from a bout of acute radiculopathy from a soft disc protrusion it is less common for him to have another attack involving the same root. This differs from lumbar disc disease, perhaps because a smaller volume of material is protruded and the body's repair mechanisms for shoring up weak areas are more effective in the neck than in the lumbar region.

6. *Associated signs and symptoms* such as weakness, numbness, or reflex change of an extremity are the usual basis for the diagnosis of radiculopathy in a patient with chronic neck and arm pain. Evidence of spinal cord dysfunction must also be carefully sought.

7. *Response to previous therapy.* Since disc syndromes often resolve, at least to some extent, response to rest and physical therapy is an important differential point. Tumors do not improve. Some acute radiculopathies are specifically aggravated by traction.

Finally, there are some odd variations in the disc syndromes such as the appearance of painless neurologic deficit. We have seen this rarely.

CLINICAL EXAMINATION

The examination begins by searching for limitation of movement of the spine, loss of its normal curve, or list. Subtle signs of muscle imbalance may be brought out by having the patient tilt his head backward, forward, and to the sides, noting limitation of motion. Specific aggravation of symptoms with hyperextension and turning the chin away from the side of the lesion (Spurling's sign) is almost pathognomonic of root compression. Tenderness of the interspinous ligaments and trigger points in tender muscle are nonspecific. Severe pain on percussion suggests a destructive lesion of the vertebra rather than a herniated disc.

The neurologic examination centers on the sensory, motor, and reflex changes characteristic of the cervical nerve root syndromes (Fig. 29.1). The areas of sensory loss do not have sharp margins. The sensory loss to any modality is never complete in monoradicular syndromes. It is best to

CERVICAL:

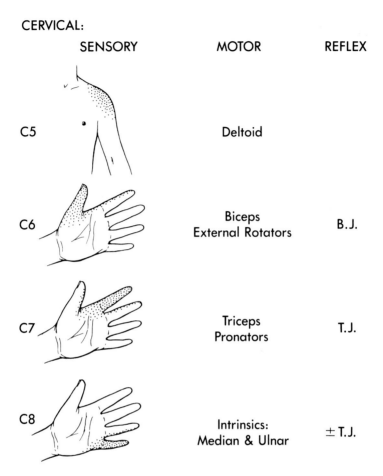

SENSORY	MOTOR	REFLEX
C5	Deltoid	
C6	Biceps External Rotators	B.J.
C7	Triceps Pronators	T.J.
C8	Intrinsics: Median & Ulnar	± T.J.

Fig. 29.1. The distribution of the more obvious sensory, motor, and reflex changes characteristic of the cervical nerve root syndromes. T1 deficit (not shown) produces a Horner's syndrome and little else except minimal weakness of the intrinsic muscles of the hand.

ask the patient if a given area "feels natural" to touch or pin scratch. The ball of the thumb or index finger are served by as much sensory cortex as the entire trunk, hence minor differences in the transmission of touch are quite noticeable. Slight subjective changes, therefore, are significant. There is, after all, no such thing as "objective" sensory change.

Motor deficit generally coincides with the sensory loss. The gross pattern is not very hard to remember: the deltoids, biceps, triceps, and the intrinsic muscles of the hand (C5, C6, C7, and C8) provide a rough survey of the lower cervical roots. Weakness of external rotation is noted in C6 loss, and the tendency of the elbow to move away from the thorax when the patient attempts to pronate his hands against resistance (C7) because he recruits internal rotators of the shoulder to assist the weak pronation. The biceps reflex is depressed in C6, the triceps in C7 lesions. A Horner's syndrome is seen in the rare T1 radiculopathy.

DIAGNOSTIC PROCEDURES

Plain X-rays

Plain films show degenerative disc disease and narrowing of the interspace, but the soft, freshly herniated nucleus often occurs at the interspace adjacent to the one with the greatest degenerative changes. Since dynamics are of interest, cervical spine x-rays should include lateral views in flexed, neutral, and extended positions.

Electromyography

Electrodiagnostic studies are useful in confirming the presence of chronic nerve root damage, i.e., damage of over 3 weeks in duration. Fibrillation seen with electromyography (EMG) is evidence of dead axons and means that the nerve root damage is severe (22). If the process seems to be progressing, this is reason to consider prompt surgical decompression. The reverse, the absence of dead axons, favors further conservative treatment. Obviously, if the pain is due chiefly to stretch of the posterior longitudinal ligament neurologic deficit will not be found by neurologic exam nor by EMG.

Myelography

This is usually reserved for those patients who have met our surgical criteria, the failure of conservative therapy, and/or serious neurologic deficit. Only rarely should this test be done simply to "rule out" a disc. Myelography often shows false-positives and the findings do not always correlate with the clinical picture. It is an important truism that one does not operate upon the x-ray but upon the patient.

Discography

Cervical discography and the disc distention tests are controversial, but may have a place in the management of certain disc problems, especially in identifying the level of discogenic pain without neurologic deficit.

Contrast Enhanced Computed Tomography Scan

We have found myelography with contrast-enhanced CT scan to be of some value. It helps differentiate the "hard" versus the "soft" disc (Figs. 29.2 and 29.3). CT scanning, however, must be quite precise and has been, in our hands, of little benefit without contrast enhancement. Two-mm cuts

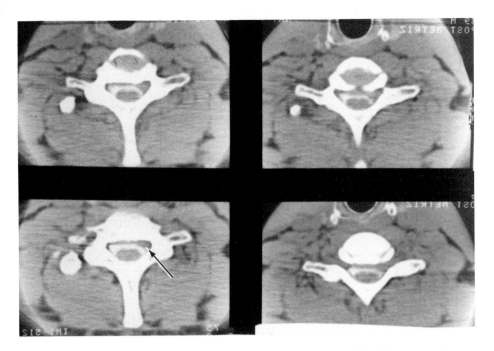

Fɪɢ. 29.2. Contrast-enhanced CT scan in a patient with an acute right C7 radiculopathy demonstrating a soft disc herniation. Note also relatively shallow cervical canal with shortening of facets, laterally placed pedicles, and relatively flat lamina. There is minimal posterior subarachnoidal space. This shallow canal was otherwise asymptomatic.

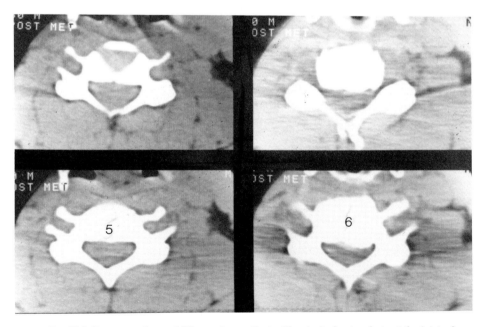

Fɪɢ. 29.3. Contrast-enhanced CT scan in a patient with a typical osteophyte at the joint of Luschka on the left in a patient with a C6 radiculopathy. The location suggests that the "soft" and "hard" discs are in different stages of the same process.

parallel to the involved disc space with sagittal reconstructions are needed.

Magnetic Resonance Imaging

We are just acquiring experience with cervical disc disease using MRI scanning. It is hoped, however, that the inflamed joint will be identified with MRI scan and conceivably could eliminate the necessity for both the myelography and discography.

Of these procedures, we have found the neurologic examination to be the most specific, and only the myelogram as sensitive, in identifying the involved root.

TREATMENT: NONOPERATIVE

Nonoperative treatment is directed at decompression of the root by traction and by measures to reduce the inflammation and edema. Often the passage of time is the first of such measures (24). Application of counterirritants, hot showers, TNS units, etc., may be helpful, especially for the reflex symptoms. During the acute phase, proper immobilization of the cervical spine by a cervical collar may also help. All nonoperative modalities should be discontinued if they increase the patient's pain or neurologic deficit.

Failure of nonoperative treatment must be specifically defined and individualized. For instance, a patient's occupation may prompt one to do surgery earlier than otherwise. Whether or not the left or the right arm is involved may be an indication for early decompression. Occupation and age may be very important. For example, left C7 paresis is most disabling to an anesthesiologist, a left C8 to a violinist or surgeon. Failure of pain control must be defined by the patient.

In the acute phase, if the pain is severe and if there is significant sensorimotor disability, very early root decompression is indicated, especially with C7 and C8 root syndromes (26–29). Otherwise an arbitrary 7–10 days at complete bedrest with traction, steroids, and analgesics should be tried. With improvement, one continues the conservative modalities, but less vigorously, decreasing the steroids or nonsteroidal anti-inflammatories.

A number of patients will plateau at a certain neurologic deficit, perhaps with significantly reduced pain. There may be a question in these patients whether or not to operate. In general, no improvement or worsening is an indication for prompt operative intervention.

TREATMENT: OPERATIVE

Selection of anterior versus posterior approach to the decompression of the root is to some extent the surgeon's choice (4–6, 25, 28, 30–33). However, discogenic pain along with claudication due to a spur at the joint of Luschka would appear to be an indication for an anterior approach. For a pure radiculopathy of acute onset, we prefer a posterior approach using a muscle splitting incision. Postoperative pain and surgical complications are negligible with this procedure, in contrast to the anterior approach (14, 25, 28, 29, 38).

In chronic radiculopathy, if the operation is for relief of pain, the surgeon needs a clear concept of the origin of that pain, *i.e.*, root, facet, disc, spur at the joint of Luschka, spur about the zygapophyseal joint, or ligaments. Here we go back to the pain history and define very carefully the pain pattern. These cases may require discography. If pain pattern is due to other than root inflammation, anterior discectomy with the microscope is preferred. We use the Cloward and Smith-Robinson techniques interchangeably. In our series of acute radiculopathies done via the posterior approach, only three of 85 have gone on to need anterior discectomy for discogenic type pain. In only one case was this at the same level. In the others, it was at the level above a previous C6–7 acute herniated nucleus pulposus. All three had the suboccipital headache syndrome, or "cervical tension syndrome."

TECHNIQUE FOR POSTERIOR MUSCLE SPLITTING APPROACH

In radiculopathy of acute soft disc herniation, we prefer the oblique muscle-splitting incision (Figs. 29.4–29.9). It allows the same exposure as a midline incision. One can, if necessary, explore three nerve roots via a Scoville-type laminotomy and hemifacetectomy. One avoids the more painful midline incision with the concomitant complications. The oblique wound is under no tension and complications are negligible (one hematoma in 85 consecutive cases). The complications of anterior fusions are numerous and well described (14) (Table 29.1).

With the patient in the lateral forward oblique position, the involved side up, the head resting on a pad, a 5-cm diagonal incision is made parallel to the trapezius fibers. The incision passes over the articulation of the desired interspace. Intraoperative x-ray may be helpful, the profile and shape of the spinous processes is quite adequate when confirmed with cervical spine films. Splitting of the trapezius fibers exposes the aponeurosis of the serratus posterior superior whose fibers are, in turn, split, exposing the splenius capitus fibers converging on the midline. These are split and the deep vertical layer of muscles, multifidus and semispinalis, are seen. Two laminae are then exposed by subperiosteal dissection and self-retaining retractors inserted. A keyhole laminotomy (Scoville) is then performed for exploration of the root and foraminotomy. The muscle layers reapproximate themselves spontaneously on removal of the retractor. Closure of

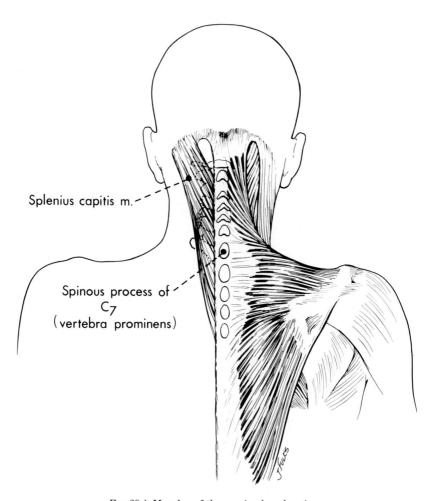

Splenius capitis m.

Spinous process of
C$_7$
(vertebra prominens)

FIG. 29.4. Muscles of the cervicodorsal region.

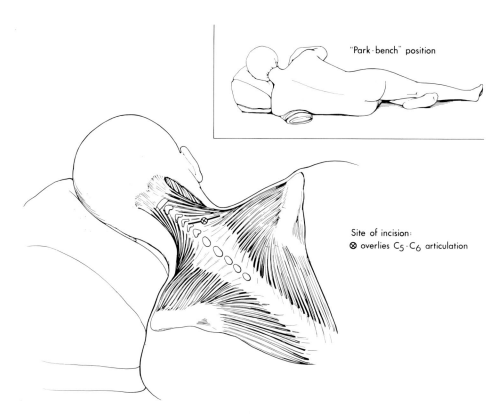

"Park-bench" position

Site of incision:
⊗ overlies C_5-C_6 articulation

FIG. 29.5. Positioning of patient for muscle split incision. AP film or intraoperative C-arm can be used at this point for localization. Injecting Indigo Carmine 0.2 ml into joint capsule is helpful if the surgeon is not comfortable with localization by palpation of the vertebral contours.

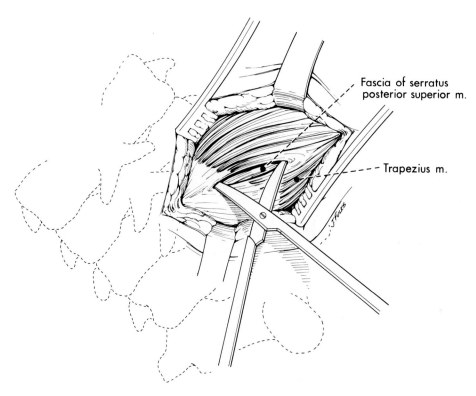

FIG. 29.6. Transverse skin incision is made. Trapezius aponeurosis and muscle fibers are split.

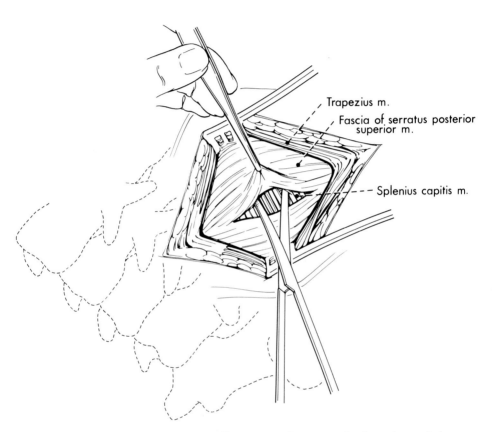

Trapezius m.

Fascia of serratus posterior
superior m.

Splenius capitis m.

FIG. 29.7. Trapezius aponeurosis and fibers retracted, aponeurosis of serratus posterior superior muscle split. The splenius capitis muscle fibers are exposed running nearly at right angles to those of the trapezius.

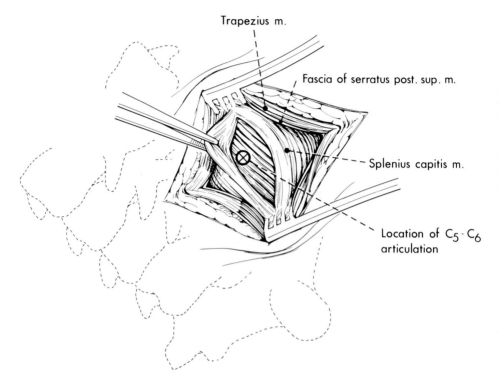

FIG. 29.8. Splenius capitis split, exposing semispinalis cervicis and multifidus muscle. These are then stripped from lamina exposing lamina and facets.

the trapezius fascia, subcutaneous tissue, and the skin is easily performed without tension (25).

THE CERVICAL MYOSPASTIC SYNDROME

A separate problem exists when the reflex cervical myospastic syndrome is present as a result of discogenic or arthrogenic pain. This phenomenon usually responds to nonoperative treatment. The diagnosis can be confirmed by response to discography. Most abnormal discs are not painful. Fusion should be confined to those which are painful after repeated but transient response to bedrest and traction, clear reproduction of the pain syndrome with discography, and temporary relief after injection of local anesthetic and steroids.

It is rare that multiple painful segments should be treated surgically, because of the multiple sources of nociceptive input that trigger the syn-

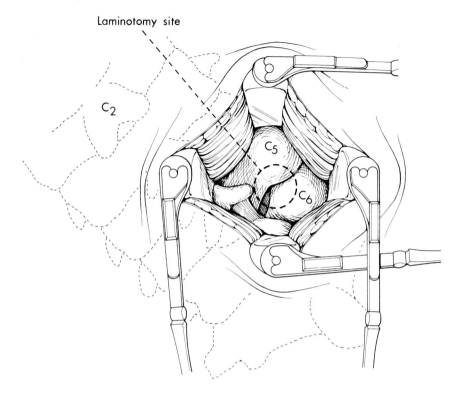

Fig. 29.9. Subperiosteal dissection of semispinalis cervicus and multifidus from laminae and facets exposes the C5–6 articulation.

TABLE 29.1

Neurologic Complications Associated with Anterior Discectomy and Fusion (Flynn) (14)

1. Horner's syndrome	13
2. Recurrent laryngeal nerve palsy	52
3. Transient radiculopathy (3 from fracture of bone graft)	14
4. Radiculopathy ("intraoperative etiology")	124
5. Progressive myelopathy increased postoperatively	1
6. Mild transient myelopathy (3 from fracture of bone graft)	6
7. Significant permanent radiculopathy	22
8. Significant permanent myelopathy	78
9. Cerebral infarction	1
	311

drome. A prompt, but unhappily transient improvement, has led to overoptimistic assessment of this operation in the past.

SUMMARY AND CONCLUSION

1. Cervical monoradiculopathy occurs most commonly at C5–6 and C6–7. It is due mostly to acute herniation of nuclear material.

2. The syndrome often responds to conservative prescription but when surgery is indicated, the results are good.

3. The neurologic examination is the most specific and sensitive clinical test.

4. Acute radiculopathies due to herniated nucleus are, in our hands, best approached via a posterior muscle-splitting incision.

5. Chronic radiculopathies due to osteophyte formation may be approached either anteriorly or posteriorly.

6. Reflex discogenic pain requiring anterior fusion exist but are less common. These patients must be carefully screened because of the functional factors involved.

REFERENCES

1. Brain, W. R. Discussion on rupture of intervertebral disc in cervical region. Proc. Roy. Soc. Med., *41:* 509–511, 1948.
2. Bucy, P. C., Heimburger, R. F., and Oberhill, H. R. Compression of cervical spine cord by herniated intervertebral discs. J. Neurosurg., *5:* 471–492, 1948.
3. Bull, J. W. D. Discussion on rupture of intervertebral disc in cervical region. Proc. Roy. Soc. Med., *41:* 513–516, 1948.
4. Cloward, R. B. Lesions of the intervertebral disc and their treatment by interbody fusion methods. Clin. Orthop., *27:* 51–77, 1963.
5. Cloward, R. B. New method of diagnosis and treatment of cervical disc disease. Clin. Neurosurg., *8:* 93–132, 1962.
6. Connolly, E., Seymour, R., and Adams, J. Clinical evaluation of anterior cervical fusion for degenerative cervical disc disease. J. Neurol., *23:* 431–437, 1965.
7. Coventry, M. B., Ghormley, R. K., and Kernohan, J. W. The intervertebral discs. J. Biol. Chem., *234:* 2951, 1959.
8. Dandy, W. E. Loose cartilage from intervertebral disk simulating tumor of spinal cord. Arch. Surg., *19:* 660–672, 1929.
9. Davidson, E., *et al.* Biochemical alterations in herniated intervertebral discs. J. Biol. Chem., *234:* 2951, 1959.
10. Davis, C. H., Jr., Odom, G. L., and Woodhall, B. Survey of ruptured intervertebral disks in cervical region. North Carolina Med. J., *14:* 61–66, 1953.
11. Epstein, J. A., Epstein, B. S., *et al.*, Cervical myeloradiculopathy caused by arthritic hypertrophy of the posterior facets and laminae. J. Neurosurg., *49:* 387–392, 1978.
12. Eyring, E. The biochemistry and physiology of the intervertebral disc. Clin. Orthop., *67:* 16–28, 1968.
13. Fager, C. A. Diagnosis of cervical nerve root compression. Med. Clin. North Am., *47:* 463–471, 1963.
14. Flynn, T. B. Neurologic complications of anterior cervical interbody fusion. Spine, *7(6):* 536–539, 1982.

15. George, R. C., and Chrisman, O. D. The role of cartilage polysaccharides in osteoarthritis. Clin. Orthop., *57:* 259–265, 1968.
16. Gower, W., and Pedrini, V. Age related variations in protein polysaccharides. J. Bone Joint Surg., *51A:* 1154–1162, 1969.
17. Hendry, N. The hydration of the nucleus pulposus. J. Bone Joint Surg., *40B:* 132–144, 1968.
18. Horack, H. M., Marvel, J. P., Jr. Cervical root syndrome. Med. Clin. North Am., *51:* 1027–1034, 1967.
19. Hunt, W. E., Paul, S. Herniated cervical and lumbar discs: a discussion of clinical findings and diagnostic procedures. Ohio St. Med. J., *65*(6): 583–587, 1969.
20. Keyes, D. C., and Compere, E. L. The normal an pathological physiology of the nucleus pulposus of the intervertebral disc. J. Bone Joint Surg., *14:* 897–938, 1932.
21. Lourie, H., Shende, N., and Stewart, D. The syndrome of central cervical disc herniation. J.A.M.A., *226:* 302–305, 1973.
22. Marinacci, A. A. A correlation between the operative findings in cervical herniated discs with the electromyograms and opaque myelograms with particular reference to simulators of post compression. Bull. Los Angeles Neurol. Soc. *30:* 118–130, 1965.
23. Markolf, K. L., and Morris, J. M. The structural components of the intervertebral disc. J. Bone Joint Surg., *56A:* 675–687, 1974.
24. Martin, G. M., and Corbin, K. B. Evaluation of conservative treatment for patients with cervical disk syndrome. Arch. Phys. Med., *35:* 87–92, 1954.
25. Miller, C. A., and Hunt, W. E. Neurological correlations in cervical monoradicular syndromes: Treatment by the muscle splitting approach. Poster Session, AANS, San Francisco, 1984.
26. Mixter, W. J., and Barr, J. S. Rupture of intervertebral disc with involvement of spinal canal. N. Engl. J. Med., *211:* 210–215, 1934.
27. Murphey, F., Simmons, J. C. H. Ruptured cervical disc: Experience with 250 cases. Am. Surg., *32:* 83–88, 1966.
28. Murphey, F., Simmons, J. C. H., *et al.* Surgical treatment of laterally ruptured cervical disc. Journal of Neurosurgery, *38:* 679–683, 1973.
29. Odom, G. L., Finney, W., Woodhall, B. Cervical disk lesions. J.A.M.A., *166:* 23–38, 1958.
30. Riley, L. Cervical disc surgery: its role and indications. Orthop. Clin. North Am., *2:* 443–452, 1971.
31. Robertson, J. T. Anterior operations for herniated cervical disc and for myelopathy. Clin. Neurosurg., *25:* 245–250, 1978.
32. Robinson, R. A. The results of anterior interbody fusion of the cervical spine. J. Bone Joint Surg., *44A:* 1569–1586, 1962.
33. Robinson, R. A., and Smith, G. W. The treatment of certain cervical-spine disorders by anterior removal of the intervertebral disc and interbody fusion. J. Bone Joint Surg., *40A:* 607, 1958.
34. Scoville, W. B. Cervical disc lesions treated by posterior operations. In *Operative Surgery,* edited by C. Rob and R. Smith, Vol. 14, ed. 2. London, Butterworths, 1971, pp. 250–258.
35. Scoville, W. B. Cervical spondylosis treated by bilateral facetectomy and laminectomy. Neurosurgery, *18:* 423–428, 1961.
36. Scoville, W. B. Types of cervical disk lesions and their surgical approaches. J.A.M.A., *196:* 479–481, 1966.
37. Scoville, W. B., Dohrmann, G. J., *et al.* Late results of cervical disc surgery. J. Neurosurg., *45:* 203–210, 1976.
38. Scoville, W. B., Whitcomb, B. B. Lateral rupture of cervical intervertebral discs. Postgrad. Med., *39:* 174–180, 1960.

39. Semmes, R. E., and Murphey, F. Syndrome of unilateral rupture of sixth cervical interver-
    tebral disk with compression of seventh cervical nerve root: report of four cases with
    symptoms simulating coronary disease. J.A.M.A., *121:* 1209–1214, 1943.
40. Simeone, F. A., and Rothman, R. H. Cervical disc disease. In: *The Spine*, Chapter 7. W.B.
    Saunders Co., Philadelphia, 1982.
41. Stookey, B. Compression of spinal cord and nerve roots by herniation of the nucleus
    pulposus in the cervical region. Arch. Surg., *40:* 417–432, 1940.

30

Surgical Treatment of Spinal Metastases

NARAYAN SUNDARESAN, M.D., GEORGE V. DIGIACINTO, M.D.,
AND JAMES E. O. HUGHES, M.D.

INTRODUCTION

Metastases to the spine represent an important cause of morbidity in cancer patients. The treatment of this clinical disorder has aroused considerable controversy in management during the past decade. A major factor for the therapeutic dilemma is the lack of controlled clinical studies evaluating the relative merits of surgery versus radiation (RT) alone. Since spinal metastases may complicate any stage of a cancer patient's illness, treatment goals vary from patient to patient. In the majority, the major goal of therapy is palliation; relief of pain, improvement of neurologic function, and preservation of autonomic function are accepted aims of therapy. In others, spinal involvement may represent the only site of disease (44–46); effective treatment in this group of patients will also have a major impact on survival. With improvements in cancer therapy, the pool of patients with spinal sites of relapse may increase and pose complex therapeutic challenges for the treating surgeon. In this review, only the literature within the past 5 years on the management of this entity is reviewed, with particular emphasis on the changing role of surgical management (3–5, 7, 8, 12, 15, 22, 23, 25, 26, 32, 35, 39, 40, 43, 47, 49).

INCIDENCE AND CLINICAL FEATURES

Autopsy data suggest that approximately 5% of cancer patients have epidural invasion of tumor, the majority resulting from extension of tumor within the vertebral body. In the clinical setting, however, precise figures for the magnitude of this problem are not available. Major oncology centers may see between 80 and 100 patients/year with this complication of cancer (17, 49). An estimate of the overall magnitude of this problem can be obtained by multiplying the expected proportion (5%) by the number of cancer deaths per year in the U.S. (14). If such estimates are accurate, the number of patients with spinal cord injury from neoplasia exceeds the number of those with traumatic injuries (29).

The socioeconomic consequences of caring for the spinal cord injury cancer patient are not important at present because the majority die within a few months. With intensive rehabilitation techniques, Murray (29) has shown that patients with partial spinal cord injuries secondary to neoplasia have the potential for longer survival. As an estimate of this problem, we have listed in Table 30.1 the five most common primary sites of cancer, including the expected incidence of osseous involvement. The higher rate of involvement of the axial skeleton by these tumors clearly underscores the important role the treatment of this complication may have in the future. Data from surgical series further suggest that 20–40% of patients undergoing surgical treatment have involvement of the spine by hematogenous spread, or by direct extension from a paraspinal focus at the time of initial diagnosis of their malignancy (36, 39, 40).

The clinical presentation of the syndrome of spinal cord compression is relatively straightforward; up to 90% of patients present with back pain with a subacute onset of symptoms. Varying degrees of motor deficit may be found on clinical examination; these deficits are appropriately classified into radiculopathy or plexopathy, cauda equina compression, or cord compression with varying degrees of paraparesis. Since restoration or maintenance of ambulation represents the most objective end point in most current series (4, 17, 18, 20, 25, 26, 34), a comparison of pre- and post-treatment ambulatory status is a major parameter that allows comparison of various modes of therapy. However, it is not clear from most published series whether assessments of neurologic deficits were made before or after high dose corticosteroid therapy. With increasing recognition of the clinical presentation by most oncologists, most patients have already received high dose steroid therapy prior to neurosurgical assessment. Response to high dose corticosteroid therapy not only influences the pretreatment evaluation, but has important prognostic significance since patients who show clinical evidence of deterioration despite steroid ther-

TABLE 30.1

Estimated New Cases and Deaths for Major Sites of Cancer—1985[a]

Site	No. of Cases	Deaths	% Spine Involvement
Lung	144,000	126,000	5–20
Colon-rectum	138,000	60,000	20
Breast	119,000	38,000	50–70
Prostate	86,000	26,000	50–70
Genitourinary	60,000	20,000	10–20

[a] From American Cancer Society. *Facts and Figures—1985.*

apy have poor outcomes regardless of treatment (2). However, despite an increasing clinical awareness of the problem, only half the patients with spinal metastases are ambulatory at the beginning of therapy; approximately 10% of patients deteriorate acutely to complete paraplegia while undergoing therapy within the hospital setting.

The need for accurate radiographic delineation by myelography to determine both the extent and the anatomic level of block is well recognized. In patients presenting with back pain alone or with referred sites of pain, complete radiologic diagnosis may require both myelography and computed tomography (CT). CT scans frequently show extensive destruction of the vertebral body when plain spine x-rays appear remarkably normal. In addition, CT scans are useful in demonstrating paraspinal masses. With the introduction of magnetic resonance imaging (MRI) scans, it is now possible to image both the spine and epidural tumor in the sagittal plane. Such scans are of value in diagnosing "segmental instability" of the spine, especially in those patients who have undergone radiation therapy.

Accurate documentation of epidural tumor by Pantopaque myelography is important for several reasons: (a) Both the upper limit and lower limit of block is marked out for appropriate radiation portals. (b) Approximately 10% of patients have multifocal sites of spine involvement. In those with poor marrow reserve, it is important to radiate only those sites of epidural encroachment. (c) On occasion, benign lesions, such as herniated discs or intradural tumors, are revealed by myelography in cancer patients. (d) The effectiveness of treatment can easily be reassessed by a refluoromyelogram. Current indications for myelography include: back pain alone with abnormal spine x-rays, or neurologic examination; or radiographic demonstration of a paraspinal mass (18, 20, 33, 34). The probability of finding epidural extension of tumor in this setting exceeds 60%.

INITIAL MANAGEMENT: RADIATION VERSUS DECOMPRESSIVE LAMINECTOMY

Until recently, the initial management of most patients who presented with an evolving motor deficit was emergency decompressive laminectomy, with removal of as much epidural tumor as was accessible through this approach. In an extensive retrospective analysis of the published literature, Gilbert et al. suggested that the results of surgical therapy were no better than that attainable by external radiation alone (17). The posttreatment ambulatory rates for both groups were slightly less than 50%; even in patients with rapidly evolving deficits (in whom surgery might have been expected to have a major role), no differences in outcome were apparent between those treated by surgery or those undergoing RT. They therefore concluded that RT should be considered the treatment of choice in most patients with neoplastic cord compression. Laminectomy was suggested for (a) tissue diagnosis when none was available, (b) patients who relapsed after receiving a course of RT, (c) patients who deteriorated while receiving RT, and (d) patients who could not receive RT because the spinal cord has previously been included in a radiation portal. Since the published results of laminectomy were not impressive, most oncologists and neurosurgeons have generally accepted these conclusions with little reservations. As a result, over the past 5 years surgery has been largely relegated to a salvage procedure.

Since the results of external radiation are still unsatisfactory, more recent attempts have focused on improved radiation techniques to improve local control either through the use of high dose fractionation or with radiation sensitizers. Obbens et al. recently reported a prospective clinical trial of 83 patients using the radiation sensitizer, metronidazole, in conjunction with a short course, high dose fractionation scheme consisting of 500 rads in 3 days followed by 400 rads in 3 days (30). No difference in outcome was seen, with response rates (for motor function) being in the range of 30–40% for both treatment and control groups. Similarly, no difference in the overall palliative index was noticed by the Radiation Therapy Oncology Groups using various dose fractionation schemes (48). Thus, although the initial improvement rate following radiation therapy varies from 50–80%, the majority of patients relapse within 6 months.

The major limiting factor with regard to further curative attempts by radiotherapy alone is the limited tolerance of the spinal cord; although the risk of radiation myelopathy is negligible in patients whose life expectancy is limited, it assumes considerable importance in those cancer patients whose overall prognosis is good. Dorfman et al. (11) recently demonstrated that even in clinically asymptomatic patients, electrophysiologic evidence of subclinical injury could be observed with the use of somatosensory potentials in patients receiving therapeutic mediastinal radiation for lung cancer. These changes were not directly related to total dose, but rather to the treatment time and the total number of fractions used. With the use of computerized treatment planning, it is now possible to deliver radiation therapy using particle beams (either proton or heavy particles) in selected patients with primary malignancies of the spine. The advantages of particle radiation as compared to photon energy include a better dose distribution with sparing of the normal tissues (i.e., the spinal cord) and a relatively enhanced radiobiological effect for heavy charged particles, such as helium. Unfortunately, these sophisticated treatment options are limited to several centers only. In addition, they are time consuming and are not generally applicable for palliative treatment in the majority of cancer patients. Attempts to improve on local control through the use of brachytherapy supplemented by radiation also have limited applications in this group of patients. In patients with malignancies involving the spine in whom curative therapy is a goal, these treatment options clearly should be considered.

More recently, we analyzed the results of decompressive laminectomy over a 5-year period in a group of 71 patients with neoplastic cord compression treated between 1979 and 1984 at Memorial Sloan-Kettering Cancer Center (26). In this group, 25 patients underwent *"de novo"* surgery followed by radiation therapy. The remaining 46 patients fit the criteria (excluding histologic diagnosis) proposed by Gilbert *et al.* (17). Pain relief was comparable in both groups (50%), although the measurement of this parameter was often confounded by the use of additional treatment modalities. Of the seven nonambulatory patients in the *"de novo"* group, six regained ambulation (85%); of the 21 nonambulatory patients in the remaining group, only seven (33%) were ambulatory postsurgery. The major finding was the significant difference in complication rates: of those undergoing *"de novo"* surgery, the overall complication rate was 16%. In those who had received prior treatment (RT or chemotherapy) the complication rate was 37%. The median survival in the *"de novo"* patients was 12 months; it was only 6 months in those who had received prior radiation. Patients who deteriorated during radiation therapy had the worst outcome, with a 30-day mortality of 21% and only one-third surviving 6 months. These findings indicate that prior therapy has an important bearing on surgical morbidity rates, although to some extent they reflect an increased risk in operating on patients with more advanced cancer. However, the use of radiation therapy clearly increased the risk of postsurgical wound breakdown in all posterior surgical approaches to the spine, both for simple laminectomy and for those patients undergoing instrumentation (42). Similar findings have been noted in a recent study published from the Mayo Clinic: Martenson *et al.* showed that patients who received corticosteroid therapy for more than 40 days had a statistically increased incidence of serious complications (27). Although the numbers in the study were small, they confirm our experience that the combined use of radiation, chemotherapy, and high dose corticosteroid therapy increases the morbidity rate in patients who subsequently undergo surgery. In addition to this complication rate, the strategy of radiation followed by surgery results in a higher incidence of recompression at the original site even in those patients who undergo maximal tumor debulking by the anterior approach.

SURGICAL CONSIDERATIONS

For surgical therapy to be successful, the approach should be directed to the site of compression of the offending tumor mass within the spinal canal. The three basic surgical approaches to the spine may be classified

as follows: (*a*) posterior approaches by laminectomy or extended posterolateral approaches, (*b*) lateral approaches to the spine by costotransversectomy in the thoracic region or a transverse process osteotomy in the
cervical and lumbar regions, and (*c*) a direct anterior approach by vertebral body resection. In addition, the restoration of stability to the spine
following tumor resection is a prerequisite for pain relief and the maintenance of early ambulation without the need for external rigid orthoses.
During the past 5 years, the need for providing stability to the spine, either
following surgical decompression or as primary therapy in those with
osseous metastases or minimal epidural disease, has been recognized in
numerous studies (6, 9, 13, 19, 21, 32, 42). However, the techniques of
stabilization vary widely and are complicated by the bewildering array of
spinal instrumentation available for both anterior and posterior spinal
surgery. In Figure 30.1, we have tabulated the relative frequencies of the
various surgical procedures carried out over a 5-year period at Memorial
Sloan-Kettering Cancer Center.

Posterior Stabilization

The clearest indication for posterior stabilization alone without decompression is in patients with metastases to the upper two cervical vertebra.

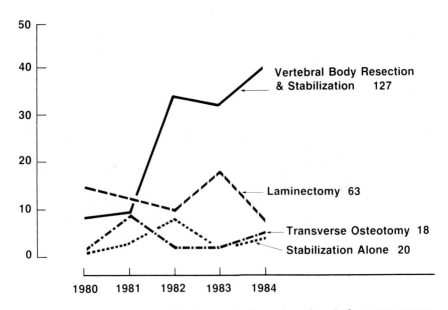

FIG. 30.1. Relative frequencies of various surgical procedures for spinal metastases over a
5-year period.

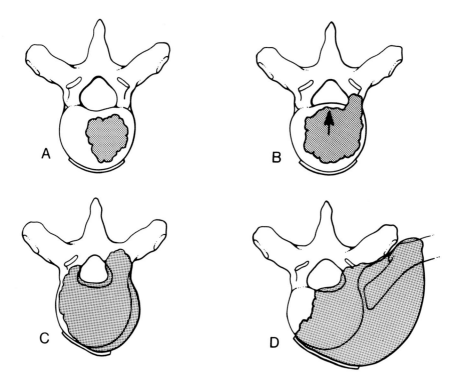

FIG. 30.2. Classification of spinal metastases by extent of involvement of the spine: (A) intraosseous tumor, (B) early epidural extension, (C) complete block, and (D) paraspinal tumor with secondary spine invasion. For curative therapy, surgery should be performed while tumor is intraosseous or has minimal epidural extension.

In these patients, atlanto-occipital or atlanto-axial instability may result secondary to tumor destruction of the anterior elements of the spine. Since a direct surgical approach involves a major transoral or transmandibular procedure, such patients are usually treated with high dose corticosteroid therapy and radiation. In our series, the majority of tumors involving this region originate either from the breast or from the lymphoreticular tissue, and thus primary radiation and steroid therapy are frequently effective in local tumor control. The clinical presentation is usually one of neck stiffness and pain, and the diagnosis can easily be missed unless displacement is marked. Plain tomography may be helpful for the examination of this region if plain radiographic findings are equivocal.

In patients without marked displacement and in those in whom myelopathy is reversed with steroid treatment, our suggested initial management is high dose corticosteroid therapy followed by external radiation (41).

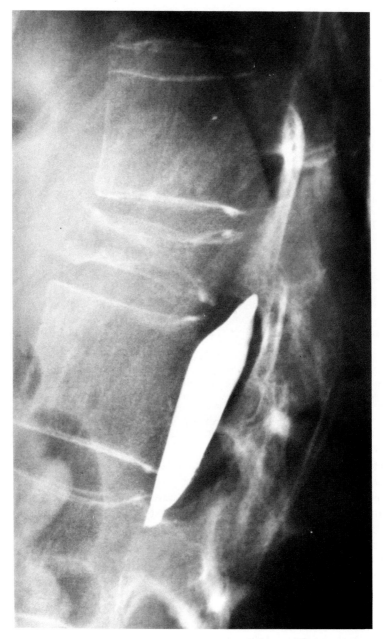

FIG. 30.3. Persistant block on refluoromyelography following laminectomy; in the presence of a collapsed vertebra with a ventral defect, an anterior approach by vertebral body resection and stabilization is the procedure of choice.

These patients only require neck immobilization with a Philadelphia collar and rarely require more rigid orthoses such as the Halo. At the end of radiation therapy, the decision for surgical stabilization may be made.

Criteria for considering surgery include persistent pain, persistent displacement, or the clinical presence of myelopathy. Posterior cervical stabilization in the upper cervical spine is best achieved by a combination of 18-gauge wires passed underneath the lamina of C1 and C2, and incorporating the entire wire matrix with methyl methacrylate. Posterior stabilization using the wire and acrylic technique can be achieved in the rest of the cervical and the thoracic regions even in those who require decompressive laminectomy by passing wires through healthy spines above and below the level of involvement and is effective in producing pain relief (6, 19). However, in the thoracic and lumbar regions, more effective posterior stabilization is achieved by instrumentation either with Harrington distraction rods or by Luque rods (9, 13, 32, 42). The advantage of Harrington instrumentation is that the height of collapsed vertebra can frequently be restored in patients with localized collapse. In addition, the rods themselves exert an anteriorly directed force vector through the facets that is frequently effective in reducing a localized kyphosis.

A major role for posterior instrumentation is the provision of rigid internal mechanical support when autologous bone grafts are used. Cusick *et al.* reported a small series of seven patients with metastatic tumor involvement in the lower thoracic and upper lumbar segments whose clinical presentation included intractable pain, minimal evidence of neurologic deficits, and persistent symptoms following radiation therapy (9). To be effective, the Harrington distraction rods should be placed such that the upper and lower hooks are at least two to three vertebral segments above and below the level of involvement. The upper hooks are generally placed into the facet joints in the thoracic region, and the lower hooks are seated on the lamina. The rods themselves are wired together with heavy 20-gauge stainless steel wire to prevent lateral displacement. In addition, methyl methacrylate is used at both the upper and lower ends to prevent displacement of the rods laterally. The immediate relief of pain in the postoperative period in Cusick *et al.*'s series suggests local segmental instability as a major cause of symptomology. In our series, pain relief was achieved in more than 80% of patients treated with instrumentation, but the neurologic deficits were less easily reversed in those who had undergone prior radiation. In addition, the combined use of both methyl methacrylate and Harrington instrumentation resulted in a significant (20%) incidence of wound breakdown in patients with advanced cancer. For these reasons, we believe that the use of Harrington instrumentation alone without major tumor resection has a limited role in the management of malig-

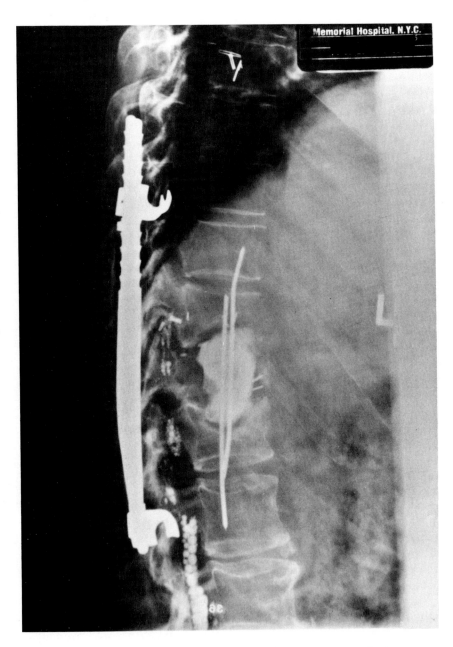

FIG. 30.4. Harrington distraction rods to supplement anterior stablization. In the presence of a kyphotic deformity secondary to tumor, anterior decompression and stabilization are preferred prior to posterior instrumentation.

nancies involving the spine. At the present time, our major indication for posterior instrumentation is to supplement anterior stabilization as well as to provide internal rigid support in patients who require autologous bone grafting.

Experience with the Luque rod system is even more limited. Flatley reported a series of seven patients with metastatic disease in whom stabilization was attempted without any attempt to resect tumor (13). The Luque system provides more physiologic and rigid fixation and is more easily adapted to junctional areas such as the cervicothoracic region or the upper thoracic segments. However, no distractional force is provided. The major advantage of Luque rods is that they offer greater protection against torsional or translational stresses on the spine. The technique of sublaminar wiring is time consuming and potentially hazardous in patients with metastatic disease. All forms of instrumentation should be considered temporary only, and in inexperienced hands they carry the potential for a high complication rate (28).

Posterolateral Approaches

Since laminectomy alone rarely allows adequate access to the anterior aspect of the cord, a number of posterolateral approaches have been described that enable more extensive tumor resection. These include resection of the facets or pedicles, costotransversectomy in the thoracic region, as well as osteotomies of the transverse process in the lumbar region. Overby and Rothman have recently described a small series of 12 patients with epidural cord compression from metastatic cancer treated by these posterolateral approaches. Neurologic improvement was seen in 75% of their patients, but the overall survival times were not mentioned (31). Although these posterolateral approaches offer better prospects for surgical palliation than the classical laminectomy, they do not allow adequate exposure for tumor resection or for anterior stabilization. For this reason, these surgical approaches should only be used in patients whose life expectancy is measured in months; in all others, local tumor recurrence is inevitable.

Vertebral Body Resection and Stabilization

Over the years, there have been sporadic reports of surgical attempts to resect tumors directly through anterior surgical approaches and provide for immediate stabilization with bone grafts or methyl methacrylate. The cervical spine is generally easily accessible through an anterior (Cloward) approach, but the majority of patients with neoplastic cord compression have involvement of the thoracic or lumbar regions. A classification of the major anterior surgical approaches used for access to the entire

TABLE 30.2

Classification of Anterior Surgical Approaches

Cervical and cervicothoracic segments (C1-T2)
  Transoral
  Transmandibular median glossotomy
  Cloward anterior cervical
  Trans-sternal
Thoracic segments (T3-T12)
  Posterolateral thoracotomy
Thoracolumbar segment (T12-L2)
  Thoracolumbar with 10–12th rib resection
Lumbar (L2-L5)
  Retroperitoneal flank
  Transabdominal

spine is shown in Table 30.2. For the majority of patients, a formal thoracotomy or retroperitoneal flank approach is required.

Several arguments have been offered for the lack of widespread use of this direct approach in patients with metastatic or primary malignancies to the spine. It has been assumed that patients with cancer and spinal involvement do not tolerate thoracotomy well, and that the resulting morbidity and mortality would be much greater than that of posterior laminec-

TABLE 30.3

Sites of Primary Cancer[a]

Site	Number	*De Novo* Surgery[b]
Lung	25	7
Kidney	15	2
Breast	14	1
Soft part sarcoma	12	5
Bone-spine	9	2
Gastrointestinal tract	4	0
Melanoma	4	0
Myeloma	4	2
Others	14	4
Total	101	23

[a] Sundaresan, N., Galicich, J. H., Lane, J. M., Bains, M. S., and McCormack, P. The treatment of neoplastic epidural cord compression by vertebral body resection. J. Neurosurg., 63: 676–684, 1985.

[b] Included patients who were given preoperative RT or chemotherapy as part of treatment protocol.

tomy approaches. In addition, it is tacitly assumed that posterolateral approaches with limited decompression provide the same degree of neurologic palliation and pain relief as the more extensive anterior approaches. Finally, while most surgeons are familiar with midline posterior approaches to the spine, anterior approaches to the spine require considerable technical expertise and may require the use of a thoracic surgeon. Since the use of radiation and/or chemotherapy results in delayed fusion if autologous bone is used, methyl methacrylate is currently the best replacement for the resected spinal segment (16, 21, 40, 43).

In view of the emphasis on radiation therapy as initial management in all patients with spinal metastases, the original indications for surgical intervention in our series were those originally described by Gilbert et al. (17). Thus, up to 80% of our patients had received prior therapy; 50% had relapsed following maximal radiation to the spine, and another 30% had been treated by surgical decompression or by laminectomy and radiation. Nevertheless, surgery was successful in restoring or maintaining ambulation in 78% of the patients in our series (46), and similar neurologic improvements were reported both by Siegal and Harrington (21, 37, 38). In our series of patients, emphasis was placed on early diagnosis and surgical intervention while patients were still ambulatory; in Siegal's series, 25% of the patients were classified as "paraplegic" prior to surgery. These differences in neurologic assessment may be due to the fact that most patients in our series were already treated with high dose steroid therapy. In addition, most of our patients underwent elective surgery after maximal benefit from steroid therapy had been attained.

A recent update of our surgical series, as well as those reported in the literature by Siegal and Harrington, is summarized in Tables 30.4 and 30.5. All three surgical series show the same remarkable degree of neurological improvement as well as pain relief, and a low morbidity and mortality rate when compared to patients treated by laminectomy. In the group of pa-

TABLE 30.4

Results of Therapy following Vertebral Body Resection and Stabilization

	Total No.	Pain Relief (%)	Motor Improvement (%)	Median Survival (Months)
Sundaresan (1985)	160	80	80	12
Siegal (1985)	61	80	80	16
Harrington (1984)	52	82	85	16

TABLE 30.5

Complication Rate following Vertebral Body Resection and Stabilization

	30-Day Mortality (%)	Morbidity (%)	Increased Neurologic Deficit (%)
Sundaresan (1985)	6	10	0
Siegal (1985)	6	11	2
Harrington (1984)	8	8	2

tients treated by *"de novo"* surgery, no mortality and minimum morbidity were encountered. These data all suggest that morbidity rates and mortality rates continue to remain much higher in patients who have received prior treatment and can be minimized by early surgery prior to radiation therapy. In addition, morbidity rates from superinfection and gastrointestinal hemorrhage are higher in those who acutely fail radiation therapy or others who relapse within 6 weeks to 3 months following treatment because of the concomitant depression of the bone marrow reserve as well as immune function by intensive medical therapy.

From a technical standpoint, the major surgical principles that are stressed in all three surgical series are the complete resection of all tumor down to the dura. The surgical approach should generally be planned on the side of a paravertebral tumor mass if one is evident on CT scans, or on the side of greater collapse and pedicle destruction if no soft tissue mass is present. Transthoracic approaches do not generally require resection of a complete rib, since closure is facilitated by preservation of all but the posterior 5–10 cm of the rib. The resected posterior segment can also be used as a lateral fusion mass to augment the methyl methacrylate stabilization procedure.

It is generally easier to plan a thoracotomy approach above the level of the involvement and to begin initial dissection in healthy, noninvolved disc spaces. The involved vertebral segments are then removed with a combination of curettes, rongeurs, and the high speed drill. In 50% of patients, more than one vertebral body may need to be resected. For additional exposure, it is possible to resect the pedicles and facets through this approach, which then allows access to the posterior aspect of the dura. In some patients, especially those with metastases from kidney or thyroid cancer, profuse vascularity and intraoperative hemorrhage may be encountered. To minimize this morbidity, we recommend preoperative angiography and embolization prior to surgery.

Following tumor resection, stabilization is best achieved by allowing

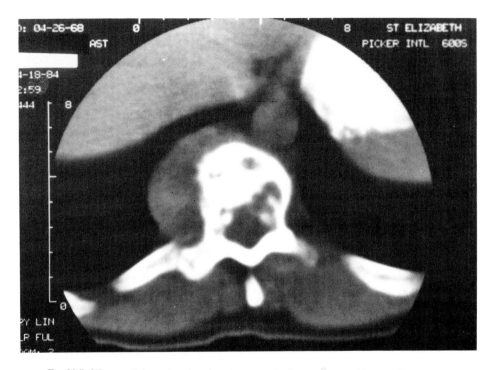

FIG. 30.5. CT scan of thoracic spine showing paraspinal tumor mass with secondary osseous destruction; the finding of a paraspinal tumor mass anteriorly indicates the need for an anterior approach, as well as the side from which the procedure should be performed.

semiliquid polymethyl methacrylate to polymerize *in situ,* while protecting the dura with Gelfoam and constant saline irrigation. To keep the methyl methacrylate in place, we favor the use of the Steinmann pin technique, wherein pins are impacted into healthy vertebra above and below the resected spinal segments (Figs. 30.6 and 30.7). This technique has the advantage of simplicity, and is applicable at all anatomic segments in the spine. Harrington has advocated the use of Knodt rods, which allow moderate anterior distraction and correction of localized kyphosis. Siegal has suggested the use of Moe sacral hooks because of their greater purchase on the vertebra (38). In our view, the technical aspects of instrumentation are less important than the necessity for complete tumor resection. It is important to realize that a one-sided approach only allows subtotal resection of the vertebral body.

For complete resection (spondylectomy), a second stage procedure through a posterior approach is necessary. At this time, the posterior

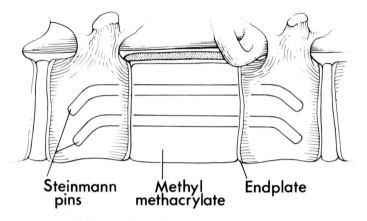

Steinmann   Methyl   Endplate
   pins   methacrylate

FIG. 30.6. Line drawing depicting technique of holding methyl methacrylate in place with Steinmann pins impacted into vertebra above and below the resected segment. For proper fixation, the end plates should be carefully stripped of all soft tissue and preserved to provide a firm base to the acrylic.

elements and removal of the remaining vertebral body and lateral masses can be performed, and posterior stabilization can be achieved with Harrington instrumentation. This two-stage procedure is indicated for curative resections of the spine for primary malignancies and for the occasional patient with a solitary metastatic focus, after curative resection of the primary tumor.

Although the majority of patients are still referred for treatment after having failed radiation, we believe that there are several important advantages of *"de novo"* surgical therapy. The mortality and morbidity of *"de novo"* surgery are currently less than 5% in experienced hands, and the operative procedure is technically safer because there is minimal or no radiation fibrosis. In addition, reduction of the tumor mass by intralesional curettage allows postoperative radiation therapy or chemotherapy to be used to eradicate microscopic foci. The value of this combined modality approach with initial surgical debulking is generally accepted as logical for other sites (10, 14), but it has yet to gain widespread acceptance for spinal disease.

Some support to the value of postoperative radiation may be seen in comparing the local recompression rates in patients who are operated on having failed radiation therapy compared to those who underwent *"de novo"* surgery in our series. Up to 50% of patients who relapse following radiation therapy develop compression at the original site in 1 year, whereas 90% of patients who were operated upon primarily continue to

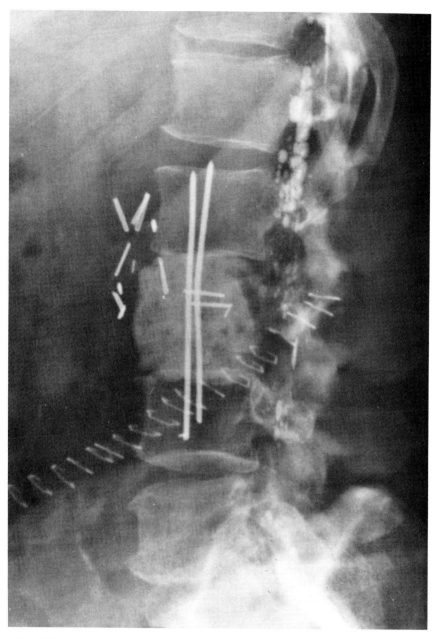

FIG. 30.7. Lateral radiograph showing completed resection and replacement of lumbar vertebra.

TABLE 30.6

Indications for Vertebral Body Resection in Malignant Disease

Pathologic compression fracture as presenting feature of
  malignancy
Solitary site of relapse
Destruction of the spine secondary to paraspinal tumor
Radioresistant tumor—kidney, melanoma, or sarcoma
Structural abnormalities of spine (collapsed vertebra,
  subluxation, or localized kyphosis)
Segmental instability following RT

remain ambulatory without tumor recompression until death or last clinical follow-up. The only exceptions to this are patients with highly radioresistant tumors, such as kidney cancer, in whom multiple staged operations to eradicate all disease within the vertebral body may be required. In view of these exciting new advances in spinal surgery, reassessment of the role of surgical therapy in the primary management of patients with primary and metastatic malignancies to the spine is indicated. A prospective study is currently under way to better define the value of surgery in patients with metastatic cancer, but the current indications for this surgical approach are summarized in Table 30.6. For this form of surgical therapy to gain acceptance as standard therapy for malignancies involving the spine, neurosurgeons must convincingly demonstrate repeatedly to their oncology colleagues the value of early neurosurgical intervention.

REFERENCES

1. American Cancer Society. *Facts and Figures, 1985.*
2. Barcena, A., Lobato, R. D., Rivas, J. J., Cordobes, F., De Castro, S., Cabrera, A., and Lamas, E. Spinal metastatic disease: analysis of factors determining functional prognosis and the choice of treatment. Neurosurgery, *15:* 820–827, 1984.
3. Bernat, J. L., Greenberg, E. R., and Barrett, J. Suspected epidural compression of the spinal cord and cauda equina by metastatic carcinoma. Cancer, *51:* 1953–1957, 1983.
4. Black, P. Spinal metastases: current status and guidelines for management. Neurosurgery, *5:* 726–746, 1979.
5. Boland, P. J., Lane, J. M., and Sundaresan, N. Metastatic disease of the spine. Clin. Orthop., *169:* 95–102, 1982.
6. Clark, C. R., Keggi, K. J., and Panjabi, M. M. Methyl methacrylate stabilization of the cervical spine. J. Bone Joint Surg., *66(A):* 40–46, 1984.
7. Constans, J. P., De Vitis, E., Donzelli, R., Spaziante, R., Meder, J. F., and Haye, C. Spinal metastases with neurological manifestations. J. Neurosurg., *59:* 111–118, 1983.
8. Costigan, D. A., and Winkelman, M. D. Intramedullary spinal cord metastasis. J. Neurosurg., *62:* 227–233, 1985.
9. Cusick, J. F., Larson, S. J., Walsh, P. R., and Steiner, R. E. Distraction stabilization in the treatment of metastatic carcinoma. J. Neurosurg., *59:* 861–866, 1983.

10. De Vita, V. T. The relationship between tumor mass and resistance to chemotherapy. Cancer, *51:* 1209–1220, 1983.

11. Dorfman, L. J., Donaldson, S. S., Gupta, P. R., and Bosley, T. M. Electrophysiologic evidence of subclinical injury to the posterior columns of the human spinal cord after therapeutic radiation. Cancer, *50:* 2815–2819, 1982.

12. Dunn, R. C., Kelly, W. A., Whons, R. N. W., and Howe, J. F. Spinal epidural neoplasia. A 15-year review of the results of surgical therapy. J. Neurosurg., *52:* 47–51, 1980.

13. Flatley, T. J., Anderson, M. H., and Anost, G. T. Spinal instability due to malignant disease. J. Bone Joint Surg., *66(A):* 47–52, 1984.

14. Fletcher, G. H. Subclinical disease. Cancer, *53:* 1274–1284, 1984.

15. Foley, K. M. The treatment of cancer pain. N. Engl. J. Med., *313:* 84–95, 1985.

16. Friedlander, G. E., Tross, R. B., Doganis, A. C., Kirkwood, J. M., and Baron, R. Effect of chemotherapeutic agents on bone. J. Bone Joint Surg., *66(A):* 602–606, 1984.

17. Gilbert, R. W., Kim, J. H., and Posner, J. B. Epidural spinal cord compression from metastatic tumor; diagnosis and treatment. Ann. Neurol., *3:* 40–51, 1978.

18. Graus, F., Krol, G., and Foley, K. Early diagnosis of spinal epidural metastasis: correlation with clinical and radiographic findings. Proc. Am. Soc. Clin. Oncol. (Abstr.), *4:* 269, 1985.

19. Hansebout, R. R., and Blomquist, G. A., Jr. Acrylic spinal fusion: a 20-year clinical series and technical note. J. Neurosurg., *53:* 606–612, 1980.

20. Harper, G. R., Rodichuk, L. D., Prevosti, L., Lininger, L., and Ruckdeschel, J. C. Early diagnosis of spinal metastases leads to improved treatment outcome. Proc. Am. Soc. Clin. Oncol. (Abstr.), *1:* 6, 1982.

21. Harrington, K. D. Anterior cord decompression and spinal stabilization for patients with metastatic lesions of the spine. J. Neurosurg., *61:* 107–112, 1984.

22. Harrison, K. M., Mus, H. B., Ball, M. R., McWhorter, M., and Case, D. Spinal cord compression in breast cancer. Cancer, *55:* 2839–2844, 1985.

23. Kaneda, A., Yamaura, I., Kamikozuru, M., and Nakai, O. Paraplegia as a complication of corticosteroid therapy. J. Bone Joint Surg., *66(A):* 783–785, 1984.

24. Kato, A., Ushio, Y., Hayakawa, T., Yamada, K., Ikeda, H., and Mogami, H. Circulatory disturbance of the spinal cord with epidural neoplasm in rats. J. Neurosurg., *63:* 260–265, 1985.

25. Levy, W. J., Latchaw, J. P., Hardy, R. W., and Hahn, J. F. Encouraging surgical results in walking patients with epidural metastases. Neurosurgery, *11:* 229–233, 1982.

26. Macedo, N., Sundaresan, N., and Galicich, J. H. Decompressive laminectomy for metastatic cancer: what are the current indications. Proc. Am. Soc. Clin. Oncol. (Abstr.), *4:* 278, 1985.

27. Martenson, J. A., Evans, R. G., and Lie, M. R. Treatment outcome and complications in patients treated for malignant epidural cord compression. J. Neuro-oncol., *3:* 77–84, 1985.

28. McAfee, P. C., and Bohlman, H. H. Complications following Harrington instrumentation for fractures of the thoracolumbar spine. J. Bone Joint Surg., *67(A):* 672–685, 1985.

29. Murray, P. K. Functional outcome and survival in spinal cord injury secondary to neoplasia. Cancer, *55:* 197–201, 1985.

30. Obbens, E. A. M. T., Kim, J. H., Thaler, H., Deck, M. D. F., and Posner, J. B. Metronidazole as a radiation enhancer in the treatment of metastatic epidural spinal cord compression. J. Neuro-oncol., *2:* 99–104, 1984.

31. Overby, M. C., and Rothman, A. S. Antero-lateral decompression for metastatic epidural spinal cord tumors. J. Neurosurg., *62:* 344–348, 1985.

32. Perrin, R. G., and Livingston, K. E. Neurosurgical treatment of pathological fracture-dislocation of the spine. J. Neurosurg., *52:* 330–334, 1984.
33. Redmond, J., Spring, D. B., Munderloh, S. H., George, C. B., Mansour, R. P., and Volk, S. A. Spinal computed tomography in the evaluation of metastatic disease. Cancer, *54:* 253–258, 1984.
34. Rodichok, L. D., Harper, G. R., and Ruckdeschel, J. C. Early diagnosis of spinal epidural metastases. Am. J. Med., *70:* 1181–1188, 1981.
35. Rodriguez, M., and Dinapoli, R. P. Spinal cord compression with special reference to metastatic epidural tumors. Mayo Clin. Proc., *55:* 442–448, 1980.
36. Saitoh, H., Hida, M., Shimbo, T., Nakamura, K., and Yamagata, J. Metastatic patterns of prostatic cancer: correlation between sites and number of organs involved. Cancer, *54:* 3078–3084, 1984.
37. Siegal, T., and Siegal, T. Vertebral body resection for epidural compression by malignant tumors: results of 47 consecutive operative procedures. J. Bone Joint Surg., *67(A):* 375–382, 1985.
38. Siegal, T., and Siegal, T. Surgical decompression of anterior and posterior malignant epidural tumors compressing the spinal cord: a prospective study. Neurosurgery, *17:* 424–432, 1985.
39. Stark, R. J., Henson, R. A., and Evans, S. J. W. Spinal metastases: a retrospective survey from a general hospital. Brain, *105:* 189–213, 1982.
40. Sundaresan, N., Galicich, J. H., Bains, M. S., Martini, N., and Beattie, E. J. Vertebral body resection in the treatment of cancer involving the spine. Cancer, *53:* 1393–1396, 1984.
41. Sundaresan, N., Galicich, J. H., and Lane, J. M. Treatment of odontoid fractures in cancer patients. J. Neurosurg., *52:* 187–191, 1981.
42. Sundaresan, N., and Galicich, J. H. Harrington rod stabilization for pathological fractures of the spine. J. Neurosurg., *60:* 282–286, 1984.
43. Sundaresan, N., and Galicich, J. H. Treatment of spinal metastases by vertebral body resection. Cancer Invest., *2:* 383–397, 1984.
44. Sundaresan, N., Bains, M. S., and McCormack, P. Surgical treatment of spinal cord compression in lung cancer. Neurosurgery, *16:* 350–356, 1985.
45. Sundaresan, N., Scher, H., Krol, G., and Whitmore, W. F., Jr. Surgical treatment of cord compression in kidney cancer. J. Clin. Oncol., in press.
46. Sundaresan, N., Galicich, J. H., Lane, J. M., Bains, M. S., and McCormack, P. The treatment of neoplastic epidural cord compression by vertebral body resection. J. Neurosurg., *63:* 676–684, 1985.
47. Tang, S. G., Byfield, J. E., and Sharp, T. R. Prognostic factors in the management of metastatic epidural spinal cord compression. J. Neuro-oncol., *1:* 21–28, 1981.
48. Tong, D., Gillick, L., and Hendrickson, F. R. The palliation of symptomatic osseous metastases: final results of the study by the Radiation Therapy Oncology Group. Cancer, *50:* 893–899, 1982.
49. Tomita, T., Galicich, J. H., and Sundaresan, N. Radiation therapy for spinal epidural metastases with complete block. Acta Radiol. Oncol., *22:* 135–143, 1983.

31

Controversies in the Surgical Management of Spasticity

DAVID L. KASDON, M.D., F.A.C.S.

INTRODUCTION

Spasticity is a disorder of motor function and tone which is characterized by a velocity-sensitive increase in resistance to passive stretch and is often accompanied by hyperactive tendon reflexes (2). The control of tone is a complicated balance of facilitation and inhibition modulated by the input of many areas of the central nervous system from the frontal lobes and nonpyramidal systems to the cerebellum and reticular activating system all the way down to the spinal cord interneurons, anterior horn cells, and Renshaw cells.

A review of the neurophysiologic abnormalities in spasticity is beyond the scope of this paper; but in order to appreciate the controversial aspects of the medical-surgical management of spasticity, certain factors must be appreciated. Davidoff's review is an excellent presentation of the medical treatment of spasticity (2). The final common pathway for all expression of tone is the anterior horn cell and myoneural junction. In addition to the alpha motor neurons that innervate the skeletal muscle, the anterior horn cells include the gamma motor neurons that innervate the intrafusal fibers of the muscle spindle. Therefore, spasticity can be expressed as alpha overactivity (alpha rigidity) or spindle overactivity (gamma rigidity). The muscle spindle responds to stretch and by its 1A and 1B fibers with their cell bodies in the dorsal root ganglion can either facilitate or inhibit alpha motor neurons by the monosynaptic stretch reflex. In addition to this reflex, a rich feltwork of interneurons provides presynaptic and post-synaptic inhibition and facilitation, which influence the activity of both the alpha and gamma motor neurons. This interneuron pool is normally under the control of descending pathways that inhibit or facilitate tone—for example, the extensor-enhancing vestibulospinal tract, the flexor-enhancing rubrospinal tract, and the reticulospinal tract. There is also considerable modulation of primary spindle afferents in the posterior or dorsal horn by neurotransmitter release. Naturally occurring substances, such as glycine and gamma aminobutyric acid, may play a major role in the presynaptic and post-synaptic inhibition of the primary spindle afferents, which in turn inhibit or facilitate both the gamma and alpha motor neurons.

EARLY TREATMENT OF SPASTICITY

Liljestrand and Magnus in 1919 demonstrated that procaine injected into the muscles of decerebrate cats could temporarily abolish their extensor tone (12). Walshe in 1924 injected procaine in the muscles of spastic patients and demonstrated temporary absence of spasticity (19). Presumably these techniques temporarily anesthetized the muscle spindle. This early work led to the technique of phenol injection, initially into the muscle and then into the peripheral nerves. Phenol injection into peripheral nerves is still the mainstay of the physiatrist's approach to the treatment of spasticity. The overwhelming advantage of phenol injection is that it is quite safe and easily performed without anesthesia or special equipment. It can be done at the bedside and is inexpensive. In addition, it can be repeated as needed. The disadvantages of peripheral phenol injection are production of considerable weakness and sensory loss and a very high recurrence rate. Virtually all patients with phenol blocks regain some degree of spasticity as the peripheral nerve undergoes repair. In patients with preservation of voluntary movement, phenol injection poses a serious risk to the muscle group supplied by the injected nerve. It does seem to have a role particularly in adductor and flexor muscles of functionally paraplegic patients.

ORTHOPAEDIC APPROACHES

The orthopaedic approach to the treatment of spasticity includes formal open neurectomy, muscle and tendon lengthening procedures, and release of contractures. The advantages of these procedures are that they are the only way to release the fixed contractures seen in chronic spasticity. The disadvantages, however, include denervation, possible vascular injury as contracted arteries are stretched, and major loss of potential voluntary motor function. Unless the underlying disorder of tone that resulted in spasticity is treated, most orthopaedic release procedures are eventual failures unless they are so radical as to produce considerable disfiguring atrophy. Neurectomy and tendon cutting also impair the possibility of functional recovery of voluntary movement in the future.

OPERATIVE ANTERIOR AND POSTERIOR RHIZOTOMY

Posterior rhizotomy was performed in patients with spasticity by Otfrid Foerster, who spared some roots in order to avoid total anesthesia. He had mixed results (4). With time, spasticity usually recurred. Freeman and

Heimburger (1948) studied a series of patients with incomplete posterior rhizotomy and were disappointed by the long-term results (5). Anterior rhizotomy was reported by Munro in 1945 in a series of 42 patients with severe lower extremity spasticity (13). All anterior roots from T11 through S1 were sectioned, and spasticity was successfully treated in 39 of the 42 patients. Munro's experience with anterior rhizotomy was duplicated by Freeman and Heimburger with successful improvement in all of their patients (6). The primary advantages of this approach were that it was long-lasting and effective, and that it spared bladder function. The major disadvantage in anterior rhizotomy is the extensiveness of the operative procedure, requiring multiple level laminectomy and the sacrifice of the potential for voluntary movement recovery. If the underlying spasticity is reduced, many patients are found to have a surprising degree of voluntary movement which had been impeded by their increased tone in antagonistic muscle groups. In addition, the potential for recovery or for the development of spinal cord regeneration or stimulation techniques makes extensive rhizotomy an undesirable choice for most patients.

CORDOTOMY

Spinal cordotomy of the anterior funiculus (presumably interrupting the facilatory vestibulospinal and reticulospinal tracts) was reported by Hyndman in 1943 (8) and Schurmann in 1949 (16). This technique was performed in an open fashion at the cervical or high thoracic region with an immediate abolition of spasticity. Unfortunately, within 2 years, spasticity had recurred in all patients. The extensor spasm component (presumably mediated by the vestibulospinal tract) usually did not recur. Myelotomy for the treatment of spasticity was reported by Bishoff in 1951 and Weber in 1955 (1, 21). The "T myelotomy" is performed through a midline incision in the dorsal cord, which is then extended in T-like fashion, anatomically interrupting the reflex arcs that connect the posterior horn and anterior horn. The advantage of this procedure is its high rate of effectiveness in reducing spasticity. Its primary disadvantage is that it is an extensive operation requiring laminectomy over several segments and is associated with frequent voiding difficulties and moderate sensory disturbance.

INTRATHECAL CHEMOTHERAPY

Treatment of spasticity with instillation of intrathecal medications has undergone a renaissance with the development of continuous flow and programmable infusion systems. Ablative chemotherapy (intrathecal phenol or alcohol) has been used for many years. Intrathecal phenol in 5% glycerin is hyperbaric and, therefore, the patient's position must be adjusted so that the appropriate target roots are in a relatively dependent position. Phenol can be combined with Pantopaque and more recently with glycerin and metrizamide in order to manipulate the neurolytic agent under fluoroscopic control (17). The disadvantages of intrathecal ablative chemotherapy are the difficulty of control in uncooperative patients, a high risk of bowel or bladder sphincter dysfunction, and production of a lower motor neuron bladder. The high risk of voluntary motor weakness carries the same disadvantages that anterior rhizotomy does. On the other hand, the advantages of intrathecal chemotherapy consist of the ease with which the "needle" procedure can be performed and the low cost of intrathecal instillation. In my experience, intrathecal phenol in glycerin is a very useful and effective treatment for spasticity, particularly in patients with multiple sclerosis who have indwelling catheters and virtually no hope of return of voluntary function.

Erickson *et al.* reported the serendipitous finding that epidural and intrathecal morphine in 1–2 mg doses, when given to patients with various pain syndromes as well as spasticity, produced relief not only from pain, but also from spasticity (3). This observation led them to treat patients with severe spasticity with morphine delivered by an implantable pump (Infusaid pump, Metalbellows Corp, Bulington, MA), which provides a continuous flow of morphine into the subarachnoid space. Three patients had prolonged control of spasticity without developing a need for progressively higher doses of morphine with this method. The advantage of this technique was that it is a small operation, which could be performed under local anesthesia and which treats the spasticity without compromising sphincter function or voluntary movement. The disadvantages include the high cost of the pump system (approximately $4,000/unit), the need for refilling the pump every several weeks, and the risk of infection over the long term.

Penn and Kroin extended the intrathecal treatment of spasticity from morphine to baclofen (Lioresal). Using a programmable pump (Medtronic model 8601, Medtronic Inc, Minneapolis, MN) connected to a catheter in the lumbar subarachnoid space, they treated six patients with severe spasticity, all of whom improved. Baclofen doses ranged from 12–400 μg/day, and the drug was given for up to 7 months in responding patients (15). The advantages of this procedure included reduction of spasms in all patients and decreased stretch reflexes in most. In addition, only one patient in six had a reduction in voluntary movement. The disadvantages are similar to those of the intrathecal morphine pump, including the need for refilling, potential drug toxicity, and the high cost of the pump. Certainly this innovative use of intrathecal neuromodulation is very promising and deserves active investigation.

SPINAL CORD STIMULATION

Spinal cord stimulation reported by Waltz and cerebellar stimulation reported by Waltz and Pani (20) and recently by Nakamura and Tsubokawa (14) have been effective in reducing spasticity in selected patients. The implantation of stimulating electrodes over the cerebellar vermis or dorsal spinal cord presumably stimulates inhibitory pathways and inhibits facilatory pathways. Long-term follow-up studies have not been encouraging perhaps because of equipment failure and electrode impairment by fibrosis. These methods have the advantages of not interrupting voluntary movement or sphincter function. Their disadvantages include high failure rate, requirement of either a posterior fossa exploration or cervical laminectomy, and the expense of the systems.

SELECTIVE RHIZOTOMY FOR TREATMENT OF SPASTICITY

Selective rhizotomy for the treatment of spasticity has been reported by Sindou *et al.* (18). This elegant procedure requires sophisticated intraoperative root stimulation, which leads to selective destruction of that portion of the motor or sensory root responsible for spasticity. This procedure appears to be highly effective and has the advantage of sparing some voluntary movement, as well as sparing bladder and sphincter function. The disadvantage of selective rhizotomy is that it requires a laminectomy under anesthesia, as well as sophisticated monitoring abilities for the intraoperative stimulation.

PERCUTANEOUS RADIOFREQUENCY RHIZOTOMY

In 1977 Kenmore reported the relief of spasticity in spinal cord and brain-injured patients utilizing a percutaneous radiofrequency rhizotomy technique (10). This procedure is performed under fluoroscopic control in the radiology department utilizing a thermister electrode placed through a large bore spinal needle (Radionics Corp., Burlington, MA). Patients with bilateral lower extremity spasticity usually have lesions made from L1 through S1 bilaterally with confirmation of needle placement by both fluoroscopy and motor stimulation parameters. Using a radiofrequency lesion generator, the stimulation threshold for each root is determined and then a heat lesion is made (usually 90°C for 120 seconds) until the postlesion stimulation threshold is elevated by at least 0.2 V.

Subsequent experience with this technique was reported by Herz *et al.* (7), and a prospective study of 25 patients was reported by Kasdon and Lathi (9). In the latter study, all or most of the prospectively identified goals were accomplished in 24 of 25 patients, with improvement persisting during an average follow-up period of 12 months. The improvement related to decreased tone was much greater than the improvement from increased range of motion.

The advantages of this procedure include a high rate of efficacy, no permanent loss of voluntary function, minimal sensory loss, and complete sparing of sphincter function. In addition, the procedure is inexpensive, does not require an open operation, and can be performed on an outpatient surgical basis. Decubitus ulcers do not prohibit its performance. Its disadvantages include variable sensory loss and a modest rate of recurrence of spasticity. Recurrent cases, however, respond well to repeat lesions.

CONCLUSION

No ideal surgical treatment exists for all cases of spasticity. An ideal procedure would be low in cost and extremely safe, requiring a small operation with complete relief of spasticity, yet total preservation of voluntary movement and normal sensation while sparing all sphincter function. At present, each patient must be individually examined and the relative merits and risks of the procedures discussed in this chapter considered. With the development of neuromodulation transmitter-like drug delivery systems, we are moving into an exciting period in spasticity treatment that hopefully will bring us closer to the "ideal treatment" for spasticity.

REFERENCES

1. Bishof, W. Die longitudinal myelotomie. Zentralbl. Neurochir., 2: 79–88, 1951.
2. Davidoff, R. A. Antispasticity drugs: mechanism of action. Ann. Neurol., 17: 107–116, 1985.
3. Erickson, D. L., Blacklock, J. B., Michaelson, M., Spurling, K. B., and Lo, J. N. Control of spasticity by implantable continuous flow morphine pump. Neurosurgery, 16: 215–217, 1985.
4. Foerster, O. On the indications and results of the excision of posterior spinal nerve roots in men. Surg. Gynecol. Obstet., 26: 463–475, 1913.
5. Freeman, L. W., and Heimburger, R. F. The surgical relief of spasticity in paraplegic patients II. Peripheral nerve section, posterior rhizotomy, and other procedures. J. Neurosurg., 5: 555–561, 1948.
6. Freeman, L. W., and Heimburger, R. F. The surgical relief of spasticity in paraplegic patients. I. Anterior rhizotomy. J. Neurosurg., 4: 435–443, 1947.
7. Herz, D. A., Parsons, K. C., and Pearl, L. Percutaneous radiofrequency foraminal rhizotomies. Spine, 8: 729–732, 1983.
8. Hyndman, O. R. Physiology of the spinal cord. II. The influence of chordotomy on existing motor disturbances. J. Nerve Ment. Dis., 98: 343–358, 1943.
9. Kasdon, D. L., and Lathi, E. S. A prospective study of radiofrequency rhizotomy in the treatment of posttraumatic spasticity. Neurosurgery, 15: 526–529, 1984.
10. Kenmore, D. E. Management of spasms and spasticity in the spinal cord and brain injured patients by percutaneous radiofrequency rhizotomy. Presented at 45th Annual Meeting of the American Association of Neurological Surgeons, Toronto, Ontario, April 24–28, 1977.

11. Kenmore, D. Radiofrequency neurotomy for peripheral pain and spasticity syndromes. Contemp. Neurosurg., 5: 1–6, 1983.
12. Liljestrand, G., and Magnus. R. Uber die wirkung des novokains auf den normalen und den tetanusstarren skelettmuskel und uber die entstehung der lokalen muskelstarre beim wunstarrkrampf. Pfluger Arch. Ges. Physiol., 176: 168–208, 1919.
13. Munro, D. The rehabilitation of patients totally paralyzed below the waist: with special reference to making them ambulatory and capable of earning their living. I. Anterior rhizotomy for spastic paraplegia. N. Engl. J. Med., 223: 453–461, 1945.
14. Nakamura, S., and Tsubokawa, T. Evaluation of spinal cord stimulation for postapoplectic spastic hemiplegia. Neurosurgery, 17: 253–259, 1985.
15. Penn, R. D., and Kroin, J. S. Continuous intrathecal baclofen for severe spasticity. Lancet, 2: 125–127, 1985.
16. Schurmann, K. Die durchschneidung der pyramidenvorderstrange und benachbarter extrapyramidaler bahen bie spastichen zustanden und unwillkurlichen bewegungsstorungen. Zentralbl. Neurochir., 9: 136–141, 1949.
17. Scott, B. A., Weinstein, Z., Chiteman, R., and Pulliam, M. W. Intrathecal phenol and glycerin in Metrizamide for treatment of intractable spasms in paraplegia. J. Neurosurg., 63: 125–127, 1985.
18. Sindou, M., Millet, M. F., Mortamis, J., and Eyssette, M. Results of selective posterior rhizotomy in the treatment of painful and spastic paraplegia secondary to multiple sclerosis. Appl. Neurophysiol., 45: 335–340, 1982.
19. Walshe, A. E. Observations on the nature of the muscular rigidity of paralysis agitans, and on its relationship to tremor. Brain, 47: 159–177, 1924.
20. Waltz, J. M., and Pani, K. C. Spinal cord stimulations in disorders of the motor system. In: Proceedings of the Sixth International Symposium on the External Control of Human Extremities, pp 545–556. Belgrade, Ygoslav Committee for Electronics and Automation, 1978.
21. Weber, W. Die behandlung der spinalen paraspastik unter besonderer berucksichtigung der longitudinalen myelotomie (Bischof). Med. Mschr., 9: 510–513, 1955.

VI

Intracranial Tumors

32

Treatment of Craniopharyngioma

JOHN SHILLITO, JR., M.D.

"Probably one of the most challenging, frustrating, and humbling benign intracranial tumors of childhood is the craniopharyngioma. Its behavior is quite different from that of the craniopharyngioma of adulthood. It appears to be a congenital rest but does not 'rest' until it has insinuated itself into available nooks from the foramen of Monro to the foramen magnum and from carotid to clivus! Lurking beneath the optic chiasm, it leads the neurosurgeon bravely on only to defeat his dissection, outmaneuver his microscope and defy his ambitions. The tumor may be difficult for several reasons. First: its site of origin in or above the sella turcica puts it in the midst of a variety of sensitive structures that will not permit injudicious dissection without leading to undesirable or disastrous consequences" (22).

It may reach amazing size and extend far from its site of origin. It probably does this by the extension of thin-walled cysts along the paths of least resistance, not only in the basal cisterns but also invaginating the third ventricle and obstructing the foramina of Monro. In these cyst walls one can see flecks of calcium. Presumably the tumor reaches these distant places in cystic form and then solidifies to form the concretions that make actual casts of the spaces occupied.

The tumor cells may appear within brain tissue including the pituitary gland, the stalk, and the hypothalamus. Finding a plane between tumor and structures that should be preserved may, on occasion, be impossible.

There is great variation in the degree of reaction incited in surrounding tissue. The adherence of tumor to brain can be negligible or marked, and the ease of removal and risk of dissection can vary accordingly. Any cells left behind will recreate the tumor.

Although disarmingly benign in its microscopic appearance, the tumor appears highly resilient and can recur from even a tiny fragment left behind unless some other measures are taken to control those fragments.

We hear frequently from proponents of total excision by radical surgery

(12, 15, 16, 19, 25). We infer that this can be carried out in all or at least almost all of the cases and this is what the operator should try to do. We have also heard from proponents of no surgery at all who advocate control of the tumor by radiation therapy alone (7). Between these two extremes of advocacy, one must pay attention to those who propose intracavitary radiation therapy for cystic tumors, and stereotactic multiple portal single dose radiation therapy for solid tumors (1–4).

In 1977, I made the following statements (23):

> "Let us consider what it is about the craniopharyngioma that makes it so challenging to the neurosurgeon and often so humbling. Can it *ever* be excised totally? Yes. Can it *always* be excised totally? No. Are there serious endocrine and neurologic deficits that may result from aggressive surgery? Certainly. Is radiation effective in halting the growth of such a benign tumor? It is. Is there hazard in its use? There is.
>
> "Especially since the advent of the CT scanner, our dilemma is occasionally compounded by the accidental discovery of an asymptomatic craniopharyngioma. The deficits acceptable when a surgeon is battling to save a child's vision or life cannot easily be tolerated when the patient is normal."

These are some of our problems. Things have changed little since these statements were made.

I would like to present the case for surgery and the attempt at total excision. Several series, reported by determined and capable surgeons, will be examined. Dr. Matson's (14, 19) series will be further updated.

We will look also at the case for nonsurgical therapy, including external radiation, special external radiation techniques, intracavitary radioactive solutions, and chemotherapy.

Finally, some suggestions for a plan of treatment will be made and I will present for the first time my own modest series of patients who have been dealt with by the suggested plan.

THE CASE FOR SURGERY

One of the first staunch advocates of attempted total excision at the first operation was Donald Matson of the Children's Hospital in Boston (19). He built a series of 51 cases between 1949 and his untimely death in 1969. He was so impressed by the bad results of problem cases referred to him after exploration, cyst aspiration, orthovoltage radiation, or a combination of these, that he made every effort to excise the tumor at the first procedure. He succeeded in total excision in 67% of such cases, but if we include the later deaths from hormone deficiencies resulting from the radical surgery, we must bring the success rate down to 55% of primary excisions as of the most recent report in 1980 (23). Of the secondary operations that he performed, he was able to achieve what he considered total excision in only 17% with an operative mortality of 25% compared to 0 in the primary series. Later deaths were more frequent and the final figure for successful total excision of the craniopharyngioma after a secondary procedure was only 17%. Another late death since 1979 lowered this figure to 12.5%. The follow-up on Matson's patients is now at least 17 years. All of his reported patients were children.

In 1975, Dr. William Sweet described a series of 37 craniopharyngioma patients (25). Nineteen of these were children. He had two operative deaths for a rate of 7%. Dr. Sweet felt that he had achieved 23 total excisions for 82% of the survivors and reoperated on four of the five whose tumors had been incompletely excised. These four subsequently died (14%). Twenty-one of the 30 were still living in 1975; a success rate of 70%. As Dr. Sweet points out, many of his cases were done after 1969 and the follow-up was, therefore, not as long as in the Matson series. The results in patients who had reoperations were not as good; 33% were still living at the time of the report. Note that the series is a mix of adult and pediatric patients.

Dr. Harold Hoffman *et al.* (12) reported in 1977 a series of 48 children with craniopharyngiomas. Sixteen of these had cysts aspirated, 15 were subjected to a subtotal resection, and 17 to a total resection of the tumor. Of the group receiving aspiration, eight had shunts, 10 were radiated, and there were only six survivors. Of the 15 subtotal excisions, six required reoperations, one shunt was performed, six were radiated, four had cyst aspirations following surgery, and there are 13 survivors.

Of the 17 attempted total excisions, there were no reoperations, no shunts performed, and no radiation therapy given. There were 15 survivors. The authors stress that there is a better quality of life after attempted total excision and indicate that the morbidity has been much less after the use of the surgical microscope was instituted.

The case for surgery pointed out by these series is that total excision at times can be achieved. However, as evidenced by Matson's series, this has been possible in approximately half of the cases. In the more recent report of Hoffman, although he indicates the desirability and possibility of total excision, he also states that there are times when this is impossible because of tumor adherence or because it was judged inadvisable even to attempt total excision.

One can only conclude that the attempt should be made but cannot succeed in all cases and the surgeon must decide when to quit so he will not hurt the patient. The surgeon must also decide what to do with the patient who harbors residual tumor.

THE CASE FOR RADIATION THERAPY

There are now many series that indicate without question the efficacy of radiation in arresting the growth of craniopharyngiomas. The bibliographies of several recent articles will lead you to earlier studies.

Cassady et al. (6) in 1983 reported from the Joint Center for Radiation Therapy, which serves Children's Hospital in Boston, a series of 40 children radiated. Some of these were our patients, but not all. Twenty-five had radiation therapy after conservative operative treatment. Four were treated without any surgery. Twenty-five are alive without evidence of active disease. Several required one or more cyst aspirations during or after x-ray therapy. Mental function appeared normal.

Fifteen were treated after more extensive surgery; five because of known residual tumor, ten because of recurrence. One died 1 year after therapy from metabolic causes; one child from Iran had been lost to follow-up. The function of Cassady's patients was usually worse after surgery and radiation than after conservative surgical procedures or none at all.

Chin et al. (8), working with Bryon Young in Lexington, Kentucky, reported improvement in the 5-year recurrence rate from 44% after surgery alone to 17% with surgery and radiation. Danoff et al. (9), reported a 16% recurrence rate after x-ray therapy, a 5-year survival rate of 73%, and a 10-year survival rate of 64%. Hoogenhout et al. (13) of the Netherlands reported, after surgery alone, a 5-year recurrence rate of 45% with 27% dead and a 10-year recurrence rate of 71% with 57% dead. Surgery plus radiation lowered these figures to 11% recurrence at 5 years and 25% at 10 years with no deaths at either time. Manaka et al. (18) in Tokyo reported that the addition of radiation to surgery alone raised the 10-year survival rate from 27% to 76%. X-ray therapy was given when total removal was impossible.

Fischer et al. (10) have summarized the Boston Children's Hospital experience with 37 patients treated by all members of the staff between 1972 and 1981. They concluded that the immediate morbidity was less with radiation therapy, but cautioned about its possible later complications.

Complications of radiation therapy in reported series have included the appearance of new tumors (17), necrosis (24), late vascular changes (20), deafness, and delayed hypopituitarism (10). A most effective method for radiating craniopharyngiomas and probably the least likely to produce complications is the utilization of multiple portals or a continuous coronal moving beam. Deleterious effects are known to be greater on younger brains.

In 1985, Liwnicz et al. (17) reported four cases of gliomas in radiated patients, one of which was a craniopharyngioma patient. Their review of the literature yielded 50 meningiomas, 24 gliomas, and 22 sarcomas developing after radiation therapy. The latency period was between 5 and 47 years.

Other methods include insertion of radioactive yttrium-90 into cystic tumors. For solid tumors, a method of single shot, multiple portal, stereotactically directed necrotizing external radiation has been advocated by Leksel and Backlund in Stockholm (2–4).

Radiation therapy has certainly saved or bought time for children with inoperable portions of their tumors or with recurrence from known or unknown missed fragments (11, 21). The less radiation any part of the brain receives the better, therefore the use of multiple portals, a moving beam, or the instillation of a beta-radiating fluid into a thin-walled cyst, or a stereotactically computerized field delivered through many portals all seem advantageous (1–4).

The sometimes distant peregrinations of a craniopharyngioma from its site of origin may complicate treatment for the radiotherapist as well as the surgeon.

THE CASE FOR CHEMOTHERAPY

In 1984, Bremer et al. (5) reported one case in which a craniopharyngioma responded to chemotherapy. The patient was 31 years old, had a recurrence following surgery, and refused more surgery or radiation. The effect of vincristine, BCNU, and procarbazine was apparent in 14 days and the tumor has been controlled for 2 years by multiple dose technique.

Takahashi et al. (26) reported in January 1985 of the use of intratumoral bleomycin in seven craniopharyngioma patients. There were four survivals and the follow-up went to 7 years.

A SMALL PERSONAL SERIES

In the 27-year period from 1958 through September, 1985 I have performed the primary operation on 20 children (Table 32.1). Their ages ranged from 11 months to 15 years, 1 month. Nineteen were explored by subfrontal craniotomy; one had a cyst tapped prior to radiation therapy because she lived far from sophisticated medical care. One child who did have a total excision died of postoperative complications within 5 days, an operative mortality of 5%. Another child thought to have had a total excision died 5 years later of hormonal insufficiency during the stress of a respiratory infection. The youngest, 10 months, with the largest tumor, died of his tumor 2 years later after three operations, cyst aspiration, and radiation. The overall death rate was, therefore, 15%. Of the three, one

TABLE 32.1

Author's Series of Primary
Craniopharyngioma Operations,
1958–1985

20 Patients
  19 Craniotomy
  1 Cyst aspiration
  1 Post op death (5%)
  1 Late death, complications surgery (5%)
  1 Death from tumor (5%)
  10 Also radiated
  7 Apparent total excision (38%)
  17 Living without active tumor (85%)

patient died from the surgery itself, one from vulnerability created by radical surgery, and the third from tumor or cyst recurrence. The first child at autopsy indeed did have a total excision; the second showed some tiny residual wisps of tumor; the last had no autopsy.

Of the seventeen living patients, seven have apparently had total excisions (39%) and have been followed 1–17 years. Ten patients received radiation therapy for inoperable tumors, known residual tumors, or for recurrence (50%). Seventeen (85%) are known to be living without evidence of active tumor.

THE SERIES

The course of the 20 patients is displayed in Table 32.2. All operations were through the subfrontal route unless otherwise indicated. The accuracy of follow-up is 100%. The dollar sign indicates gainful employment, "at home" indicates inability to become independent, usually for lack of incentive but also because of recent memory problems. All patients received their primary treatment by the author. Patients seen after surgery elsewhere and who had secondary treatment are not included. No living patient has as yet shown evidence of active residual tumor.* A brief paragraph about each patient follows.

Case 1. R.G.

Excision was considered total. The chiasm was prefixed. The boy was maintained on thyroid, vasopressin, and phenytoin; was hyperna-

---
* See Addendum, p. 545.

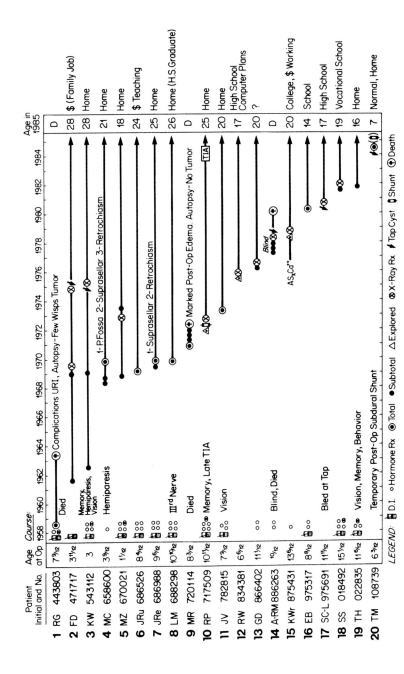

tremic and hyperosmolar; had behavior problems; and was considered uneducable. The patient died during a mild respiratory infection while in an ambulance on the way to the hospital. At autopsy, only a few wisps of tumor showed but destruction of parts of the hypothalamus and the fornices was evident.

Case 2. F.D.

This patient underwent a subtotal operation with reoperation 7 years later followed by radiation therapy. The patient needs vasopressin but will not take it nor any other hormones. He complains of feeling "tired." This 28-year-old now works for his father.

Case 3. K.W.

This girl was felt to have had a total excision. Hemiparesis developed on fifth postoperative day. Second operation for recurrence was performed 7 years later. Radiation therapy was given 7 years after second operation for recurrent tumor, partly cystic. Urgent cyst aspiration for failing vision during radiation therapy; residual field defects persist. The patient attended special classes after 8th grade. She is now 28 years old, living at home, and working in a special workshop.

Case 4. M.C.

Patient presented with ataxia, head tilt, vomiting, lethargy, and lower cranial nerve signs. Pneumoencephalography showed a mass in the left posterior fossa and the suprasellar region. Operating first where symptoms and signs pointed, we found a craniopharyngioma cyst in the posterior fossa. It was drained and biopsied. At a second operation the typical suprasellar cyst and its extension downward were removed from anterior to the chiasm. She too developed a hemiparesis after this operation. Eighteen months after her first operation she was found on lateral tomograms to have a finely calcified cyst wall in the third ventricle, not appreciated earlier. This was removed through the lamina terminalis. She is at home, requires no replacement therapy of any kind. She was never radiated and is now 21 years old.

Case 5. M.Z.

The next youngest patient in the series, at 13 months, this child had a subtotal excision. Follow-up studies including pneumoencephalography documented the residual tumor and repeat studies showed its growth 4 years after operation. At that point, radiation therapy was given. Her lack of cooperation made visual examination so inaccurate that we were led to explore her to rule out optic chiasm compression. A cystic residual tumor was partly removed. Vision was stabilized; she is at home, now 18 years old.

Case 6. J.Ru.

This boy had total excision of a rock-hard tumor from anterior to the chiasm. Sixteen years later he shows no evidence of tumor. He has graduated from college and teaches algebra and computer science. He is now 24 years old.

Case 7. J.Re.

This patient underwent two operations; first, anterior to the chiasm and second, posterior to the chiasm for a missed third ventricular component. She is on replacement therapy and is happy at home at age 25 years.

Case 8. L.M.

Patient underwent a total excision and developed third nerve palsy. The patient graduated from high school, lives at home, and works in a workshop. She is 26 years old.

Case 9. M.R.

This girl died from cerebral edema after total excision. Three decompression operations failed. At autopsy no tumor was found. This case was the only operative mortality.

Case 10. R.P.

Calcified mass extended from sella to foramina of Monro. It was explored but we desisted because of its firmness and tenacious adherence to surroundings. The patient was shunted and radiated. Memory problems and insecurity preclude employment. Recently, he has had several transient neurologic deficits with hemiparesis and altered consciousness 13 years after radiation. These presumed TIAs from late vascular changes could not be documented because of sensitivity to dye and lack of permission. The patient is 25 years old and living at home. (See Addendum, p. 545.)

Case 11. J.V.

This patient underwent a total excision operation. She lives at home in South America and is on replacement therapy. At age 17, she stopped school this year because of feeling "too tired."

Case 12. R.W.

This patient was explored because of failing vision. A solid, adherent tumor with a prefixed chiasm was discovered. No attempt at removal was made. The patient was radiated while on dexamethasone (Decadron; Merck, Sharp, Dohme). Vision returned. He is 17 years old, has graduated from high school, and is taking computer courses.

Case 13. G.D.

He underwent a subtotal excision; wisps were left on brain stem and one optic nerve. The patient was radiated and placed on minor replacement therapy at home. A moving single parent makes follow-up details spotty. Boy is now 20 years old, recently located again.

Case 14. A.-R.M.

This was the youngest patient in the series at 10 months old. An immense tumor extended almost to the vertex. The patient was too young to radiate. A subtotal operation was carried out. Five months later regrowth of tumor caused sudden blindness. After a second craniotomy radiation therapy was given. Two months after the second craniotomy a cyst was aspirated. The child returned to Iran where doctors allegedly reported regrowth of tumor, mostly cyst fluid. He then returned to the United States and was hospitalized because of progressive respiratory difficulties; subsequently, the patient died in hospital. The parents refused further surgery and autopsy. Death from regrowth of tumor and reaccumulation of cyst fluid was presumed.

Case 15. K.Wr.

Calcification near the optic chiasm was a surprise finding on skull films taken for headache. Calcified area was 4×6 mm in size. Pneuomocephalography defined its location as just below the optic chiasm. Since there was a family history of tuberculosis and she had positive skin tests, she was placed on antituberculous drugs and the lesion watched periodically for about a year. Thirteen months later it was conclusively bigger. Exploration identified a barely visible yellow-green mass stuck to the undersurface of her normally functioning optic chiasm. One-quarter milliliter of characteristic fluid was aspirated. It was elected to desist and give her radiation lest her vision be jeopardized. Vision remains normal. She is on only estrogens. The tumor remains static. She is a senior at college, majoring in psychology, and has four part-time jobs! (See Addendum, p. 545.)

Case 16. E.B.

Oculomotor signs led to the discovery of an uncalcified unenhancing suprasellar mass. On exploration it proved to be a craniopharyngioma and it was possible to excise it totally. After a long period of anorexia she is now normal, back at school, and has had no sign of tumor for 5 years. She is now 14 years old.

Case 17. S.C.-L.

This girl lives in the Caribbean. She had a large cystic tumor. We elected to aspirate and give radiation therapy as the method of treatment least likely to produce deficits which would be difficult to handle at home. As aspiration was being completed, arterial blood appeared from the needle and she dilated one pupil! Immediate CT scan showed no gross blood. She recovered promptly and had radiation therapy. Five years later, she is a senior in high school at age 17 with plans to go on to a university. She is on no medication.

Case 18. S.S.

Partial excision was performed of a tenacious tumor with prefixed chiasm. Two cysts were drained, one of which had been obstructing the third ventricle. Total removal was judged dangerous. The patient was radiated. On replacement medication, she is now attending vocational school. Tumor shrank and remains static 4 years later. She is now 19 years old.

Case 19. T.H.

A difficult total excision was performed. The chiasm was prefixed with dissection carried out under the optic nerve. No radiation therapy was given. T.H. has visual deficit, poor memory, behavior problems, and she requires replacement therapy. No residual has been seen at 4-year follow-up. She is 16 years of age and living at home.

Case 20. T.M.

A rather acute loss of vision led to a CT scan that showed an immense suprasellar cyst, some of the rim of which was calcified (Fig. 32.1). On the day of arrival the cyst was aspirated through a drill hole in the skull. Craniotomy a few days later permitted total excision of the cystic tumor which was only lightly adherent to its surroundings. One month later, a bulging bone flap heralded a subdural fluid collection which was shunted to the peritoneum for 2 months. The shunt was then removed. The boy's vision is normal. He has no need for replacement medication and has no loss of olfaction. It is now only 15 months since operation with no sign of tumor. He is 7 years, 5 months old.

Those radiated have shown no regrowth of tumor with the possible exception of the young boy in Case 14, who may have had regrowth of solid tumor as well as the known reaccumulation of cyst fluid. He and

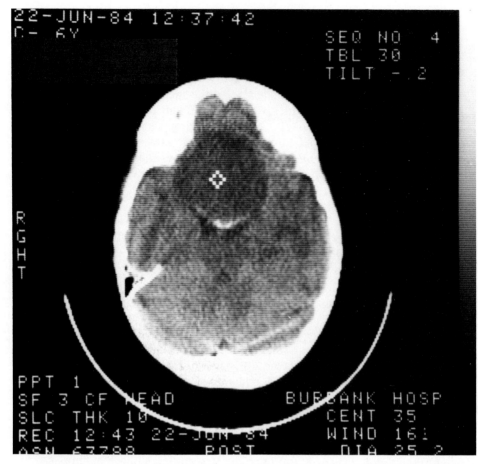

FIG. 32.1. Unenhanced CT scan of the patient in case 20 showing large cyst with slight calcification in its lower wall.

Case 3 required cyst aspirations for fluid accumulating during or after radiation therapy. There have been no new tumors seen in the path of radiation nor radiation necrosis, as yet. Seven total excisions are believed to have been achieved. (See Addendum, p. 545.)

SUGGESTIONS FOR TREATMENT

There is no single "treatment of craniopharyngioma." There must be a plan customized for each patient. That plan could include surgery unless, or until, it can be demonstrated that surgery is either unnecessary for decompression, will be inadequate, or is too risky to achieve a total excision.

This decision may, at times, be made from diagnostic studies alone, but in most cases exploration of the tumor and the testing of its adherence to its surroundings will be the only thorough and fair way to determine whether it can be totally excised or not.

When it becomes apparent to the careful surgeon that his dissection is likely to produce more trouble than he wants, he should stop and rely upon some of these other methods to control the residual tumor.

To sum it up in a word: **INDIVIDUALIZE**.

ADDENDUM

Since preparation of this manuscript two patients have developed what appears to be a new tumor, intrinsic to the brainstem and within the field of radiation previously received.

Case 10, R.P., nearly 15 years after his radiation therapy, developed odd sleep patterns, a fixed hemiparesis, and cranial nerve deficits. CT and MRI scans indicated recurrence of a craniopharyngioma with enhancement pushing against the brainstem but also a low density lesion intrinsic to the right thalamus and upper brainstem. Stereotactic biopsy of these two areas was undertaken. From the area which appeared to be recurrent craniopharyngioma we did indeed find craniopharyngioma cells, this time with mitoses which had not been seen before. From the area suggesting an intrinsic glioma of the brainstem, tissue was obtained which was not diagnostic of tumor. It was elected to radiate these areas. He began to improve markedly after two treatments, and after 2700 rad all of the deficits have regressed and he is close to normal neurologically.

Case 15, K.W.R., developed a hemiparesis and lower cranial nerve deficits within a few weeks. This occurred 8 years after her radiation therapy for craniopharyngioma. A CT and MRI scan showed changes consistent with an intrinsic glioma of the brainstem on the appropriate side. Her neurological deficits were remarkably reduced by more radiation, but only transiently. The area was not biopsied. Recurrent deficits are being treated with intra-arterial BCNU.

REFERENCES

1. Backlund, E. O. Studies on craniopharyngiomas. I. Treatment past and present. Acta Chir. Scand., *138:* 743–747, 1972.
2. Backlund, E. O., Johansson, L., and Sarby, B. Studies on craniopharyngiomas. II Treatment by stereotaxis and radiosurgery. Acta Chir. Scand., *138:* 749–759, 1972.
3. Backlund, E. O. Studies on craniopharyngiomas. III. Stereotaxic treatment with intracystic yttrium-90. Acta Chir. Scand., *139:* 237–247, 1973.
4. Backlund, E. O. Studies on craniopharyngiomas. IV. Stereotaxic treatment with radiosurgery. Acta Chir. Scand., *139:* 344–351, 1973.
5. Bremer, A. M., Nguyen, T. Q., and Balsys, R. Therapeutic benefits of combination chemotherapy with vincristine, BCNU, and procarbazine on recurrent cystic craniopharyngioma. A case report. J. Neurooncol. *2:* 47–51, 1984.

6. Cassady, J. R., Eifel, P., and Belli, J. R. Progress and problems of the treatment of brain stem glioma, medulloblastoma, and craniopharyngioma in childhood. In: *Recent Trends in Radiation Oncology and Related Fields*, edited by Amendola and Amendola, Elsevier Science Publishing Co., 1983, pp. 89–94.
7. Cavazzuti, V., Fischer, E. G., Welch, K., Belli, J. A., and Winston, K. R. Neurological and psychophysiological sequelae following different treatments of craniopharyngioma in children. J. Neurosurg., *59:* 409–417, 1983.
8. Chin, H. W., Maruyama, Y., and Young, B. The role of radiation treatment in craniopharyngioma. Strahlentherapie, *159:* 741–744, 1983.
9. Danoff, B. D., Cowchock, F. S., and Kramer, S. Childhood craniopharyngioma: survival, local control, endocrine and neurologic function following radiotherapy. Int. J. Radiat. Oncol. Biol. Phys. *9:* 171–175, 1983.
10. Fischer, E. G., Welch, K., Belli, J. A., Wallman, J., Shillito, J., Winston, K. R., and Cassady, R. Treatment of craniopharyngiomas in children: 1972–1981. J. Neurosurg., *62:* 496–501, 1985.
11. Hoff, J. T., and Patterson, R. H. Craniopharyngiomas in children and adults. J. Neurosurg., *36:* 299–302, 1972.
12. Hoffman, H. J., Hendrick, E. B., Humphreys, R. P., *et al.* Management of craniopharyngioma in childhood. J. Neurosurg., *47:* 218–227, 1977.
13. Hoogenhout, J., Otten, B. J., Kajem, I., Stoelinga, G. B. A., and Walder, A. N. D. Surgery and radiation therapy in the management of craniopharyngiomas. Int. J. Radiat. Oncol. Biol. Phys., *10:* 2293–2297, 1984.
14. Katz, E. L. Late results of radical excision of craniopharyngiomas in children. J. Neurosurg., *42:* 86–90, 1975.
15. Konovalov, A. N. Microsurgery of tumors of diencephalic region. Neurosurg. Rev., *6:* 37–41, 1983.
16. Symon, L. Radical excision of craniopharyngioma. J. Neurosurg., *62:* 174–181, 1985.
17. Liwnicz, B. H., Berger, T. S., Wiwnics, R. G., and Aron, B. S. Radiation associated gliomas: a report of four cases and analysis of postradiation tumors of the central nervous system. Neurosurgery, *17:* 436–445, 1985.
18. Manaka, S., Teramoto, A., and Takakura, K. The efficacy of radiotherapy for craniopharyngioma. J. Neurosurg., *62:* 643–656, 1985.
19. Matson, D. D., and Crigler, J. F. Management of craniopharyngioma in childhood. J. Neurosurg., *30:* 377–390, 1969.
20. Mori, K., Taketschi, J., Ishikawa, M., Handa, H., Toyama, M., and Yamaki, T. Occlusive arteriopathy and brain tumor. J. Neurosurg., *49:* 22–35, 1978.
21. Richmond, I. L., Wara, W. M., and Wilson, C. B. Role of radiation therapy in the management of craniopharyngiomas in children. Neurosurgery, *6:* 513–517, 1980.
22. Shillito, J., Jr. Treatment of craniopharyngioma of childhood. In: *Current Controversies in Neurosurgery*, edited by T. P. Morley. WB Saunders, Philadelphia, 1976, pp. 332–336.
23. Shillito, J., Jr. Craniopharyngiomas: the subfrontal approach or none at all? In: *Clinical Neurosurgery*, edited by P. W. Carmel, Vol. 27, Chapter 12, Williams & Wilkins, Baltimore, 1980, pp. 188–205.
24. Sundaresan, N., Galicich, J. H., Deck, M. D. F., *et al.* Radiation necrosis after treatment of solitary intracranial metastases. Neurosurgery, *8:* 329–333, 1981.
25. Sweet, W. H. Radical surgical treatment of craniopharyngioma. In: *Clinical Neurosurgery*, edited by E. B. Keener, Vol. 23, Chapter 5, Williams & Wilkins, Baltimore, 1976, pp. 52–79.
26. Takahashi, H., Nakazama, S., and Shimura, T. Evaluation of postoperative intratumoral injection of bleomycin for craniopharyngioma in children. J. Neurosurg., *62:* 120–127, 1985.

CHAPTER

33

Treatment Options in the Management of Prolactin-Secreting Pituitary Tumors

MARTIN H. WEISS, M.D.

Remarkable advances in neurochemistry, receptor physiology, imaging capacities, and neuroendocrine assessment during the past decade have dramatically altered the clinical management of patients harboring prolactin-secreting pituitary adenomas. These tumors comprise the majority of functional pituitary tumors that present to the clinician. The options available to the practitioner who is challenged by these problems provide an unusual opportunity for integrating multiple modalities of therapy. These options provide an extraordinarily high potential for effective treatment that assures resolution of clinical symptomatology as well as intracranial mass effect.

In the experience of our group at the University of Southern California, it is best to think of classification for pituitary tumors. The classification evolved with the clinical presentation of such lesions. This so-called staging process compartmentalizes these lesions into specific categories that fit specific therapeutic modalities to effect a cure. Stage I tumors are those that are less than 1 cm in diameter and have not infiltrated the overlying dura or bone of the sella turcica. Stage II tumors are greater than 1 cm in size with or without suprasellar extension but without invasion of overlying dura or sella turcica. Stage III tumors represent those lesions that locally invade the dura and floor of the sella. Stage IV tumors diffusely invade the sella and surrounding structures with or without extension into the anterior, middle, or posterior fossae or any combination of these. This classification system proves useful because surgical cure of stage I and stage II lesions can be accomplished with a high degree of confidence, whereas the latter stages (III and IV) usually defy cure by any single modality and, therefore, frequently require a combination of therapeutic ventures to effect the desirable result.

A brief review of the physiology of prolactin release is requisite to develop the practical principles of treatment that will be discussed subsequently. Prolactin is the only hormone of the anterior pituitary to be exclusively regulated by a mechanism of tonic inhibition effected by neurotransmitter release from the hypothalamus. As best defined by present-day

standards, the neurotransmitter regulating release of prolactin has dopaminergic characteristics and may be dopamine itself, although precise
definition awaits further confirmation. On the other hand, although there is
no known or defined prolactin-releasing factor or hormone, TRH (thyroid-
releasing hormone) does have the capacity to stimulate release of prolactin from adenohypophysial lactotrophs, a capacity that becomes clinically
significant in the patient with primary hypothyroidism who is found to
have an elevated prolactin along with pituitary hyperplasia that may mimic
a pituitary adenoma but responds to the restoration of a euthyroid state.
Since maintenance of a normal prolactin is dependent upon transmission
of the dopaminergic substance from the hypothalamus to the anterior
pituitary via the portal vasculature, interruption of this pathway may lead
to aberrant release of prolactin causing measurable hyperprolactinemia
because of this "stalk section effect." Resolution of the symptomatology
engendered by the latter two processes is dependent upon correction of
the underlying causal factor and, therefore, will not be addressed further
in this discussion.

Recognition of the transmitter interaction between the hypothalamus
and anterior pituitary allowed pharmacologists to address the issue of
developing a dopaminergic compound whose side-effects would be infrequent enough to allow broad application to a large population. This search
led to the release of bromocryptine by the Food and Drug Administration
(FDA) in August 1978 after extensive clinical trials indicated the efficacy
of this compound in Great Britain, Canada, and the United States. Bromocryptine is an ergot derivative with dopaminergic characteristics, which
has proven tolerable to the vast majority of patients treated with the agent;
only about 8% of patients are unable to tolerate its administration because
of undesirable side-effects. It is extraordinarily effective in suppressing
prolactin secretion and will restore normal prolactin levels in better than
95% of patients who are able to tolerate a therapeutic dose. In addition,
numerous investigators have demonstrated that bromocryptine will significantly reduce the size of large prolactin-secreting pituitary tumors in at
least 50% of patients harboring prolactin-secreting macroadenomas (1).
Thus, this agent proves to be a powerful tool in our armamentarium for
treatment of these disorders.

At the time of its original release by the FDA, bromocryptine was approved for use *only* in patients harboring "physiological hyperprolactinemia." A specific admonition against its use in the presence of a pituitary
tumor was enclosed in the literature describing its utilization. However,
extensive experience with the use of bromocryptine in patients harboring
prolactin-secreting adenomas has engendered a modification of the guidelines for the use of bromocryptine, allowing its utilization in patients with

pituitary tumors so long as great care is taken in patients who become pregnant while harboring a prolactin-secreting pituitary tumor. These lesions have an accelerated growth rate during pregnancy. It may be stated, therefore, that bromocryptine is an acceptable alternative modality available to the practitioner for management of prolactin-secreting pituitary adenomas.

On the other hand, this agent does not provide the final word with respect to this management problem. Bromocryptine is not curative in that it does not obliterate or eliminate the underlying pituitary tumor. It is still necessary to administer the medication, as we best understand it, for the remainder of the patient's life to suppress the aberrant clinical symptomatology generated by hyperprolactinemia. Withdrawal of the drug is followed by a rapid return of hyperprolactinemia and a return to, at the least, the original size of the tumorous mass. The foregoing results have been demonstrated in those patients who have undergone involution of the tumor under treatment. Although most patients will "tolerate" the medication, symptoms of dizziness and a mild degree of nausea while under treatment frequently compel the patient to tell you that they just "don't feel normal" and would prefer to be off the medication if a viable alternative existed. Finally, recent preliminary reports indicate that patients harboring microadenomas who have been treated with bromocryptine for more than 6–12 months and who subsequently wish to have their pituitary tumors surgically extirpated have a lower cure rate. This presumably relates to some alteration in tumor characteristics that adversely influences surgical resection.

With these background factors in mind, we may now turn to an assessment of specific circumstances in which the previous considerations may be applied. The stage I or pituitary microadenoma offers the highest opportunity for surgical cure while at the same time presenting an ill-defined need for specific therapeutic intervention. In our own series (1), slightly more than 15% of these lesions followed for 10 years with no treatment will show progressive enlargement; there is obviously no "rush" to treat these lesions with concern for tumor mass. The two principal causes for treatment of these lesions are the desire for pregnancy on the part of the patient harboring a prolactin-secreting microadenoma or concern for the genesis of premature osteoporosis in the young woman who is amenorrheic and hypoestrogenemic as a consequence of her systemic hyperprolactinemia. The former consideration is a frequent and significant clinical factor; concern for premature osteoporosis is genuine but at present more of a hypothetical concern awaiting clinical confirmation. Assuming that you are confronted with a patient harboring a pituitary microadenoma in whom a decision to undertake treatment has been made, what are your options? In our experience, the following considerations apply whether the patient is contemplating pregnancy or not. Surgical resection of these lesions, in our hands, carries an 84% chemical cure rate at 1 year following surgery. Mortality in these circumstances is zero and morbidity (including cerebrospinal fluid leak, meningitis, cranial nerve palsies, and hormonal dysfunction) is less than 1%. None of our patients who have had serum prolactins under 10 ng per ml at 6 weeks postsurgery have had any evidence of recurrence of disease. On the other hand, some 20% of patients whose prolactins at 6 weeks postoperatively range between 10 and 20 ng per ml have developed systemic hyperprolactinemia again when followed for 5 years postoperatively. This compares with recent reports of a 20–50% incidence of recurrent hyperprolactinemia in the absence of demonstrable tumor by sophisticated imaging technique in these patients. We have found that measurement of serum prolactin shortly after surgery (within the first week) is not as reliable. An index of the status of prolactin secretion is that measured at the 6-week follow up visit, and we rely upon this latter value as an index for need for further therapeutic intervention where that proves necessary.

Bromocryptine, on the other hand, will restore normal serum prolactin in virtually 100% of those patients with pituitary microadenomas who are able to tolerate the drug. We have treated more than 50 patients who wished to become pregnant and who harbored prolactin-secreting microadenomas with bromocryptine. Of the 35 completed pregnancies that ensued, all resulted in normal children. Only one tumor grew sufficiently during the course of the pregnancy to warrant reinstitution of treatment with bromocryptine, which proved satisfactory for management of this problem until completion of a full-term pregnancy.

Obviously, either surgery or bromocryptine provides a viable opportunity to maximize the potential for pregnancy in the infertile female harboring a prolactin-secreting microadenoma. In addition, we have not seen any significant growth of these lesions in any patient taking bromocryptine chronically. The choice of therapy clearly remains with the patient based upon personal preference and concern about the need for chronic treatment required with medical management.

Stage II tumors present similar options to the patient and treating physician, although the results of surgery generally do not match the chemical results from administration of bromocryptine in virtually every large series that has been reported. The advantage of surgery lies in its ability to reduce tumor size with a chemical cure rate of approximately 50% in our hands. Although treatment with bromocryptine will usually restore normal serum prolactins in better than 90% of these patients, those tumors which are cystic or low density on contrast-enhanced high-resolution computed tomography (CT) scans fail to show reduction in size in our experience. Such lesions are best approached by an initial attempt at surgical extirpation with reservation of bromocryptine for treatment of that group in which systemic hyperprolactinemia remains postoperatively. Simple follow-up without any therapeutic intervention is unacceptable in this group since these tumors have already demonstrated a biologic propensity for growth and, therefore, demand therapeutic intervention. In those tumors that significantly enhance on the CT scan, either surgical extirpation or chronic treatment with bromocryptine are viable alternatives assuming that the patient understands the complexities and complications of both therapeutic modalities.

Stage III and IV prolactin-secreting pituitary tumors virtually defy cure by any single modality. Best efforts with moderately invasive tumors yield a 25% chemical cure rate in these aggressive tumors. Those tumors that are diffusely invasive with extension into adjacent fossae have a chemical cure rate approaching zero utilizing surgery as the only form of therapy. On the other hand, these tumors frequently have very high levels of prolactin which require administration of large quantities of bromocryptine in order to effect a reduction in tumor mass and systemic hyperprolactinemia. Under such circumstances, the incidence of clinically significant side-effects increases as the dose of bromocryptine increases. We have, therefore, adopted a program of combined therapy for the management of these problems recognizing that this offers the patient the best opportunity for symptom-free control of their pituitary tumors. Our first step is to place the patient on bromocryptine in increasing doses until a serum prolactin of less than 20 ng per ml is established. Two weeks after reaching this objective, a CT scan is obtained to determine the influence of bromocryptine on tumor mass. In those patients in whom there is no reduction of tumor size at this time, a repeat scan is obtained 4 weeks later for further assessment. If there continues to be no effect on tumor size, surgical extirpation of the lesion is attempted, usually followed by a course of post-operative radiation therapy to complete this therapy. If this type of lesion should present with visual compromise, which appears progressive even after institution of treatment with bromocryptine, surgical intervention is undertaken sooner. Our experience has shown that those patients whose tumor masses respond positively to bromocryptine treatment will generally appreciate an improvement in their visual compromise shortly after institution of therapy.

If the CT scan taken 2 weeks following restoration of normal prolactin values does indeed indicate a positive effect on tumor mass, medication is continued for another 6 weeks when maximum impact will have been achieved. We have seen extensive tumors reduced to the point that the sella appears empty after only medical management while others were reduced only approximately 30%.

At this point, once again, there is an option of further treatment. It is reasonable to simply continue the patient on bromocryptine, recognizing that he or she may well have to take large doses of this medication for the remainder of his or her life. At this point, a viable alternative proven effective in our hands is an attempt at tumor extirpation. We have, to our delight, found that those tumors that are significantly reduced in size may lend themselves to chemical cure with a higher frequency under these circumstances, although the majority of the extensively invasive tumors still have some degree of systemic hyperprolactinemia. However, following such tumor reduction, one is frequently able to utilize lower doses of bromocryptine to maintain a therapeutic effect and, therefore, allow the patient to feel better while under chronic therapy. Under circumstances of need for chronic bromocryptine maintenance, a repeat scan is obtained at 3 months and 9 months postoperatively in addition to yearly thereafter. If the scans at 3 and 9 months postoperatively fail to show any evidence of progression of tumor and prolactin remains suppressed on the medication (as has been our usual experience), no radiation therapy is utilized to augment the therapy.

No single therapeutic modality is either ideal or unacceptable in the management of these problems. We are fortunate that the management of stage I and stage II tumors lends itself well to surgical intervention as a definitive and brief endeavor that does not require a life-long commitment to a medical regimen whose side-effects are appreciable. At the same time, both we as practitioners and the patient are fortunate to have a set of therapeutic options available that frequently are not competitive but are complementary, allowing us to reduce or eliminate tumor mass and restore normal endocrine function.

REFERENCE

1. Weiss, M. H., Wycoff, R., Yadley, R., Gott, P., and Feldon, S. Bromocryptine treatment of prolactin secreting tumors: surgical implications. Neurosurgery, *12:* 640–642, 1983.

34

Controversies in the Management of Cushing's Disease

WILLIAM F. CHANDLER, M.D., and DAVID E. SCHTEINGART, M.D.

Since Harvey Cushing first described pituitary-dependent hypercortisolemia in 1931 (3), the diagnosis and treatment of Cushing's disease has remained a major challenge to endocrinologists and surgeons. Although it has become clear over the past 20 years that the great majority of patients with hypercortisolemia have an adrenocorticotrophic hormone (ACTH)-secreting pituitary adenoma as an etiology, many controversies surround their identification and subsequent treatment.

DIAGNOSIS

Clinical

The clinical manifestations of hypercortisolemia (Cushing's syndrome) have proven consistent over the years and are usually easily recognized by the educated physician. Occasionally, the more striking physical signs of obesity, "moon facies," dorsal fat pad, purple striae, and hirsuitism are subtle and patients present primarily with muscle weakness, hypertension, osteoporosis, or mental disorders. These clinical manifestations result from the metabolic effects of excessive amounts of pituitary and adrenal hormones. These manifestations involve many organ systems and biochemical processes depending on the severity and duration of the hypercortisolemia and the presence of other pituitary or adrenal hormones such as ACTH, prolactin, androgens, and mineralocorticoids, all of which can contribute to the patient's symptomatology. While patients with Cushing's syndrome may present with manifestations exhibited by obese patients without primary glucocorticoid excess (hypertension, diabetes, androgen-type hirsutism, acne), the following findings are specific for Cushing's syndrome: (*a*) symptoms and signs of protein catabolism; (*b*) trunkal obesity; (*c*) lanugal hirsutism; (*d*) tinea versicolor; (*e*) wide purple striae; and (*f*) hyperpigmentation. Pituitary ACTH-dependent Cushing's syndrome occurs ten times more commonly in women than men while the ectopic ACTH syndrome occurs twice as often in men than women. Cushing's disease also has been well-documented in children and adolescents (20).

Endocrine

Patients with ACTH-dependent Cushing's syndrome exhibit increased secretion of ACTH and cortisol. In addition, the feedback relationship between the pituitary and the adrenal glands is abnormal. This abnormality includes the loss of normal negative feedback regulation of ACTH release and the loss of normal circadian rhythm of ACTH and cortisol secretion. Thus, patients with Cushing's disease demonstrate high baseline urinary 17-hydroxycorticoids and free cortisol as well as high-plasma ACTH and cortisol levels. Cushing's patients with typical testing responses to metyrapone, an 11-beta-hydroxylase inhibitor, suppress cortisol levels and increase ACTH secretion. They also show a lack of normal suppression of cortisol secretion with *low* doses of dexamethasone but suppress cortisol secretion with *high* doses of dexamethasone to values below 50% of baseline levels. There is controversy on the significance of atypical test responses, especially nonsuppressible pituitary ACTH-dependent Cushing's syndrome. In these, the patients fail to suppress on the high dose of dexamethasone.

Lamberts *et al.* (11) have suggested that nonsuppressible Cushing's syndrome is usually of hypothalamic origin and is accompanied by pituitary hyperplasia rather than pituitary adenoma. However, some patients with pituitary adenomas fail to suppress on the high dose of dexamethasone. It is possible that in these patients, dexamethasone metabolism has been accelerated by the intake of microsomal hydroxylating enzyme-inducing drugs. In those cases, the high dose of dexamethasone produces a lower dexamethasone level than that which is normally seen and which is required for effective suppression. Another possibility is that patients with nonsuppressible Cushing's syndrome have ectopic corticotrophic releasing factor (CRF)-secreting tumors, which in turn stimulate the pituitary gland to secrete excessive amounts of ACTH. Recent reports in the literature of ectopic ACTH-secreting tumors show that these patients do not nonsuppress with high doses of dexamethasone. However, the biochemical behavior of patients with ectopic ACTH-CRF syndrome covers a spectrum of responses, from lack of suppressibility to normal suppression with high dose dexamethasone. In the absence of dexamethasone suppressibility, an exaggerated response to metyrapone may point toward pituitary ACTH-dependent Cushing's syndrome. It has recently been suggested that stimulation of ACTH secretion with CRF can specifically separate classical pituitary ACTH-dependent Cushing's syndrome from ectopic-ACTH syndrome. However, this test needs to be better validated before it can be reliably used in this differential diagnosis. Another type of patient with Cushing's syndrome in whom a diagnosis may be confusing is the one presenting with periodic hormonogenesis (19). These patients have unusual patterns of ACTH and cortisol secretion as a result of which diagnostic biochemical changes are present intermittently.

Oldfield *et al.* (15) recently reported the value of bilateral simultaneous inferior petrosal sinus sampling for ACTH to help localize the laterality of a pituitary microadenoma. The value of this test stems from the fact that the hormonal secretion from a laterally placed microadenoma drains preferentially into the ipsilateral inferior petrosal sinus. Of the 10 microadenomas reported by the authors, seven were found at surgery to have microadenomas on the side of the higher ACTH levels. Another three patients were in remission by hemiresection of the pituitary on the side of the ACTH gradient, even though no tumor could be identified during surgery. This would appear to be a particularly valuable test for patients with endocrine evidence of pituitary ACTH-dependent hypercortisolism, but with a nonlocalizing CT scan.

Imaging

Imaging techniques available to evaluate the presence, size, and consistency of pituitary lesions have changed dramatically in the past 5 years. If Cushing's disease is suspected clinically and/or endocrinologically, a high-resolution computed tomographic (CT) scan of the pituitary is currently the initial study of choice. This should include direct coronal views as well as standard axial views and sagittal reconstruction. Most all macroadenomas will be imaged and, in our experience since 1980, seven of 21 or 35% of microadenomas were demonstrated. All seven of these correlated well with the surgical findings. The CT image of the adenoma may be hypodense, isodense, or hyperdense relative to the surrounding pituitary. Thus, although CT scanning is extremely useful when positive, a negative scan by no means rules out a microadenoma.

CT scanning has replaced standard tomography and plain sellar x-rays, and is the study of choice for preoperative evaluation of the surgical anatomy of the sphenoid sinus. Pneumoencephalography, angiography, contrast cisternography, and cavernous sinus venography currently have no role in the imaging of ACTH secreting adenomas. The value of magnetic resonance imaging is yet to be demonstrated, but may well add significantly to our ability to identify and localize microadenomas.

Differential Diagnosis

Part of the difficulty in effecting a remission in patients with hypercortisolemia is that several etiologies exist other than the ACTH secreting pituitary adenoma. Of patients with noniatrogenic Cushing's syndrome, 60–80% have a pituitary origin, with the remainder equally divided between an adrenocortical origin and extrapituitary "ectopic" neoplasms producing ACTH. Adrenal Cushing's syndrome is more common in children, where adrenal carcinoma is found in over 50% of children under the age of 15 years (4). As mentioned above, ectopic Cushing's syndrome is much more common in adult males, as opposed to pituitary Cushing's which is 10 times more common in females. Bronchial carcinoid or other forms of lung cancer are the most common source of ectopic ACTH secretion. We have identified one case in which a lung carcinoid secreted both ACTH and CRF. A few other reports exist of ectopic CRF secretion, and one report of a CRF-secreting hypothalamic gangliocytoma (8). In instances in which immunohistochemically demonstrated pituitary corticotrophic hyperplasia is present, concern remains that hypersecretion of CRF by the hypothalamus may exist. This etiology currently remains unproven and controversial. We have also documented a case of a true ACTH-secreting pituitary adenoma located within the "ectopic" pituitary tissue commonly found within the sphenoid sinus. This tumor was removed and a complete remission resulted.

TREATMENT

Surgical

Surgical treatment of hypercortisolism includes procedures directed at the pituitary, the adrenal, and the various ectopic sources. Little controversy exists with regard to the surgical resection of an ectopic lesion once identified. We believe it is important to perform immunohistochemical staining of the tissue resected to verify the presence of ACTH- and/or CRF-secreting cells. The remission rate is high if the neoplastic tissue is totally resected, and the ultimate prognosis is related to the activity of the primary malignancy. Likewise if an adrenocortical neoplasm (unilateral) or adrenal nodular hyperplasia (bilateral) is identified and appropriate unilateral or bilateral adrenalectomy performed, the remission rates should be high. In cases of metastatic adrenal carcinoma, medical therapy such as mitotane must be used.

The surgical treatment of pituitary ACTH-dependent Cushing's disease includes the microsurgical removal of microadenomas, macroadenomas, and total hypophysectomies. Since most macroadenomas are identified preoperatively by CT or magnetic resonance imaging (MRI) scanning, little other work-up remains, and the surgical challenge is to remove as much ACTH secreting tumor as possible. Even with considerable suprasellar extension this is usually performed transsphenoidally. If the tumor is invasive into the dura, total resection may be impossible, but the overall reported remission rates are surprisingly good. Boggan et al. (1) reported remissions in 45% of 22 macroadenomas, Salassa et al. (16) in 61% of 18, Hardy (6) in 63% of 8, Leudecke (12) in 75% of 16 and Kuwayama and

Kageyama (9) in 100% of 12. Recurrence rates of hypercortisolism in patients with macroadenomas, however, is reported to be higher than after microadenoma resection (9).

The microsurgical transsphenoidal selective resection of ACTH-secreting pituitary microadenomas is currently the most common treatment of hypercortisolism and comes closest to the ideal form of treatment for this disease. If a microadenoma can be identified and totally resected, the remaining pituitary tissue remains functional and patients can enjoy a remission without loss of endocrine function. It is common, however, that after selective adenoma resection, patients experience transient (6 months to 2 years) adrenal insufficiency requiring maintenance hydrocortisone replacement. In our experience, as well as others', if the cortisol levels only return to the normal range, a recurrence is more likely (12).

Since less than 50% of microadenomas can be imaged preoperatively, the surgical exploration becomes an extremely critical part of the treatment. Our findings support those of others that the majority of microadenomas are located laterally in the sella, usually within the gland (1, 12, 16). The adenoma tissue is virtually always more white and much softer than the surrounding gland. Although some microadenomas are obvious upon opening the dura, many require painstaking dissection around and within the pituitary to be located. Some microadenomas, like macroadenomas, will invade the dura laterally and defy total resection. There are also collections of ACTH-secreting cells that are so small that only a "soft spot" may be recognized during surgery, and yet a complete remission is effected by its removal even with negative pathologic examination.

These patients with surgically identifiable but pathologically unconfirmed microadenomas comprise 6–21% of reported series of microadenomas including our own (1, 9, 16). A corollary to this fact is that the surgeon cannot rely heavily on the pathologists' interpretation of small bits of tissue sent for frozen section. These specimens can be very difficult if not impossible to distinguish from normal pituitary. In an effort to improve the accuracy of frozen sections, we have been utilizing a new rapid staining method which takes advantage of the difference in fibrovascular stromal patterns in adenomas versus normal pituitary (14). Fluoriceinated *Ricinus communis* agglutinin is used which rapidly binds to the vascular stroma of fresh frozen surgical specimens. In adenoma, the normal acinar pattern is lost and the stromal pattern becomes a collection of disconnected fragments.

The incidence of finding microadenomas in reported *surgical* series ranges from 60–75% (1, 6, 9, 12, 16), and our experience is 23 of 32 patients or 72%. The remission rates in patients who have undergone microadenoma resection is reported to be from 87–96% (1, 6, 9, 12, 16) and in our experience was 20 of 23 or 87%.

If a specific adenoma cannot be identified during surgery, then a decision must be made whether to perform a partial or total hypophysectomy. If preoperative inferior petrosal sinus sampling has been carried out and is clearly lateralizing, then an appropriate hemiresection of the hypophysis should be performed. If the endocrine studies strongly indicate a pituitary origin, but the petrosal sinus sampling is not lateralizing and the patient does not wish to have children, then a total hypophysectomy should be considered. This should only be performed after a lengthy preoperative discussion with the patient regarding this possibility. If the patient wishes to have children, then alternative forms of therapy including adrenalectomy must be considered.

Medical

Various drugs have been used for the treatment of Cushing's disease. Some of these drugs act on neurotransmitters and decrease the secretion of ACTH. Cyproheptadine, a serotonin-antagonist, and bromocriptine, a dopamine receptor agonist, have been reported to suppress ACTH and cause remission of Cushing's syndrome (7). However, cyproheptadine can suppress ACTH secretion in patients with Nelson's syndrome and in some patients with ectopic ACTH syndrome. It is not clear if, in these cases, cyproheptadine directly suppresses ACTH secretion or acts by some other local mechanism which involves a neurotransmitter mediated hormone secretion. Cyproheptadine has not been found consistently to suppress ACTH and cortisol levels and when it does, its effects are only temporary, lasting while the drug is being administered. Recurrence of the disease occurs after interruption of therapy. Undesirable weight gain has been reported as a consistent side-effect of cyproheptadine therapy. Metyrapone, in doses of 1.5–3 gm daily, can promptly suppress cortisol secretion and induce remission of Cushing's syndrome while other more permanent forms of treatment are being pursued.

Mitotane (o,p'-DDD) is the only drug that both inhibits cortisol biosynthesis and destroys adrenocortical cells secreting cortisol without interfering with aldosterone production to the same extent (18). In combination with radiation therapy, mitotane has been found to induce remission of Cushing's syndrome in 80% of patients. The limiting factor with mitotane therapy are its side-effects which include anorexia, nausea, diarrhea, somnolence, pruritus, hyperlipoproteinemia, and hyperuricemia. A combined treatment with pituitary radiation and mitotane chemotherapy can be given when transphenoidal pituitary surgery fails to bring about remission of the disease. Since there is evidence that mitotane also suppresses ACTH release, chemical adrenal ablation with this drug is not usually associated with the development of Nelson's syndrome.

Compounds with antiglucocorticoid effects, which act at the cell receptor level, are presently being tested. The use of these drugs will probably be limited to those cases in which excessive cortisol production cannot be controlled by either surgery or radiation therapy. The degree of control of Cushing's syndrome with most medical approaches, the incidence of recurrence of the disease, and of complications of therapy are still subject to investigation.

Radiation

Although we believe selective pituitary microsurgical resection is the primary treatment of choice, various forms of radiation therapy remain available for surgical failures or for patients who are not surgical candidates. Conventional high-voltage radiotherapy of pituitary lesions provides a remission in only 20–50% of adults, but perhaps up to 80% of children (4). Shortcomings of this therapy include the risk of loss of function of the normal pituitary tissue and the lag time of up to 18 months for a drop in cortisol levels. Focused heavy particle proton beam radiation has been utilized over the past decade at two institutions in the United States with perhaps slightly greater remission rates, but with the same drawbacks. Rahn and colleagues in Stockholm have used the Leksell focused cobalt radiosurgical unit recently to treat 126 pituitary Cushing's patients, but their remission rates are not yet available (5). Implants of yttrium-90 or gold-198 are moderately successful, but require transsphenoidal implantation and also may result in hypopituitarism.

Overall, we have reserved radiation therapy for pituitary macroadenomas or microadenomas that have failed surgical therapy. Medical therapy is often combined with this to provide more immediate relief of symptoms. The highly focused radiotherapy of Rahn is promising, but must await analysis of both the rate remission and postradiation pituitary hypofunction. A drawback of this therapy is that it is currently available only in Stockholm, and will likely remain very limited in access.

PATHOLOGY

With the extraordinarily accurate immunologic labeling methods at the light and electron microscopic levels available, little controversy remains regarding the precise cellular make up of pituitary, adrenal, and even ectopic lesions. Pituitary adenomas contain predominantly ACTH- and B-endorphine-secreting cells and are usually negative for GH, prolactin, and the other common hormones. As mentioned above, ectopic tumors occasionally contain CRF as well as, or rarely in place of, ACTH.

One remaining controversy is whether or not "hyperplasia" of pituitary ACTH secreting cells exists. Although Wilson's group did not identify a single case of hyperplasia in his series of 100 patients (1), scattered well-documented case reports of hyperplasia can be found in the literature. McKeever in 1982 reported a case in which serial section of the entire pituitary revealed eight separate abnormal areas characterized by expanded but intact acinar patterns containing mostly (90%) but not exclusively corticotrophs (13). He proposed the following criteria for hyperplasia: (a) multifocal areas positive for ACTH-secreting cells; (b) inclusion in these areas of minor populations of other normal secreting cells; and (c) expanded fibrovascular stroma with preservation of the acinar configuration. Schnall et al. (17) also performed serial sections on the entire hypophysis of a Cushing's patient who was in remission posthypophysectomy and found only corticotroph hyperplasia. Lamberts et al. (10) reported a case believed to represent multiple nests of corticotrophs, but the entire pituitary was not available for study.

Overall, it appears that corticotroph hyperplasia does exist in a small percentage of cases, and may explain the failure of partial microresection to effect remission in selected cases. The question of whether a hypothalamic abnormality with elevated CRF is the ultimate etiology in some of these cases remains to be proven. As noted above, ectopic tumors may secrete CRF which would be expected to create corticotroph hyperplasia. The pathologic criteria set forth by McKeever et al. (13) with particular attention to the stromal pattern, may help to identify these cases of hyperplasia.

TREATMENT OF SURGICAL FAILURES AND RECURRENCES

The treatment of patients who fail to demonstrate remission after pituitary exploration is dependent upon the findings at surgery. During transsphenoidal surgery a microadenoma or macroadenoma is identified and resection attempted, or no pathology is found and biopsies are taken. If remission is not evident after selective microadenoma resection, several treatment options are available. Since, as mentioned above, multiple microadenomas remain a possibility, reoperation with partial or complete hypophysectomy is an option in selected patients. If the original microadenoma did not appear invasive and the patient does not desire pregnancy, then total hypophysectomy is a viable choice. If the patient wishes pregnancy, then either medical treatment or adrenalectomy is offered. If the tumor appeared invasive, then pituitary radiation is often an effective treatment.

If remission does not result from an attempted removal of a macroadenoma, then radiation is clearly in order. This may be combined with medical therapy to provide a more rapid remission.

If no tumor is identified during surgery or on biopsy, then a search for an ectopic or adrenal source must be renewed. If further work-up including petrosal sinus sampling confirm a pituitary origin, then either total hypophysectomy or radiation therapy must be considered. The danger of adrenalectomy in this situation is, of course, the risk of developing Nelson's syndrome secondary to continued pituitary tumor growth.

If hyperplasia is confirmed by biopsy then a rare ectopic tumor secreting CRF must be ruled out. If this is not identified then either radiation, hypophysectomy, or medical or surgical adrenalectomy must be considered. If CRF hypersecretion by the hypothalamus exists, there is no currently known specific treatment.

Treatment of recurrences likewise is dependent upon the original pathology, and has been successfully treated both by re-exploration and/or radiation therapy (1, 2, 9).

REFERENCES

1. Boggan, J. E., Tyrrell, J. B., and Wilson, C. B. Transsphenoidal microsurgical management of Cushing's disease. J. Neurosurg., 59: 159–200, 1983.
2. Caplan, R. H., and Annis, B. L. Recurrent Cushing's disease: successful treatment by pituitary irradiation of transsphenoidal hypophysectomy in two cases. Neurosurgery, 7: 160–165, 1980.
3. Cushing, H. The basophil adenomas of the pituitary body and their clinical manifestations (pituitary basophilism). Bull. Johns Hopkins Hosp., 50: 137–195, 1932.
4. Gold, E. M. The Cushing syndromes: changing views of diagnosis and treatment. Ann. Intern. Med., 90: 829–844, 1979.
5. Granholm, L. Personal communication, 1985.
6. Hardy, J. Cushing's disease: 50 years later. Can J. Neurol. Sci., 9: 375–380, 1982.
7. Krieger, D. T., Amorosa, L., Linick, F. Cyproheptadine-induced remission of Cushing's disease. N. Engl. J. Med. 293: 893, 1975.
8. Kuwayama, A., Kageyama, N. Current management of Cushing's disease. Part 1. Contemp. Neurosurg., 7(2): 1–6, 1985.
9. Kuwayama, A., Kageyama, N. Current management of Cushing's disease. Part II. Contemp. Neurosurg., 7(3): 1–6, 1985.
10. Lamberts, S. W. J., Stefanko, S. Z., DeLange, S. A., Fermin, H., Van Der Vijver, J. C. M., Weber, E. F. A., and DeJong, F. H. Failure of clinical remission after transsphenoidal removal of a microadenoma in a patient with Cushing's disease: multiple hyperplastic and adenomatious cell nests in surrounding pituitary tissue. J. Clin. Endocrinol. Metabol., 50: 793–795, 1980.
11. Lamberts, S. W., Delange, S. A., and Stefanko, S. Z. Adrenocorticotropin-secreting pituitary adenomas originate from the anterior or the intermediate lobe in Cushing's disease: differences in the regulation of hormone secretion. J. Clin. Endocrinol. Metabol. 54: 286, 1982.
12. Luedecke, P. Management of Cushing's disease. Presented at the 8th International Congress of Neurological Surgery, Toronto, July 11, 1985.
13. McKeever, P. E., Koppelman, M. C. S., Metcalf, D., Quindlen, E., Kornblith, P. O., Strott, C. A., Howard, R., and Smith, B. H. Refractory Cushing's disease caused by multinodular ACTH-cell hyperplasia. J. Neuropath. Exper. Neurol., 41: 490–499, 1982.
14. McKeever, P. E., Laverson, S., Oldfield, E. H., Smith, G. H., Gadille, D., Chandler, W. F.

Stomal and nuclear markers for the rapid identification of pituitary adenomas at biopsy. Arch. Pathol. Lab. Med., *109:* 509–514, 1985.

15. Oldfield, E. H., Chrousos, G. P., Shulte, H. M., Schaaf, M., McKeever, P. E., Krudy, A. G., Cutler, G. B., Loriaux, D. L., and Doppman, J. L. Preoperative lateralization of ACTH-secreting pituitary microadenomas by bilateral and simultaneous inferior petrosal venous sinus sampling. N. Engl. J. Med., *312:* 100–103, 1985.

16. Salassa, R. M., Laws, E. R., Carpenter, P. C., and Northcutt, R. C. Cushing's disease—50 years later. Am. Clin. Climatol. Assoc. (transactions), *94:* 122–129, 1982.

17. Schnall, A. M., Kovacs, K., Brodkey, J. S., Pearson, O. H. Pituitary Cushing's disease without adenoma. Acta Endocrinol., *94:* 297–303, 1980.

18. Schteingart, D. E., Tsao, H. S., Taylor, C. I., *et al.* Sustained remission of Cushing's disease with Mitotane and pituitary irradiation. Ann. Intern. Med. *92:* 613, 1980.

19. Schteingart, D. E., and McKenzie, A. K. Twelve hour cycles of ACTH and cortisol secretion in Cushing's disease. J. Clin. Endocrinol. Metabol. *51:* 1195, 1980.

20. Styne, D. M., Grumbach, M. D., Kaplan, S. L., Wilson, C. B., and Conte, F. A. Treatment of Cushing's disease in childhood and adolescence by transsphenoidal microadenomectomy. N. Engl. J. Med., *310:* 889–893, 1984.

35

The Role of Radiation Therapy in the Treatment of Low-Grade Gliomas

GLENN E. SHELINE, M.D., PH.D.

There have been many reports, often conflicting, regarding the role of radiotherapy for treatment of well-differentiated or "low-grade" astrocytomas. To date, however, there has been no randomized trial addressing this issue. Based on a limited retrospective review, Lindgren thought that some astrocytomas are sensitive to irradiation and that the clinical response may be very marked (11). Levy and Elvidge (10) had a 5-year survival rate of 36% with irradiation versus 26% without. Bouchard (2) and Bouchard and Pierce (3) reported a 49% 5-year survival rate for "adequately irradiated" patients; compared to the 26% reported by Levy and Elvidge for patients operated during the same calendar years, but not irradiated, this led Bouchard and Pierce (3) to conclude that irradiation was beneficial. Uihlein *et al.* (15) found no difference in 3- and 5-year survival rates for irradiated and nonirradiated patients with grade 1 and 2 astrocytomas. Schultz *et al.*, in 1968 (14) considered the "mature" astrocytomas to be radioinsensitive. In none of these reports were patient selection factors, patient characteristics, or the radiation therapy adequately described. Lack of suitable control groups and use of different classification systems also contributed to the problems of interpretation.

In 1975, we (9) presented the results for surgery with and without radiation therapy obtained at the University of California, San Francisco (UCSF). However, before summarizing that and other more recent reports, I would like to emphasize several of the prognostic factors noted by Leibel *et al.* at UCSF (9) and by Scanlon and Taylor (13) and, especially, Laws *et al.* (8) of the Mayo Clinic. It is now evident that these factors should be considered when preparing or interpreting any report on low-grade astrocytomas. One of the most important prognostic factors is age; younger patients do better than older ones. In the recent report by Laws *et al.*, (Table 35.1) the 5-year survival rate was 83% for patients less than 20 years of age, 35% for ages 20–49 years, and 12% for those older than 50 years. The functional status of the patient also plays a significant role. With no postoperative performance deficit, no alteration of consciousness, and no per-

TABLE 35.1

Selected Prognostic Factors* (Laws et al.)

Prognostic Factor	5 Year Survival, %
Ages, years: ≤19	83
20–49	35
>50	12
Functional Status	
Performance deficit:	
None vs. moderate to severe	42 vs. 9
Altered consciousness: No vs. Yes	38 vs. 10
Personality change: No vs. Yes	40 vs. 16
Removal: Total	61
Less than Total	32
Date of Surgery	
1949 or earlier	24
1950–1969	42
1970–1975	38

* Differences significant with $p < 0.01$ to < 0.0001.

sonality change, the overall 5-year survival rates ranged from 38–42%. These rates decreased to 9–16% when one of these features was present. Interestingly, age and functional status also were two of the main prognostic factors found for malignant gliomas in the large randomized trials of both the Brain Tumor Study Group (BTSG) (4) and the Radiation Therapy Oncology Group (RTOG) (5). That a patient in poor functional condition because of an advanced tumor might have a poor prognosis is readily understood but it is unclear why age should play such a significant role in both the low- and high-grade gliomas.

Several studies, including those of Leibel *et al.* (9) Fazekas (7), and Laws *et al.* (8), have shown that when total resection can be achieved, the survival rate is increased; in the Mayo material, for example, the 5-year survival rates were 61% with total resection versus 32% without. At UCSF they were 100% with complete resection and 46% or 19%, depending upon whether or not radiation therapy was given, with incomplete resection. Another important factor demonstrated in the Mayo Clinic material was the calendar date of the surgery. Excluding surgical deaths, the 5-year survival rates were 24% before 1950 and approximately 40% thereafter. Laws pointed out that the quality of the surgery improved with time. It should be noted that the quality of radiation therapy also has improved. In their 1966 report, Uihlein *et al.* (15) stated that 10–15 years earlier radiation therapy at the Mayo Clinic seldom exceeded a maximum of 1200 R given over 5–6 days repeated once or twice at 6- to 8-week intervals. Thus, the maximum tumor dose was only 2000–3500 R delivered over several months with long interruptions of therapy. At the time of the 1966 report many patients still received only 3500–4000 R. In 1985 most radiation oncologists would consider either of these radiation therapy techniques inadequate. It is likely that in all major clinics the quality of surgery, radiation therapy, and patient management have improved with time.

Thus, in order to evaluate the relative merits of various approaches to treatment of low-grade astrocytomas: (a) studies should be stratified at least by the important prognostic variables such as age, functional capacity, and extent of resection; (b) the quality of each form of therapy should be considered; and (c) treatment groups to be compared should be managed concurrently. Furthermore, if patients are selected for, rather than randomly assigned to, a particular form of therapy, the selection factors must be clearly stated. Unfortunately, these basic requirements are not met in any published study of low-grade astrocytomas.

Before turning to a comparison of the UCSF and Mayo Clinic experiences, which constitute the main emphasis of this presentation, a few other reports that have appeared since the mid 1970s will be summarized. Marsa et al. (12) (Table 35.2), presented the Stanford experience with 40 patients of mixed ages with hemispheric cerebral astrocytomas. The 5- and 10-year survival rates were 41% and 22%, respectively. This study contained no nonirradiated control patients, and pertinent selection factors were not described; hence, it provides little insight into the value of radiotherapy. Bloom (1) reported the experience at the Royal Marsden Hospital in London (Table 35.3) for 120 adult patients with supratentorial low-grade lesions. Bloom found greater survival rates at both 5 and 10 years for grade 1, as compared with grade 2, astrocytomas but also had no nonirradiated controls.

Fazekas (7) (Table 35.4) analyzed the Geisinger Medical Center results for 68 patients with grades 1 or 2 astrocytoma. Radiation therapy was given to about two-thirds of patients with each grade of tumor. Although

TABLE 35.2

Marsa et al.—1975

Irradiated cerebral astrocytomas
All ages—40 patients

Actuarial survival
  5 years—41%
  10 years—22%

No nonirradiated controls

TABLE 35.3

Bloom—1982

Adults—supratentorial—120 patients*		
Survival	Grade 1	Grade 2
5 years	33%	21%
10 years	10%	6%

* No nonirradiated controls.

some of his patients were irradiated and others were not, Fazekas used unclear selection factors to determine which patients received radiotherapy. Most (three-quarters) of the Geisinger patients were operated upon by one neurosurgeon, and it seems reasonable to assume that selection played an important role in determining which patients were to be referred for radiotherapy. According to the grading system, as used at the Geisinger Medical Center, grade 2 lesions were more than four times as common as

TABLE 35.4

Fazekas—1977—68 Patients

Patient Characteristics

	No. of Patients	≤16 Years of Age	Gross Excision	Irradiated
Grade 1 (20%)†	12			58%
Grade 2 (53%)†	56			68%
Irradiated	45	22%	29%	
Nonirradiated	23	74%	39%	

† ( ) = 5-year survival rate

Life-Table Survival Rates

Treatment	No. of Patients	Survival, % 5 Years
Irradiated	45	54
Nonirradiated	23*	32
Gross Excision	22	90
Incomplete Excision	45	31
Irradiated	31	41
Nonirradiated	14	13

* Includes 7 childhood posterior fossa astrocytomas; all survived disease free 3–16 years.

grade 1 lesions. Unexpectedly, the 5-year survival rate for grade 1 lesions was 20% versus 53% for grade 2. This raises questions as to the prognostic value of the grading system, at least as applied at the Geisinger Clinic. Prognostically, the nonirradiated group represented a more favorable mix of patients than did the irradiated group because it contained a greater percent of patients ≤ 16 years of age, 74% versus 22%, and gross excision was accomplished more frequently, 39% versus 29%. Nevertheless, the 5-year survival rate for patients receiving radiation therapy was better than for those not receiving it; namely, 54% versus 32%, respectively. This difference in favor of the irradiated group occurred in spite of the fact that the nonirradiated group not only had better prognostic factors but also included seven children, with posterior fossa astrocytoma; all of whom were disease free at the time of reporting. Patients with gross total excision did better than those with an incomplete excision, 90% versus 31%. Most important for present considerations is the fact that in patients with incomplete excision the 5-year survival rate was 41% with radiotherapy and 13% without, even though the irradiated patients appear to have been a less favorable group.

In a report from the Cross Cancer Institute on 107 patients with supratentorial astrocytomas, Weir and Grace (16) suggested that the main determinants of prolonged survival are young age, clinical status at the time of surgery, and the use of radiation therapy. The influence of radiation therapy on survival occurred primarily in the first 3 years postirradiation, after which the survival curves tended to converge. Incomplete recording of prognostic variables, failure to describe selection criteria, and lack of information regarding radiation technique, including fractionation, total dose, and treatment volume, make this study difficult to interpret.

DeWit et al. (6) (1984) recently reported a group of 35 children, less than 15 years of age. All 35 received radiation therapy. The large majority, 30 of 35, had infratentorial lesions, which were thought to be totally resected in 10. They were predominantly grade 1 (31 of 35). In the 30 patients with infratentorial astrocytoma, there was no recurrence in the 10 with totally resected tumors versus four in the 20 incompletely resected. Three of the five supratentorial lesions recurred. As expected in children with predominantly grade 1 infratentorial lesions, relapse-free survival rates were very good, being 87% at 5 years and 70% at 10 years. The authors concluded that low-grade astrocytoma in childhood is a malignant disease and warrants aggressive treatment. Their current treatment policy is to give radiation therapy for incompletely resected cerebellar lesions, cystic or noncystic, and for all noncerebellar lesions. They advocate 5000–5500 rads and the use of generous sized radiation fields.

Factors relative to patients treated at the Mayo Clinic and at UCSF are

TABLE 35.5

Comparison of Patients: UCSF vs. Mayo Clinic

	Scanlon & Taylor	Laws *et al.*	Leibel *et al.*
Period	1960–1969	1915–1975	1942–1967
Site	Intracranial	Cerebral hemisphere	Intracranial
Age			
<20	53 (40%)	52 (12%)	38 (31%)
≥20	81 (60%)	409 (88%)	84 (69%)
Therapy*	S + RT	S & S + RT	S & S + RT
Grade 1	42 (31%)	123 (27%)	82 (67%)
2	92 (69%)	338 (73%)	40 (33%)
Total	134	461	122

* S = surgical resection; RT = radiotherapy.

compared in Tables 35.5 and 35.6. The report by Laws *et al.* (8) covered the period 1915–1975 and was limited to patients with cerebral hemisphere astrocytomas. Scanlon and Taylor (13) reported on an intermediate period, 1960–1969, and included lesions primarily of the cerebrum and cerebellum. Leibel *et al.* (9) from UCSF, also included both cerebral and cerebellar astrocytomas as well as a few, 6%, that arose in the brain stem. While 30–40% of the patients of Scanlon and Taylor (13) and of Leibel *et al.* (9) were less than 20 years of age, only 12% of Laws' patients were in this age group.

TABLE 35.6

Comparison of Therapy: UCSF vs Mayo Clinic

Scanlon & Taylor		
All irradiated; doses given in "ret"		
Included 94 supratentorial tumors		
*Laws et al.**		
"Nonirradiated"	(0–<4000 rads)	252 (55%)
Adequately irradiated	(4000–7900 rads)	74 (16%)
Unknown irradiation		135 (29%)
Leibel et al.		
"Complete" resection alone		14 (12%)
Incomplete resection alone		37 (30%)
Incomplete resection plus radiation		71 (58%)

* 105 (23%) had total (57) or radical subtotal (48) resection.

According to Scanlon and Taylor (13) and Laws *et al.* (8), grade 2 lesions were two to three times as common as grade 1. In contrast, Leibel *et al.* (9) found grade 1 occurred twice as frequently as grade 2. It should be noted that normally at UCSF, the grading system is not used; in this instance it was applied retrospectively in an effort to facilitate comparison of our data with other data in the literature. For this purpose the pathology slides of all patients were reviewed, without knowledge of the clinical outcome, by Dr. Surl L. Nielson (Leibel *et al.*; Nielson, personal communication, 1985) who attempted to follow the criteria laid down by Kernohan and the Mayo Clinic group. Tumors showing only increased cellularity and possibly slight nuclear enlargement were classified as grade 1. With increased cellularity, irregular nuclear outline or hyperchromasia, the lesion was classed as grade 2. There is a considerable degree of subjectivity in defining grades 1 and 2; nevertheless, it is difficult to explain the marked difference in relative frequency of the two grades as reported from various clinics.

Although Scanlon and Taylor (13) included 94 patients with supratentorial tumors irradiated at the Mayo Clinic between 1960 and 1969, when presumably good radiation therapy was available, Laws *et al.* (8) reported only 74 patients with supratentorial tumors given "adequate radiation therapy" over six decades, including the decade reviewed by Scanlon and Taylor (Table 35.6).

Other differences occurred between the UCSF and Mayo material (Table 35.7). At UCSF, 12% had total resection. These patients received surgery only and were excluded from the comparison between surgery with and surgery without radiation therapy. On the other hand, 23% of the Mayo Clinic cases reported by Laws *et al.* had either a total or radical subtotal resection and it is unclear which of these patients were included in the various treatment groups. Inclusion or exclusion of patients with complete resection from a treatment group could significantly effect the relative survival rates of the irradiated and nonirradiated patients.

Scanlon and Taylor (13) reported radiation doses in terms of "ret" rather than rads. This statement of dose, designed to reduce different radiation dose schedules to a common denominator, makes use of a formula derived for acute reactions in skin. In all probability this formula is neither valid for evaluating the response of low-grade astrocytomas nor for predicting brain tolerance to radiation. Furthermore, an unknown proportion (see comment of Dr. Julian T. Hoff at the end of the Scanlon and Taylor paper) of the Mayo Clinic patients received nonstandard split-course radiation therapy in which one portion of the radiation therapy was given before and the other portion following an interruption of a few weeks.

Laws *et al.* divided their patients into three groups. The largest group,

55% of the total patient population, received either no radiation therapy or radiation doses up to 3999 rads; these patients, even though they may have had nearly 4000 rads, constituted the main group against which the "adequately irradiated" group was compared. Approximately one-third of the patients had radiotherapy at medical facilities other than the Mayo Clinic and details of their therapy are unknown. Only one-sixth (16%) of the patients were considered to have been adequately irradiated at the Mayo Clinic. It is unclear how this relatively small portion of the entire patient population was selected. By definition, the adequately irradiated group received between 4000 and 7900 rads but, as with the Scanlon and Taylor report, the fractionation, the site at which dose was calculated and the use of split-course radiotherapy are unspecified. Based on experience with virtually all other human tumors, 4000 rads would be expected to be inadequate for a low-grade astrocytoma. Furthermore, 7900 rads probably exceeds brain tolerance and, of itself, leads to decreased survival.

At UCSF, astrocytoma patients were divided into three groups. One group of 14 had complete resection; none of these was irradiated. Eleven of the 14 tumors occurred in the cerebellum and nine of the 11 were in patients less than 20 years of age. Patients with incompletely resected tumors were subdivided into those who did or did not receive postoperative radiation therapy. Radiation therapy was given in the conventional manner as a single continuous course. Dose was calculated as the minimum dose within the tumor. Most patients, approximately two-thirds, received a total tumor dose of 5000–5500 rads given in five fractions per week over 5½–6 weeks. Five patients received doses between 5500 and 6000 rads and 21 received smaller doses. The lower doses were used primarily during the earlier portion of the study period when the treatment regimen had not yet been standardized.

It is evident that important factors such as age distribution, tumor sites included, application of the grading system, frequency of total resection, therapy selection factors, radiation therapy techniques, radiation doses, and methods of data analysis differ widely between the two reports from the Mayo Clinic and between the Mayo Clinic reports and UCSF. Nevertheless, an attempt will be made to reconcile the data from these studies.

Tables 35.7–35.9 compare survival rates reported from the Mayo Clinic and UCSF. Scanlon and Taylor (Table 35.7) had a 5-year survival rate of 64% versus 36.5% overall survival rate by Laws et al. The better survival rate of Scanlon and Taylor is limited to the older patients. Below 20 years of age the 5-year survival rates were similar, 80% and 83%. From 20 years upward, the results of Scanlon and Taylor are better. The better survival reported by Scanlon and Taylor persists when grade 1 and grade 2 are considered separately. The survival differences between these two Mayo

TABLE 35.7

Survival—Mayo Clinic

| | Age, Years | 5-Year Survival, % | | |
		Grade 1	Grade 2	Grades 1 & 2
Scanlon & Taylor	0–79	76	58	64
	0–19			80
	20–39			61
	40–59			42
	60–79			16
Laws *et al.*	0–≥50	44	34	36.5
	0–19			83
	20–49			35
	≥50			12

TABLE 35.8

Survival—Laws et al.

	No. of Cases	Survival 5 Years	
0–<4000 rads	252	34 ⎫	
Unknown irradiation	135	35 ⎬ $p = 0.05$	
≥4000–7900 rads	74	49 ⎭	
Grade 1	123	44 ⎫ $p = 0.1$	
Grade 2	338	34 ⎭	

TABLE 35.9

Survival

| | Leibel *et al.* | | | Laws *et al.* |
| | | Incomplete Resection | | All Cases |
Interval Years	Complete Resection	Alone	Plus RT	
3	100%	27%	59%	~50%
5	100%	19%*	46%**	36.5% (~99%)†
10	100%	11%	35%	~21% (~95%)
15	89%	4%	25%	16% (~90%)
20	88%	0	23%	16%

† ( ) = expected survival; ~ = data from graphs.
* 25% for grade 1 and 0 for grade 2.
** 58% for grade 1 and 25% for grade 2.

series are not fully understood but may be due, in part at least, to differences in selection and treatment factors. In addition, all of the Scanlon and Taylor patients had radiotherapy, whereas only 16% of those of Laws *et al.* were known to have had at least 4000 rad irradiation, and it may be that this consistent use of radiotherapy by Scanlon and Taylor played a significant role.

Table 35.8 gives the survival data of Laws *et al.* as functions of the treatment given and of tumor grade. Patients who received either no irradiation or up to 4000 rads had a 5-year survival rate of 34%. The group that received unknown radiotherapy had a similar 5-year survival rate, namely 35%. The rate for patients with 4000 or more rads was 49%. The difference between the first two groups and the adequately treated group has a *p*-value of 0.05. Laws *et al.* concluded from a multivariate regression analysis that "radiation therapy was of clear benefit, primarily in older patients with incompletely removed tumors."

Table 35.9 presents survival data for the UCSF series together with selected comparison data from Laws *et al.* At UCSF patients thought to have had a complete resection did well. The only death, up to 20 years, occurred in a patient 70 years of age who died of congestive heart failure 12 years after therapy without evidence of recurrence. At UCSF at all time intervals from 3–20 years patients with incomplete resection plus postoperative radiation therapy did better than those who had incomplete resection alone. The overall survival rates for the patients of Laws *et al.* fall between those for incomplete resection alone and incomplete resection plus radiotherapy at UCSF, even though the Mayo series includes and the UCSF series excludes patients with complete resection.

At UCSF, patients with grade 1 lesions did better than grade 2 and, in each grade, postoperative irradiation appeared beneficial.

The column on the right with numbers in parenthesis (Table 35.9) gives expected survival rates, based on life table analysis, for a population with age and sex composition similar to that of Laws *et al.* (8). At 5 years, the survival rate for astrocytoma patients is about one-third of that calculated for a normal population. By 15 years it is down to about one-fifth of that expected. Although Laws *et al.* identified a relatively good risk group with a 15-year survival rate of 87%, in general these so-called low-grade, often termed benign, tumors are highly lethal. It seems evident that, at least for patients not in the Laws' good-risk group, better therapy than any developed to date is needed.

In summary, the available data are such that it is difficult to take a categorical position regarding the use of postoperative radiation therapy for low-grade astrocytomas. Nevertheless, decisions must be made and they must be made on the evidence available. Except for a selected group, including those with resected juvenile pilocytic astrocytoma of the cerebellum and the good risk group of Laws *et al.*, I believe present evidence supports the position that postoperative radiation therapy is beneficial for patients with incompletely resected astrocytomas. Although these astrocytomas are generally lethal, they tend to be slowly progressive. Thus, the therapy should be relatively conservative so that it does not of itself lessen life expectancy or produce excessive morbidity. With conventionally fractionated radiotherapy, we advocate doses in the 5000–5500 rad range, reduced for children under 2 or 3 years of age. It is expected that this will control some tumors, or at least significantly delay their recurrence, with a minimum risk of radiation injury.

Very young children and infants pose a special problem in that an adequate radiation dose is likely to lead to unacceptable late sequelae. Therefore, in such patients, we delay initiation of radiotherapy as long as possible. Unless there is evidence that immediate irradiation is necessary, close clinical observation together with repeated high quality CT and/or MRI scans are used to gauge disease progression. Radiotherapy is withheld until there is evidence of clinically significant tumor growth.

What is needed is a prospective and controlled study properly designed to determine which patients and which tumors should be irradiated as part of the primary treatment. Due to the slowly progressive nature of these tumors, such a study will require long observation.

REFERENCES

1. Bloom, H. J. G. Intracranial tumors: response and resistance to therapeutic endeavors, 1970–1980. Int. J. Radiol. Oncol. Biol. Phys. *8:* 1083–1113, 1982.
2. Bouchard, J. Central nervous system. In *Textbook of Radiotherapy*, 2nd ed. edited by G. Fletcher. Philadelphia, Lea and Feibiger, 1973, pp. 366–418.
3. Bouchard, J., and Peirce, C. B. Radiation therapy in the management of neoplasms of the central nervous system, with a special note in regard to children—twenty years' experience, 1939–1958. A. J. R., *84:* 610–628, 1960.
4. Byar, D. P., Green, S. B., and Strike, T. A. Prognostic factors for malignant glioma. In *Oncology of the Nervous System*, edited by M. D. Walker, Martinus Nijhoff Publishers, Netherlands, 1983, pp. 379–395.
5. Chang, C. H., Horton, J., Schoenfeld, D., Salazer, O., Perez-Tamayo, R., Kramer, S., Weinstein, A., Nelson, J. S., and Tsukada, Y. Comparison of postoperative radiotherapy and combined postoperative radiotherapy and chemotherapy in the multidisciplinary management of malignant gliomas. Cancer, *52:* 997–1007, 1983.
6. Dewit, L., Van Der Schueren, E., Ang, K. K., Van Den Bergh, R., Dom, R., and Brucher, J. M. Low-grade astrocytoma in children treated by surgery and radiation therapy. Acta Radiol., *23:* 1–8, 1984.
7. Fazekas, J. T. Treatment of grades I and II brain astrocytomas. The role of radiotherapy. Int. J. Radiol. Oncol. Biol. Phys., *2:* 661–666, 1977.
8. Laws, E. R., Jr., Taylor, W. F., Clifton, M. B., and Okazaki, H. Neurosurgical management of low-grade astrocytoma of the cerebral hemispheres. J. Neurosurg., *61:* 665–673, 1984.

9. Leibel, S. A., Sheline, G. E., Wara, W. M., Boldrey, E. B., and Nielsen, S. L. The role of radiation therapy in the treatment of astrocytomas. Cancer, *35:* 1551–1557, 1975.

10. Levy, L. F., and Elvidge, A. R. Astrocytoma of the brain and spinal cord—a review of 176 cases, 1940–1949. J. Neurosurg., *13:* 413–443, 1956.

11. Lindgren, M. Roentgen treatment of gliomata. Acta Radiol., *40:* 325–334, 1953.

12. Marsa, G. W., Goffinet, D. R., Rubinstein, L. J., and Bagshaw, M. A. Megavoltage irradiation in the treatment of gliomas of the brain and spinal cord. Cancer *36:* 1681–1689, 1975.

13. Scanlon, P. W., and Taylor, W. F. Radiotherapy of intracranial astrocytomas: analysis of 417 cases treated from 1960 through 1969. Neurosurgery, *5:* 301–308, 1979.

14. Schulz, M. D., Wang, C. C., Zinninger, G. F., and Tefft, M. Radiotherapy of intracranial neoplasms. Prog. Neurol. Surg. *2:* 318–370, 1968.

15. Uihlein, A., Colby, M., Jr., Layton, D., Parsons, W., and Carter, T. Comparison of surgery and surgery plus irradiation in the treatment of supratentorial gliomas. Acta Radiol., *5:* 67–78, 1966.

16. Weir, B., and Grace, M. The relative significance of factors affecting postoperative survival in astrocytomas, grades one and two. Le J Canadien des Sci Neurol., *3:* 47–50, 1976.

36

The Neurosurgical Management of Low-Grade Astrocytoma

EDWARD R. LAWS, JR., M.D., WILLIAM F. TAYLOR, PH.D., ERIK J.
BERGSTRALH, HARUO OKAZAKI, M.D., and MARVIN B. CLIFTON, M.D.

The management of low-grade astrocytomas of the brain remains a controversial issue (9, 11, 30, 35). Because patients with these tumors have favorable courses in so many instances, it is difficult to determine with certainty the benefit of any specific form of therapy (1, 2, 4, 5, 8, 16–21, 26, 30, 31). These tumors are rather heterogeneous as well, and careful analysis of natural history and results of therapy demands many levels of stratification and long-term follow-up. For these reasons, a retrospective analysis of all patients with grade 1 and grade 2 astrocytomas treated at the Mayo Clinic between 1915 and 1976 was undertaken.

HISTORICAL PERSPECTIVE

This review covers six decades during which medicine in general and neurosurgery in particular have made great progress. The patients studied were operated upon by one of 14 staff neurosurgeons or by residents supervised by them. The basic surgical philosophy did not change over time and was generally one of removing as completely as possible all resectable brain tumors (17). As medical care has become more sophisticated and modern transportation has made the Mayo Clinic more accessible, patients with astrocytomas are seen earlier in the course of the disease, and fewer patients are in critical or moribund condition at the time of surgery. Our analysis shows that there has been no change over time in the proportions of low- to high-grade astrocytomas seen, nor has there been a change in the proportions of low-grade tumors represented at the various sites within the brain. The proportions of patients in various age categories has not changed; neither has the sex distribution (22).

Until the recent advent of computer-assisted stereotactic surgery, biopsy was utilized sporadically in the surgical management of these tumors. Biopsy was relatively common until the 1950s and, thereafter, was only infrequently utilized. The concept of radical subtotal removal, *i.e.*, the removal of all but microscopically detectable tumor in inaccessible margins, was not utilized until the 1950s.

Although some patients received radiation therapy before 1940, modern concepts of radiotherapy date from the end of World War II. Radiation dosages in excess of 4000 rads were not given until the 1950s. In recent decades, the proportion of surgically treated low-grade astrocytoma patients referred for postoperative radiation therapy has remained relatively constant.

Because many of the patients treated live at some distance from the Mayo Clinic, more than half of those who had postoperative radiation therapy received it elsewhere, making details of therapy other than total dose in rads difficult to obtain.

A prior epidemiologic study indicated (27) that astrocytomas grades 1 and 2 (as distinct from glioblastomas) accounted for 251 (8%) of the 3210 primary brain tumors and 18% of all 1418 astrocytomas detected in a 30-year period between 1935 and 1964. There were 1167 glioblastomas (astrocytoma grades 3 and 4) during the same period (36% of the total primary brain tumors). In another careful study, low-grade astrocytomas represented 32% of Weir's total of surgically managed astrocytoma cases seen in the 10-year period, 1960–1970 (35).

LIMITATIONS OF THE STUDY

The Mayo Clinic is a nonurban referral center, and patterns of referral and follow-up care are in some cases different from other major medical centers. Although about 80% of Mayo Clinic patients come from within a radius of 400 miles, many come from other areas in the United States and from other countries as well. These facts should influence neither the disease nor the outcome with regard to survival.

Survival alone is a less than ideal end-point in studying a disease or its therapy, however, in a sample this size it is impractical and imprecise to estimate either quality of survival or time to recurrence, two important aspects of the outcome. Information on survival as determined by death certificates places time of death accurately, but does little to document extent of disease. The death certificates are helpful, however, in identifying those patients who died of causes other than the astrocytoma.

The radiotherapy data were handled in an arbitrary fashion. The selection of well-documented therapy totaling between 4000 and 7900 rads as the definition of the adequately treated group seemed reasonable, based on previous studies of radiation therapy for gliomas (3, 10, 23, 25, 32–34). Many patients who were treated by radiation therapy in their local medical facilities were placed in the "unknown" category because of uncertainty over the dose given, thus creating a bias in the radiation therapy data favoring the methods used at the Mayo Clinic (7, 25, 32).

In considering results of radiation therapy, another selection bias must be acknowledged. Those patients referred for postoperative radiation tended to be those with difficult, infiltrative, incompletely removed tumors, and there is no satisfactory control group.

CHARACTERISTICS STUDIED

In addition to basic descriptive data for each patient analyzed, information was systematically collected and recorded for a large number of features. Important variables analyzed included: neurologic symptoms and signs, time from onset of symptoms to diagnosis, preoperative neurologic state (0–4) and performance state (0–4), type of surgery ("total," radical subtotal, subtotal, biopsy only), use of lobectomy, size of tumor, presence of a cyst, postoperative neurologic and performance status, postoperative radiation therapy and dose, therapy for recurrent tumor, grade of recurrent tumor, and the occurrence of postoperative complications such as infection.

MATERIALS AND METHODS

A search was made of Mayo Clinic records in order to detect every case of low-grade astrocytoma. Several approaches were taken. (a) The Medical Diagnostic Index provided identification of patients with brain tumors for whom the diagnosis of astrocytoma or glioma was coded. This located the majority of cases. (b) The Tissue Registry was searched, reviewing all cases recorded after 1915 which might have been low-grade astrocytoma. (c) Finally, accurate data for recent years were available from operative notes within the Department of Neurosurgery. The assessment of acceptability of cases and abstracting of needed data was then done by a scrutiny of the individual patient records.

In order to be included in the study, pathologic confirmation at the Mayo Clinic was required. All cases had been examined by neuropathologists at least twice and grading was carried out according to the standard system described by Kernohan (14, 24, 28) (the majority of the cases had been reviewed and graded initially by Kernohan himself). No systematic analysis of other histologic features of the tumors was undertaken. Each of the medical records was reviewed by two neurosurgeons, and data were recorded on a standardized form. Current follow-up data were obtained on all but 13 of the cases by communicating with patients, families, referring physicians, and State vital statistics departments. Eight of these 13 cases were followed more than 5 years. Twelve were kept in the study as "alive when last known"; one lost within 30 days was included in the total but was excluded from further analysis.

Death certificates were obtained for every patient known to be deceased, and autopsy reports were obtained whenever possible.

From the search described above, 851 cases of low-grade astrocytoma other than optic glioma were accepted for study. The site of origin of the tumor was judged to be supratentorial in 500 patients: 208 in the frontal lobe, 207 temporal, 77 parietal, and 8 occipital. There were 74 "deep" tumors involving the basal ganglia or thalamus, 190 tumors of the cerebellum, 81 brain stem gliomas, three in the corpus callosum, and three "others." A separate study of 104 optic nerve gliomas has previously been reported (29).

Deaths occurring within 30 days of initial surgical treatment are commonly related to the surgery. There were 69 of these among the 851 cases studied herein.

SURVIVAL ANALYSIS

Survival tables and the corresponding survival curves are based on the Kaplan-Meier method (13). Significance tests for comparing survival of various subgroups are log rank tests or, on occasion, likelihood ratio tests based on the observation that most of the survival curves are nearly exponential for the first 5 years. In the figures the curves have been smoothed for simplicity and plotted (logarithmically) so that parallel curves indicate equal risk of death. The choice of "time zero" equal to date of surgery plus 30 days was made to exclude the biasing effect of surgical deaths, which occurred much more often in cases before 1950. Death from any cause was defined as the end-point. Patients still living at last follow-up were withdrawn from the analysis as of the date last known alive. The 12 other patients lost to follow-up were also withdrawn at the date last known.

RESULTS

The analysis in this study has had the following strategy. Predictor variables were sought from the data first by examining the survival of patients classified by each variable one at a time. Then subsets of variables were studied by multiple regression methods as described by Cox (6). This was done for the total and for several calendar periods within the 1915–1975 period (Tables 36.1 and 36.2).

The analyses of treatment variables for surgery and radiation therapy are given in Tables 36.3–36.10. Total resection surgery was related to much higher survival than any of the others. However, survival beyond 5 years was as good for radical subtotal surgery, but not for biopsy or subtotal resection. Radiation, on the other hand, was not strongly associated with survival. At doses over 4000 rads results with regard to survival were generally better than for lesser or unknown doses. This, too, varied after 5 years with the unknown group continuing to have poorer survival than the others.

TABLE 36.1

Number of Patients and 5-Year Survival by Various Characteristics of Patients: Low-Grade Astrocytoma—Mayo Clinic 1917–1975 (Supratentorial Sites, Survivors of 1st 30 Days after Surgery)

Characteristics of Brain Tumor Patients	No.	Survivors to 5 Years %	p-Value	Survivors to 15 Years if Alive at 5 Years %	p-Value
Total	461	36.5		44.3	
Calendar period					
<1949	124	24]		47⌉	
1950–69	231	42⌉	<0.0001	43	0.9
1970–75	106	38⌋		53⌋	
Age					
0–19	52	83]		86]	
20–49	322	35]	<0.0001	30⌉	<0.0001
>50	87	12]		38⌋	
No. months onset symptoms to surgery					
0–2	79	34] ⌝		65⌉	
3–5	50	18] ⌟		89⌋	
6–11	66	36⌉	0.0002	31⌉	0.03
12–59	181	39 ⌟		40	
>60	85	44⌋		36⌋	
Seizure					
Yes	305	40]	0.0009	42⌉	0.4
No	156	29]		50⌋	
Headache					
Yes	205	27]	<0.0001	47⌉	0.9
No	256	44]		43⌋	
Nausea/vomiting					
Yes	44	23]	0.01	75⌉	0.3
No	417	38]		42⌋	
Papilledema					
Yes	101	27]	0.009	43⌉	0.8
No	360	39]		44⌋	
Altered consciousness					
Yes	30	10]	<0.0001	67⌉	0.8
No	431	38]		44⌋	
Personality change					
Yes	75	16]	<0.0001	34⌉	0.06
No	386	40]		45⌋	
Language deficit					
Yes	65	22]	0.0004	49⌉	0.3
No	396	39]		44⌋	
Visual loss					
Yes	75	27]	0.02	60⌉	0.3
No	386	38]		42⌋	

TABLE 36.1 (*Continued*)

Characteristics of Brain Tumor Patients	No.	Survivors to 5 Years		Survivors to 15 Years if Alive at 5 Years	
		%	p-Value	%	p-Value
Motor deficit					
Yes	122	30]	0.007	53]	0.5
No	339	39]		41]	
Sensory loss					
Yes	50	26]	0.04	49]	0.9
No	411	38]		44]	
Preoperative neurologic deficit					
None	159	47]	<0.0001	33]	0.2
Unknown	55	60]		72]	
Mild	190	25]		48]	
Moderate/severe	57	23]		52]	
Preoperative performance deficit					
None	291	38]	<0.0001	37]	0.1
Unknown	55	60]		72]	
Mild	84	21]		54]	
Moderate/severe	31	23]		57]	
Surgery					
Biopsy/subtotal	356	32]	<0.0001	37]	0.1
Radical subtotal	48	44]		52]	
Total	57	61]		59]	
Site					
Frontal	190	33]	0.6	35]	0.01
Temporal	192	37		40]	
Parietal	71	44		67]	
Occipital	8	38]		100]	
Grade					
1	123	44]	0.1	54]	0.04
2	338	34]		40]	
Diameter of tumor (cm)					
Unspecified	332	35]	0.06	43]	0.4
<5	70	32]		44]	
>5	59	47		47]	
Cyst					
Single only	92	51]	0.009	56]	0.05
None or multiple	369	33]		40]	
Infection					
Yes	13	23]	0.03	100]	0.3
No	448	37]		44]	
Radiation treatment					
None or <4000	252	34]	0.05	54]	0.01
Unknown	135	35]		29]	
>4000 rads	74	49]		43]	

TABLE 36.1 (*Continued*)

Characteristics of Brain Tumor Patients	No.	Survivors to 5 Years		Survivors to 15 Years if Alive at 5 Years	
		%	*p*-Value	%	*p*-Value
Postoperative neurologic deficit					
None	127	49		37	
Unknown	88	44	<0.0001	69	0.2
Mild	153	33		45	
Moderate/severe	93	16]		33	
Postoperative performance deficit					
None	227	42		42	
Unknown	89	44	<0.0001	69	0.4
Mild	112	27		36	
Moderate/severe	33	9		33	

Characteristics showing little or no indication of association with survival

Sex	*p* = 0.5
Side of brain	0.2
Lobectomy	0.4

All of the above statements reflect a very conservative use of *p*-values as indicators of significance. Because so many variables were tested, we chose a *p* value of 0.005 as our level of significance. "Highly significant" values are quoted only for *p*-values under that level. Since some 30 variables were tested we might have used $0.05 \div 30 = .0017$ with some justification, but decided 0.005 was a sufficient safeguard for our purposes here.

The items above were all considered singly. Obviously they are correlated and some may be completely explained by others. In an effort to detect these relationships, they were examined simultaneously in a step-down regression analysis based on the Cox proportional hazards mode (6) utilizing the first 5 years of survival. Six variables were clearly dominant for supratentorial tumors and together predicted survival significantly better than the others. Adding any of the other variables did not yield significant improvement. By far the most powerful of these six variables was age. The second was postoperative neurologic deficit. The others were altered consciousness, personality change, type of surgery, calendar period, and site.

The importance of neurologic deficit was surprising in that it was a somewhat vague and qualitative summary of patient records done by a staff surgeon as a quick overview. On the other hand, it may not be surpris-

TABLE 36.2

Number of Patients and Surgical Deaths by Various Characteristics Supratentorial Low-Grade Astrocytomas ("Surgical Deaths" are Deaths Occurring within 30 Days of Surgery)

Characteristics of Brain Tumor Patients	No.	Surgical Deaths No.	%	p-Value
Total	499	38	7.6	
Calendar period				
<1949	148	24	16.2	
1950–69	243	12	4.9	<0.0001
1970–75	108	2	1.9	
Altered consciousness				
No	460	29	6.3	0.0002
Yes	39	9	23.1	
Months from onset to treatment				
0–2	94	15	16.0	
3–11	128	12	9.4	0.0005
12+	277	11	4.0	
Headache				
No	268	12	4.5	0.004
Yes	231	26	11.3	
Preoperative performance deficit				
None	305	14	4.6	
Mild	98	14	14.3	0.004
Moderate/severe	96	10	10.4	
Lobectomy				
No	407	37	9.1	0.009
Yes	92	1	1.1	
Diameter of tumor				
Unknown	367	35	4.1	
<5 cm	73	3	9.5	0.02
≥5 cm	59	0	0	
Seizures				
No	175	19	10.9	0.04
Yes	324	19	5.9	
Motor deficit				
No	361	22	6.1	0.04
Yes	138	16	11.6	

TABLE 36.3
Longevity Related to Type of Surgery

Type of Surgery	No. of Patients	5-year Survival (%)	10-year Survival (%)
Biopsy only	147	48.0	34.2
Subtotal removal	391	41.9	26.7
Radical subtotal removal	80	54.8	42.8
"Total" removal	151	77.6	68.6

TABLE 36.4
Longevity following Lobectomy in Low-Grade Astrocytoma of the Cerebral Hemispheres

Lobectomy	No. of Patients	5-year Survival (%)	10-year Survival (%)
Yes	92	38.8	27.2
No	382	36.6	18.2

TABLE 36.5
Longevity Related to Radiation Therapy: Low-Grade Astrocytoma— All Cases

Radiation Therapy	No. of Patients	5-year Survival (%)	10-year Survival (%)
None	463	49.9	40.4
Adequate dose (4000–7900 rads)	122	62.3	38.3
Unknown	197	47.7	31.1

TABLE 36.6
Longevity Related to Radiation Therapy: Low-Grade Astrocytomas—Cerebellar Tumors

Radiation Therapy	No. of Patients	5-year Survival (%)	10-year Survival (%)
None	119	84.8	81.2
Adequate dose (4000–7900 rads)	12	76.2	63.5
Unknown	36	80.1	71.5

TABLE 36.7

Longevity Related to Radiation Therapy: Low-Grade Astrocytomas—
Deep Supratentorial Tumors

Radiation Therapy	No. of Patients	5-year Survival (%)	10-year Survival (%)
None	29	54.8	47.2
Adequate dose (4000–7900 rads)	24	91.3	80.8
Unknown	14	57.1	49.0

TABLE 36.8

Longevity Related to Radiation Therapy: Low-Grade
Astrocytomas—Brainstem Tumors, Surgically Proven

Radiation Therapy	No. of Patients	5-year Survival (%)	10-year Survival (%)
None	46	47.3	31.1
Adequate dose (4000–7900 rads)	10	56.0	37.3
Unknown	12	65.6	65.6

TABLE 36.9

Longevity Related to the Presence of a Single Cyst

	Single Cyst	No. of Patients	5-year Survival (%)
All tumors	Yes	235	72.4
	No	547	42.3
Cerebellar astrocytoma	Yes	119	87.2
	No	48	74.7
Supratentorial astrocytoma	Yes	93	53.0
	No	381	33.2

TABLE 36.10

Low-Grade Astrocytoma: Management of Recurrent Tumor

Treatment of Recurrence	No. of Patients	6-month Survival (%)	12-month Survival (%)
None	10	63.4	47.6
Surgery or surgery plus other modalities	105	58.1	45.7
Nonsurgical therapy	36	63.4	46.1

ing when one realizes that this summary takes into account many of the symptoms listed above. The variable seems to serve well in place of several individual symptoms.

The usefulness of altered consciousness is lessened when we note that for only 31 (7%) of the patients was this symptom found. When it occurred, survival was dismal. Personality change occurred more often, and when it did survival was also very poor.

Survival was poorer before 1950 than after. As mentioned earlier, we believe this reflects a less sophisticated state of development of surgical and diagnostic procedures.

Variation by site within the supratentorial region was not strong when considered individually. However, it turned out to be of importance in the multiple analysis.

The regression analysis provided, in addition to the definition of the important variables, weights for these variables. These were simplified and a numerical score was developed and tested as a prognostic indicator for survival. This has previously been reported (15).

TUMOR RECURRENCE

There were 151 patients with recurrent tumor (Table 36.10) documented either at subsequent surgery or at autopsy. Among the supratentorial tumors, initial tumor grade was 1 in 15 patients and grade 2 in 64 patients. A change to astrocytoma grade 3 or 4 occurred in 39 patients (49%). This indicates that, over time, about one-half of the low-grade tumors tend to remain true to grade. The 49% who progressed may be explained either by sampling error at the initial biopsy or by dedifferentiation or malignant transformation of the tumor as part of its natural history.

SURGICAL DEATHS

Deaths within 30 days of surgery are defined here as "surgical deaths." In the 499 cases of supratentorial astrocytoma with adequate follow-up, there were 38 (7.6%) such deaths. Analysis by calendar period demonstrates a very strong decrease in surgical mortality from the early period before 1950 up into the 1970s. The early percentage of surgical deaths was 16%, the most recent was only 2%. The second most important variable in the analysis of operative mortality is altered consciousness which is also one of the strong variables with respect to total survival (Table 36.2). Surgical deaths accounted for 23% with this characteristic, and only 6% without it. The other three most significant characteristics were months from onset to treatment, headaches, and preoperative performance deficit.

DISCUSSION

The analysis of survival data from these patients with low-grade astrocytoma confirms and re-emphasizes characteristics of gliomas which have become increasingly apparent with more recent studies of this neoplasm. The age of the patient at the time of diagnosis has an overwhelming effect on outcome, eclipsing all other variables and all forms of management. The reasons for this phenomenon are not clear, but it is evident that this tumor is quite different in its biologic behavior when it appears in a young host.

It was not surprising to confirm the lack of sex difference in survival and the fact that there was little difference between astrocytomas grade 1 and grade 2. The presence of a single cyst, thought to be a highly favorable feature, had a consistently favorable influence on survival. Lobectomy, which is thought to improve survival in malignant astrocytomas (12), had little influence on the outcome of supratentorial low-grade astrocytomas.

The fact that survival is better in the most indolent tumors with longer symptomatic periods prior to therapy, seizures as a symptom, and less in the way of performance or neurologic deficits is no surprise. Conversely, the poor survival accompanying patients who present with signs and symptoms of increased intracranial pressure, altered consciousness, personality change, and significant performance deficits can be anticipated.

With regard to therapeutic intervention, the data generally support a philosophy of radical surgical removal whenever possible. This conclusion may be biased, however, in that there is a tendency for the most favorable lesions to be treated with radical surgery and the less favorable (deep, infiltrative, noncystic) to be treated with more limited approaches.

Despite the consideration of multiple variables, it was difficult to prove a beneficial effect for postoperative radiation therapy except in patients over 40 years of age (those with many poor prognostic features).

"Modern" neurosurgery is capable of dealing effectively with low-grade astrocytomas, confirming the diagnosis, reducing or eliminating tumor burden, and having a very low operative mortality rate. The long-term (15-year) survival rate for supratentorial low-grade astrocytomas ranges from 87% for favorable patients with tumors "totally" removed to 16% for the average case. Further improvement in the outcome for these patients will most likely rest with advances in our understanding of the basic biology and pathogenesis of gliomas.

ACKNOWLEDGMENTS

The authors are grateful to Mrs. Constance Hoeft for her expert assistance in preparation of the manuscript, to Mrs. Verna Hoverman, Mrs. Shirley Christensen, and Mrs. Susanne Daood for assistance with data analysis.

REFERENCES

1. Adson, A. W., Svien, H. J., and Dodge, H. W. Jr. Brain tumors. A study of postoperative results and survival periods. Postgrad. Med., *9:* 198–210, 1951.
2. Alpers, B. J., and Rowe, S. N. The astrocytomas. Am. J. Cancer, *30:* 1–18, 1937.
3. Bailey, P. Further remarks concerning tumors of the glioma group. Bull. Johns Hopkins Hosp., *40:* 354, 1927.
4. Bailey, P., and Cushing, H. *A Classification of the Tumors of the Glioma Group on a Histogenetic Basis with a Correlated Study of Prognosis.* J.B. Lippincott Co., Philadelphia, 1926.
5. Betty, M. J. Quality of survival in treated patients with supratentorial gliomata. J. Neurol. Neurosurg. Psychiatr., *27:* 556–561, 1964.
6. Cox, D. R. Regression models and life tables. J. R. Stat. Soc. (B), *2:* 187–220, 1972.
7. Eagan, R. T., Childs, D. S. Jr., Layton, D. D. Jr., Laws, E. R. Jr. *et al.* Dianhydrogalactitol and radiation therapy: treatment of supratentorial glioma. J.A.M.A., *241:* 2046–2050, 1979.
8. Elvidge, A., Penfield, W., and Cone, W. The gliomas of the central nervous system. A study of 210 verified cases. Res. Publ. Assoc. Nerv. Ment. Dis., *16:* 107–181, 1937.
9. Gol, A. The relatively benign astrocytomas of the cerebrum. A clinical study of 194 verified cases. J. Neurosurg., *18:* 501–506, 1961.
10. Hochberg, F. H., Linggood, R., Wolfson, L., *et al.* Quality and duration of survival in glioblastoma multiforme: combined surgical, radiation and lomustine therapy. J.A.M.A., *241:* 1016–1018, 1979.
11. Horrax, G. Benign (favorable) types of brain tumor. The end results (up to 10 years) with statistics of mortality and useful survival. N. Engl. J. Med., *250:* 981–984, 1954.
12. Jelsma, R., and Bucy, P. C. Glioblastoma multiforme: its treatment and some factors effecting survival. Arch. Neurol., *20:* 161–171, 1969.
13. Kaplan, E. L., and Meier, P. Nonparametric estimation from incomplete observations. J. Am. Statist. Assoc., *53:* 457–481, 1958.
14. Kernohan, J. W., Mabon, R. F., Svien, H. J., *et al.* Symposium on new and simplified concept of gliomas; a simplified classification of gliomas. Proc. Mayo Clin., *24:* 71–75, 1949.
15. Laws, E. R. Jr., Taylor, W. F., Clifton, M. B., and Okazaki, H. Neurosurgical management of low-grade astrocytoma of the cerebral hemispheres. J. Neurosurg., *61:* 665–673, 1984.
16. Levy, L. F., and Elvidge, A. R. Astrocytomas of the brain and spinal cord. A review of 176 cases, 1940–1949. J. Neurosurg., *19:* 365–374, 1956.
17. MacCarty, C. S. Surgical treatment of gliomas of the brain. J. Int. Coll. Surg., *23:* 290–297, 1955.
18. Matsukado, Y., MacCarty, C. S., and Kernohan, J. W.: The growth of glioblastoma multiforme (astrocytomas, grades 3 and 4) in neurosurgical practice. J. Neurosurg., *18:* 636–644, 1961.
19. Mercuri, S., Russo, A., and Palma, L. Hemispheric supratentorial astrocytomas in children: long-term results in 29 cases. J. Neurosurg., *55:* 170–173, 1981.
20. Miller, R. H., Craig, W. M., and Kernohan, J. W. Supratentorial tumors among children. Arch. Neurol. Psychiatr., *68:* 797–814, 1953.
21. Nakissa, N., and Pleuk, H. Radiation therapy of astrocytomas grades I-IV. Int. J. Radiat. Oncol. Biol. Phys., *4(Suppl 2):* 229–230, 1978.
22. Percy, A. K., Elveback, L. R., Okazaki, H., *et al.* Neoplasms of the central nervous system: epidemiologic considerations. Neurology, *22:* 40–48, 1972.
23. Salcman, M., Kaplan, R. S., Ducker, T. B., *et al.* Effect of age and reoperation on survival in the combined modality treatment of glioblastoma multiforme. Neurosurgery, *10:* 454–463, 1982.

24. Sayre, G. P. The concept of grading gliomas of the central nervous system. J. Int. Coll. Surg., *26:* 440–447, 1956.
25. Scanlon, P. W., and Taylor, W. F. Radiotherapy of intracranial astrocytomas: Analysis of 417 cases treated from 1960 through 1969. Neurosurgery, *5:* 301–308, 1979.
26. Scherer, H. J. The forms of growth in gliomas and their practical significance. Brain, *63:* 1–35, 1940.
27. Schoenberg, B. S., Christine, B. W., and Whisnant, J. P. The descriptive epidemiology of primary intracranial neoplasms: the Connecticut experience. Am. J. Epidemiol., *104:* 499–510, 1976.
28. Svien, H. J., Mabon, R. F., Kernohan, J. W., *et al.* Symposium on a new and simplified concept of gliomas: astrocytomas. Proc. Mayo. Clin., *24:* 54–64, 1949.
29. Tenny, R. T., Laws, E. R. Jr., Younge, B. R., *et al.* The neurosurgical management of optic glioma: Results in 104 patients. J. Neurosurg., *57:* 452–458, 1982.
30. Thomas, D. G. T., Graham, D. I. (editors). *Brain Tumors: Scientific Basis, Clinical Investigation and Current Therapy,* Butterworths, London, 1980.
31. Tooth, H. H. Some observations on the growth and survival period of intracranial tumors; based on the records of 500 cases with special reference to the pathology of the gliomata. Brain, *35:* 61, 1912.
32. Uihlein, A., Colby, M. Y., Layton, D. D., *et al.* Comparison of surgery and surgery plus irradiation in the treatment of supratentorial gliomas. Acta Radiol. [Ther] (Stockh), *5:* 67–78, 1966.
33. Walker, M. D., Alexander, E. Jr., Hunt, W. E., *et al.* Evaluation of BCNU and/or radiotherapy in the treatment of anaplastic gliomas: a cooperative clinical trial. J. Neurosurg., *49:* 333–343, 1978.
34. Walker, M. D., Green, S. B., Byar, D. P., *et al.* Randomized comparisons of radiotherapy and nitrosoureas for the treatment of malignant glioma after surgery. N. Engl. J. Med., *303:* 1323–1329, 1980.
35. Weir, B., and Grace, M. The relative significance of factors affecting postoperative survival in astrocytomas, grades one and two. Can. J. Neurol. Sci., *47:* 50, 1976.

VII

Infections

37

Brain Biopsy for Encephalitis

M. J. SCHLITT, M.D., RICHARD B. MORAWETZ, M.D., J. M. BONNIN, M.D., H. E. ZEIGER, M.D., and R. J. WHITLEY, M.D.

Brain biopsy performed for diagnosis on encephalitis remains a controversial subject (46). Renewed interest and concern have developed as relatively nontoxic antiviral drug therapies have become widely available, and the acquired immune deficiency syndrome (AIDS) threatens to reach epidemic proportions. This paper will discuss the use of brain biopsy in the management of four groups of patients: (*a*) patients thought to have herpes simplex encephalitis; (*b*) patients thought to have Creutzfeldt-Jakob disease; (*c*) patients who are in an iatrogenic state of immunocompromise for prevention of rejection of transplanted organs; and (*d*) patients with AIDS who develop focal lesions of the central nervous system.

Of considerable interest to neurosurgeons is the risk to the members of the operating room team of contracting the disease they are attempting to diagnose by brain biopsy, or, in the circumstance of patients with AIDS, the risk of becoming infected with the HTLV-III retrovirus. The risk of contracting Creutzfeldt-Jakob disease has been a concern for many years, and the developing epidemic of patients infected with the HTLV-III virus has augmented those concerns. Therefore, an assessment has been made of this risk to the operating neurosurgeon and the members of the operating room team of exposure to the brain tissue and blood of patients who fall into the four categories listed above. Also, an assessment of the relative hardiness of the infectious agent involved will be presented, together with recommendations regarding special techniques for sterilization of instruments and clean-up of the operating room where applicable.

HERPES SIMPLEX ENCEPHALITIS

Herpes simplex encephalitis is the most common fatal sporadic encephalitic illness in humans (27). The only effective treatment for this disease currently available involves the use of nucleoside analogs, and clinical trials to assess the efficacy of these agents have depended largely upon brain biopsy to establish diagnosis with certainty (6, 10, 11, 15, 21, 29, 32, 36, 41, 46–51). Herpes simplex is not the most common viral encephalitis in adults; arboviral and enteroviral infections occur more frequently (19), and their initial presentation can be quite similar to that of herpes simplex encephalitis with the appearance of acute or subacute neurologic dysfunction with fever and/or lymphocytic pleocytosis in the cerebrospinal fluid. Experience in the treatment of patients with herpes simplex encephalitis indicates that the appearance of an abnormality within the temporal lobe of the patient's brain as seen on computed tomographic (CT) scanning predicts a very poor prognosis for that patient (29). If therapy is to be effective, it must be initiated as early as possible in the course of this disease, as viral replication time for the herpes simplex virus in the central nervous system is about 18 hours, and over a period as short as 24 hours a patient's brain disease can worsen such that meaningful recovery is no longer possible.

With the advent of relatively nontoxic antiviral agents that can be administered in small volumes of intravenous fluid, some workers have recommended treating patients suspected of having herpes simplex encephalitis with those pharmacologic agents without confirming the diagnosis by brain biopsy and viral culture. However, even with the information provided by the sophisticated neurodiagnostic procedures currently available, brain biopsy will reveal conditions other than herpes simplex encephalitis that may respond to either medical or surgical treatment in as many as 20% of cases. Examples are tuberculous and cryptococcal meningitis and subdural empyema. Brain biopsy in the hands of an experienced neurosurgeon carries a very low risk of morbidity and mortality (29). One cubic centimeter of tissue should be taken from the anterior portion of the inferior temporal gyrus on the side determined by clinical data such as localizing seizures, and/or by neurodiagnostic tests such as electroencephalography (EEG) and CT scanning. To date, we have not utilized magnetic resonance imaging (MRI) scanning in the assessment of these patients because they are often confused and occasionally combative at the time of work-up. Antiviral therapy should be initiated at the first suspicion that a patient may have herpes simplex encephalitis, and brain biopsy should be performed within 24 hours. There is no evidence to suggest that this has produced false negative biopsies (48). This is not surprising in that replication time for herpes simplex virus is about 18 hours, and for at least 24 hours after initiation of drug therapy intact viral particles will be present in quantities greater than can be inhibited by accumulated drug. The risk to the operating team of obtaining a brain biopsy for patients with herpes simplex encephalitis appears minimal.

Access of herpes simplex virus to the central nervous system is not well understood. Transmission could occur either along olfactory pathways or via trigeminal fibers, to lead to the characteristic frontotemporal distribution of lesions. Recent experimental evidence tends to implicate the olfactory pathways (41, 43). The infrequency of herpes simplex encephalitis, relative to the frequency of trigeminal system infection (3), remains a puzzle. It is possible that ophthalmic infection could occur following conjunctival inoculation by splash from the wound of an infected patient, particularly if a member of the operating team was receiving chronic immunosuppressive therapy. The virus envelope is disrupted by detergent, enabling easy inactivation.

CREUTZFELDT-JAKOB DISEASE

For many years, absolute diagnosis of Creutzfeldt-Jakob disease has depended on examination of brain tissue obtained at brain biopsy or at autopsy. The disease is caused by a kuru-like agent, occurs worldwide, and is uniformly fatal (16). Its incidence is estimated at one case per million population per annum. The disease should be described as subacute spongiform encephalopathy rather than encephalitis. Although the clinical diagnosis is generally not difficult except in its early stages, confusion with Alzheimer's disease (20, 43), toxic or metabolic encephalopathy, meningeal carcinomatosis, and other subacute diseases of the central nervous system occurs occasionally (1). Increasing attention is being given to kuru-like agents as the possible etiologic agent in certain cases of dementing disease, including patients labeled as having Alzheimer's disease (43).

Documented cases of iatrogenic transmission of subacute spongiform encephalopathy have occurred via corneal transplantation (12), the donor having suffered from the disease and from the use of inadequately sterilized depth electrodes in successive patients following use in a patient with Creutzfeldt-Jakob disease (5). Gibbs discusses other cases in which infection at surgery may have occurred (16). Since kuru, a form of subacute spongiform encephalopathy identified among the Fore people of the New Guinea highlands, has been shown to have been transmitted by cannibal ingestion of the infected brain tissue of diseased relatives, and since subacute spongiform encephalopathy has been transmitted from primate to primate, including human to chimpanzee, chimpanzee to chimpanzee, and chimpanzee to other primates, the operating neurosurgeon and the members of the operating room team as well as patients are believed to be at risk for contraction of this disease (5). The potential for contamination of the surgeon's corneas by irrigant splashed from the wound, mandates protective eyewear. The agent can be transmitted to primates by inoculation of tissues other than brain, such as lung, liver, and kidney (16) from infected humans; inoculation of cerebrospinal fluid from patients with

Creutzfeldt-Jakob disease into the brains of primates has transmitted the disease as well (16). Transmission of the disease through the use of human growth hormones obtained from pooled human pituitary glands obtained at autopsy has been documented recently (8). According to Gibbs the agent has not yet been isolated from human blood, urine, or feces (16).

Decontamination of instruments used for brain biopsy in patients suspected of harboring Creutzfeldt-Jakob disease agent can be accomplished by autoclaving at 121°C for 1 hour, immersion in 1 N NaOH or 2.5% NaOCl for 15 minutes, or immersion in 0.1 N NaOH or 0.5% to 1.0% NaOCl for 1 hour (17). Gibbs and his co-workers have recently shown that steam autoclaving for 1 hour at 2 atm pressure and 121°C, or dry heat for 1 minute at ambient pressure and 240°C, inactivated Creutzfeldt-Jakob disease agent (9). However, infected material can be stored in 10–20% formaldehyde at room temperature for long periods without significant loss of titer, and the agent resists most antiseptics (16). Therefore, care should be taken to sterilize instruments and the operating room environment carefully where necessary.

Brain biopsy is currently employed to establish the diagnosis of Creutzfeldt-Jakob disease with certainty in those situations where such information is deemed important. In the future, if medical therapy is developed for this disease, brain biopsy may well be a part of experimental protocols, as has been the case in the development of drug therapy for herpes simplex encephalitis.

TRANSPLANTATION PATIENTS

Patients who are in an iatrogenically induced state of immunocompromise are at risk for the development of central nervous system infections and malignancies. The outlook in these patients may be considerably better, however, since in many cases their state of immunocompromise can be reversed or lessened by cessation of or reduction in the dosage of immunosuppressive drugs. The acute or subacute appearance of neurologic abnormality of either focal or diffuse nature should prompt immediate evaluation of such patients. Although many of the central nervous system (CNS) infections seen in such patients can be diagnosed by means other than brain biopsy, disorders such as progressive multifocal leukoencephalopathy (PML), reticulum cell sarcoma, and early fungal brain abscess may require brain biopsy for their diagnosis. Their differentiation without diagnostic tissue may be impossible, and appropriate treatment may depend on prompt and precise diagnosis.

PML was first recognized as a distinct entity by Åstrom et al. in 1958 (2), and to date more than 200 cases have been reported (13, 24, 33, 49).

Causative agents have been demonstrated to be polyomaviruses, specifically JC and SV 40-PML (7, 9, 25, 31, 33, 38, 39, 43, 45, 52). Currently, diagnosis can be established only by brain biopsy. The authors have had experience with three patients who developed PML, two of whom were in an iatrogenically induced state of immunocompromise following renal transplantation and one of whom was receiving chemotherapy for poorly differentiated lymphocytic lymphoma (39). Each patient presented with neurologic signs, which were focal in the two transplant recipients (39). All patients underwent a battery of neurodiagnostic studies, including lumbar puncture, EEG, and CT scanning of the head. Although none of the studies was diagnostic, the CT scan precisely localized white matter lesions in areas appropriate to the neurologic deficit. To establish diagnosis 1 cm^3 of brain tissue was taken from such an area of involvement, using stereotactic biopsy in the most recent case. Diagnosis was by light and electron microscopy (Figs. 37.1 and 37.2).

In order to minimize artifact and allow complete pathologic examination, tissue samples should be placed into 10% buffered formalin and in glutaraldehyde within minutes of removal. Viral cultures specific for polyomavirus are utilized infrequently because of difficulties associated with them. JC polyomavirus will grow only in primary human fetal glial cell cultures and only very slowly (22, 34, 44, 52). Primary human fetal glial cell cultures are difficult to maintain and difficult to utilize, making histopathologic studies the most practical method of diagnosis. Electron microscopic study of infected tissues shows intranuclear particles in the 30–40 nm range, an appearance specific for polyomavirus (Fig. 37.1) (1, 2, 5, 9, 13, 26, 28, 31, 38, 39, 43, 45, 48).

The method of transmission of PML is unknown. Transmission of the disease from an immunocompromised to a normal host is extremely unlikely. Precautions taken in dealing with these patients, including normal contact isolation procedures, are primarily designed to prevent transmission of the disease to other patients who are immunocompromised. Routine operating room procedures for handling patients and for sterilization of instruments appear adequate for protection of both the members of the operating team and patients.

AIDS

The emergence of an epidemic of patients with AIDS has provided a totally new challenge for neurosurgeons. As many as a million people may have been infected with the HTLV-III virus (7, 17, 22, 23), although only a small percentage thus far have developed the state of immunocompromise known as AIDS that places these patients at risk for secondary infection of the central nervous system (24). Most of today's practicing neurosurgeons

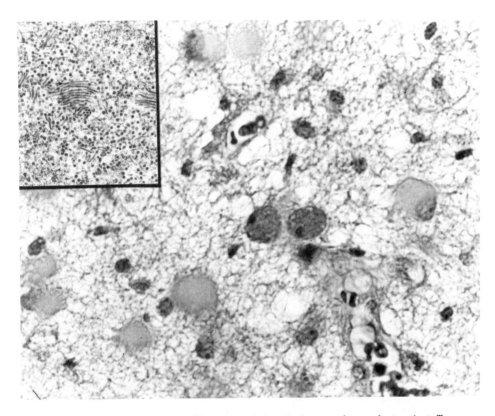

FIG. 37.1. Progressive multifocal leukoencephalopathy in a renal transplant patient. Two enlarged oligodendrocytes with a typical nuclear appearance in a field displaying intense reactive proliferation of astrocytes. Hematoxylin and eosin, 132×. *Inset,* round and tubular forms of the JC virus in the nucleus of an oligodendrocyte. Electron micrograph, 22000×.

have not had experience with an epidemic in which a fatal infectious disease kills large numbers of previously healthy people (22). Historical perspective on the effect of epidemics of infectious disease on human history can be gained from the book *Rats, Lice, and History,* written by Hans Zinser and published in 1935 (51).

Opportunistic infections of the central nervous system are demonstrated in about 30% of patients with AIDS at some point in their management (24). A recent study of a group of patients with AIDS documented that the average lifespan of that group of patients following initial hospitalization for their first opportunistic infection was 224 days. Levy *et al.* (24) documented mean survival in eight patients of 9 months after first presentation, and 4.4 months after appearance of central nervous system disease,

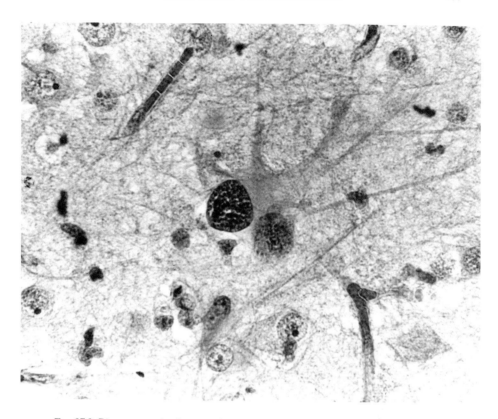

FIG. 37.2. Bizzare, neoplastic-appearing astrocytes with large hyperchromatic nuclei in a patient with progressive multifocal leukoencephalopathy. Hematoxylin and eosin, 132×.

indicating the rapidity of progression of the disease once established (22). The period from exposure to the virus to development of symptoms is estimated as ranging from 4–62 months. At the time of submission of this chapter, no real progress had been reported in attempts to develop a vaccine for prevention of this viral disease.

CNS infections documented in patients with AIDS include toxoplasmosis, cytomegalovirus, *Pneumocystis carinii*, *Candida albicans* abscess, herpes simplex encephalitis, tuberculosis, PML, cryptococcosis, and others. These must be distinguished from the intracerebral malignant lymphomas that these patients are also at risk to develop. Polymicrobial infections have also been documented (14), making brain biopsy necessary for diagnosis and appropriate treatment. Some workers (35) have suggested a trial of therapy for toxoplasmosis in patients with AIDS who have CNS mass lesions without confirmation by brain biopsy. Though *Toxoplasma gondii* is quite common in these patients, many other possibilities must be considered as noted above, and the presence of toxoplasmosis in association with tuberculosis has been documented in a patient with AIDS (14). There is a risk, therefore, that treatment for toxoplasmosis may lead to transient improvement followed by worsening as other microbes assert themselves. Currently (24), biopsy of CNS lesions presenting in patients with AIDS represents the best means of designing appropriate therapy for these patients. The use of CT stereotaxis and intraoperative ultrasound has increased the safety of such biopsies.

At present little information is available concerning the risk to neurosurgeons who operate on patients infected by the HTLV-III virus, including patients who have AIDS. The risk of nosocomial infection with HTLV-III virus in health care workers in contact with AIDS patients and with specimens from those patients is being studied. A recent report documenting follow-up of 85 individuals with nosocomial exposure (including 31 victims of needle stick blood exposure, 9 endoscopists involved in the care of AIDS patients, and 8 pathologists and 20 laboratory workers handling AIDS specimens) was reassuring in that not a single HTLV-III seroconversion was observed among health care workers exposed to the virus (18). The mean interval between accident and serologic testing was 8 months (range 0.5 to 20 months). Particularly reassuring to surgeons and other members of the surgical team is the lack of seroconversion among those who were victims of needle stick accidents. Recent reports, however, indicate that three victims of needle stick exposure to the HTLV-III virus have undergone seroconversion. This information suggests that a needle stick to a member of the operating team occurring during an operation for brain biopsy in a patient with AIDS carries a lower risk of infection than a similar accident occurring during operation on a patient with hepatitis B, estimated at 10–15% if the exposed individual is negative for hepatitis B antibody and the patient is positive for hepatitis B surface antigen (24). While adequate follow-up of individuals with nosocomial exposure will require years, available evidence suggests that operations on patients with AIDS probably carry less risk to members of the operating team than was originally feared. The results of these studies suggest that isolation procedures currently recommended for AIDS are adequate.

The HTLV-III virus is felt to be relatively fragile, and current procedures for routine sterilization of instruments used in the operating room are adequate for inactivation of the HTLV-III virus. When patients with known AIDS undergo operation, operative precautions and clean-up procedures should be the same as those employed when patients with known active hepatitis B undergo operation.

SUMMARY

Brain biopsy is justified in patients suspected of having encephalitis or viral encephalopathy because those patients are most likely to be helped if a diagnosis is made rapidly and with the greatest certainty possible. Neurosurgeons are occasionally reluctant to undertake brain biopsy because the procedure is diagnostic rather than therapeutic in intent. However, using currently available techniques a 1 cm^3 sample of brain tissue can be taken with very low risk of morbidity or mortality (29, 46). We recommend that the sample be taken from the anterior portion of the inferior temporal gyrus on the more affected side in patients with herpes simplex encephalitis, and from an area of maximum demonstrated involvement in other situations, using stereotactic techniques and intraoperative ultrasound as necessary. The risk to the operating surgeon and to the other members of the operating team appears very low in all of the situations discussed in this chapter. However, the authors feel that every patient should be approached as if he carries the hepatitis B virus. As indicated, the incidence of contracting hepatitis B after sustaining needle stick exposure to blood from persons positive for hepatitis B surface antigen is 10–15%. Conjunctival contamination by splash from the wound is a known method of inoculation of surgeons with hepatitis B virus and is a possible means for transmission of other viral diseases. We recommend that every patient be approached as if he has hepatitis B, not because the agent diseases discussed are known to be as infectious as hepatitis B, but because constant vigilance and careful technique offer the best protection to the surgeon and the members of the operating team in most situations, and because one can never be certain what agent diseases a given patient may harbor.

With the exception of the Creutzfeldt-Jakob virus, the agents responsible for all of the viral diseases discussed are inactivated by standard procedures for sterilization of operating room instruments. Procedures necessary to inactivate the Creutzfeldt-Jakob disease virus have been presented.

In the report documenting transmission of Creutzfeldt-Jakob disease through human growth hormone preparations the authors state, "We are once again dramatically reminded that human tissues are a source of infectious disease, and that any therapeutic transfer of tissue from one person to another carries an unavoidable risk of transferring the infection. In this context, we must continue to worry about such products as follicle stimulating hormone, luteinizing hormone, prolactin and human interferon, as well as skin, bone, bone marrow, dura mater, blood vessel, and nerve grafts and organ transplantation" (8).

REFERENCES

1. Adams, R. D., and Victor, M. *Principles of Neurology*, 3rd edition. McGraw-Hill, New York, 1985.
2. Åstrom, K-E., Mancall, E. L., and Richardson, E. P., Jr. Progressive multifocal leukoencephalopathy. Brain, *81:* 93–111, 1958.
3. Baringer, J. R., and Swoveland, P. Recovery of herpes-simplex virus from human trigeminal ganglions. N. Engl. J. Med., *288:* 648–652, 1973.
4. Barza, M., and Pauker, S. G. The decision to biopsy, treat, or wait in suspected herpes encephalitis. Ann. Intern. Med., *92:* 641–649, 1980.
5. Bernoulli, C., Siegfried, J., Baumgartner, G., Regli, F., Rabinowicz, T., Gajdusek, D. C., and Gibbs, C. J., Jr. Danger of accidental person-to-person transmission of Creutzfeldt-Jakob disease by surgery. Lancet, *1:* 478–479, 1977.
6. Braun, P. The clinical management of suspected herpes virus encephalitis. A decision-analytic view. Am. J. Med., *69:* 895–902, 1980.
7. Broder, S., and Gallo, R. C. A pathogenic retrovirus (HTLV-III) linked to AIDS. N. Engl. J. Med., *311:* 1292–1297, 1984.
8. Brown, P., Gajdusek, C., Gibbs, C. J., and Asher, D. M. Potential epidemic of Creutzfeldt-Jakob disease from human growth hormone therapy. N. Engl. J. Med., *313:* 728–731, 1985.
9. Brown, P., Gibbs, C. J., Jr., Amyx, H. L., Kingsbury, D. T., Rohwer, R. G., Sulima, M. P., and Gajdusek, D. C. Chemical disinfection of Creutzfeldt-Jakob disease virus. N. Engl. J. Med., *306:* 1279–1282, 1982.
10. Dayes, L. A., Cushman, A., Boche, R., Miller, D., Peterson, D., and Quilligan, J. J. Herpes simplex encephalitis and its neurosurgical implications: report of five cases. Int. Surg., *66:* 255–258, 1981.
11. DeSclafani, A., Kohl, S., and Ostrow, P. T. The importance of brain biopsy in suspected herpes simplex encephalitis. Surg. Neurol., *17:* 101–106, 1982.
12. Duffy, P., Wolf, J., Collins, G., DeVoe, A. G., Streeten, B., and Cowen, D. Possible person-to-person transmission of Creutzfeldt-Jakob disease. N. Engl. J. Med., *290:* 692–693, 1974.
13. England, J. D., Hsu, C. Y., Garen, P. D., Goust, J. M., and Biggs, P. J. Progressive multifocal leukoencephalopathy occurring with the acquired immune deficiency syndrome. South. Med. J., *77:* 1041–1043, 1984.
14. Fischl, M. A., Pitchenik, A. E., and Spira, T. J. Tuberculous brain abscess and Toxoplasma encephalitis in a patient with the acquired immunodeficiency syndrome. J.A.M.A., *253:* 3428–3430, 1985.
15. Garcia, J. H., Colon, L. E., Whitley, R. J., and Wilmes, F. Diagnosis of viral encephalitis by brain biopsy. Semin. Diagn. Pathol. *1:* 71–81, 1984.
16. Gibbs, C. Creutzfeldt-Jakob disease. Neurosurgery, *253:* 1994–2001, 1985.
17. Goedert, J. J., Sarngadharan, M. G., Biggar, R. J., Weiss, S. H., Winn, D. M., Grossman, R. J., Greene, M. H., Bodner, A. J., Mann, D. L., Strong, D. M., Gallo, R. C., and Blattner, W. A. Determinants of retrovirus (HTLV-III) antibody and immunodeficiency conditions in homosexual men. Lancet, *2:* 711–6, 1984.
18. Hirsch, M. S., Wormser, G. P., Schooley, R. T., Ho, D. D., Felsenstein, D., Hopkins, C. C.,

Joline, C., Duncanson, F., Sarngadharan, M. G., Saxinger, C., and Gallo, R. C. Risk of nosocomial infection with human T-cell lymphotropic virus III (HTLV-III). N. Engl. J. Med., *312:* 1–4, 1985.

19. Ho, D. D., and Hirsch, M. S. Acute viral encephalitis. Med. Clin. North. Am., *69:* 415–429, 1985.

20. Kirschbaum, W. R. *Jakob-Creutzfeldt disease.* American Elsevier, New York, 1968.

21. Kohl, S., and James, A. R. Herpes simplex virus encephalitis during childhood: importance of brain biopsy diagnosis. J. Pediatr., *107:* 212–215, 1985.

22. Landesman, S. H., Ginzburg, H. M., and Weiss, S. H. Special report. The AIDS epidemic. N. Engl. J. Med., *312:* 521–525, 1985.

23. Laurence, J., Brun-Vezinet, F., Schutzer, S. E., Rouzioux, C., Klatzmann, D., Barre-Sinoussi, F., Chermann, J. C., and Montagnier, L. Lymphadenopathy-associated viral antibody in AIDS. Immune correlations and definition of a carrier state. N. Engl. J. Med., *311:* 1269–1273, 1984.

24. Levy, R. M., Pons, V. G., and Rosenblum, M. L. Central nervous system mass lesions in the acquired immunodeficiency syndrome (AIDS). J. Neurosurg., *61:* 9–16, 1984.

25. Manz, H. J., Dinsdale, H. B., and Morrin, P. A. F. Progressive multifocal leukoencephalopathy after renal transplantation: demonstration of Papova-like virions. Ann. Intern. Med., *75:* 77–81, 1971.

26. Marriott, P. J., O'Brien, M. D., Mackenzie, I. C. K., and Janota, I. Progressive multifocal leukoencephalopathy: remission with cytarabine. J. Neurol. Neurosurg. Psychiatry, *38:* 205–209, 1975.

27. Meyer, H. M., Jr., Johnson, R. T., Crawford, I. P., Dascomb, H. E., and Rogers, N. G. Central nervous system syndromes of "viral" etiology. Am. J. Med., *29:* 334–347, 1960.

28. Miller, J. R., Barrett, R. E., Britton, C. B., Tapper, M. L., Bahr, G. S., Bruno, P. J., Marquardt, M. D., Hays, A. P., McMurtry, J. G., 3rd, Weissman, J. B., and Bruno, M. S. Progressive multifocal leukoencephalopathy in a male homosexual with T-cell immune deficiency. N. Engl. J. Med., *307:* 1436–1438, 1982.

29. Morawetz, R. B., Whitley, R. J., and Murphy, D. M. Experience with brain biopsy for suspected herpes encephalitis: a review of forty consecutive cases. Neurosurgery, *12:* 664–657, 1983.

30. Nahmias, A. J., Whitley, R. J., Visintine, A. N., Takei, Y., and Alford, C. A., Jr. Herpes simplex virus encephalitis: laboratory evaluations and their diagnostic significance. J. Infect. Dis., *145:* 829–836, 1982.

31. Narayan, O., Penney, J. B., Jr., Johnson, R. T., Herndon, R. M., and Weiner, L. P. Etiology of progressive multifocal leukoencephalopathy. N. Engl. J. Med., *289*(24): 1278–1282, 1973.

32. Padgett, B. L., and Walker, D. L. Virologic and serologic studies of progressive multifocal leukoencephalopathy. In: *Polyomaviruses and Human Neurological Diseases,* edited by J. L. Sever and D. L. Madden, pp 107–117. Liss, New York, 1983.

33. Padgett, B. L., Walker, D. L., ZuRhein, G. M., EcKroade, R. J., and Dessel, B. H. Cultivation of papova-like virus from human brain with progressive multifocal leukoencephalopathy. Lancet, *1:* 1257–60, 1971.

34. Padgett, B. L., Walker, D. L., ZuRhein, G. M., Hodach, A. E., and Chou, S. M. JC Papovavirus in progressive multifocal leukoencephalopathy. J. Infect. Dis., *133:* 686–690, 1976.

35. Pitchenick, A. E., Fischl, M. A., and Walls, K. W. Evaluation of cerebral mass lesions in acquired immunodeficiency syndrome. N. Engl. J. Med., *308:* 1099, 1983.

36. Rappel, M., Dubois-Dalcq, M., Sprecher, S., Thiry, L., Lowenthal, A., Pelc, S., and Thys, J. P. Diagnosis and treatment of herpes encephalitis. A multidisciplinary approach. J. Neurol. Sci., *12:* 443–458, 1971.

37. Raws, W. E. Herpes simplex virus types I and II and herpes virus simiae. In: *Diagnostic Procedures for Viral, Rickettsial, and Chlamydia 5 Infections*, edited by E. H. Lennette and N. J. Schmidt. American Public Health Association, Washington, DC, 1979, pp 309–374.

38. Saxton, C. R., Gailiunas, P., Jr., Helderman, J. H., Farkas, R. A., McCoy, R., Diehl, J., Sagalowsky, A., Murphy, F. K., Ross, E. D., Silva, F. R., and Walker, D. L. Progressive multifocal leukoencephalopathy in a renal transplant recipient. Increased diagnostic sensitivity of computed tomographic scanning by double-dose contrast with delayed films. Am. J. Med., *77:* 333–337, 1984.

39. Schlitt, M., Morawetz, R. B., Bonnin, J., Chandra-Sekar, B., Curtis, J. J., Diethelm, Jr., A. G., Whelchel, J. D., and Whitley, R. J. Progressive multifocal leukoencephalopathy: three patients diagnosed by brain biopsy with prolonged survival in two. Neurosurgery, *18:* 407–414, 1986.

40. Schlitt, M., Lakeman, A. D., Wilson, E. R., To, A., Acoff, R. W., Harsh, G. R., Whitley, R. J. A rabbit of focal herpes simplex encephalitis. J. Infect. Dis. *153:* 732–735, 1986.

41. Skoldenberg, B., Forsgren, M., Alestig, K., Bergstrom, T., Burman, L., Dahlqvist, E., Forkman, A., Fryden, A., Lovgren, K., Norlin, K., Norrby, R., Olding-Stenkvist, E., Stiernstedt, G., Uhnoo, I., and de Vahl, K. Acyclovir versus vidarabine in herpes simplex encephalitis. Lancet, *2:* 707–711, 1984.

42. Stroop, W. G., Schaefer, D. C. Production of encephalitis restricted to the temporal lobes by experimental reactivation of herpes simplex virus. J. Infect. Dis. *153:* 721–731, 1986.

43. Traub, R., Gajdusek, D. C., and Gibbs, C. J., Jr. Transmissible virus dementia: The relation of transmissible spongiform encephalopathy to Creutzfeldt-Jakob disease. In: *Aging and Dementia*, edited by W. L. Smith and M. Kinsbourne, pp. 91–154. Spectrum Publications, Jamaica, NY, 1977.

44. Warren, J. Papovavirus infections. In: *Diagnostic Procedures for: Viral, Rickettsial and Chlamydial Infections*, edited by E. H. Lennette and N. J. Schmidt, ed. 5, pp. 1000–1005. American Public Health Association, Washington, DC, 1979.

45. Weiner, L. P., Hearndon, R. M., Narayan, O., Johnson, R. T., Shah, K., Rubinstein, L. J., Preziosi, T. J., and Conley, F. K. Isolation of virus related to SV40 from patients with progressive multifocal leukoencephalopathy. N. Engl. J. Med., *286:* 385–390, 1972.

46. Weisz, R. R. Brain biopsy in herpes simplex encephalitis. N. Engl. J. Med., *303:* 700, 1980.

47. Whitley, R. J., Soong, S-J., Dolin, R., Galasso, G. J., Ch'ien, L. T., and Alford, C. A. Adenine arabinoside therapy of biopsy-proved herpes simplex encephalitis. N. Engl. J. Med., *297:* 289–294, 1977.

48. Whitley, R. J., Soong, S-J., Hirsch, M. S., Karchmer, A. W., Dolin, R., Galasso, G., Dunnick, J. K., and Alford, C. A. Herpes simplex encephalitis: vidarabine therapy and diagnostic problems. N. Engl. J. Med., *304:* 313–318, 1981.

49. Whitley, R. J., Soong, S-J., Linneman, C., Jr., Liu, C., Pazin, G., and Alford, C. A. Herpes simplex encephalitis. Clinical Assessment. J.A.M.A., *247:* 317–320, 1982.

50. York, G. K. Herpes simplex encephalitis: biopsy of treatment? Ann. Intern. Med., *93:* 506–507, 1980.

51. Zinzer, H., *Rats, Lice and History.* Boston Atlantic Monthly Press, Little Brown & Co., 1935.

52. ZuRhein, G. M., and Chou, S. M. Particles resembling papova viruses in human cerebral demyelinating disease. Science, *148:* 1477–1479, 1965.

CHAPTER

38

Controversies in the Management of Brain Abscesses

MARK L. ROSENBLUM, M.D., THOMAS J. MAMPALAM, M.D.,
and VINCENT G. PONS, M.D.

INTRODUCTION

Sir William Macewen was the first physician to diagnose, localize, and suggest surgical treatment of a brain abscess in a patient (41). That accomplishment, in 1876, and his classic treatise *Pyogenic Infective Diseases of the Brain and Spinal Cord* (42), published in 1893, establish Macewen as the father of modern-day brain abscess management. The therapy he recommended for these lesions was drainage of the infective process and treatment of the underlying sinusitis. In 1926, Dandy recommended aspiration as the primary surgical modality (20). Finally, in 1936, Vincent became the first to advocate complete surgical extirpation of these lesions (61).

Technologic advances over the last two decades have greatly improved the diagnosis and treatment of many neurosurgical conditions. Advances that have played a major role in the management of brain abscesses include the use of the operating microscope, improved microbiological techniques for identifying infective agents, more effective antibiotic regimens, the development of the computed tomographic (CT) brain scan, and, most recently, the use of stereotactic surgical techniques guided by CT scanning or real-time ultrasound imaging.

Nevertheless, the management of brain abscesses is still a controversial subject. In this chapter, we will discuss the issue of surgical versus nonsurgical treatment, the choice of a surgical procedure, the selection and timing of antibiotic regimens, and the utility of corticosteroids. First, however, let us review what is known of the pathogenesis of brain abscesses and examine how this knowledge affects the diagnosis of these lesions.

PATHOGENESIS AND DIAGNOSIS OF BRAIN ABSCESSES

In 1908, Harvey Cushing said, in reference to brain abscesses, "The clinical history is of paramount importance in these cases, for there are no absolutely diagnostic signs" (19). Approximately 80% of patients with a brain abscess have a known predisposing factor that has contributed to the development of the intracranial infection (1, 17, 52, 55). The most common of these are introduction of organisms as a result of head trauma or surgical procedures; contiguous spread of infection from sinusitis or mastoiditis; hematogeneous spread of organisms from pulmonary infections, bacterial endocarditis, or other sources of septicemia; and vascular shunts between the right and left sides of the heart (*e.g.*, in congenital cyanotic heart disease and pulmonary arteriovenous fistulas) that permit bacterial access to cerebral vessels because the normal pulmonary "bacterial filter system" is bypassed. In the past, brain abscesses frequently occurred through the spread of an infection from an adjacent air-containing sinus; however, earlier and more effective treatment of purulent sinus and mastoid infections has significantly reduced the number of brain abscesses from this source. More recently, deficiencies in cell-mediated immunity stemming from immunosuppressive therapy for organ transplant procedures and from the acquired immunodeficiency syndrome (AIDS) have resulted in an increasing incidence of brain abscesses, particularly those caused by *Toxoplasma gondii*, cytomegalovirus, and *Mycobacterium* sp. (13, 38, 40).

Unfortunately, 10–20% of patients with brain abscesses have no identifiable predisposing factor at the time of diagnosis (17, 52, 55). In these cases, it is not known whether the previous infection was so minor as to cause no clinically evident infection or whether it had resolved before the brain abscess became manifest.

The development of brain abscesses has been clearly delineated by Britt and Enzmann in their classic experimental and clinical studies. Using a canine model of streptococcal abscess, they identified four stages in the encapsulation process: early cerebritis on days 1–3, late cerebritis on days 4–9, early capsule formation on days 11–13, and late capsule formation after day 14 (14). This pattern has been confirmed by studies in other animal models (26), as well as by clinical observations (52, 64) suggesting that it takes approximately 2 weeks from the implantation of the infective organism for a well-formed abscess to develop in the majority of patients who have the capacity to mount a host response to the infection.

The symptoms of a brain abscess are those of a rapidly expanding intracranial mass lesion and include seizures, focal neurologic deficits, and headaches. Meningismus associated with ventricular or meningeal enhancement on CT scans, and a low-grade fever or an elevated crythrocyte sedimentation rate without a demonstrated systemic cause, support the possibility that a brain abscess is present. Fevers higher than 38.5°C occur in less than 50% of patients (52, 55).

The CT brain scan has remarkably improved the ability to diagnose and localize pyogenic brain abscesses and has led to a decrease in the mortality rate among patients with these infections (52). The classic appearance on contrast-enhanced CT scans is a lesion with a smooth, thin, regular wall; there is decreased density both in the center of the lesion (representing pyogenic material) and in the surrounding white matter (representing edema). On noncontrast scans, the wall may be isodense or denser than normal brain. Additional CT findings that make the diagnosis of brain abscess likely include the presence of gas within the lesion when there is little probability of a dural fistula, and ventricular or meningeal enhancement, especially when associated with symptoms and signs of meningitis.

The differential diagnosis of a lesion resembling a bacterial abscess on the CT scan includes primary and metastatic tumors, infarctions, hematomas, and radiation necrosis, as well as fungal, parasitic, and tuberculous infections. Figures 38.1–38.6 are CT scans from patients in whom a presumptive diagnosis of pyogenic brain abscess had been made preoperatively. The final diagnoses in these cases were glioblastoma multiforme (Fig. 38.1), metastatic adenocarcinoma (Fig. 38.2), tuberculous granuloma (Fig. 38.3), cysticercosis (Fig. 38.4), primary cerebral lymphoma (Fig. 38.5), and resolving intracerebral hematoma (Fig. 38.6). It is apparent from these and other examples that a bacterial brain abscess cannot be diagnosed unequivocally from CT scan findings alone.

Britt and Enzmann and their colleagues have suggested that the diagnosis of a brain abscess would be improved by performing serial CT scans after the injection of contrast material (12, 24). Increased density in the center of the ring would indicate a lesion in the cerebritis phase; if the wall itself retained rather than lost its density in 45- to 90-min delayed scans, the abscess would most likely be poorly encapsulated. We believe that increased density in the wall of an abscess on unenhanced scans probably reflects the presence of a significant amount of collagen and suggests a well-encapsulated lesion. CT scans obtained before and after the injection of contrast material in a patient with a multiloculated brain abscess are shown in Figure 38.7.

SURGICAL VERSUS NONSURGICAL TREATMENT

The controversy over whether all brain abscesses require surgical treatment began in 1971, when Heinemann and Baude reported the nonsurgical cure of six patients with cerebritis and suggested that early infective lesions might be amenable to medical management (28). In 1973, Black and colleagues aspirated large abscesses in patients being treated with antibiotics and determined the concentration of drugs within the lesions as well as the ability of the organisms to grow in culture (7). Several antibiotics were found in concentrations greater than the minimum inhibitory concentrations for the organisms cultured. The demonstration that bacteria

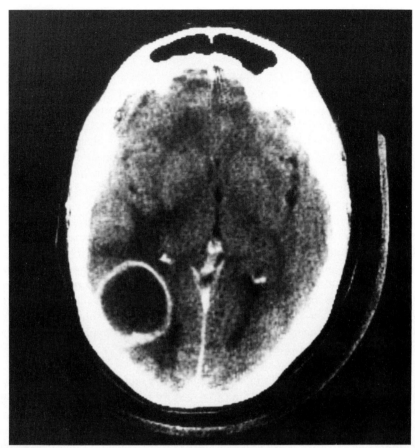

Fig. 38.1

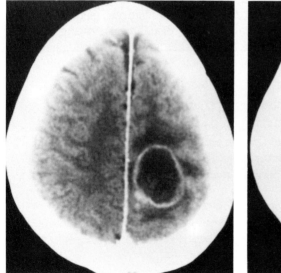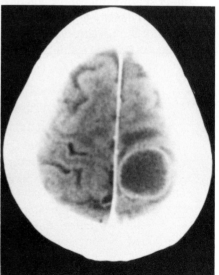

Fig. 38.2

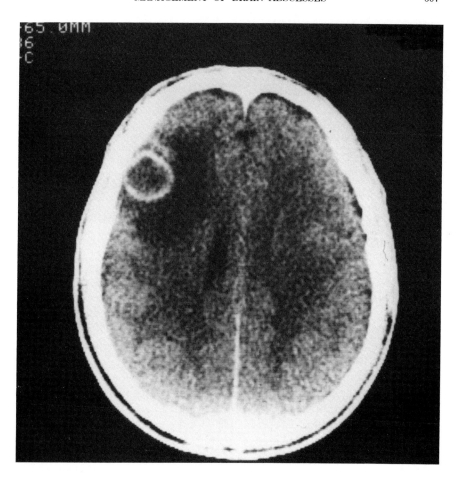

FIG. 38.3. CT brain scan of a 43-year-old man thought to have a brain abscess. Tuberculous granuloma was subsequently diagnosed at surgery.

FIG. 38.1. CT brain scan of a 52-year-old woman thought to have a brain abscess. Glioblastoma multiforme was subsequently diagnosed at surgery.

FIG. 38.2. CT brain scans of a 45-year-old man thought to have a brain abscess. Metastatic adenocarcinoma was subsequently diagnosed at surgery.

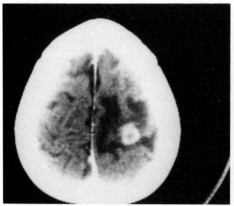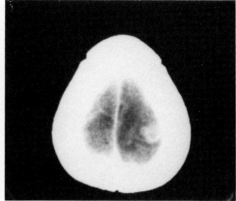

FIG. 38.4. CT brain scans of a 25-year-old man thought to have a brain abscess. Cysticerco-sis was subsequently diagnosed at surgery.

were nevertheless able to grow from the aspirated contents led to the conclusion that something within the abscess prevents antibiotics from inhibiting bacterial multiplication and that all brain abscesses should be drained surgically. Their study, however, included only six patients and in some cases the duration of antibiotic therapy was very short. Moreover, the lesions were large, averaging more than 5 cm in diameter (P. Black, personal communication, 1980). Very large abscesses provide an environment that might inhibit the microbicidal activity of antibiotics; such lesions probably harbor too many bacteria for the leukocytes and antibiotics to eradicate (Z. Werb, personal communication, 1985).

In 1975, Chow and colleagues reported the first nonsurgical cure of an apparently well-encapsulated brain abscess (18). In 1978, Berg and associates documented the resolution of brain abscesses in four patients without surgery and suggested that such lesions could be treated medically (6). It appears likely, however, that these four patients had cerebritis. In 1980, Rosenblum and colleagues presented eight patients with presumed brain abscesses who were treated with antibiotics only (51). Serial CT scans demonstrated shrinkage or resolution of the lesions in all eight cases. Four of these abscesses were probably in the cerebritis phase and four were in the encapsulated phase.

In 1981, Britt and associates studied the pathologic correlates of evolving experimental brain abscesses and demonstrated that a ring-enhancing lesion on the CT scan could be present in the late cerebritis phase and did not necessarily prove that the lesion was encapsulated (14). This finding suggests that the outcome of nonsurgical management might, in certain

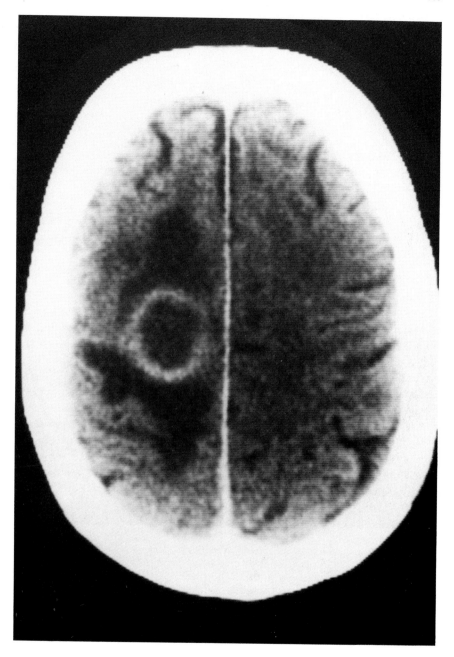

Fig. 38.5. CT brain scan of a 32-year-old man with the acquired immunodeficiency syndrome shows a primary cerebral lymphoma. The diagnosis was verified at operation.

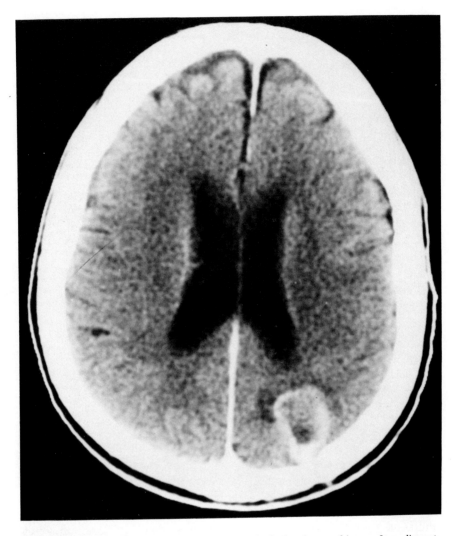

FIG. 38.6. CT brain scan of a 54-year-old woman who had undergone biopsy of a malignant brain stem tumor and placement of a ventriculostomy catheter 2.5 months previously. The patient did not receive antibiotics after the biopsy. The scan shows a lesion in the track of the catheter that was thought to be an abscess. At operation, a lesion with a thick, hemosiderin-stained capsule was removed. No organisms were identified by Gram's stain or culture. Histologically, the abscess contained hemosiderin-stained necrotic debris and only a few chronic inflammatory cells. No antibiotics were given postoperatively, and the lesion has not recurred. Resolving hematoma was the final diagnosis.

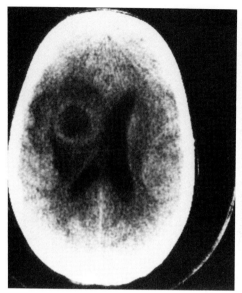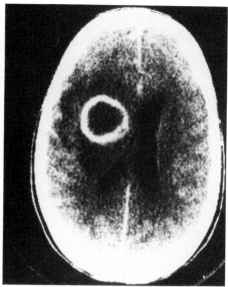

FIG. 38.7. CT brain scans before (*left*) and after (*right*) injection of contrast medium in a patient who had a surgically documented streptococcal brain abscess. The unenhanced scan shows a ring; the contrast-enhanced scan shows a homogeneously enhancing regular ring around the lesion, except in the location nearest the ventricle.

cases, reflect the treatment of cerebritis rather than of a well-formed abscess. Dobkin and colleagues also demonstrated the nonspecificity of ring enhancement on CT scans in cases of "medically cured" brain abscesses (23).

There is little doubt, however, that well-developed abscesses can shrink and possibly disappear without the need for operative intervention. CT scans from a patient who had multiple brain abscesses, including lesions in both cerebral hemispheres and in the pons, attributable to a severe pulmonary infection are shown in Figure 38.8. Neurological abnormalities had been present for more than 2 weeks before admission to the hospital, and the patient presented with symptoms and signs of ventriculitis. She was treated with antibiotics specific for the organism cultured from her lungs, and the contrast-enhancing lesions gradually resolved. Five years later, she is well and has no neurologic symptoms.

Our search of the literature yielded 23 articles published between 1975 and 1985 that included 67 cases of brain abscesses that were treated without surgery (4, 6, 9, 10, 15, 16, 18, 21, 27, 30, 32–34, 43, 46, 49, 51, 53, 55, 59, 60, 62, 64). The cases that were described in detail are summarized in

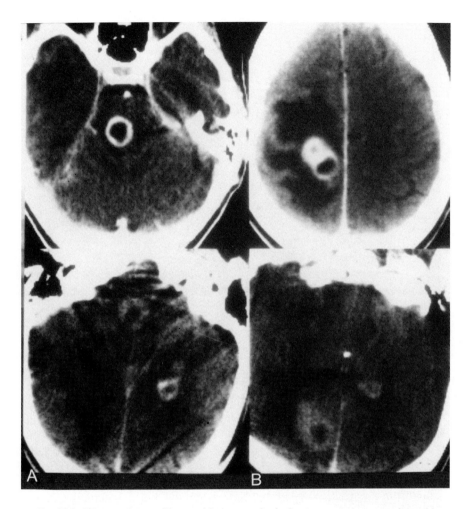

FIG. 38.8. CT scans from a 54-year-old woman who had cataract surgery complicated by pneumonia and a pleural empyema caused by a streptococcal species. The infections were treated with ampicillin and gentamycin. Three weeks later, she became ataxic and lethargic. A CT scan demonstrated multiple ring-enhancing lesions. Two weeks later, she was transferred to UCSF. She was febrile, lethargic, and had meningeal signs. The admission CT scans (A, B, and C) showed ring-enhancing lesions in both parietal lobes and in the pons, as well as evidence of ventriculitis. Therapy with high-dose intravenous penicillin was started; chloramphenicol was added 2 weeks later. The lesions decreased in size on serial CT scans obtained at 2 weeks (D), 5 weeks (E), 13 weeks (F), and 9 months (G) after her treatment at UCSF was started. Five years later, the patient is well and neurologically intact.

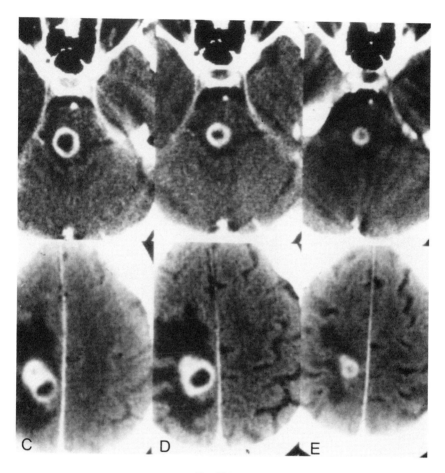

FIG. 38.8*C-E*

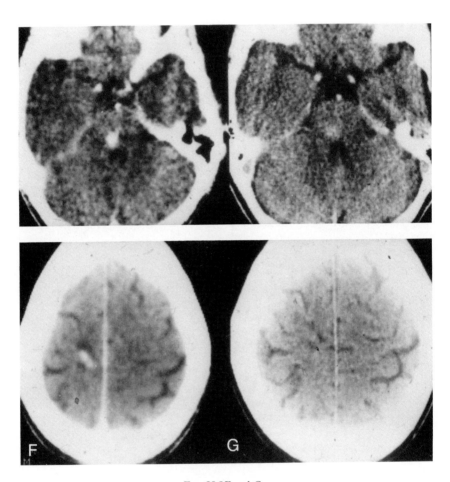

FIG. 38.8F and G

TABLE 38.1

*Neurological Grade at Admission and at Hospital Discharge
in 53 Patients with Brain Abscesses Treated Successfully
without Surgery**

Grade	Examination	Initial	Discharge
0	Alert, no deficits	2	45
I	Alert, slight deficits	19	8
II	Lethargic, moderate deficits	21	
III	Obtunded, marked deficits	9	
IV	Coma	2	

* Cases are from references 4, 6, 8, 10, 15, 16, 18, 30, 32–34, 43, 46, 49, 51, 53, 54, 59, 60, 62, and 64.

Tables 38.1–38.4. The number of patients is different for each analysis because we included only those whose characteristics were clearly delineated. Table 38.1 describes the admission and discharge clinical status for 53 successfully treated patients. The majority of these patients were either alert and had slight neurologic deficits (40%) or were lethargic and had moderate deficits (40%). A significant number of patients (20%), however, were obtunded and had marked deficits or were comatose; in many cases, the more severe neurologic deficits reflected abscesses within the brain stem. At discharge, all of these patients were alert and had no or minimal neurologic deficits.

The causative organism was presumed or known from a positive culture obtained from blood, CSF, or other bodily fluids (19 cases) and from aspiration of one of multiple abscesses (9 cases) in approximately two-

TABLE 38.2

*Identification of Organisms Responsible for Brain Abscess: 39 Cases with
Known, Presumed, or Unknown Organisms**

		Multiple Abscesses	
	Single Abscess	Nonsurgical Treatment Only	Aspiration of One Abscess
Known	NA	NA	9
Presumed from culture elsewhere	10	9	0
Unknown	7	4	0

* Cases are from references 4, 6, 8, 10, 15, 16, 18, 21, 27, 30, 32–34, 43, 46, 49, 51, 53, 54, 60, and 64.

TABLE 38.3

*The Source and Type of Organisms Presumed to be Responsible for Abscess
Development in 32 Cases**

Source		Organism	
Aspiration of different abscesses	9	*Staphylococcus/Streptococcus* sp.	14
Blood	12	*Fusobacterium*	2
Lung	2	*Bacteroides*	2
Cerebrospinal Fluid	3	Other	9
Other	1	Not Specified	7
Not specified	5		

* Multiple organisms were found in two patients. Cases are from references 6, 8, 15, 16, 18, 22, 27, 30, 33, 34, 43, 46, 49, 51, 53, 54, 62, and 64.

thirds of all cases (Table 38.2). The most common source of identified organisms was from the blood in patients with septicemia and from aspiration of one of the lesions in patients with multiple abscesses (Table 38.3). *Streptococcus* and *Staphylococcus* sp. were found most often. Antibiotics were administered for at least 6 weeks in most cases and were specific for the organism cultured in 28 of 39 patients.

The first decrease in the size of the lesions was documented by CT scanning 1 week to 6 months after the start of antibiotic therapy (Table 38.4). Determining how quickly the abscess began to shrink, however, depends on the frequency of follow-up CT scans. Because some patients

TABLE 38.4

*Timing of CT Brain Scan Changes in 42 Patients
Treated without Surgery**

	First Decrease in Lesion Size	All Contrast-enhancing Lesions Disappeared†
1 week	4	
2 weeks	6	
3–4 weeks	5	1
5–8 weeks	7	10
2–6 months	20	10
>6 months		18

* Cases are from references 6, 8, 10, 15, 16, 27, 30, 32, 33, 43, 46, 49, 51, 53, 54, 60, 62, and 64.

† In three cases, the time at which all contrast lesions disappeared was not stated.

probably had CT scans at infrequent intervals, the values listed in Table 38.4 represent maximum estimates. Although most of the abscesses began to decrease in size during the first 2 months and disappeared within 6 months, contrast-enhancing abnormalities often persisted for more than 6 months. This phenomenon has been well-documented. However, CT scan abnormalities need not disappear before antibiotic therapy is discontinued in order to achieve a successful clinical outcome (51, 64).

We reviewed the five largest series of patients whose abscesses were treated nonsurgically (8, 51, 54, 62, 64) to determine the outcome of cases in which we assumed that the lesion was well encapsulated when antibiotic therapy was started (Table 38.5). This assumption was based on the CT findings, the presence of symptoms for at least 2 weeks before the start of therapy, or subsequent pathologic evaluation. Because of the possible inaccuracy of this method, our conclusions must be considered only estimates of the potential success of medical therapy alone. From our 1980 series, we included four patients whose lesions were treated successfully and four patients who required surgical ablation after both an initial operation and prolonged treatment with antibiotics proved unsuccessful (51). One patient with congenital cyanotic heart disease had a localized abscess rupture without diffuse ventriculitis and probably died of a primary cardiac cause. Thus, in our small series, medical therapy led to a decrease in the size of the abscess on CT scans in 50% of patients, and one patient died. Similar results were obtained by Whelan and Hilal (64) and by Weisberg (62). In two later series, Rousseaux and colleagues (54) and Bloom and Tuazon (8) reported that 21 of 22 "encapsulated" abscesses were cured without surgery, and only one patient died. The better results in these two series might be attributable to improved patient selection criteria for nonsurgical management (51). Overall, medical treatment was successful in 37 of 50 patients (74%) in these five series, and there were two deaths (4%).

TABLE 38.5

Results of Medical Therapy for "Encapsulated" Abscesses in 50 Patients

Study	Year	No. of Patients	Success	Deaths
Rosenblum *et al.* (51)	1980	8	4	1
Whelan and Hilal (64)	1980	13	7	0
Weisberg (62)	1981	7	5	0
Rousseaux *et al.* (54)	1985	15	14	1
Bloom and Tuazon (8)	1985	7	7	0
Total		50	37 (74%)	2 (4%)

The series of Rousseaux and colleagues (54) merits examination in detail, for although theirs was not a randomized study, the cases were well described and carefully followed. The 31 patients, treated from 1979 to 1982 in Lille, France, were divided into three groups: 15 were treated with antibiotics alone (group 1); four with aspiration and antibiotics (group 2); and 12 with surgical excision and antibiotics (group 3). Ten of the 15 patients in group 1 had multiple abscesses, compared with none of four in group 2 and two of 12 in group 3. The patients treated with antibiotics alone tended to have deeper lesions; seven patients had deep abscesses, including three in the brain stem. In contrast, none of the patients in group 2 and only one in group 3 had deep lesions. A further difference between the three groups was the size of the abscesses. The mean diameter of the lesions on CT scans was 2.1 cm (range, 1–4 cm) in group 1, 4.5 cm (range, 4–5 cm) in group 2, and 3.7 cm (range, 2.5–5 cm) in group 3. The preoperative neurologic status was approximately the same in all three groups. Group 1, for example, included five patients who were at least lethargic with marked neurologic deficits before therapy with antibiotics was started.

Infective organisms were identified positively or were presumed, from cultures of other bodily fluids, to be the source of infection in approximately half of the cases. Antibiotics were administered for a mean of 16 weeks in group 1, 10 weeks in group 2, and 6 weeks in group 3. There was one death in the antibiotic treatment group and none in the aspiration group; two patients whose abscesses were removed surgically died. The follow-up period was at least 9 months in 12 cases in group 1, four cases in group 2, and eight cases in group 3. The neurologic status improved almost equally in all treatment groups; approximately half of the patients had persistent neurologic deficits, but none had a recurrent abscess. Thus, in this series of patients with comparable neurologic status before treatment, the outcome of antibiotic therapy alone was similar to that of surgical therapy. Overall, the patients treated with antibiotics alone had smaller abscesses in deeper locations and received antibiotics for a longer period.

Although Rousseaux and colleagues have achieved impressive results, we do not agree with their suggestion that all brain abscesses should be treated with antibiotics alone. Our reservation applies particularly to patients who have significant neurologic deficits, those with large abscesses (more than 3 cm in diameter), and those with multiple lesions in surgically accessible locations. Because initial neurologic status is strongly associated with outcome in patients treated surgically (11, 17, 52, 55), a maximum attempt must be made to confirm the diagnosis, identify the organism, and remove or aspirate the lesions in patients with severe neurological deficits. As we emphasized in our previous article, nonsurgical treatment should be reserved for patients who have small (less than 3 cm in diameter) or multiple lesions and those who are poor candidates for surgery (51). Antibiotics should be administered intravenously for at least 6–8 weeks. If serial CT scans show growth of the abscess at any time during treatment with antibiotics, or no decrease in the size of the lesion within 4 weeks, a surgical procedure should be performed to confirm the diagnosis, to obtain a sample for culture, and to remove as much purulent material as possible.

The primary advantage of nonsurgical treatment has been that it avoids the risks of surgery and anesthesia. Now, however, stereotactic aspiration procedures guided by CT scanning or ultrasound imaging can be performed under local anesthesia. Moreover, a surgical approach permits confirmation of the diagnosis, allows immediate decompression of mass lesions, reduces the duration of antibiotic therapy and consequently results in a shorter hospital stay, and increases the likelihood of cure. Surgery must be performed when drug-resistant organisms are identified or presumed to be the cause of the abscess or when a wound must be débrided (e.g., if a foreign body is present).

We believe that the success of nonsurgical therapy for brain abscesses has two major implications. First, it confirms the potential for cure of cerebritis with antibiotics. Second, it provides a rational approach to the treatment of patients with multiple brain abscesses. In such cases, one of the lesions should be aspirated or removed to confirm the diagnosis and identify the responsible organism(s) so that appropriate, specific antibiotic therapy can be devised to treat the remaining lesions. The one absolute contraindication for surgical treatment is a poorly controlled bleeding diathesis; medical therapy can be instituted in such patients if a bacterial brain abscess is strongly suspected. However, before nonsurgical treatment is attempted in other patients, the diagnosis must be firmly supported by the identification of a predisposing factor and by imaging studies that strongly suggest the presence of an abscess, the patient must be alert and clinically stable, the lesions must be small and deep, the patient must represent a major risk for surgery and anesthesia, and the organism must be identified presumptively from culture elsewhere.

The question one must ask in determining how to manage patients with pyogenic brain abscesses is this: "Which treatment is more conservative?" We believe a surgical approach is usually the more conservative one. However, if nonsurgical management is to be pursued, the patients must be carefully selected, and CT scans must be obtained frequently. It is particularly important that the primary physician be a neurosurgeon who is prepared to operate at the first sign of failure of medical therapy.

SURGICAL PROCEDURES

Various surgical procedures have been advocated for the treatment of brain abscesses, including drainage, aspiration, and total removal. Drainage has been replaced by aspiration and resection and is now seldom used. Aspiration has the advantages of speed and decreased morbidity, especially with the use of stereotactic techniques; surgical removal affords a greater likelihood of cure and shortens the duration of antibiotic therapy. In choosing between these alternatives, various factors, including surgical morbidity, success rate, and sequelae such as recurrence and seizure disorders, also must be considered.

Abscesses have the potential to recur, particularly when a foreign body is present. At one extreme, recurrences have been reported as long as 36 years and 51 years after foreign body implantation (50, 58). It is more common for abscesses to recur months after surgery, presumably from an organism harbored within the capsule itself; however, recurrences of this type have been observed as late as 11 and 13 years after aspiration (5, 31).

In 1951, Jooma and colleagues studied the long-term sequelae of surgery in 295 patients who had undergone aspiration, drainage, or excision of a brain abscess (31). Their findings are summarized in Table 38.6. The recurrence rate among 184 patients whose lesions were aspirated or drained was 8%, whereas none of 111 patients whose lesions were excised had a recurrence. There was no significant difference between the three surgical modalities in the percentage of patients who had seizures postoperatively, which ranged 43–55%. This study also showed that before CT scanning became available, the mortality rate was lowest among patients whose abscesses were excised and that the results of all three procedures improved after penicillin became available. In 1973, Legg and colleagues performed a similar study in 70 patients whose abscesses were treated

TABLE 38.6

*Sequelae of Aspiration, Drainage, or Excision in 295 Patients with Brain Abscesses**

	Aspiration	Drainage	Excision	Total
No. of patients	95	89	111	
Mortality	58/95 (61%)	45/89 (50%)	15/111 (13%)	
Without penicillin	37/50 (74%)	32/57 (56%)	8/38 (21%)	77/145 (53%)
With penicillin	21/45 (44%)	14/32 (41%)	7/73 (9%)	41/150 (27%)
Seizures†	15/31 (48%)	21/38 (55%)	36/83 (43%)	
Recurrence†	7/88 (8%)		0/96 (0%)	

* Data are from Jooma and colleagues (31).

† For 173 patients followed for at least 1 year.

surgically (36). Like Jooma, they noted the high incidence of seizures after aspiration (67%) and excision (78%), and, in addition, documented the long delay that is occasionally seen in the development of epilepsy in such cases. The onset of seizures occurred within 1 year after surgery in 41% of patients, after 2–5 years in 41%, and after 6–15 years in 18%.

We conclude that multiple abscesses and those in deep or critical locations should be aspirated. In the case of multiple lesions, the one that is most accessible and has the largest low-density center should be aspirated so as to increase the likelihood of obtaining a positive culture. Multiloculated abscesses and those that are superficial or contain a foreign body should be removed. The observation that fungal organisms may involve the wall of the abscess suggests that surgical extirpation is also necessary in these cases (1, 57).

ANTIBIOTIC SELECTION

The choice of antibiotics for treatment of infections of the central nervous system involves several controversial issues. In general, the factors that determine efficacy of any antibiotic agent include the drug concentration in the area of infection, the bacteriostatic versus the bacteriocidal effect of the agent on the infecting microorganism, and the duration of therapy.

Early studies by Wellman and colleagues (63) and Kramer and colleagues (35) to determine antibiotic penetration and concentration in normal brain tissue showed that the tissue: blood concentration ratios tended to vary widely for different antibiotics. The concentration of antibiotics achieved in human brain abscesses has been studied by Black and associates (7) and DeLouvois and colleagues (22). These and other studies were reviewed by Everett and Strausbaugh (25). The data suggest that antibiotics known to cross the blood-cerebrospinal fluid (CSF) barrier also cross the blood-brain barrier, presumably because these barriers share a similar anatomic basis, the tight junctions at the microvascular endothelium. Hence, antibiotics like chloramphenicol, metronidazole, sulfonamides, isoniazid, rifampin, and flucytosine, which penetrate well into normal brain and CSF, have potential utility for the treatment of brain abscesses.

When the permeability of the blood-brain barrier is altered by inflammatory conditions such as cerebritis and abscesses, antibiotics that usually do not penetrate into CSF or brain tissue, such as the penicillins and the cephalosporins, can penetrate well. Studies of the aminoglycoside antibiotics (e.g., gentamicin) in experimental brain abscess have demonstrated variable penetration (44). Aminoglycosides have traditionally been labeled as poor penetrators, especially into CSF, and cannot be used alone intravenously to treat Gram-negative meningitis in adults. However, for these and other antibiotic compounds labeled as poor penetrators of brain and CSF, their clinical efficacy in the treatment of brain abscesses has not been adequately correlated with their penetration capabilities, as has been done for meningitis. For example, one of these antibiotics, vancomycin, was evaluated in a case of staphylococcal brain abscess. Penetration of this drug was excellent; the concentration in abscess fluid was approximately 80% of the simultaneously obtained serum concentration (39). In patients with meningitis, the concentration of vancomycin in CSF is only 10% to 20% of the serum concentration. Therefore, penetration of vancomycin into an abscess may be greater than that into CSF. However, the correlation between penetration of an antibiotic into the infected area and the success of therapy has not been well established. Although vancomycin was found in the abscess fluid of the case mentioned above, it failed to sterilize the abscess cavity. As noted above, Black and associates reported in vitro growth of organisms obtained by aspiration of abscesses in which adequate concentrations of antibiotic were present (7). These observations suggest that achieving a concentration sufficient to inhibit growth of the organism in culture does not guarantee the cure of a brain abscess.

In selecting an appropriate antibiotic for treatment of brain abscesses, the mode of action of the drug must also be considered. Winn and colleagues reported that the bacteriostatic agent chloramphenicol was inferior to the bacteriocidal agent penicillin in the treatment of *Staphylococcus aureus* abscesses in rats (65). Others have also suggested that bacteriostatic agents should not be utilized alone in the treatment of brain abscesses. It must be emphasized, however, that some antibiotics generally considered to be bacteriostatic may have a bacteriocidal effect on certain organisms (*e.g.*, chloramphenicol activity against *Bacteroides* sp., pneumococci, and *Hemophilus influenzae*).

A further consideration in the choice of antibiotic is the possibility that bacteria will develop resistance to the agent being administered (3). Sole treatment with drugs such as rifampin and chloramphenicol might result in the emergence of resistant organisms. Thus, although chloramphenicol penetrates CSF and abscess cavities well, it may be ineffective against certain Gram-negative bacteria because it is a bacteriostatic agent and because resistent organisms may emerge during therapy (3).

Should antibiotics be given preoperatively? The advantages of preoperative antibiotics are that the patient would receive earlier treatment and that such treatment would prevent the spread of infection during aspiration or surgical removal of the abscess. The disadvantage is the possibility of obtaining false-negative cultures, particularly from smaller lesions. Since the success of nonsurgical treatment has confirmed the potential for the cure of cerebritis, which in its very early phase would include any operative spillage of organisms, preoperative antibiotics would not be recommended. Furthermore, if an abscess is large enough at the time of diagnosis that brain herniation or ventricular rupture is imminent, we recommend immediate surgical treatment instead of delaying surgery while a preoperative course of antibiotics is being administered. The advantage of obtaining a positive organism culture and knowing the specific antibiotics to give over a long period of time, particularly with the possibility of complications from such treatment (*e.g.*, bone marrow suppression from chloramphenicol), strongly suggests that antibiotics not be given before operative intervention.

Whenever possible, the antibiotics should be specific for the organism cultured. If no organism is identified, then the antibiotic should be selected according to the bacterial etiology presumed to have caused the lesion. Etiology-based therapy is partially based on the predisposing cause, the anatomic location of the abscess, and the likely organisms involved in that area, and is reviewed elsewhere (11, 22). We believe that the best antibiotics for the treatment of abscesses are those that cross the blood-CSF and blood-brain barriers, including agents that can do so in the presence of inflammation. However, there have been no detailed experimental or clinical studies correlating the penetration and concentration of an antibiotic with the efficacy of therapy for these lesions.

CORTICOSTEROIDS

To understand the possible effects of corticosteroids on the development and treatment of brain abscesses requires knowledge of host response to an infected wound. This process is illustrated in Figure 38.9, which is based on information from the wound healing literature (29, 37, 56, 57) and supported by many studies in patients with systemic infected and noninfected wounds (T. Hunt, D. Hohn, D. Bainton, Z. Werb, personal communications, 1985). The white blood cells vital to the body's defense against infection are produced by stem cells in the bone marrow. Within 1 hour after the introduction of infective organisms into the brain parenchyma, polymorphonuclear leukocytes are attracted into the wound by a process called chemotaxis; they continue to be attracted for 24 hours and remain within the wound for 1–2 days. These leukocytes kill bacteria in both an oxygen-dependent and in a less important oxygen-independent fashion. From day 1 through the first week, monocytes are attracted to the wound, where they exist for several weeks as activated macrophages. Macrophages are responsible for the majority of the bacteriocidal action of white blood cells within abscesses and are the primary cells capable of killing obligate intracellular pathogens. Macrophages also cooperate with the lymphocytes to identify foreign antigens and kill pathogenic organ-

HOST DEFENSES

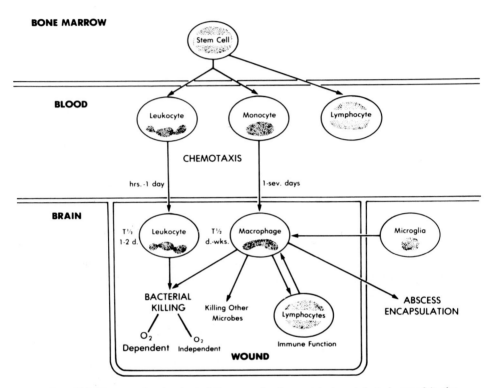

Fig. 38.9. Diagram showing host defense mechanisms against an infected wound in the brain. See text for details.

isms. The microglial cells that normally reside within the brain are thought to be the brain's "resident macrophages" and are presumably also attracted into the infected wound, where they perform functions similar to those of macrophages derived from blood monocytes.

Macrophages also play an important role in abscess encapsulation. This process is illustrated in Figure 38.10. The macrophages that are attracted into the wound produce wound angiogenesis factor (WAF) and macrophage-derived growth factor (MDGF). WAF and MDGF are responsible for the migration and proliferation of fibroblasts, which produce procollagen. WAF and MDGF also result in capillary budding and endothelial proliferation. Once oxygen is delivered to the region around the abscess

ABSCESS ENCAPSULATION

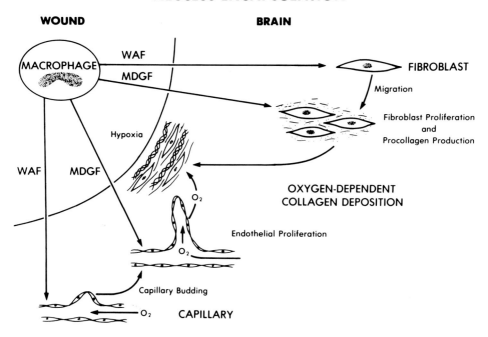

FIG. 38.10. Diagram of the process of abscess encapsulation. See text for details.

through the new capillaries, the procollagen is deposited as collagen around the lesion, and the walling-off process is complete.

The administration of corticosteroids early in the process of brain abscess development (cerebritis) results in decreased chemotaxis of both leukocytes and monocytes. With fewer of these cells present, the eradication of bacteria by leukocytes and cooperative immune processing by macrophages are reduced. In addition, corticosteroids interfere directly with the production of WAF and MDGF. Thus, it appears that corticosteroids significantly inhibit the host defenses involved with the walling-off and cure of brain abscesses. This assumption has been confirmed by studies in various animal models.

In experimental studies of *S. aureus* brain abscess in cats, Bohl and colleagues found that steroids decreased remote edema and inflammation as well as abscess encapsulation (9). Neuwelt and colleagues induced *Escherichia coli* abscesses in rats and reported that steroids decreased the number of macrophages in the lesions and inhibited gliosis. Finally, Quartey and associates showed in both streptococcal and staphylococcal brain abscesses in rabbits that steroids limit white blood cell access, organism killing, and capsule formation (48).

We believe corticosteroids have a beneficial effect in reducing brain edema associated with abscesses (2), but decrease the attraction of white blood cells to the site and retard encapsulation. Therefore, corticosteroids should only be used to reduce mass effect caused by abscess and edema when necessary to prevent progressive decline in neurologic function. An abscess that produces a neurologic deficit, but is too small to pose a threat of herniation (*e.g.*, small lesions in the motor strip), might be treated with corticosteroids to improve clinical function; however, the potentially deleterious effects of such treatment on the ultimate outcome must be recognized. The overall benefit of decreasing focal neurologic deficits in these circumstances is unclear. If possible, administration of corticosteroids should be avoided in the early stages of brain abscess development so that leukocytes and macrophages will be attracted in sufficient numbers to initiate bacterial killing and speed encapsulation.

Another factor to be considered is the effect of corticosteroids on follow-up CT scans during treatment (45). Whelan and Hilal reported that administration of corticosteroids decreased enhancement of the abscess wall on CT scans and that withdrawal of steroid occasionally resulted in increased enhancement, despite clinical stability and eventual cure (64). Britt and Enzmann also found that steroids decrease wall enhancement, but only in the cerebritis stage of abscess development (12, 24). Thus, it may be safely assumed that administration of corticosteroids can affect the intensity of wall enhancement of brain abscesses on CT scans. For this reason, a change in the volume of the abscess is a more reliable indication of the effectiveness of therapeutic maneuvers in patients receiving steroids.

CONCLUSIONS AND SUGGESTED THERAPEUTIC PROTOCOL

We recommend that surgery be performed for diagnosis and for therapy in most cases of presumed brain abscess. The few exceptions have been outlined in the section on surgical versus nonsurgical treatment. Corticosteroids should be used to reduce a mass effect that causes significant neurologic deficit and poses a threat of herniation. Preoperative administration of antibiotics appears to be of little benefit and should be avoided. Antibiotic therapy should include agents that are specific and bacteriocidal for the organism obtained and, if possible, that cross the blood-brain and blood-CSF barriers. Antibiotics should be given parenterally for 4–8 weeks, depending on the type of surgical procedure. Follow-up CT scans are essential in all cases of brain abscess, regardless of the treatment. These studies should be obtained at least every 2 weeks during treatment

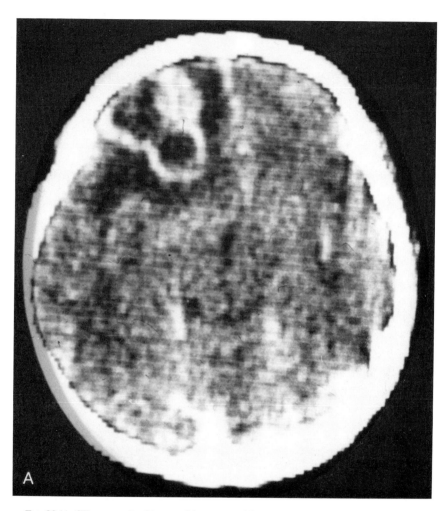

FIG. 38.11. CT scans of a 24-year-old woman with congenital cyanotic heart disease. In 1976, a right frontal brain abscess was surgically drained (A). In 1982, a new medial left parietal multiloculated abscess was documented (B).

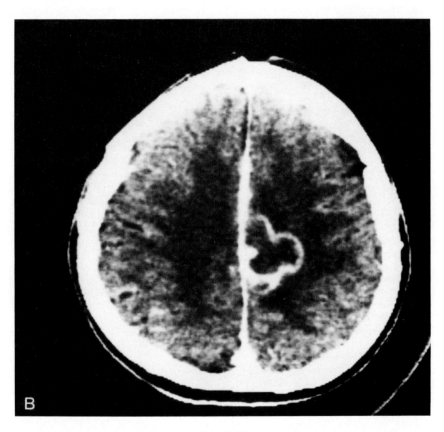

FIG. 38.11B.

and monthly for 4–6 months or until the lesion is no longer present on contrast-enhanced scans, whichever comes first. The physician must be on the alert for recurrence of the abscess, particularly when foreign bodies remain within the brain parenchyma or when a predisposing condition persists. CT scans should be performed whenever new neurological symptoms or signs are detected. As Cushing stated in 1908, "The most important of all therapeutic measures is prophylaxis" (19). For example, persistent right-to-left cardiac shunts should be corrected to prevent the development of new abscesses from this source (Fig. 38.11). Clinicians must be mindful that any change in the therapy of brain abscesses must provide a significant advantage over the improved results that have been obtained recently (52). Finally, the neurosurgeon must play the pivotal role in deciding which treatment carries the lowest risk for the patient and is most likely to result in a cure.

ACKNOWLEDGMENT

This chapter is dedicated to the memory of Dr. Richard Britt for his pioneering work on the pathogenesis of brain abscesses. Dr. Rosenblum is supported, in part, by Teacher Investigator Development Award No. 1K07 NS 00604 from the National Institute of Neurological and Communicative Diseases and Stroke and by grants CA-13525 and CA-31882 from the National Cancer Institute. The authors thank Stephen Ordway for his excellent editorial assistance.

REFERENCES

1. Adams, J. Parasitic and fungal infections of the nervous system. In *Greenfield's Neuropathology*, edited by W. Blackwood, and J. A. N. Corsellis. E. Arnold, Edinburgh, 1976, pp. 269–291.
2. Alderson, D., Strong, A. J., Ingham, F. R., and Selkon, J. B. Fifteen-year review of the mortality of brain abscesses. Neurosurgery, *8:* 1–5, 1981.
3. Barriere, S. L., Conte, J. E., Jr. Emergence of multiple antibiotic resistance during the therapy of *Klebsiella pneunomia* meningitis. Am. J. Med. Sci., *279:* 61–65, 1980.
4. Barsoum, A. H., Lewis, M. C., and Canillo, K. I. Nonoperative treatment of multiple brain abscesses. Surg. Neurol.; *16:* 283–287, 1981.
5. Beller, A. J., Saher, A., and Praiss, I. Brain abscess: review of 89 cases over 30 years. J. Neurol. Neurosurg. Psychiatr., *36:* 758–768, 1973.
6. Berg, B., Franklin, G., Cuneo, R., Boldrey, E., and Shemling, B. Nonsurgical cure of brain abscess: early diagnosis and follow-up with computed tomography. Ann. Neurol., *3:* 974–978, 1978.
7. Black, P., Graybill, J. R., and Charache, P. Penetration of brain abscess by systemically administered antibiotics. J. Neurosurg., *38:* 705–709, 1973.
8. Bloom, W. H., and Tuazon, C. U. Successful treatment of multiple brain abscesses with antibiotics alone. Rev. Infect. Dis., *7:* 189–199, 1985.
9. Bohl, I., Wallenfang, T., Bothe, H., and Schürmann, K. The effect of glucocorticoids in the combined treatment of experimental brain abscess in cats. Adv. Neurosurg., *9:* 235–133, 1981.
10. Brand, B., Caparosa, R. J., and Lubic, L. Otorhinological brain abscess therapy—past and present. Laryngoscope, *94:* 483–487, 1984.

11. Britt, R. H. Brain abscess. In: *Neurosurgery*, edited by R. H. Wilkins, and S. S. Rengachary. McGraw-Hill, New York, 1985, pp. 1928–1956.
12. Britt, R. H., and Enzmann, D. R. Clinical stages of human brain abscesses on serial CT scans after contrast infusion: computed tomographic, neuropathological, and clinical correlation. J. Neurosurg., *59:* 972–989, 1983.
13. Britt, R. H., Enzmann, D. R., and Remington, J. S. Intracranial infection in cardiac transplant recipients. Ann. Neurol., *9:* 107–119, 1981.
14. Britt, R. H., Enzmann, D. R., and Yeager, A. S. Neuropathological and computerized tomographic findings in experimental brain abscess. J. Neurosurg., *55:* 590–603, 1981.
15. Bronitsky, R., Craig, R. H., and McGee, Z. A. Multiple brain abscesses: combined medical and neurosurgical therapy. South. Med. J., *75:* 1261–1263, 1982.
16. Burke, L. P., Ho, S. U., Cerullo, L. J., Kim, K. S., and Harter, D. H. Multiple brain abscesses. Surg. Neurol., *16:* 452–454, 1981.
17. Carey, M. E., Chan, S. N., and French, L. A. Experience with brain abscesses. J. Neurosurg., *36:* 1–9, 1972.
18. Chow, A. W., Alexander, E., Mongomerie, J. Z., and Guze, L. B. Successful treatment of non-meningitic listerial brain abscess without operation. West. J. Med., *122:* 167–171, 1975.
19. Cushing, H. Surgery of the head. In: *Surgery: Its Principles and Practice*, edited by W. W. Keen. W. B. Saunders, Philadelphia, 1908, pp. 174–182.
20. Dandy, W. E. Treatment of chronic abscess of the brain by tapping: Preliminary note. J.A.M.A., *87:* 1477–1478, 1926.
21. Davini, V., Rivano, C., Borzone, M., Capuzzo, T., and Altomonte, M. Bilateral brain abscesses—report of 2 cases. Zentralbl. Neurochir., *45:* 329–334, 1984.
22. deLouvois, J., Gortavi, P., and Hurley, R. Bacteriology of abscesses of the central nervous system. A multicentre prospective study. Br. Med. J., *2:* 981–984, 1977.
23. Dobkin, J. F., Healton, E. B., Dickinson, T., and Brust, J. C. M. Nonspecificity of ring enhancement in "medically cured" brain abscesses. Neurology, *34:* 139–144, 1984.
24. Enzmann, D. R., Britt, R. H., and Placoney, R. Staging of human brain abscess by computed tomography. Radiology, *146:* 703–708, 1983.
25. Everett, E. D., and Strausbaugh, L. J. Antimicrobial agents and the central nervous system. Neurosurgery, *6:* 691–714, 1980.
26. Falconer, M. A., McFarlan, A. M., and Russell, D. S. Experimental brain abscesses in the rabbit. Br. J. Surg., *30:* 245–260, 1943.
27. George, B., Roux, F., Pillon, M., Thurel, C., and George, C. Relevance of antibiotics in the treatment of brain abscesses. Acta Neurochir., *47:* 285–291, 1979.
28. Heineman, H. S., and Baude, A. I. Intracranial suppurative disease. J.A.M.A., *218:* 1542–1547, 1971.
29. Hohn, D. Host defences: the phagocytes. In: *Surgical Infectious Diseases*, edited by R. L. Simmons, and R. J. Howard. Appleton-Century-Crofts, New York, 1982, pp. 242–252.
30. Hutchinson, R., and Heyn, R. M. Listerial brain abscess in a patient with leukemia: successful nonsurgical management. Clin. Pediatr., *22:* 312, 1983.
31. Jooma, O. V., Pennybacker, J. B., and Tutton, G. K. Brain abscesses: aspiration, drainage or excision. J. Neurol. Neurosurg. Psychiatr., *14:* 308–313, 1951.
32. Kamin, M., and Biddle, D. Conservative management of focal intracerebral injection. Neurology, *31:* 103–106, 1981.
33. Kermani, N., Tuazon, C. U., Ocuin, J. A., Thompson, A. M., Kramer, N. C., and Geelhoed, G. W. Extensive cerebral nocardosis cured with antibiotic therapy alone. Case report. J. Neurosurg., *49:* 924–928, 1978.

34. Kottas, L., and Smith, G. A possible new approach to the management of brain abscesses. Infection, *1 & 2:* 81–83, 1978.

35. Kramer, P. W., Griffith, R. S., and Campbell, R. L. Antibiotic penetration of the brain. A comparative study. J. Neurosurg., *31:* 295–302, 1969.

36. Legg, N. J., Gupta, P. C., and Scott, D. F. Epilepsy following cerebral abscess: A clinical and EEG study of 70 patients. Brain, *96:* 259–268, 1973.

37. Leibovich, S. J., and Ross, R. The role of the macrophage in wound repair. Am. J. Pathol., *78,* 71–100, 1975.

38. Levy, R. M., Bredesen, D. E., and Rosenblum, M. L. Neurological manifestations of the acquired immunodeficiency syndrome (AIDS): experience at UCSF and review of the literature. J. Neurosurg., *62:* 475–495, 1985.

39. Levy, R. M., Gutin, P. H., Baskin, D. S., and Pons, V. G. Vancomycin penetration of a brain abscess: case report and review of the literature. Neurosurgery, *18:* (In press, 1986).

40. Levy, R. M., Pons, V. G., and Rosenblum, M. L. Central nervous system mass lesions in the acquired immunodeficiency syndrome (AIDS). J. Neurosurg., *61:* 9–16, 1984.

41. Macewen, W. Intracranial lesions, illustrating some points in connection with the localisation of cerebral affections and the advantages of antiseptic trephaning. Lancet, *2:* 581–583, 1881.

42. Macewen, W. *Pyogenic Infective Diseases of the Brain and Spinal Cord,* J. Maclehose and Sons, Glasgow, 1893.

43. Mathiesen, G. E., Meyer, R. D., George, W. L., Cirton, D. M., and Finegold, S. M. Brain abscess and cerebritis. Rev. Infect. Dis., *6:* 101–106, 1984.

44. Neuwelt, E. A., Baker, D. E., Pagel, M. A., and Blaak, N. K. Cerebrovascular permeability and delivery of gentamicin to normal brain and experimental brain abscess in rats. J. Neurosurg., *61:* 430–439, 1984.

45. New, P. F. J., Davis, K. R., and Ballantine, H. T., Jr. Computed tomography in cerebral abscess. Radiology, *121:* 641–646, 1976.

46. Norden, C. W., Ruben, F. L., and Selker, R. Nonsurgical treatment of cerebral nocardiosis. Arch. Neurol., *40:* 594–595, 1983.

47. North, R. J. The action of cortisone acetate on cell-mediated immunity to infection: suppression of host cell proliferation and alteration of cellular composition in infective foci. J. Exp. Med., *134:* 1485–1500, 1971.

48. Quartey, G. R. C., Johnston, J. A., and Rozdilsky, B. Decadron in the treatment of cerebral abscess: an experimental study. J. Neurosurg., *45:* 301–310, 1976.

49. Rennels, M. B., Woodward, C. L., Robinson, W. L., Gumbinas, M. T., and Brenner, J. J. Medical cure of apparent brain abscesses. Pediatrics, *72:* 220–224, 1983.

50. Robinson, E. F., Moiel, R. H., and Gol, A. Brain abscess 36 years after head injury. J. Neurosurg., *28:* 166–168, 1968.

51. Rosenblum, M. L., Hoff, J. T., Norman, D. A., Edwards, M., and Berg, B. Nonoperative treatment of brain abscesses in selected high-risk patients. J. Neurosurg., *52:* 217–225, 1980.

52. Rosenblum, M. L., Hoff, J. T., Norman, D., Weinstein, P. R., and Pitts, L. H. Decreased mortality from brain abscesses since advent of computerized tomography. J. Neurosurg., *49:* 658–668, 1978.

53. Rotherman, E. B., and Kessler, L. A. Use of computerized tomography in nonsurgical management of brain abscess. Arch. Neurol., *36:* 25–26, 1979.

54. Rousseaux, M., Lesoin, F., Destee, A., Jomin, M., and Petit, H. Long-term sequelae of hemispheric abscesses as a function of treatment. Acta Neurochir., *74:* 61–67, 1985.

55. Samson, D. S., and Clark, K. A current review of brain abscesses. Am. J. Med., *54:* 201–210, 1973.

56. Sandberg, N. Time relationship between administration of cortisone and wound healing in rats. Acta Chir. Scand., *127:* 446–455, 1964.

57. Steinberg, G. K., Britt, R. H., Enzmann, D. R., Finlay, J. L., and Arvin, A. M. Fusarium brain abscess. J. Neurosurg., *58:* 598–601, 1983.

58. Swann, B. M. Brain abscess: A world record? Delaware Med. J., *42:* 363–366, 1970.

59. Vallee, B., Bessen, G., Garre, M., Le Guyader, J., and Garre, H. Cure by medical treatment of a brain stem abscess in a case of multiple encephalic suppuration. Neurochirurgie, *26:* 401–403, 1980.

60. Vaquero, J., Cabezudo, J. M., and Leunda, G. Nonsurgical resolution of a brain stem abscess. Case report. J. Neurosurg., *53:* 726–727, 1980.

61. Vincent, C. Sur une méthode de traitement des abcès subaigus des hémisphères cérébraux: large décompression, puis ablation en masse sans drainage. Gaz. Med. Fr., *43:* 93–96, 1936.

62. Weisberg, L. A. Nonsurgical management of focal intracranial infection. Neurology, *31:* 575–580, 1981.

63. Wellman, W. E., Dodge, H. W., Jr., Heilman, F. R., and Petersen, M. C. Concentration of antibiotic in the brain. J. Lab. Clin. Med., *43:* 275–279, 1954.

64. Whelan, M. A., and Hilal, S. K. Computed tomography as a guide in the diagnosis and followup of brain abscesses. Radiology, *135:* 663–671, 1980.

65. Winn, H. R., Mendes, M., Moore, P., Wheeler, C., and Rodeheaver, G. Production of experimental brain abscess in the rat. J. Neurosurg., *51:* 685–690, 1979.

Antibiotic Prophylaxis in Neurosurgery

STEPHEN J. HAINES, M.D.

INTRODUCTION

There is little disagreement that the prevention of postoperative neurosurgical infections is important. There continues to be a good deal of controversy, however, regarding specific techniques of infection prevention. The use of antibiotics for the purpose of preventing rather than treating infections has been an area of controversy for many years. The purpose of this review is to examine the scientific evidence regarding antibiotic prophylaxis in neurosurgery that has accumulated since the last comprehensive review of the subject (11).

Before examining that evidence, it is perhaps appropriate to respond to the assertion that the limited application of antibiotic prophylaxis is so inexpensive and risk-free that it is not necessary to insist on sound scientific evidence to support the practice. I believe that this view is incorrect for a number of reasons. There are known risks to the individual receiving even a single systemic dose of antibiotic. These include potentially lethal anaphylactic reactions, very uncomfortable manifestations of allergy in the case of certain antibiotics such as vancomycin, hypotensive episodes, and the local complications of infusion. It has been estimated that approximately 8% of patients receiving penicillin will suffer some adverse reaction (29). The long-term effects of the selective pressure of a short-term, broadly applied prophylactic antibiotic program are expected to be minimal but are unknown. Past expectations of minimal long-term effects have proven to be unreliable.

The expense of even a short perioperative antibiotic protocol using a relatively inexpensive drug when applied as a matter of policy to neurosurgical procedures throughout the country is considerable. Figures from the National Center for Health Statistics from 1981 indicate that somewhat more than 800,000 operations were performed on the central nervous system in this country in that year (19). These figures include many diagnostic procedures but exclude nearly 200,000 operations on intervertebral discs and between 50,000–100,000 carotid endarterectomies. If we use the estimate of 800,000 neurosurgical operations per year and postulate a three-dose perioperative prophylactic antibiotic regimen, approximately 2.4 million antibiotic doses will be given prophylactically. I have been quite surprised to learn that the cost to the patient of a single intravenous dose of cefazolin, which costs the pharmacist approximately $3.25 can be inflated by diluent, supplies, and professional dispensing fees to as high as $37.00 per dose at some institutions. Using a conservative estimate of $10.00 per dose, we arrive at a figure of $24 million per year.

All of these potential liabilities are quite minor for each individual patient. However, if we are to advocate antibiotic prophylaxis as a matter of policy, the risks and liabilities become important and it is appropriate to require a sound basis for the institution of such a policy.

The ensuing discussion will be divided into two parts. First, the issue of prophylaxis for clean procedures without implantation of foreign body will be discussed. This will be followed by a discussion of prophylaxis for cerebrospinal fluid shunt surgery.

ANTIBIOTIC PROPHYLAXIS FOR CLEAN NEUROSURGICAL PROCEDURES

Five years ago there were very little data to support the hypothesis that perioperative antibiotic administration prevented the development of postoperative wound infection. Since that time more information has been produced to support the concept, although none of it can be considered definitive. The remarkable experience that Malis reported in 1979 using a combination of systemic vancomycin and tobramycin with topical streptomycin has continued to the present time, with a series of patients in excess of 5000 experiencing only two primary wound infections according to his definition (15). In my view, the strength of such a remarkable experience is its virtual elimination of infection. Had this experience been repeated at other institutions, there would be little room to argue against its use. However, subsequent reports by Quartey and Polyzoidis (21) and from the University of Pittsburgh (13) using this regimen indicated an expected infection rate of approximately 1%. While this is a low infection rate, one expects clean operations to have infection rates below 2% and, therefore, the effect is not sufficiently dramatic to overcome the inherent variation in infection rates between the surgeons, institutions, and over time.

Savitz and Katz reported using a short perioperative course of cephalothin resulting in a series of 1000 patients without primary wound infection (23). Once again, other institutions using a very similar regimen continued to experience infection and this experience, while it may be considered supportive of the value of antibiotic prophylaxis, cannot be considered definitive. One must keep in mind that it is possible to attain very low infection rates with very strict antiseptic techniques in the absence of systemic antibiotic administration.

Two studies have attempted to obtain information in a more controlled setting. Our own retrospective case control study of risk factors for infection, reported at this meeting last year, supports the concept that antibiotic administration may reduce infection rates (17). The infection experience in 9202 clean neurosurgical procedures performed at the University of Minnesota between 1970 and 1984 was reviewed. During this time there was no fixed policy regarding the use of perioperative antibiotics. One hundred and one infections were identified in this group of operations for a crude infection rate of 1.1%. An attempt was made to identify controls for each of the infected patients matched by surgeon, diagnosis, procedure, age, gender, and year of operation. It was possible to identify 89 matches. These were perfectly matched for surgeon, diagnosis, and procedure. Age, gender, and mean year of surgery were extremely close in the two groups (Table 39.1). When the use of perioperative antibiotics was examined in these matched pairs we found 50 pairs in which both the infected patient and the control either received or did not receive antibiotics. These 50 pairs provide no useful information regarding the benefit of antibiotics. Of the remaining 39 pairs where antibiotic use differed, in 33 pairs the uninfected control received perioperative antibiotics while the infected patient did not (Table 39.2). This suggests that the risks of developing infection when perioperative antibiotics were used was about 20% of the risk of developing infection when they were not used. This association was statistically significant.

Unfortunately, there are factors, such as severity of illness, which we were not able to control, and the lack of any standard prophylactic protocol in the study makes it extremely difficult to recommend a particular method of prophylaxis. This information must be considered strongly supportive but not definitive.

TABLE 39.1

Characteristics of Patient Population: University of Minnesota Wound Infection Study

	Control Patients	Infected Patients
Diagnosis		
Procedure	Exact match	
Surgeon		
Mean age in years	42.3	42.0
(standard deviation)	(19.1)	(20.8)
Sex (% male)	60	64
Year of operation (mean)	1974.8	1975.2

TABLE 39.2

Use of Perioperative Antibiotics: University of
Minnesota Wound Infection Study

		Antibiotic Used in Control Patient?		
		Yes	No	Total
Antibiotics used in	Yes	11	6	17
infected patient?	No	33	39	72
	Total	44	45	89

Odds Ratio   0.18 : 1
95% Confidence Interval   0.07–0.45
McNemar's Chi Square   17.33, 1 d.f. $p = 0.0001$

In 1984, Geraghty and Feely published a prospective clinical trial of the gentamycin, vancomycin, and streptomycin protocol (10). They included 402 patients in the trial who were alternately allocated to receive antibiotics or not. Apparently no placebo or blinding procedure was used. The total duration of the study is unclear and, in general, the report is too brief to provide much detail about the conduct of the study. The number of infections was eight, and seven of these occurred in the control group. When tested with a one-sided significance test the difference is significant by traditional standards. This test, however, ignores the possibility that the antibiotic group might do worse than the control group, a phenomenon that has been reported in some retrospective studies. However, using the more conservative two-sided test, the results do not attain significance and the number of end-points is so small that a single misclassification error or missed infection in the treated group would render the results of the study insignificant. When such tenuous significance is coupled with the lack of blinding and an open, nonrandom allocation procedure, the results of the study cannot be considered conclusive.

Where do we stand? Most experts outside the field of neurosurgery continue to recommend against systemic antibiotic prophylaxis in procedures where the expected risk of infection is less than 2%, a category for which the value of antibiotic prophylaxis has never been conclusively demonstrated. On the other hand, the supportive evidence for the value of antibiotic prophylaxis in clean neurosurgical procedures is growing in quantity and quality. I feel that a study of sufficient size and careful design to allow a definitive conclusion, either pro or con, to be drawn is both justifiable and feasible.

ANTIBIOTIC PROPHYLAXIS IN CEREBROSPINAL FLUID SHUNT SURGERY

One would think that it would be easier to demonstrate the value of antibiotic prophylaxis in shunt operations than in clean operations without shunt placement. Shunt operations are more liable to infection and, therefore, benefit should be more easily demonstrated. Even more surgeons are convinced about the value of prophylaxis in these operations than for clean, nonforeign-body procedures. In addition, benefit has been demonstrated for procedures with implantation of other foreign bodies, such as total hip arthroplasty. Unfortunately, it is exceedingly difficult to demonstrate from available data that antibiotics have any impact on the incidence of infection following shunt operations.

I shall attempt to deal with the large volume of uncontrolled data expeditiously and treat the published controlled clinical trials in more detail. The uncontrolled data may be useful primarily in three ways. First, if these data are highly consistent and show very little overlap in infection rate between patients treated with antibiotic prophylaxis and those not so treated, it may be possible to draw satisfactory conclusions. Second, if the use of antibiotics is associated with the virtual elimination of infection the case would be quite strong. Third, if the data show a strong trend in infection rate over time that is associated with the use of antibiotic prophylaxis, conclusions may be drawn.

I have collected reported infection rates in a series of shunt operations including 48 patients or more from 1957 to the present (1–3, 5, 7–9, 12, 14, 16, 18, 20–22, 24, 26–28, 30, 34, 35). Figure 39.1 shows a plot of these infection rates on the Y axis with the final year of entry into the series or year of the report on the X axis. We note immediately that there is a very large amount of variation in infection rate. There is a suggestion of a trend toward reduction of infection rate over time. Second, we see that no report suggests that infection can be completely eliminated although there are a number of recent series with infection rates below 5%. Figure 39.2 shows those series for which antibiotic use can be identified. In some cases, the control and treatment arms of the controlled study are plotted as separate points. In other cases, the entire series was treated one way or the other. We see that there is scatter and overlap between the series treated with and without antibiotics, that while the antibiotic series do tend to have lower infection rates than the untreated series, the difference is not so great that it overcomes the variation and overlap and that the trend to lower infection rates in recent years appears to be of about the same magnitude in both groups. We also see two series of patients not given antibiotics that have extraordinarily high infection rates. These happen to be the control groups of the only two randomized trials that have shown therapeutic benefit of antibiotic prophylaxis.

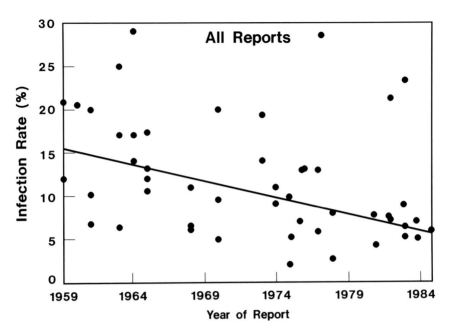

FIG. 39.1. Shunt infection rates by year of report for series including at least 48 patients.

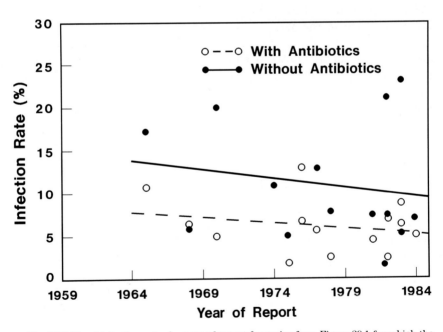

FIG. 39.2. Shunt infection rates by year of report for series from Figure 39.1 for which the use of antibiotic prophylaxis could be identified.

From these uncontrolled data I think that one can draw the conclusion that there is a suggestion of lower infection rates in the antibiotic-treated patient but that there is sufficient variation that this difference cannot be proven from such data. Additionally, the trend of approximately one-third of a percent reduction in the infection rate per year simply with the passage of time indicates that the historical comparisons of infection rates must be considered very suspect.

In an attempt to obtain better controlled information, Walters and others have performed a case control analysis of the experience at the Hospital for Sick Children in Toronto (31). Thirty-two shunt infections and 32 shunt operations without infection were randomly selected from their files. The patients were comparable in diagnosis, age, and sex. The risk of infection in patients operated upon without antibiotic prophylaxis was found to be more than three times greater than in those operated under antibiotic coverage (Table 39.3). These results must be interpreted with the usual cautions regarding retrospective studies and with the understanding that no particular antibiotic protocol was followed throughout the study.

I am aware of seven randomized clinical trials of antibiotic prophylaxis in shunt operations. These can be discussed in three groups. The first two studies, by Weiss and Raskind (33) and by Bayston (3) include so few infections (one in the Weiss and Raskind study, and three in Bayston study) that they provide no useful information. Three studies fail to find a statistically significant difference between the antibiotic treated and control patients. Our study, performed using methicillin, found the infection rate in the antibiotic group to be half that in the placebo group, but the difference was not statistically significant (12). Wang *et al.*, again at the Hospital for Sick Children, used cotrimoxazole and found virtually identi-

TABLE 39.3

*Contingency Table for Antibiotic Use among Cases and Controls: Toronto Study**

	Infected Cases	Noninfected Controls	Total
No antibiotics	28	18	46
Antibiotics	4	14	18
Total	32	32	64

$p = 0.01$ (Fisher's Exact Test, 2-tailed)
Summary Odds Ratio (Mantel-Haentzel) = 3.27

* Used with kind permission of Dr. Walters.

cal infection rates in the treated and control groups (32). Schmidt *et al.*
used methicillin and actually found a higher infection rate in the antibiotic
group than in the control group (25). The difference was not statistically
significant. The difficulty with each of these three negative studies is that
none was large enough to have a reasonable chance of finding even a 50%
reduction in infection rate in the treated group. Therefore, while they offer
little evidence supporting the practice of prophylaxis, they provide no
evidence that the practice is not effective.

The last two controlled trials did document a significant reduction in
infection rate in the antibiotic treated group. Epstein reported the results
of his study at the American Association of Neurological Surgeons meeting
in 1982 (6). Cephalothin was used intravenously and intraventricularly.
There were 78 patients in the trial with one infection in the treated group
(2.6%) and eight infections in the placebo group (21.1%). Blomstedt reported the study of 122 shunt operations randomized between cotrimoxazole and placebo. The infection rate was 6% in the antibiotic group and
23% in the placebo group (4). In both studies, the differences were statistically significant.

As mentioned before, the infection rates in the control groups in both
these studies were remarkably high. Indeed, they had the highest infection
rates ever reported in a series of patients known not to have received
antibiotic prophylaxis and they were exceeded in only two series in which
the use of antibiotics is unknown. Because of this, one must be concerned
that these studies are making a false comparison, *i.e.*, that some additional
factor placed the control patients in these trials at unusual risk. One might
argue that this was the result simply of closer observation in the setting of
an organized trial; however, such high infection rates were not seen in
other organized trials. Neither trial identified an unusual risk factor, although the patients in Epstein's trial did receive a placebo injection into
the shunt system at the end of the operation.

What conclusions can be drawn from these controlled trials? First, despite suggestive and supportive evidence of prophylactic benefit, the value
of antibiotic prophylaxis in shunt operations with a baseline infection rate
below 20% has never been demonstrated. Second, surgeons afflicted with a
shunt infection rate exceeding 20% should be using antibiotic prophylaxis.
Such an infection rate should also prompt a very careful review of aseptic
procedure.

The reasons for failure to demonstrate a benefit of antibiotic prophylaxis may be many. It is possible that the wrong drugs are being studied
and that they are being given at the wrong dosages and time intervals. It is
well-documented that the presence of a foreign body alters host defenses
against infection and it may be that a completely different set of antibiot-

ics, more effective in this altered environment, may be required. Possibly other modes of administration or other measures altogether will be required to protect shunted patients satisfactorily from infection. At this time, the question remains open. Further study both of existing prophylactic regimens and of innovative regimens is clearly indicated. Such studies must be of sufficient size and quality to have a reasonable chance of detecting the differences that they seek.

REFERENCES

1. Agir, F., Levin, B., and Duff, T. A. Effect of prophylactic methicillin on cerebrospinal fluid shunt infections in children. Neurosurgery, 9: 6–8, 1981.
2. Bayston, R., and Lari, J. Sources of infection in colonized shunts. Dev. Med. Child. Neurol., 16 (Suppl 32): 16–22, 1974.
3. Bayston, R. Antibiotic prophylaxis in shunt surgery. Dev. Med. Child Neurol., 17 (Suppl 35): 99–103, 1975.
4. Blomstedt, G. C. Results of trimethoprim-sulfamethoxazole prophylaxis in ventriculostomy and shunting procedures. A double-blind randomized trial. J. Neurosurg., 62: 694–697, 1985.
5. Bruce, A. M., and Lorber, J., Shedden, W. Y. H., and Zachary, R. B. Persistent bacteremia following ventriculo-caval shunt operations for hydrocephalus in infants. Dev. Med. Child Neurol., 5: 461–470, 1963.
6. Epstein, M. H., Kumor, K., Hugues, W., and Lietman, P. The use of prophylactic antibiotics in pediatric shunting operations—A double-blind prospective randomized study, presented at Annual Meeting, American Association of Neurological Surgeons, Honolulu, Hawaii. April, 1982.
7. Forrest, D. M., and Cooper, D. J. W. Complications of ventriculoatrial shunts. A review of 455 cases. J. Neurosurg., 29: 506–512, 1968.
8. Gardner, B. P., and Gordon, D. S. Postoperative infection in shunts for hydrocephalus: Are prophylactic antibiotics necessary? Br. Med. J., 284: 1914–1915, 1982.
9. George, R., Leibrock, L., and Epstein, M. Long term analysis of cerebrospinal fluid shunt infection. A 25 year experience. J. Neurosurg., 51: 804–811, 1979.
10. Geraghty, J., and Feely, M. Antibiotic prophylaxis in neurosurgery. A randomized control trial. J. Neurosurg., 60: 724–726, 1984.
11. Haines, S. J. Systemic antibiotic prophylaxis in neurological surgery. Neurosurgery, 6: 355–361, 1980.
12. Haines, S. J., and Taylor, F. Prophylactic methicillin for shunt operations: Effects on incidence of shunt malfunction and infection. Child's Brain, 9: 10–22, 1982.
13. Haines, S. J., and Goodman, M. L. Antibiotic prophylaxis of postoperative neurosurgical wound infection. J. Neurosurg., 56: 103–105, 1982.
14. Luthardt, T. Bacterial infections in ventriculoauricular shunt systems. Dev. Med. Child Neurol., 12 (Suppl 22): 105–109, 1970. (This article lists 14 series included in Figure 39.1)
15. Malis, L. I. Personal communication. 1985.
16. McCullough, D. C., Cane, J. G., Presper, J. H., and Wells, M. Antibiotic prophylaxis in ventricular shunt surgery. I. Reduction of operative infection rates with methicillin. Child's Brain, 7: 182–189, 1980.
17. Mollman, H. D., and Haines, S. J. Risk factors for postoperative neurosurgical wound infection: a case-control study. J. Neurosurg., 64: 902–906, 1986.

18. Morrice, J. J., Young, D. J. Bacterial colonization of Holter valves: a 10 year study. Dev. Med. Child Neurol., *16* (Suppl 32): 85–90, 1974.

19. Nat. Ctr. for Health Statistics, Pokras, R. Utilization of short stay hospitals vital and health statistics, Series 13, 72 DHHS Publication (PHS)83–1733. 1983.

20. Overton, M. C., Snodgrass, S. R. Ventriculovenous shunts for infantile hydrocephalus. A review of 5 years experience with this method. J. Neurosurg., *23:* 517–521, 1965.

21. Quartey, J. R. C., and Polyzoidis, K. Intraoperative antibiotic prophylaxis in neurosurgery: a clinical study. Neurosurgery., *8:* 669–671, 1981.

22. Raimondi, A. J. Robinson, J. S., and Kuwamura, K. Complications of ventriculoperitoneal shunt and a critical comparison of the three-piece and one-piece systems. Child's Brain, *3:* 321–342, 1977.

23. Savitz, M. H., and Katz, S. S. Rationale for prophylactic antibiotics in neurosurgery. Neurosurgery, *9:* 142–144, 1981.

24. Schimke, R. T., Black, P. H., Mark, V. H., and Swartz, M. N. Indolent staphylococcus albus or aureus bacteremia after ventriculoatriostomy. Role of foreign body in its initiation and perpetuation. N. Engl. J. of Med., *264:* 264–270, 1961.

25. Schmidt, K., Gjerris, F., Osgaard, O., Hvidberg, E. F., Kristiansen, J. E., Dahlerup, B., and Kruse-Larsen, C. Antibiotic prophylaxis in cerebrospinal fluid shunting: A prospective randomized trial in 152 hydrocephalic patients. Neurosurgery, *17:* 1–5, 1985.

26. Schoenbaum, S. C., Gardner, P., and Schillito, J. Infection of cerebrospinal fluid shunts: epidemiology, clinical manifestations and therapy. J. Inf. Dis., *131:* 543–552, 1975.

27. Shurtleff, D. B., Christie, D., and Foltz, Z. C. Ventriculo-auriculostomy—associated infection. A 12 year study. J. Neurosurg., *35:* 686–694, 1971.

28. Slight, P. H., Gundling, K., Plotkin, S. A., Schut, L., Bruce, D., and Sutton, L. A trial of vancomycin for prophylaxis of infections after neurosurgical shunts (letter). N. Engl. J. Med., *312:* 9–21, 1985.

29. Smith, J. W., Johnson, J. E., and Cluff, L. E. Studies on the epidemiology of adverse drug reactions. II. Evaluation of penicillin allergy. N. Engl. J. of Med., *274:* 998–1002, 1966.

30. Venes, J. L. Control of shunt infection. Report of 150 consecutive cases. J. Neurosurg., *45:* 311–314, 1976.

31. Walters, B. C., Hoffman, H. J. Hendricks, E. B., and Humphreys, R. P. Decreased risk of infection in cerebrospinal fluid shunt surgery using prophylactic antibiotics: a case-control study. Z. Kinderchir., *40 (Suppl 1):* 15–18, 1985.

32. Wang, E. E. L., Prober, C. G., Heindrick, B. E., Hoffman, H. J., and Humphreys, R. P. Prophylactic sulfamethoxazole and trimethoprim in ventriculoperitoneal shunt surgery. A double-blind, randomized, placebo control trial. J.A.M.A., *251:* 1174–1177, 1984.

33. Weiss, S. R., and Raskind, R. Further experience with the ventriculoperitoneal shunt. Int. Surg., *53:* 300–303, 1970.

34. Welch, K. The prevention of shunt infection. Zeits Kinderchirurg, *22:* 465–475, 1977.

35. Yu, H. C., and Patterson, R. H. Prophylactic antimicrobial agents after ventriculoatriostomy for hydrocephalus. J. Pediatr. Surg., *8:* 881–885, 1973.

VIII

Neurosurgical Treatment of Vertigo

40

Neurosurgical Treatment of Vertigo by Microvascular Decompression of the Eighth Cranial Nerve

PETER J. JANNETTA, M.D., MARGARETA B. MØLLER, M.D., PH.D., AAGE R. MØLLER, PH.D., and LALIGAM N. SEKHAR, M.D.

Symptoms of vertigo, dysequilibrium, and tinnitus are common, and the cause, in the vast majority of patients, is not known. As a result of extrapolation from other cranial nerve problems that are known to be caused by neural compression from blood vessels and can be treated by moving the blood vessels away from the involved nerve (3–5, 8), it was reasonable to assume that eighth cranial nerve symptoms could be caused by vascular compression and that the symptoms could be treated by decompression of the nerve using microsurgical techniques (5–7, 9). Blood vessels cause compression of cranial nerves as a consequence of the aging process because of elongation of the arteries at the base of the brain and caudal displacement of the hindbrain in the posterior fossa. Symptoms in younger people are more frequently caused by veins around the pontomedullary junction than by arteries.

In the literature, it is frequently stated that these symptoms are "multifactorial" in origin. In a sense, this is correct. But the multiple factors which cause and modify the symptoms are related to the neurovascular relationships. These factors include, among others, the size of the causative blood vessel, the velocity with which the blood vessel comes into contact with the nerve, the severity of the compression, the duration of the compression, the location of the vessel on the nerve, and the number of blood vessels involved.

In this paper, after a brief historical survey, we will discuss the indications for operation, the preoperative evaluation of patients, a few details of operative technique, including electrophysiologic monitoring, operative findings, and operative results, and complications.

The history of surgery of the otovestibular system reflects once again the proclivity for neurosurgeons to develop something in their area (a new perspective, a new operative technique, etc.) and give it away to other specialists. In the premodern era, Prosper Ménière was the first person to begin the development of a useful categorization of eighth nerve symptoms (2, 11–14). It must be appreciated that, although the observations by Ménière were incomplete (as are many observations!) and the ideas regarding pathogenesis in error, the need for some categorization was important. From the original papers evolved a hierarchy of diseases and syndromes including such entities as: Ménière's disease, Ménière's syndrome, vestibular or cochlear Ménière's disease, benign paroxysmal positional nystagmus or vertigo (BPPN), undiagnosable disease of the vestibular system, idiopathic sensorineural hearing loss, labyrinthitis, vestibular neuritis, vestibular neuronitis, etc. My colleagues and I have perhaps further added to this *potpourri* of diagnoses by coining the term disabling positional vertigo (DPV) for a certain subset of these patients (9). We identified a specific group of patients, whose symptoms are caused by cross-compression of the eighth cranial nerve (CN VIII). These patients with DPV, in lack of understanding of the pathology by their primary physicians, have received one or many of the above diagnoses. Most common is "vestibular Ménière's" or "uncompensated vestibular neuronitis."

The modern era in the surgery of vertigo began as early as 1927, as reported in Dandy's 1928 article on Ménière's disease (2) (Fig. 40.1). Dandy's patient number 8 in his series of nine who underwent posterior fossa section of the auditory nerve was a clinic patient at the Johns Hopkins Hospital. In his description of the operation, Dandy included the following information:

". . . It is worthy of note that 1 year before the operation, the eighth nerve was explored and an anomalous artery lying on the nerve was 'clipped.' A unilateral decompression resulted. No improvement followed."

ARCHIVES OF SURGERY

VOLUME 16	JUNE, 1928	NUMBER 6

MÉNIÈRE'S DISEASE

ITS DIAGNOSIS AND A METHOD OF TREATMENT *

WALTER E. DANDY, M.D.

BALTIMORE

FIG. 40.1. Dandy's first article on Ménière's disease, published in 1928. In this paper, a case of vascular decompression of the auditory nerve is briefly mentioned (2).

ANOMALOUS VASCULAR LESION IN CEREBEL-LOPONTILE ANGLE

SEVERE NEURALGIC PAIN IN THE EAR AND PROFOUND NERVOUS DISTURBANCE; OPERATION AND RECOVERY

HAROLD I. LILLIE, M.D.

AND

WINCHELL McK. CRAIG, M.D.

ROCHESTER, MINN.

FIG. 40.2. The 1936 article by Lillie and Craig, a case report concerning an 18-year-old girl with lancinating ear pain (glossopharyngeal neuralgia) and ipsilateral hearing loss. This appears to be the first reported case in whom vascular decompression of a cranial nerve was performed (10).

Of course, no one knows who performed this prior operation, which may have been the first cranial nerve decompression operation. It failed for reasons now obvious but not appreciable without the use of the microscope: Blood vessels on the auditory nerve peripheral to the brain stem, although common, do not cause vertigo.

Another case report is of major significance in the history of surgery of the cranial nerves. In 1936, Lillie and Craig (10) discussed an 18-year-old girl with intractable sharp stabbing pain in the left ear (Fig. 40.2). This case report is focused primarily on the ear pain but the title is significant. Intertwined with the history of the patient's otalgia are statements concerning increasing deafness in the left ear or "profound nerve deafness on the left." The progressive nature of the deafness suggested a cerebellopontine angle lesion and, at operation, significant compression of the auditory nerve by an "anomalous" artery, presumably the anterior inferior cerebellar artery or one of its branches, which could be seen looping over the eighth nerve (*rostral and posterior*) and *anterior to* the ninth nerve (Fig. 40.3). The authors went on to say:

". . . The artery could not be elevated until the ninth nerve had been sectioned. After this was done, we were able to slip the arterial loop from its position between the eighth and the ninth nerve, thus relieving the pressure on the eighth nerve . . .

"At the time of her dismissal, no apparent change had taken place in the hearing in the left ear, but 6 weeks later, she wrote that her left ear had returned to normal and that she could hear a watch tick and could use the telephone without pain and with apparently normal hearing."

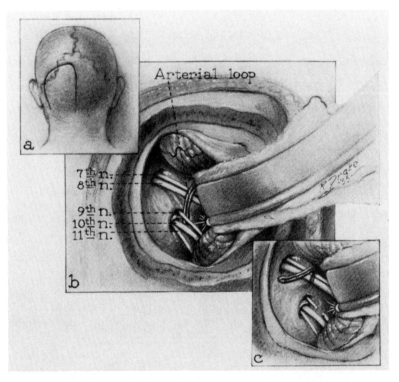

Arterial loop

7th n.
8th n.

9th n.
10th n.
11th n.

a

b

c

FIG. 40.3. "Drawings of the craniotomy, with *a* showing the incision; *b* exposure of the cranial nerves and the position of the arterial loop, and *c* division of the ninth nerve and elevation and displacement of the arterial loop, thereby relieving pressure on the eighth nerve" (10).

This rather obscure 1936 case report, which dealt primarily with glossopharyngeal neuralgia and was discovered in the bibliography of an old article concerning glossopharyngeal neuralgia, is to our knowledge the first validly reported cranial nerve vascular decompression. One can wonder why the concept was not extended and developed by the authors and others. Many answers can be given. One answer, which may be most reasonable, is that available technology was not sufficient to prove or disprove a generalization of the observation. Magnification techniques especially were necessary. In any event this case, in retrospect, was an important observation in the development of cranial nerve surgery.

Two points should be made now. First the criteria for each diagnosis have been altered over the years. Ménière's original patients, for instance, would not be classified as Ménière's disease or syndrome today. The criteria have varied as new diagnostic tests have been applied to patients with vertigo, etc. The authors' contemporary perspective is to look at these symptoms and signs as a continuum related to the multiple factors noted above and thoroughly dependent upon them. The problem in doing this for the uninitiated reader is that such a perspective demands an apparent "jump" in logic: one must first accept the principle of compressing blood vessels as causative of the symptoms and signs. Second, patients followed for any period of time shift quite clearly from one diagnostic category to another. This is reflected in the medical records of many of our patients who had been followed carefully for long periods of time by one or several physicians. At any given point in their course, the symptoms, signs, and testing results might indicate a specific diagnostic category (as noted above). The treating physician might note the change from his prior impression but frequently would ignore the differences and adhere to his prior diagnosis.

The indications for operation in patients with vertigo, disequilibrium, and tinnitus are collated in Table 40.1. Operation is considered only in those who are disabled by their symptoms or at least so impaired that they cannot function at home, socially, or in the workplace. Obvious causes of their symptoms, which are treatable by other techniques (*i.e.*, removal of a tumor) or for whom there is no useful treatment (*i.e.*, noise-induced tinnitus and hearing loss) must be excluded. The patients should have had extensive medical treatment by those medications which have been proved useful to relieve vertigo. If tinnitus alone is the symptom, they should have been treated with a masker. The brain stem evoked responses (BSERs) and/or hearing tests should demonstrate the presence of unilateral disease of the eighth nerve and absence of peripheral pathology, or at least unilateral preponderance if there has been a history of bilateral sequential disease. A frank positional history is most helpful but not necessary. Most patients do report worsening of their symptoms when lying on the ipsilateral side. Additional symptoms are varied and complex, with

TABLE 40.1

Auditory Nerve: Indications for Operation

1. Disabling symptoms of vertigo, tinnitus, and/or dysequilibrium refractory to medical treatment
2. Unilateral disease or consecutive bilateral disease
3. Positional history, symptoms usually exacerbated when symptomatic side down (one exception)
4. Abnormal brain stem auditory evolved potentials, usually a T-+++ delay

nausea predominating (Table 40.2). By adhering to these criteria we have assuredly restricted surgery to the "worst case" group of patients. This is in some ways unfortunate because the worse the symptoms, the greater the duration, the more severe the functional loss, especially in tinnitus patients, the worse the ability of the auditory nerve to return to normal or near-normal function. This audiovestibular correlation with severity has been sadly most significant in our results of operation on tinnitus in that the patients most disturbed by their symptoms are least likely to improve after microvascular decompression (MVD).

Preoperative evaluation following detailed history and physical examination, repeat otoneurology consultation (M.M.), routine laboratory work, and roentgenograms of chest and skull should include computed tomography (CT) and repeat of the otovestibular testing done on the initial examination. Special and general medical consultations are obtained as required.

The preoperative otoneurologic testing in our series consists of evaluation for the presence of spontaneous or positional nystagmus and for abnormal function as shown by the results of the Romberg and tandem Romberg tests (Table 40.3). Preoperative and postoperative evaluation of hearing includes pure-tone and speech audiometry, measurement of thresholds for the crossed acoustic middle-ear reflexes at 500, 1000, and 2000 Hz, and recording of BSERs (15). These tests were performed in all

TABLE 40.2

Symptoms and Signs

Symptoms

Spinning, whirling sensation; vertigo, worse in certain head positions
Off-balance; dysequilibrium; bumps into things
Blurred vision; objects moving
Staggering; prefer support when walking; "walking like a drunk"
"Queasy"; nausea; occasional vomiting
Rocking sensation; occasionally better when in motion
Tinnitus (hissing or pulsatile)
Occasional ear pain (sharp—stabbing)
Occasional twitching around the eye
Symptoms are fluctuating; worse when physically active, better or
    asymptomatic at bed rest

Signs

Spontaneous or positional nystagmus
Romberg and tandem Romberg tests positive
Abnormal gait
Occasional titubation

TABLE 40.3

Preoperative Evaluation

Acoustic Nerve Dysfunction Work-up

Plain skull roentgenograms
Otovestibular testing
Brain stem auditory evoked responses (BSER)
CT with and without contrast
Otolaryngology consultation

Test Results

Hearing loss, unilateral, of sensorineural type
Abnormal middle ear acoustic reflexes (elevated threshold or poor growth of responses)
Abnormal BSER (increased interpeak latency wave I to III on the affected side or increased latency wave V contralateral ear)
Abnormal vestibular tests

patients except the first series for whom middle-ear reflexes and BSERs were not yet available.

Tests of vestibular function include the recording of spontaneous and positional nystagmus (six head positions and bilateral Hallpike maneuvers if possible) and alternate or simultaneous bithermal caloric testing. In addition, rotational tests and posturography were performed in four patients (18).

OPERATIVE PROCEDURE

Under general endotracheal anesthesia, the patient is placed in the contralateral lateral decubitus position. A three-point head holder is positioned so that it holds the neck in modest traction and the head slightly flexed and turned to the operative (up) side. The auditory nerve and adjacent brain stem are exposed through a retromastoid craniectomy 3–3.5 cm in diameter, utilizing craniectomy and microsurgical techniques that have been described previously (3, 4, 7, 8). In more recent patients the craniectomy has been smaller (about 2.5 cm in diameter) (Fig. 40.4*A*).

By means of a surgical binocular dissecting microscope and a narrow-bladed, self-retaining retractor, the flocculus of the cerebellum is elevated rostrally off the glossopharyngeal and vagus nerves on which it rests (Fig. 40.4*B*). This dissection is carried to the brain stem, exposing the lateral pontomedullary junction and the adjacent cranial nerves, including the facial, auditory, abducens, glossopharyngeal, and vagus nerves. The cerebellum is similarly retracted caudally from above, to visualize the trigeminal nerve. Small arteries or veins (or both) of the posterior circulation may be found to be compressing the nerve at their junctional area with the

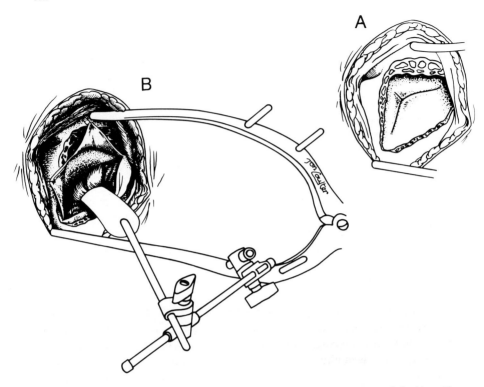

FIG. 40.4A and B. Drawing of low, lateral retromastoid craniectomy on left side with patient in lateral position. (A) Craniectomy extends to sigmoid sinus and to occipital floor. Mastoid air cells are waxed if entered. (B) Retractor arrangement for exposure of auditory nerve. Initial maneuver is that of elevation of inferolateral cerebellum from caudal to rostral.

brain stem in patients with hyperactive dysfunction symptoms of the appropriate nerve (e.g., trigeminal neuralgia, blood vessel causing pulsatile compression of trigeminal nerve; hemifacial spasm, blood vessel causing pulsatile compression of facial nerve). Vascular decompression is performed by gently mobilizing the offending arterial loop(s) or vein(s) away from the junctional area of the nerve and interposing small pledgets of soft plastic felt between the vessel, in its new position, and the brain stem and adjacent nerve. Smaller veins (under 3 mm in diameter) may be coagulated, using precise bipolar radiofrequency current, and divided. The arteries are vital and must be preserved. We believe that the pathologic neurovascular compression is a result of the aging process—i.e., mild arterial elongation and looping, as well as mild caudal displacement of the hindbrain in the posterior fossa.

Auditory function is monitored during the operation by recording BSERs and compound action potentials directly from the exposed auditory nerve. The recording electrode used for direct auditory nerve monitoring is shown in Figure 40.5 (16, 17). The operative findings and procedure are recorded on videotape and 35-mm color slides. Offending arterial loops, including anterior or posterior inferior cerebellar arteries and their branches, are usually visualized with relative ease. The frequency of intrinsic surface veins, which lie generally in the pia around the pontomedullary junction and can cause the symptoms and signs, cannot be overemphasized. They are often found in conjunction with arterial compression. They are usually covered by the flocculus except in the regions rostral and caudal to the auditory nerve. The choroid plexus of the fourth ventricle can also cover a causative vein. Arteriolar loops may cause or contribute to the neural compression. The locations of compressing blood vessels causing vertigo and tinnitus are shown in Figure 40.6A and B. A clear clinical-pathologic correlation exists which is helpful in planning the operation (Table 40.4). Operative results are tabulated in Tables 40.5 and 40.6. Illustrative cases are shown in Figures 40.7–40.9. Results of audiometry and BSER recording in three patients are shown in Figures 40.10–40.12.

Vertigo generally responds rapidly; dysequilibrium, less rapidly; and tinnitus, slowly to microvascular decompression. The more nerve function that is lost, the less likely function will return to normal. This is especially true in tinnitus. Many of our patients with disabling positional vertigo as

TABLE 40.4

Operative Results

The Clinical-Pathologic Correlation of Eighth Nerve
Vascular Compression

Location of Vessels
  Brain stem vs. distal
  Auditory vs. vestibular vs. both
Correlations: Location of compression
  Vertigo—Vestibular portion at or on brain stem
  Dysequilibrium (without vertigo)
    Vestibular portion adjacent to brain stem
  Decreased Vestibular Function
    Vestibular portion anywhere
  Tinnitus—Cochlear portion anywhere
  Hearing Loss—Cochlear portion anywhere
Therefore, if both vertigo and tinnitus—compression must be at brain
  stem if one vessel is causal
Problem—Multiple vessels are frequent

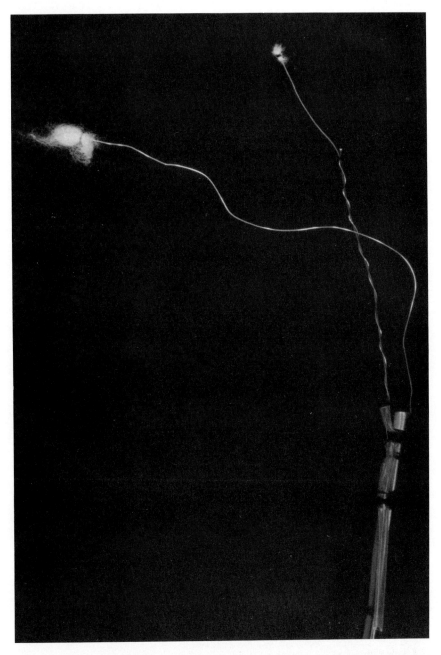

FIG. 40.5. Fine silver wire electrode used for direct recording of auditory nerve compound action potentials. The electrode is attached to a post of an angulated Weitlaner retractor (V. Mueller and Co., Chicago, IL) via a connecting rod and joint. The wire is insulated with Teflon except for the tip, which is bent backward and covered by a small cotton wick. The larger wick is the indifferent electrode which is placed in the wound periphery. We now use a separately placed wire and needle electrode.

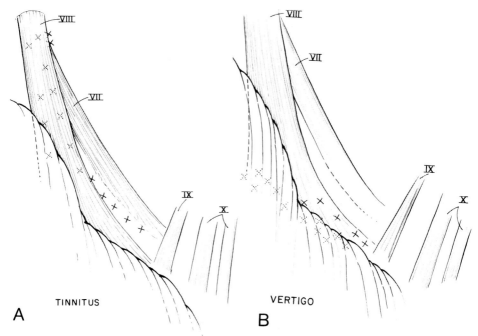

A TINNITUS   B VERTIGO

Fig. 40.6. Drawing of caudal right cerebellopontine angle, patient in lateral position. The facial and auditory nerves rise at an angle and blend into the caudal pons to the level of the pontomedullary junction which is located at the level of the rostral aspect of the glossopharyngeal nerve. The blended area is shown as though discrete. It is variable, as seen anatomically, although it is physiologically constant. The junction of auditory nerve with pons is usually hidden by the flocculus and not infrequently by the choroid plexus of the lateral recess of the fourth ventricle. (*A*) The locations of vascular compression causing tinnitus (indicated by *x*), which are anywhere on the cochlear portion of the nerve and adjacent caudal brain stem. (*B*) The locations of vascular compression causing vertico (*x*), which are anywhere on the vestibular portion at the brain stem. VII denotes the facial nerve, VIII the auditory nerve, IX the glossopharyngeal nerve, and X the vagus nerve. (Modified from N. Engl. J. Med. *310:* 1700–1705, 1984, with permission)

TABLE 40.5

Tinnitus—Operative Results

Results of Microvascular Decompression (1983–1985)
Total operated upon = 100
Total with adequate follow-up = 64

Category	Excellent	Good	No Change	Worse	Hearing Loss	Totals
Disabling positional vertigo	13 (32%)	23 (57%)	6		(1)	42
"Acoustic neuroma syndrome"	2	3				5
Ménière's syndrome	5	1				6
Tinnitus	1	3	5	2	(1)	11
Totals	21	30	11	2	(2)	64

TABLE 40.6

*Tinnitus Patients—November
1981 to July 1985*

Patients (No.)	22
Abnormal BSER	22
Abnormal audiogram	16
Abnormal acoustic reflex	14
Results	
Excellent	3
Improved	6
No change	10
Worse (1 deaf)	3

their primary problem have tinnitus which is mild, not accompanied by serious hearing loss, and not a major complaint. These patients frequently have complete relief of their tinnitus. Patients with severe tinnitus as their primary problem, however, have usually had their symptoms for many years. They usually have pronounced sensorineural hearing loss. This group usually does not do as well as the others.

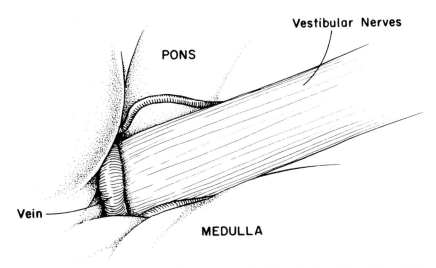

FIG. 40.7. The first microvascular decompression for vertigo. Performed December, 1972 in a 55-year-old woman. Right cerebellopontine angle, sitting position. Vein compressing superior and inferior nerves at brain stem. Flocculus was dissected away from posterior aspect of auditory nerve to the brain stem to gain this exposure.

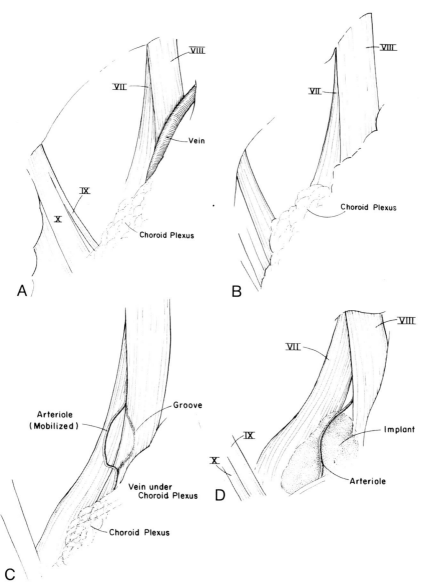

Fig. 40.8. The first patient with recurrent symptoms who was reoperated upon, a 49-year-old man. First operation, for dysequilibrium, performed in January, 1982. Second operation, for vertigo, performed in February, 1983. Left cerebellopontine angle, lateral position. (*A*) First operation. Vein on superior and inferior vestibular nerves just distal to brain stem and adjacent to flocculus causing severe dysequilibrium and occasional vertigo. (*B*) Same. Vein has been coagulated and divided. (*C*) Second operation. Vein on brain stem under choroid plexus of lateral recess of fourth ventricle, arteriole mobilized. (*D*) Same. Vein has been coagulated and divided and arteriole held away from N VIII by small implant of shredded Teflon felt.

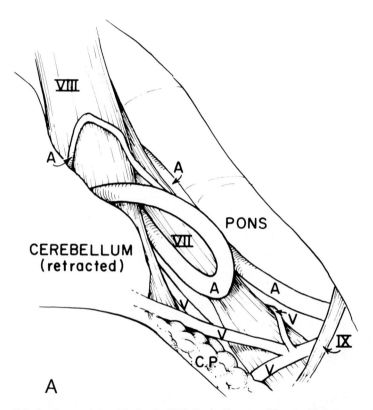

FIG. 40.9. Our first patient with classical Ménière's disease, a 35-year-old woman operated upon in 1982. Right side, lateral position. (*A*) Drawing of neurovascular relationships before decompression. (*B*) Photograph of same (16×). (*C*) Photograph of same after coagulation and division of small veins and placement of implant of shredded Teflon felt to decompress arterial loops. Abbreviations: *A.*, artery; *V.*, vein; *C.P.* choroid plexus; *VII*, facial nerve; *VIII*, auditory nerve; *IX*, glossopharyngeal nerve.

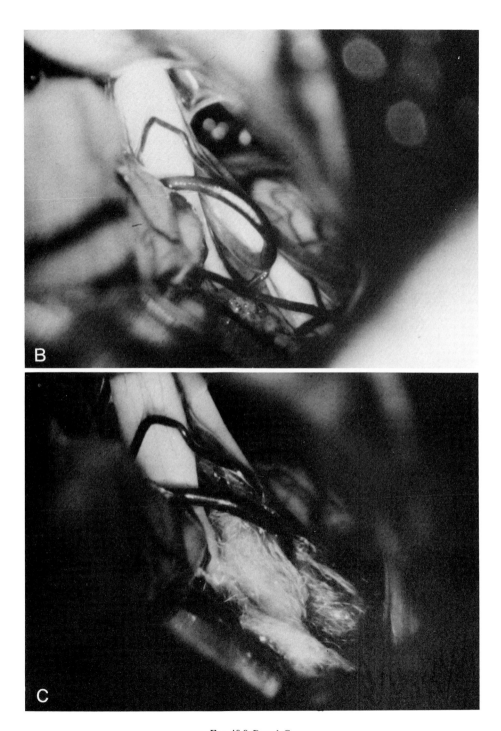

FIG. 40.9.*B* and *C*.

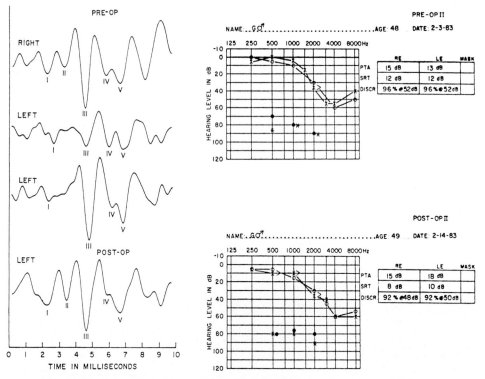

Fig. 40.10. Results of audiometry and brain stem auditory evoked responses (BSER) pre- and postoperatively in a patient with left-sided dysequilibrium and some vertigo. BSER from the left ear show absent wave II, reduced amplitude of wave III, and prolonged latencies of waves IV and V, preoperatively. The patient underwent microvascular decompression (MVD) of NVIII and was asymptomatic for 1 year and then had recurrent vertigo and tinnitus in the left ear. Lower two tracings show the BSER recorded from the left ear before and after the second operation. Wave II is absent while waves III to V are normal. After this second operation the BSER became normal and the patient is asymptomatic.

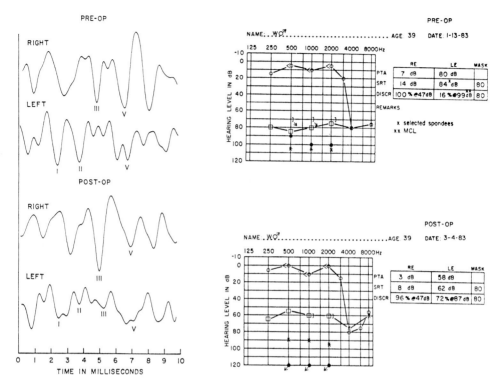

FIG. 40.11. Results of audiometry and BSER pre- and postoperatively in a patient with disabling vertigo, tinnitus, and hearing loss in the left ear. The BSER from the left ear show increased latency of wave II (0.3 msec) and absent wave III but normal latency of wave V. Postoperatively, wave I and II are normal but latencies of waves II, III, and V are abnormal. Speech reception threshold (SRT) improved from 84 dB to 62 dB and the discrimination score increased by 56% postoperatively. In addition, the threshold for the acoustic middle ear reflex returned to normal postoperatively (postoperative test were done 4 weeks after microvascular decompression of the left audiovestibular nerve).

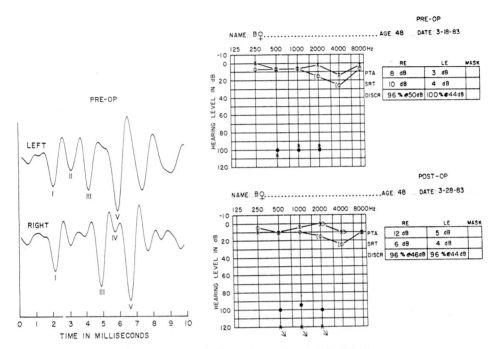

FIG. 40.12. Results of audiometry and BSER recorded pre- and postoperatively in a patient with disabling positional vertigo, right side. Preoperatively, wave II is broad and with reduced amplitude and the latency of wave III is prolonged by 0.7 msec. The interpeak latency (IPL) of waves III to V is normal. The audiogram shows a mild sensorineural deficit in the right ear which is unchanged postoperatively. The patient underwent microvascular decompression (MVD) of the right audiovestibular nerve during which an artery was found to be compressing the caudal portion of the vestibular nerve.

We have had no operative mortality in MVD operations upon the auditory nerve. There have been no wound infections or meningitis. Two patients operated upon for vertigo and disequilibrium and three operated upon for tinnitus suffered postoperative ipsilateral deafness and this is our most serious complication of these procedures. Auditory nerve MVD patients have more immediate postoperative nausea than those who undergo similar procedures upon the other cranial nerves. The incidence of postoperative delayed headache with meningismus ("posterior fossa syndrome," "aseptic meningitis") occurs in 15% of patients and is relieved by lumbar puncture and a brief course of steroids. One of our tinnitus patients who was not relieved of his symptoms recently committed suicide 4 months postoperatively after a surgeon in another city told him that the operation was a failure and that there was nothing that could be done for his symptom. It was too soon to tell.

Cross-compression of the cranial nerves at their root entry zone can occur because as arteries elongate with increasing age they may become frankly tortuous. They may also become ectatic as a result of atherosclerosis or deterioration of vascular collagen or both. In addition, the hindbrain appears to sag caudally with age. Because the arteries supplying blood to the posterior portion of the brain arise anteriorly and extend posterolaterally around the brain stem, elongation of the arteries or sagging of the brain may lead to the formation of abnormal neurovascular contacts. The relations between neural structures and veins, both intrinsic surface veins and those bridging the dural venous sinuses, may also be altered. Very slight changes in the relationships of these structures can lead to abnormal neurovascular contacts which, in turn, cause hyperactivity or hypoactivity, depending on the site of contact and the rate at which the development of such contact occurs, etc. In general, gradually progressive pulsatile compression of neural tissue at or proximal at the point where peripheral myelin (Schwann cells) gives way to the proximal portion of the nerve and adjacent brain stem, which is invested by central-nervous system myelin (oligodendroglia), causes symptoms of hyperactivity. Later, symptoms and signs of progressive loss of function also appear.

Abnormal impulse activity in the vestibular nerve resulting from pulsatile cross-compression could explain the symptoms of positional vertigo. The mechanism may be similar to or the same as the kindling phenomenon. The auditory nerve is unusually long (2.5 cm) and a considerable part of it is covered by central myelin. It is probable that somewhere along its length an offending blood vessel could disturb the impulse activity in such a way that severe symptoms result. Citron and Hallpike (1) reported one case of benign paroxysmal positional vertigo in a patient who underwent intracranial section of the eighth nerve to relieve the symptoms of positional vertigo. During the operation a large convoluted vein crossing and lying in close contact with the eighth nerve was noticed, but the vein was not thought to have contributed to the symptoms.

Although the permanent morbidity in our series of cranial nerve MVD patients has been modest and mortality rates minimal, we consider MVD of the cranial nerves a major operative procedure. Our overall mortality rate in over 2000 such operations is 0.25% (five patients) with no mortality since 1980. A fully trained team, meticulous attention to detail, use of advanced monitoring techniques, and a fully trained microsurgeon with both experience in the surgery of the cerebellopontine angle and specific training in microvascular decompression of the auditory nerve are all important if the operations are to be performed safely and effectively. Some level of recurrent symptoms will occur in up to 20% of patients with trigeminal neuralgia and 5–10% of those with hemifacial spasm. Because many recurrences of trigeminal neuralgia are due to recollateralization of pontine surface intrinsic veins, and because compression by intrinsic pontomedullary surface veins are a common cause of vertigo and tinnitus, we believe that the rate of recurrence of these symptoms over the years will approach the rate in trigeminal neuralgia. The operation is certainly technically more difficult to perform than an auditory nerve section. The results regarding quality of life are incomparable. This nondestructive physiologic procedure is recommended as the first procedure in those in whom an operation is indicated.

REFERENCES

1. Citron, L., and Hallpike, C. S. A case of positional nystagmus of the so-called benign paroxysmal type and the effects of treatment by intracranial division of the VIII nerve. J. Laryngol. Otol., 76: 28–33, 1961.
2. Dandy, W. E. Ménière's disease. Its diagnosis and a method of treatment. Arch. Surg., 16: 1127–1152, 1928.
3. Jannetta, P. J. Cranial rhizopathies. In: Neurological Surgery, edited by J. Youmans, Vol. 6. W. B. Saunders, Philadelphia, 1982, pp. 3589–3603.
4. Jannetta, P. J. Hemifacial spasm. In: The Cranial Nerves, edited by M. Samii, and P. J. Jannetta. Springer-Verlag, Heidelberg, 1981, pp. 484–493.
5. Jannetta, P. J. Neurovascular compression in cranial nerve and systemic disease. Ann. Surg., 192: 518–525, 1980.
6. Jannetta, P. J. Neurovascular cross-compression in patients with hyperactive dysfunction symptoms of the eighth cranial nerve. Surg. Forum, 26: 467–469, 1975.
7. Jannetta, P. J. Neurovascular cross-compression of the eighth nerve in patients with vertigo and tinnitus. In: The Cranial Nerves, edited by M. Samii, and P. J. Jannetta. Springer-Verlag, Heidelberg, 1981, pp. 552–555.
8. Jannetta, P. J. Treatment of trigeminal neuralgia by micro-operative decompression. In: Neurological Surgery, edited by J. Youmans, Vol. 6, 1982, pp. 3589–3603.
9. Jannetta, P. J., Møller, M. B., and Møller, A. R. Disabling positional vertigo. N. Engl. J. Med., 310: 1700–1705, 1984.

10. Lillie, H. I., Craig, W. McK. Anomalous vascular lesion in cerebellopontine angle: severe neuralgic pain in the ear and profound nervous disturbance; operation and recovery. A.M.A. Arch. Otolaryngol., *23:* 642–645, 1936.
11. Ménière, M. Bull. Acad. de med., Paris, *26:* 241, 1861.
12. Ménière, M. Malaise de l'oreille interne offrant les symptons de la congestion cerebral apoplectiforme. Gazz. med. de Paris, *16:* 29, 55, 68, 1861.
13. Ménière, M. Nouveaux documents relatifs aux lesions del'oreille interne characterisees par des symptons de congestion cerebral apoplectiforme. Gazz. med. de Paris, *16:* 239, 379, 597, 1861.
14. Ménière, M. Sur une forme particuliere de surdite grave dependant d'une lesion de l'oreille interne. Gazz. med. de Paris, *16:* 29, 1861.
15. Møller, A. R. Improving brain stem auditory evoked potential recordings by digital filtering. Ear Hear., *4:* 108–113, 1983.
16. Møller, A. R., and Jannetta, P. J. Monitoring auditory functions during cranial nerve microvascular decompression operations by direct recording from the eighth nerve. J. Neurosurg., *59:* 493–499, 1983.
17. Møller, A. R., and Jannetta, P. J. Monitoring auditory nerve potentials during operations in the cerebellopontine angle. J. Otolaryngol., Head Neck Surg., *92:* 434–439, 1984.
18. Wall, C., III, and Black, F. O. Postural stability and rotational tests: their effectiveness for screening dizzy patients. Acta Otolaryngol. (Stockh.), *95:* 235–246, 1983.

41

Microsurgical Vestibular Nerve Section for Intractable Ménière's Syndrome— Technique and Results

EDWARD C. TARLOV, M.D.

A sinking feeling on the part of the neurosurgeon is common when asked to evaluate a patient with dizziness, although, fortunately, we are not often in this position. Our forefathers in neurosurgery, Dandy (2, 3), McKenzie (16), and Falconer (4), knew well the gratification that came with relieving episodic vertigo by vestibular nerve section in patients with severe Ménière's syndrome. However, preservation of hearing was usually not an issue in the era before microsurgery. Many of these patients were deaf before operation, but even those not already deaf could usually not expect to have the cochlear nerve preserved. Facial palsy was also an occasional consequence of the procedure. In subsequent years, the neurosurgical operation for intracranial vestibular nerve section became all but forgotten in most neurosurgical units and was replaced by otolaryngologic procedures, including labyrinthectomy, which is applied only to patients who are already deaf, and endolymphatic shunting, which frequently does not relieve vertigo (5, 7, 8, 10, 13).

With present microsurgical methods, selective intracranial section of the vestibular nerve can be carried out safely with preservation of hearing and facial nerve, and this extremely effective operation can be used to relieve the disabling vertigo of Ménière's syndrome. For vestibular nerve section to be successful, however, accurate preoperative diagnosis of Ménière's syndrome is essential. The operation is not likely to succeed in relieving vertigo from other causes, just as the operations for classic tic douloureux can only be expected to bring more misery to both patient and surgeon when carried out for atypical facial pain.

ALTERNATIVE THEORIES

Jannetta (14), who did much to advance the surgical treatment of tic douloureux, expanded his theory of vascular compression in cranial rhizopathies to include some patients with complaints of dizziness. Which patients, however, is the question. How are the dizzy patients for whom he recommends microvascular decompression to be identified? They are apparently a specific group and not among those with Ménière's syndrome discussed here. A new syndrome, "disabling positional vertigo," was identified in a recent report by Jannetta *et al.* (15). The nine patients they described with this condition experienced constant positional vertigo or dysequilibrium so severe that they were constantly nauseated and disabled. These patients had no hearing disturbance and no loss of vestibular function. Typically, they had been seen by a number of physicians. The vertigo, although described as constant, was precipitated by changes in head position. In two of the nine patients it was post-traumatic. All but one patient had specific changes in brain stem auditory evoked responses, resembling those in patients with acoustic nerve tumors and consisting of a latency shift of wave II and an abnormal amplitude and shape of wave III. To relieve the condition, Jannetta *et al.* (15) used microvascular decompression of one vestibular nerve.

The appropriateness of preoperative diagnosis is essential to the success of this operation, but it seems difficult to identify these patients and to know which vestibular nerve to explore. Evidently, we must rely on the brain stem auditory evoked responses, but the described findings appear to be subtle. Neurosurgeons are in agreement about the criteria for diagnosing typical tic douloureux and hemifacial spasm, but vertigo with changes in position can occur from peripheral causes (vestibular neuronitis and benign positional vertigo), from central diseases (brain stem and cerebellar demyelinating diseases, trauma, and arteriosclerosis), and from functional disturbances. The latter is an especially worrisome category in view of the lack of clear-cut clinical findings in the patients for whom Jannetta *et al.* (15) recommended operation.

In other related conditions operation is seldom seriously considered. Benign paroxysmal positional vertigo, similar to but apparently not the same as the condition Jannetta *et al.* (15) described, is a self-limited clinical entity in which the patient experiences vertigo on tilting the head back to look up or in lying on or rolling over onto the affected ear. The finding of calcium concretions in the semicircular canal at postmortem examination has led to naming this condition cupolithiasis. The condition rarely lasts 1 year. The patient is advised to avoid the provocative position. If the condition persists longer than 1 year, the branch of the vestibular nerve to the posterior canal can be divided through the tympanic membrane via the internal auditory canal with relief of symptoms (6) but at considerable risk to hearing.

Jannetta *et al.* (15) recommended microvascular decompression for patients who had disabling positional vertigo continuously in the upright position. This description may stretch and confuse the term positional vertigo. Their concept of neural hyperactivity due to vascular compression of the cranial nerves at their root entry zone requires continuing attention and evaluation. Yet, in tic douloureux, even when the strongest case for a vascular compressive mechanism can be made, several phenomena are unexplained (1).

In patients with tic douloureux obvious sensory loss is rare, but in hemifacial spasm mild facial weakness is common. However, with a large acoustic neuroma, facial weakness is late in developing despite gross distortion of facial nerve by a large acoustic neuroma whereas sensory loss from distortion of the trigeminal nerve occurs much sooner despite the fifth nerve being farther from the tumor. Therefore, the effects of distortion by an acoustic neuroma are at variance with the theory of Jannetta *et al.* (15) and with the findings in hemifacial spasm and tic douloureux.

The superior cerebellar artery is frequently near the root exit zone of the motor root of the fifth nerve, yet masseter spasm is incredibly rare. Why do we not see a syndrome affecting the motor root of the fifth nerve similar to hemifacial spasm if the mechanism is the same? By the same token one might expect neuralgia of the nervus intermedius to be common with hemifacial spasm, yet this does not seem to occur. Also, although the anterior-inferior cerebellar artery frequently passes between the facial nerve and the root entry zone of the eighth nerve, eighth nerve symptoms are not reported with hemifacial spasm or vice versa.

A strange and striking feature of tic douloureux is that remissions occur almost as a rule, yet they rarely occur in hemifacial spasm. It is difficult to explain why remissions occur in tic douloureux if vascular compression is indeed the underlying pathologic condition. Further questions arise in the absence of symptoms in patients with vascular compression and in the absence of vascular compression in patients with symptoms.

In other situations symptoms have never been attributed to vessels. The spinal nerve roots frequently have vessels intimately related at their entry or exit from the spinal cord. The third, fourth, and sixth cranial nerves have many vessels. The third nerve passes between the superior cerebellar artery and the posterior cerebellar artery just beyond the point that it leaves the midbrain. Yet in none of these approximately 130 nerve roots have symptoms been attributed to vascular compression. Clearly, all the answers are not in.

DIAGNOSIS AND TREATMENT

Intractable Ménière's syndrome is less difficult to define. It is found in a small portion of patients with complaints of dizziness and is characterized by fluctuating hearing loss, tinnitus, and bouts of violent vertigo (17).

Vertigo is usually the most disabling feature. Most patients with Ménière's syndrome are managed by otolaryngologists. Use of diuretic agents, restriction of salt in diet, and administration of vestibular sedatives are ordinarily the initial treatments. In the 123 years since Ménière first described the syndrome, a variety of surgical treatments have been used when medical measures have failed, and their multiplicity attested heretofore to the lack of a satisfactory surgical cure. Endolymphatic shunting operations carried out in an effort to relieve tinnitus and hearing loss have been disappointing for relief of vertigo (9). Labyrinthine destructive procedures that can relieve vertigo invariably destroy hearing, which is a disadvantage because the disorder may become bilateral in about 20% of patients. Selective vestibular nerve section, however, can relieve the vertigo and, if desired, can be combined with endolymphatic shunting operations (19, 20).

The diagnosis of true Ménière's syndrome is not common among the spectrum of patients with complaints of dizziness. The incidence of the disorder is estimated at one per 100,000 population. Strict clinical criteria for diagnosis should be used. In most instances the onset is between the ages of 30 and 60 years with the young and old rarely affected. Recurring attacks usually increase in frequency. Ultimately, hearing loss is almost always permanent in untreated patients, and vertigo may continue after deafness is complete.

Vertigo is the first symptom in the majority of patients, and it is usually the most disabling feature of the disease. Tinnitus is almost always present and in unilateral cases may be the most reliable indicator of the labyrinth involved. The stage of fluctuating hearing loss may last from a few weeks to several years before the loss becomes fixed. Hearing fluctuations and deafness are usually associated with the bouts of vertigo. A premonitory aura with fullness in the head of the affected ear is common. Drop attacks ("the otolithic crisis of Tumarkin") occasionally occur as the result of loss of tonic influences of the otoliths. In severe attacks the patient may be thrown to the ground or if seated as when dining may suddenly become disoriented with respect to gravity. Nystagmus may accompany the attacks, but its direction is not of localizing value.

Findings of electronystagmography with caloric testing are usually abnormal and may demonstrate canal paresis with diminished responses to warm and cold water or air on the affected side. Occasionally, directional preponderance or spontaneous nystagmus to the side opposite the diseased labyrinth occurs. On audiologic testing the majority of patients show low-frequency perceptive hearing loss with fairly good discrimination, loudness recruitment, and negative tone decay on impedance audiometry.

Brain stem auditory evoked response testing demonstrates normal latencies.

The most important differential diagnosis is between Ménière's disease and acoustic neuroma. The latter tends not to cause as severe vertigo as Ménière's syndrome. The loss of vestibular function is usually slow, producing mild ataxia rather than paroxysmal disturbances. Computed tomographic (CT) scanning, including CT pneumography if necessary in suspicious cases, is helpful in excluding the possibility of an acoustic neuroma. Brain stem auditory evoked response testing can identify an eighth nerve lesion but is not specific for its nature.

Pathologic examination of the temporal bones in a patient who died after operation for Ménière's syndrome showed dilatation of the endolymph spaces at the expense of the perilymph spaces (11). This was thought to have caused the symptoms because equal perilymph and endolymph pressures are required for normal cochlear and vestibular function. The situation is similar to hydrocephalus or glaucoma in that the accumulation of excess endolymph is probably caused by deficient reabsorption.

Because of the relatively high incidence of bilateral involvement, attempts at preserving existing hearing or improving hearing have considerable importance. Nevertheless, destruction of the labyrinth has continued as a standard otologic operation when hearing preservation is not a consideration. This may be performed as a transmastoid or a permeatal procedure. It results in a total loss of hearing and is not a desirable form of treatment in patients with unilateral Ménière's syndrome if there is useful hearing in the affected ear or if there is loss of hearing on the other side from other causes. It is also not desirable in bilateral Ménière's syndrome if both ears are affected early in the disease, if one labyrinth has been destroyed before disease appears in the other ear, or if hearing is poor in one ear and is rapidly failing in the other.

A variety of operations to relieve the excess pressure of endolymph have been carried out, principally aimed at preserving or improving hearing and relieving tinnitus. A series of shunting operations creating fistulas from the endolymphatic sac to the mastoid cavity or the subarachnoid space has been the standard alternative, but controversy about the efficacy of these procedures has existed. Glasscock et al. (9) in a recent review of results of shunting procedures found among 112 patients that 66% were relieved of further vertigo and 47% were relieved of tinnitus. Thirty-five percent had decreased hearing, and 45% had stable hearing after shunting. The natural course of the illness is characterized by remissions, and because the hearing loss fluctuates, lengthy and careful follow-up is required to determine the effect of the therapy on hearing. The endolymphatic to subarachnoid shunt has been described by House (12) and the endolymphatic sac to mastoid shunt by Shea (18). At this time, however, the value of shunting procedures alone for Ménière's syndrome is unproved.

The pioneer neurosurgeons had a large experience with vestibular nerve section in Ménière's syndrome, and the operation proved to be reliable in their hands. Dandy (3) refined the operation to the extent that only two deaths occurred among his 587 patients. Vertigo was relieved entirely in 90%, was unchanged in 5%, and was worse in 5%. In the majority of these 587 patients the entire eighth nerve bundle was sectioned with total loss of auditory as well as vestibular function. Fifty-four of the patients had facial paralysis, which was permanent in 17. Of 95 patients in whom only the vestibular portion of the nerve was sectioned, nine had improved hearing, 27 had unchanged hearing, 46 had loss of hearing, and 13 were totally deaf. Falconer (4), in a later era, was able to preserve hearing on the operated side to some degree in his eight patients. The microsurgical technique described here permits consistent postoperative hearing preservation.

MICROSURGICAL PROCEDURE

Selective microsurgical vestibular nerve section is indicated when hearing preservation is a consideration and when the vertiginous attacks are severe. Hearing preservation is a consideration when hearing is normal or nearly normal in the affected ear, when hearing is useful in the affected ear, or when there is any evidence of bilateral involvement—in effect, whenever hearing has not already been lost. This procedure permits exposure of the endolymphatic sac and the vestibular nerve at one operation. The morbidity of the operation has been low, and it has proved to be effective for control of whirling vertigo with this disabling symptom eliminated in almost all patients. The procedure can be carried out as a combined neurosurgical-otologic operation.

Approach

The vestibular nerve can safely be exposed via three routes. In an extradural approach along the floor of the middle fossa, the vestibular nerve may be sectioned in the internal auditory canal. In the most lateral portion of the canal, the superior and inferior vestibular nerves are separate. Theoretical considerations might make it seem desirable to section only the superior vestibular nerve in order to reduce postoperative imbalance. However, my experience has been that postoperative imbalance from sectioning of the entire vestibular nerve is minimal. The middle fossa approach does not permit simultaneous exposure of the endolymphatic sac as can be achieved through the posterior fossa. Some degree of retraction on the temporal lobe is necessary with this approach. For these reasons, I have not employed the middle fossa exposure of the vestibular nerve.

Extradural transmastoid exposure may be performed by an approach anterior or posterior to the sigmoid sinus (Fig. 41.1). As the extradural transmastoid exposure of the endolymphatic sac is most familiar to otologists, it is worthwhile to review advantages and disadvantages of the anterior approach compared with the posterior exposure that I have begun to use routinely. In exposure through the mastoid anterior to the sigmoid sinus, the mastoid is burred away exposing the sigmoid sinus, the large mastoid emissary vein is skeletonized, and a wide bony removal over the

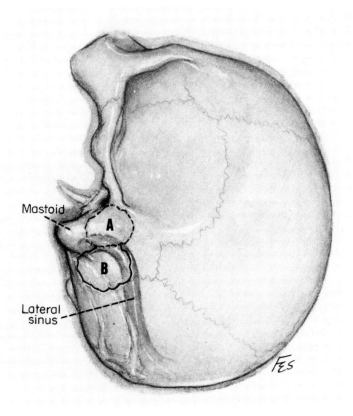

FIG. 41.1. View of skull by surgeon with patient in supine position and head turned to the opposite side. The two approaches anterior (A) and posterior (B) to the sigmoid sinus are indicated. The posterior approach is more familiar to most neurosurgeons.

sigmoid sinus is carried out (Fig. 41.2). Because the operation is performed with the patient in the supine position, I have never had difficulties with air embolization or with handling the sigmoid sinus. The wide bony removal over the sigmoid sinus permits gentle downward extradural retraction of the sigmoid sinus and cerebellar hemisphere to facilitate a less tangential angle of visualization of the vestibular bundle as it passes into the internal auditory meatus (Fig. 41.3). The endolymphatic sac is exposed extradurally, and a strip of absorbable gelatin foam (Gelfoam) can be placed into the lumen of the endolymphatic sac or an Arenberg shunt may be positioned from the endolymphatic sac to the mastoid cavity. In carrying out an endolymphatic sac to mastoid shunt I believe it to be undesirable to use extensive bone waxing over the mastoid air cells as this would eliminate the shunting pathway.

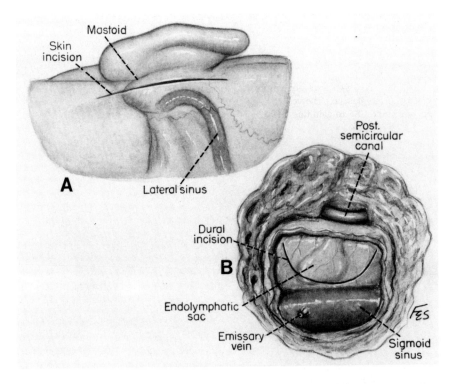

FIG. 41.2. (A) Skin incision at level of mastoid for exposure anterior to sigmoid sinus. (B) Dural incision anterior to sigmoid sinus. The mastoid emissary vein has been skeletonized. The dura is sloping away from the surgeon and is very thin. The posterior semicircular canal limits the anterior portion of the exposure.

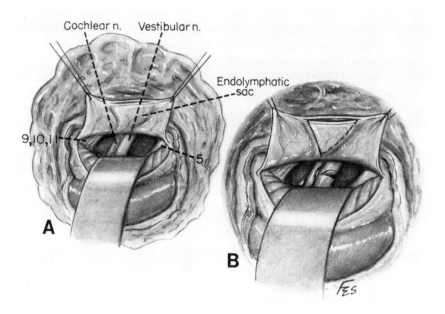

Cochlear n.   Vestibular n.

Endolymphatic
--sac

9,10,1

5

A

B

FIG. 41.3. (A) Exposure anterior to sigmoid sinus providing view of the cochlear and vestibular bundles. (B) The vestibular nerve has been sectioned. It is important to aspirate subarachnoid CSF to gain this exposure.

Depending on the shape of the lateral wall of the posterior fossa, which is somewhat variable, exposure of the dura anterior to the sigmoid sinus is nearly tangential, and tight dural closure is difficult. Another disadvantage is that the dural opening is made in a small area bounded anteriorly by the internal auditory meatus and posteriorly by the sigmoid sinus. In a patient with a short muscular neck or a thick mastoid, there is little leeway to alter or vary the surgeon's line of visualization of the intradural structures. The exposure of the eighth nerve bundle, although adequate to section the vestibular nerve, is limited. For orientation it is helpful to gain a view of the trigeminal nerve superiorly and of the ninth, tenth, and eleventh nerves inferiorly. I have not encountered any difficulties requiring hemostatic control of adjacent vessels, but if this were necessary the exposure anterior to the sigmoid sinus would be somewhat limited to accomplish it.

The wider exposure through the posterior fossa facilitates positive identification of the eighth nerve complex because it permits confirmation of proximity of the eighth nerve to the flocculus; visualization of the fifth nerve rostrally and the ninth, tenth, and eleventh nerve complex below; and identification of the bony internal auditory meatus. The posterior approach avoids the difficulties of dural closure of the very thin, tangentially exposed dura anterior to the sigmoid sinus. With the anterior approach, we have seen several instances of leakage of cerebrospinal fluid (CSF), a problem that is not infrequent with transmastoid or translabyrinthine exposure of the posterior fossa.

We modified the operation in the manner to be described and have found exposure posterior to the sigmoid sinus to be simple and expeditious. The difference between the two exposures, anterior and posterior to the sigmoid sinus, is somewhat analogous to the difference between other anterior and posterior approaches. By the anterior exposure visualization is limited whereas from behind the sigmoid sinus a wide view of the posterior fossa is obtained. With the patient in the supine position with the head turned contralaterally it is striking how little cerebellar retraction is necessary after CSF has been aspirated. When the procedure is carried out in this manner the structures behind the endolymphatic sac are well seen from within the dura, morbidity has been minimal, and dural closure over a patch graft has not been a problem.

Position

I formerly considered the sitting position to have virtually indispensable advantages in posterior fossa surgery. However, during development of microsurgical approaches to tic douloureux, particularly in elderly patients, I have found that the cerebellopontine angle can be exposed safely and widely with the patient in the supine position. The view obtained when the surgeon becomes familiar with use of this position is almost identical to that obtained with the sitting position, except that the surgical field is rotated 90°. Although I consider the sitting position to be safe based on the very low incidence of problems with it over many years, I have been using the supine position increasingly for all surgery at the cerebellopontine angle.

The supine position eliminates the hazards of the sitting position, principally related to hypotension and air embolism, without losing most of its advantages. The head of the operating table is slightly elevated, which considerably reduces venous pressure, and the patient's neck is rotated contralaterally and moderately flexed. Two fingers can be inserted beneath the chin when the neck is in proper position. When CSF has been aspirated from the cisterna magna, almost no cerebellar retraction is needed, and no arterial or central venous line is necessary. The surgeon is seated behind the patient's head, and the operating microscope is brought in from the surgeon's left side to permit easy access by the scrub nurse to his or her

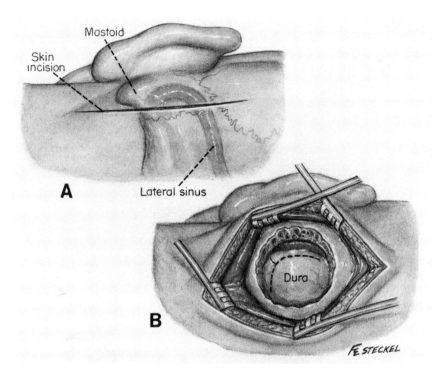

FIG. 41.4. (A) Incision posterior to sigmoid sinus. (B) Dura exposed as in exposure of the trigeminal nerve in tic douloureux. (Reproduced with permission from Tarlov, E., and Oliver, P. Selective vestibular nerve section combined with endolymphatic sac to subarachnoid shunt for intractable Ménière's syndrome: surgical technique. Contemp. Neurosurg., *4:* 4, 1983.

right hand. The position of the patient's head from the surgeon's viewpoint is shown in Figure 41.4A.

Technique

I prefer a Mayfield three-point fixation unit that permits the use of the Leyla self-retaining retractor system. A paramedian incision is made about 1 cm posterior to the mastoid prominence (Fig. 41.4A), which requires minimal hair shaving, and a craniotomy is carried out laterally extending over the junction between the transverse and sigmoid sinuses (Fig. 41.4B). In a deep posterior fossa we skeletonize part of the sigmoid sinus, which facilitates exposure of the endolymphatic sac, and the dura is at first opened inferiorly.

Ordinarily, the cerebellar hemisphere is somewhat full at this stage. With the cottonoid over the cerebellar hemisphere, a ribbon retractor is used to elevate the cerebellar hemisphere gently and to expose the cisterna magna (Fig. 41.5). The arachnoid over the cisterna magna is punctured with the suctioning device and cerebrospinal fluid is aspirated until no more can be obtained, which results in slackening of the cerebellar hemisphere. The force of gravity provides most of the necessary cerebellar retraction from here on. Petrosal veins are identified at this point, the arachnoid is swept medially off the junction of petrosal veins with the petrosal sinus, and the veins are coagulated. They are then divided with curved microscissors, leaving the usual cuff adjacent to the petrosal sinus for safety.

The retractor is used to place the arachnoid over the internal auditory meatus on a slight stretch, largely to protect the cerebellar hemisphere. As the redundant arachnoid now forms a cistern, it can be swept medially and left intact over much of the cerebellopontine angle cistern system.

Tortuous vessels in the region of the eighth nerve complex have not infrequently been observed during the course of operations for tic

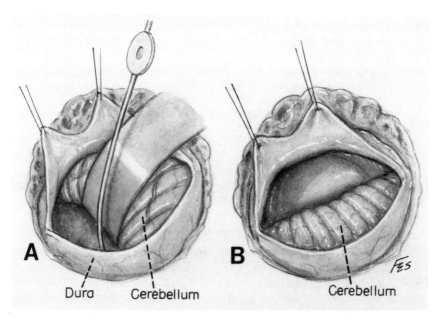

FIG. 41.5. (A) CSF being aspirated from cisterna magna. (B) Cerebellum becomes very slack. Virtually no cerebellar retraction is required. (Reproduced with permission from Tarlov, E., and Oliver, P. Selective vestibular nerve section combined with endolymphatic sac to subarachnoid shunt for intractable Ménière's syndrome: surgical technique. Contemp. Neurosurg., 4: 4, 1983.)

douloureux in patients without eighth nerve signs or symptoms. However, I have not encountered them during operations for Ménière's syndrome. No causative relationship between extreme vascular compression and the symptoms of Ménière's syndrome has, in my opinion, ever been proved. Thus, I would not presently consider it advisable to carry out vascular decompression in severely symptomatic patients with Ménière's syndrome although the microvascular decompression operation has, I believe, proved its value in the treatment of many patients with tic douloureux.

Once the retractor has been positioned correctly, a wide view of the eighth nerve complex from the internal auditory meatus to the brain stem is obtained. The vestibular portion of the eighth nerve occupies the superior half of the combined bundle. It is usually slightly grayer than the more inferiorly lying cochlear division. At the level of the internal auditory meatus a plane of cleavage between the vestibular and cochlear divisions may be visible. Gently depressing the vestibular portion of the nerve inferiorly allows visualization of the much whiter facial nerve lying anterosuperiorly.

Vessels coursing along the eighth nerve bundle must be preserved if hearing preservation is to be accomplished. Frequently there are few or no vessels to contend with, but it is occasionally necessary to dissect carefully around a small vessel coursing across the vestibular nerve and to separate it from the nerve sharply. When a clear plane of cleavage between the vestibular and cochlear nerves cannot be visualized, I section the superior half of the combined cochlear and vestibular bundle. As the cochlear nerve and its blood supply are delicate, no manipulation of the cochlear portion is carried out. After section of the vestibular nerve (Fig. 41.6), no vestibular function on the operated side has been demonstrable postoperatively by caloric testing.

In an effort to determine its value in guiding the surgeon to preserve cochlear nerve function, I have used brain stem auditory evoked response testing intraoperatively. With capability for this testing, the procedure itself is simple enough. A special microphone is placed on the ipsilateral ear. Once the appropriate scalp leads have been positioned, satisfactory intraoperative tracings can be obtained. Even with rapid averaging techniques, however, the time needed for interpretation is too long to permit immediate feedback to the surgeon carrying out the manipulations. The test may demonstrate that some surgical manipulation previously carried out has caused a change in the evoked response latency, but this information would only be helpful if it were available during the course of each movement, which it is not. Nevertheless, brain stem auditory evoked response testing may be helpful in preserving cochlear function.

After vestibular nerve section the otologic portion of the operation, if any, is carried out. The angulation of the microscope can be adjusted to visualize the dura over the posterior face of the petrous bone. The endo-

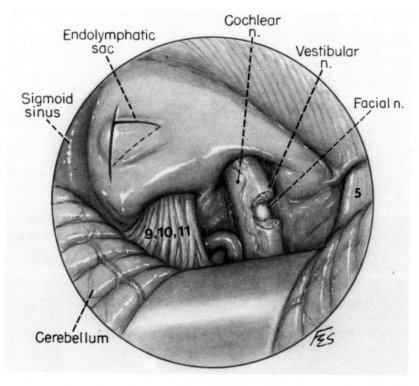

FIG. 41.6. View of the vestibular nerve and the ninth, tenth, and eleventh bundles below. The vestibular nerve has been sectioned, and the facial nerve lying anteriorly can be visualized. The endolymphatic sac lies posteriorly, approximately midway between the sigmoid sinus and the internal auditory meatus. An otologic procedure can be carried out if indicated.

lymphatic sac that lies approximately midway between the posterior rim of the internal auditory meatus and the sigmoid sinus can be exposed, and the dura can be inspected and palpated. The endolymphatic sac is usually not immediately obvious, but once it has been identified, an incision entirely through both layers of the dura can be carried out. The otologic surgeon can then proceed, and the lumen of the endolymphatic sac is entered; the fenestration is shown in Figures 41.7 and 41.8. In occasional instances when disease is long-standing, the endolymphatic sac may be fibrotic and placement of a shunt may not be possible. There is no doubt that some failure of endolymphatic shunting is related to fibrosis of the endolymphatic sac system.

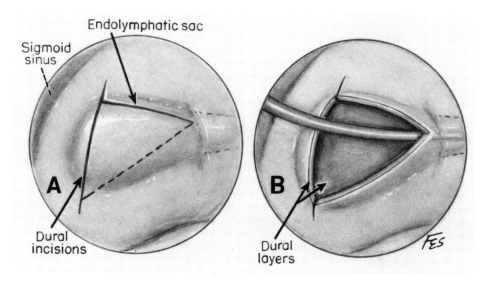

FIG. 41.7. Shunting technique for fenestrating endolymphatic sac. The inner layer of dura is excised so that the sac can communicate further with the subarachnoid space. (Reproduced with permission from Tarlov, E., and Oliver, P. Selective vestibular nerve section combined with endolymphatic sac to subarachnoid shunt for intractable Ménière's syndrome: surgical technique. Contemp. Neurosurg., *4:* 6, 1983.)

A pericranial graft taken in the initial phase of the procedure is used for a patulous dural closure. The muscles, subcutaneous tissues, and skin are then closed in layers, and a dressing is applied (Fig. 41.9).

As would be expected, vertigo after operation seems to be proportional to the extent of preoperative vestibular function as determined by electronystagmography. Patients with the most severe vestibular impairment before operation have been the least disturbed in the early postoperative period. However, all of our patients have been discharged within 1 week and have had minimal residual ataxia at 1 month. With this posterior approach, leakage of CSF has not been a problem. By contrast, our earlier transmastoid exposures anteriorly did lead to leakage of CSF, and reclosure of the wound was necessary on several occasions because of the thinness of the dura anterior to the sigmoid sinus and its oblique angle from the surgeon's view. No facial weakness has occurred with the posterior exposure, and the procedure can be carried out without producing loss of hearing.

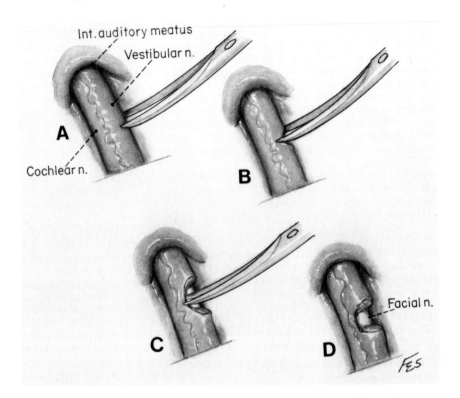

FIG. 41.8. Steps in sectioning the vestibular portion of the nerve. The cochlear nerve appears slightly whiter than the vestibular nerve. As the vestibular nerve is sectioned, the facial nerve lying anteriorly comes into view. The vestibular nerve occupies the rostral half of the combined vestibular and cochlear bundle. The left nerve is visualized with the patient in the supine position. The internal auditory meatus lies superiorly.

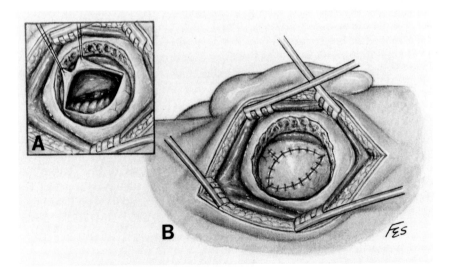

FIG. 41.9. Insert *A* shows slack cerebellum after CSF has been aspirated. Vestibular and cochlear nerves visible above cerebellum. *B*. Dural closure with patch graft.

RESULTS

Twenty-four patients have undergone elective microsurgical vestibular nerve section via the posterior fossa for intractable vertigo with follow-up times ranging from 6 months to 6 years. Twenty patients had bona fide Ménière's syndrome. The vestibular nerve was microsurgically sectioned sparing the cochlear nerve and its blood supply. Postoperative studies in these patients revealed no vestibular function on the operated side. Eighteen of the 20 patients have had no repeat attack of vertigo, one has had several minor attacks relieved by medication, and the other has had attacks presumably due to development of Ménière's involvement of the opposite side. Hearing preservation was possible in all of the patients. The operation was carried out on the only hearing ear in three patients and in several patients with normal hearing preoperatively and postoperatively. Three patients had had a contralateral labyrinthine operation; even these did not have disabling ataxia postoperatively. Death due to cerebellar swelling occurred in one patient, 1 day postoperatively.

Three patients in whom vestibular neuropathy was suspected preoperatively underwent the operation. These patients were not believed to have Ménière's syndrome. The vestibular nerve was sectioned in two of these patients, of whom one has had no further attacks and one has continued symptomatic as before. The third patient had decompression of a vascular loop compressing the vestibular bundle, and the operation had no lasting benefit.

One patient who underwent exploration for a suspected acoustic neuroma had vestibular nerve section. The operation did not abolish his dizziness.

Vestibular nerve section is most likely to be successful in patients with bona fide Ménière's syndrome. Its results have been unpredictable when the preoperative diagnosis was not typical Ménière's syndrome. Further experience with the category of patients described by Jannetta et al. (15) may indicate the possible value of microvascular decompression in disabling positional vertigo, but this is not advisable in patients with Ménière's syndrome. For patients with Ménière's syndrome, vestibular nerve section is associated with little or no important postoperative deficit and can be carried out with preservation of hearing. I strongly prefer vestibular nerve section to vascular decompression in patients with Ménière's syndrome. In the majority of patients, relief of whirling attacks of dizziness, the most disabling feature of Ménière's syndrome, has persisted in the follow-up period. The procedure appears to be promising in the surgical treatment of intractable Ménière's syndrome when relief of vertigo with hearing preservation is desired.

ACKNOWLEDGMENT

I wish to express appreciation to *Contemporary Neurosurgery* for permission to use portions of text and figures from my previous article.

REFERENCES

1. Adams, C. B. T. Personal communication, 1985.
2. Dandy, W. E. Treatment of Ménière's disease by section of only the vestibular portion of the acoustic nerve. Bull. Johns Hopkins Hosp., *53:* 52–55, 1933.
3. Dandy, W. E. Ménière's disease: its diagnosis and a method of treatment. Arch. Surg., *16:* 1127–1152, 1928.
4. Falconer, M. A. Treatment of Ménière's disease, letter. Br. Med. J., *2:* 179, 1963.
5. Flur, E., and Tovi, D. Microscopic intracranial section of the vestibular nerve in Ménière's disease: a preliminary report. Acta Otolaryngol. (Stockh.), *59:* 604–606, 1965.
6. Gacek, R. R. Singular neurectomy update. Ann. Otol. Rhinol. Laryngol., *91:* 469–473, 1982.
7. Glasscock, M. E., and Miller, G. W. Middle fossa vestibular nerve section in the management of Ménière's disease. Laryngoscope, *87:* 529–541, 1977.
8. Glasscock, M. E. III, Hughes, G. B., Davis, W. E., and Jackson, C. G. Labyrinthectomy versus middle fossa vestibular nerve section in Ménière's disease. A critical evaluation of the relief of vertigo. Ann. Otol. Rhinol. Laryngol., *89:* 318–324, 1980.
9. Glasscock, M. E. III, Miller, G. W., Drake, F. D., and Kanok, M. M. Surgical management of Ménière's disease with the endolymphatic subarachnoid shunt: a five-year study. Laryngoscope, *87:* 1668–1675, 1977.
10. Green, R. E. Surgical treatment of vertigo, with follow-up on Walter Dandy's cases. Neurologic aspects. Clin. Neurosurg., *6:* 141–152, 1959.
11. Hallpike, C. S., and Cairns, H. Observations on the pathology of Ménière's syndrome. J. Laryngol. Otol., *53:* 625–654, 1938.
12. House, W. F. Subarachnoid shunt for drainage of hydrops. A report of 63 cases. Arch. Otolaryngol., *79:* 338–354, 1964.
13. House, W. F., and Fraysse, B. Revision of the endolymphatic subarachnoid shunt for Ménière's disease. Review of 59 cases. Arch. Otolaryngol., *105:* 599–600, 1979.
14. Jannetta, P. J. Microsurgical approach to the trigeminal nerve for tic douloureux. Prog. Neurol. Surg., *7:* 180–200, 1976.
15. Jannetta, P. J., Møller, M. B., and Møller, A. R. Disabling positional vertigo. N. Engl. J. Med., *310:* 1700–1705, 1984.
16. McKenzie, K. G. Intracranial division of the vestibular portion of the auditory nerve for Ménière's disease. Can. Med. Assoc. J., *34:* 369–381, 1936.
17. Schuknecht, H. F. Ménière's disease: a correlation of symptomatology and pathology. Laryngoscope, *73:* 651–665, 1963.
18. Shea, J. J. Teflon film drainage of the endolymphatic sac. Arch. Otolaryngol., *83:* 316–319, 1966.
19. Silverstein, H., and Norrell, H. Vestibular nerve section in Ménière's syndrome. Presented at the meeting of the Neurosurgical Society of America, Key West, Florida, May 1983.
20. Tarlov, E., and Oliver, P. Selective vestibular nerve section combined with endolymphatic sac to subarachnoid shunt for intractable Ménière's syndrome: Surgical technique. Contemp. Neurosurg., *4:* 1–6, 1983.

Index